# Medical Ethics

## Accounts of Ground-Breaking Cases

*SEVENTH EDITION*

Gregory E. Pence

University of Alabama at Birmingham

Mc
Graw
Hill
Education

MEDICAL ETHICS: ACCOUNTS OF GROUND-BREAKING CASES, SEVENTH EDITION

Published by McGraw-Hill Education, 2 Penn Plaza, New York, NY 10121. Copyright © 2015 by McGraw-Hill Education. All rights reserved. Printed in the United States of America. Previous editions © 2011, 2008, and 2004. No part of this publication may be reproduced or distributed in any form or by any means, or stored in a database or retrieval system, without the prior written consent of McGraw-Hill Education, including, but not limited to, in any network or other electronic storage or transmission, or broadcast for distance learning.

Some ancillaries, including electronic and print components, may not be available to customers outside the United States.

This book is printed on acid-free paper.

1 2 3 4 5 6 7 8 9 0 DOC/DOC 1 0 9 8 7 6 5 4

ISBN 978-0-07-803845-7
MHID 0-07-803845-6

Senior Vice President, Products & Markets: *Kurt L. Strand*
Vice President, General Manager, Products & Markets: *Michael Ryan*
Vice President, Content Production & Technology Services: *Kimberly Meriwether David*
Managing Director: *William R. Glass*
Brand Manager and Managing Editor: *Sara Jaeger*
Executive Director of Development: *Lisa Pinto*
Associate Marketing Manager: *Alexandra Schultz*
Content Project Manager: *Jessica Portz*
Buyer: *Susan Culbertson*
Cover Design: *Studio Montage, St. Louis, MO*
Cover Image: © *Lawrence Lawry/Getty Images RF*
Media Project Manager: *Jennifer Bartell*
Composition: *Cenveo® Publisher Services*
Typeface: *10/12 Palatino LT Std*
Printer: *R. R. Donnelley*

All credits appearing on page or at the end of the book are considered to be an extension of the copyright page.

**Library of Congress Cataloging-in-Publication Data**

Pence, Gregory E., author.
[Classis cases in medical ethics]
 Medical ethics : accounts of ground-breaking cases / Gregory E. Pence, professor of philosophy, School of Medicine and Department of Philosophy, University of Alabama at Birmingham.—Seventh edition.
 pages cm
 Editions 1-5 published under: Classic cases in medical ethics.
 Audience: Grade 9 to 12.
 Includes bibliographical references and index.
 ISBN 978-0-07-803845-7 (alk. paper)
 1. Medical ethics—Case studies. I. Title.
R724.P36 2015
174.2—dc23                                   2013043702

The Internet addresses listed in the text were accurate at the time of publication. The inclusion of a website does not indicate an endorsement by the authors or McGraw-Hill Education, and McGraw-Hill Education does not guarantee the accuracy of the information presented at these sites.

www.mhhe.com

# *Preface*

I am proud that this text will be 25 years old in 2014. I worked hard in 2013 to make the 7th edition the best ever. This new edition retains in-depth discussion of famous cases, while providing updated, detailed analysis of issues those cases raise. Each chapter also focuses on a key question that could be debated in class.

Unique to this text is a single, authorial voice integrating description of the cases and their issues with historical overviews. The text is the only one that follows cases over decades to tell readers what did and, often, what *did not*, happen. Written by a professor who helped found bioethics and who has published in the field for 40 years, the text gives students a sense of mastery over this exciting, complex field. After they have read the book, I hope that students and will feel that they have learned something important and that time studying the material has been well spent.

## New to the 7th Edition

New research was added to each chapter, and a new list of topics to debate was included on the inside cover of the book. Every chapter has been rewritten, tightened, and augmented; issues have been clarified. Highlights of the new edition are outlined here.

**Chapter 1, Ethical Reasoning, Moral Theories, Principles, and Bioethics—** Moved from the end to the beginning of the book. A new section was added on good and bad reasoning in bioethics.

**Chapter 5, Abortion: The Trial of Kenneth Edelin—**New efforts of states to close abortion clinics after conviction in Philadelphia of an African-American doctor.

**Chapter 9, Medical Research on Animals—**Now includes updated information on the cessation of the use of chimpanzees in research.

**Chapter 10, Medical Research on Vulnerable Human Subjects—**New section was added on a collaborative model for medical research with people in developing countries.

**Chapter 11, Surgeon's Desire for Fame: Ethics of the First Transplants—**More "firsts" involving transplants of face, arms, hands, fingers, and trachea.

**Chapter 12, Just Distribution of Organs: The God Committee and Personal Responsibility**—More emphasis on whether bad health behavior should disqualify patients for organ transplants.

**Chapter 14, Ethical Issues of Intersex and Transgender Persons**—Includes material on gender re-assignment surgery, the fetal dex controversy, and treatment of people who are transsexuals and intersex.

**Chapter 15, Involuntary Psychiatric Commitment: The Case of Joyce Brown**—Updates on the death of Joyce Brown.

**Chapter 16, Ethical Issues in Testing for Genetic Disease**—Includes a new case focusing on Angelina Jolie's radical mastectomy.

**Chapter 17, Ethical Issues in Stopping the Global Spread of AIDS**—Progress in stopping the global spread of HIV is covered in this revised chapter.

**Chapter 18, Ethical Issues with the Affordable Care Act**—This new chapter analyzes ethical issues of the Affordable Care Act (aka "Obamacare"), including estimated costs and problems of implementation.

**Chapter 19, Ethical Issues in Medical Enhancement**—This new chapter focuses on use of doping and steroids in sports and whether use of any enhancement is a form of cheating.

As usual, I updated chapters about assisted dying, Dr. Anna Pou and her tragic situation during Hurricane Katrina in New Orleans (Chapter 3), reproductive human cloning (Chapter 7), stem cells (Chapter 7), allocating organs (Chapter 12), and Baby Jane Doe as a living adult (Chapter 8). Herein also is the latest on the Octamom, the Gosselins (Chapter 6), elderly women gestating babies (Chapter 6), and comatose patients in minimally conscious states.

The 7th edition features an Online Learning Center at www.mhhe.com/pence7e with content written and curated by Gregory Pence. It includes Learning Objectives for each chapter and suggests movies to show in class. For instructors, there is a password-protected section that gives suggested exam questions, also written by Gregory Pence. The supplementary readings listed on the next page are available on the Online Learning Center and tied to chapter content from the 7th edition. Certain topics in the 7th edition of *Medical Ethics* (left side) correlate with more in-depth ethical supplementary readings from Pence's *Elements of Bioethics* text (right side):

*MEDICAL ETHICS 7e*

*ELEMENTS OF BIOETHICS*

Chapter 3—Requests to Die: Terminal
Patients

Chapter 9—Is There A Duty To Die?

Chapter 5—Abortion: The Trial of Kenneth
Edelin

Chapter 7—Are Genetic Abortions
Eugenic?

Chapter 6—Assisted Reproduction,
Multiple Births, and Elderly
Parents

Chapter 5—Emotivism and Banning Some
Conceptions

Chapter 8—The Ethics of Treating Impaired
Babies

Chapter 7—Are Genetic Abortions
Eugenic?

Chapter 10—Medical Research on
Vulnerable Human Subjects

Chapter 8—Can Research Be Just on
People with Schizophrenia?

Chapter 12—Just Distribution of Organs:
The God Committee and
Personal Responsibility

Chapter 2—Kant on Whether Alcoholism
is a Disease

Chapter 12—Just Distribution of Organs:
The God Committee and
Personal Responsibility

Chapter 3—Kant's Critique of Adult
Organ Donation

Chapter 15—Involuntary Psychiatric
Commitment: The Case of
Joyce Brown

Chapter 8—Can Research Be Just on
People with Schizophrenia?

If you have suggestions for improvement, please email me at: pence@uab.edu.

# About the Author

Gregory E. Pence is a professor and chair of the Department of Philosophy at the University of Alabama at Birmingham. Between 1977 and 2011, he was responsible for Medical Ethics teaching at the University of Alabama Medical School. He continues to direct its Early Medical School Acceptance Program.

In 2006, and for achievement in medical ethics, Samford University awarded him a Pellegrino Medal. He testified about human cloning before committees of the U.S. Congress in 2001 and the California Senate in 2003.

He graduated cum laude with a B.A. from the College of William and Mary in 1970 and earned a Ph.D. from New York University in 1974.

In 2010, his UAB team was national champion of the Intercollegiate Ethics Bowl. In 2011, his UAB team was national champion of the Bioethics Bowl at the National Undergraduate Bioethics Conference at Duke University. At UAB, he has won the Ingalls and President's Awards for excellence in teaching.

- He has written five trade books, including *Who's Afraid of Human Cloning?* (1998), *Re-Creating Medicine: Ethical Issues at the Frontiers of Medicine* (2000), *Designer Food: Mutant Harvest or Breadbasket of the World?* (2002), *Cloning After Dolly: Who's Still Afraid?* (2004), and *How to Build a Better Human: An Ethical Blueprint* (2012).

- He has edited three books of general essays, *Classic Works in Medical Ethics* (1995), *Flesh of My Flesh: The Ethics of Cloning Humans* (1998), and *The Ethics of Food: A Reader for the Twenty-First Century* (2002).

- He has published 54 op-ed essays in national publications: two each in the *New York Times, Los Angeles Times, Newsweek, and Chronicle of Higher Education*; one each in the *Los Angeles Times, Atlanta Journal-Constitution*, and *Philadelphia Inquirer*; and 35 in the *Sunday Birmingham News*. His reader, *Brave New Bioethics*, collects these essays from 1974 to 2002.

**Books By Gregory Pence**

*Ethical Options in Medicine,* 1980

*Classic Cases in Medical Ethics,* 1990, first edition

*Seven Dilemmas in World Religions* (with G. Lynn Stephens), 1994

*Classic Cases in Medical Ethics,* 2nd edition, 1995

*Who's Afraid of Human Cloning?* 1998

*Classic Works in Medical Ethics: Core Philosophical Readings,* 1998

*Flesh of My Flesh: The Ethics of Cloning Humans: A Reader,* 1998

*Classic Cases in Medical Ethics,* 3rd edition, 2000

*Recreating Medicine: Ethical issues at the Frontiers of Medicine,* 2000

*Designer Food: Mutant Harvest or Breadbasket of the World?* 2002

*The Ethics of Food: A Reader for the 21st Century,* 2002

*Brave New Bioethics: A Collection of Essays,* 2002

*Classic Cases in Medical Ethics,* 4th edition, 2004

*The Elements of Bioethics,* 2006

*Cloning After Dolly: Who's Still Afraid?* 2004

*Classic Cases in Medical Ethics,* 5th edition, 2008

*Medical Ethics: Accounts of Ground-Breaking Cases,* 6th edition, 2011

*How to Build a Better Human: An Ethical Blueprint,* 2012

# Acknowledgments

Several people helped in preparing the 7th edition of this text. As ever, Rachael Rosales, now at Harvard Medical School, began the summer of 2013 as a perfect research assistant. Michelle Chang, now at UAB Medical School, took over from Rachael and performed superbly in the summer of 2013, researching updates and proofing chapters. Aditi Jani, a senior BS/MD student at UAB, finished the project and did a lot of heavy lifting when it came to proofing and improving the flow of the text, as well as spotting inconsistencies.

Users of this text also improved the new edition with their suggestions and corrections. In particular, Charles Cardwell, Pellissippi State Community College in Tennessee, and David Court Lewis, Owensboro Community College, Kentucky, improved the chapters in many ways. Charles Cardwell has my ongoing gratitude as any textbook author's best friend and careful critic.

For helpful suggestions, I also thank Scott McCandliss of Southern Polytechnic University; Frank Chessa, Tufts University Medical Center; Kenneth Schaffner, University of Pittsburgh; John Huss, University of Akron; student Courtney Ormsby, New York; Jasper Hopkins, University of Minnesota; John Ryan, Community College of Vermont; Patricia Schankin of Trinity Health in Michigan; and UAB surgeon David Joseph.

Working for McGraw-Hill, Maureen Allaire Spada was the perfect editor and helped me take this text to a higher level. I also appreciated the following reviewers for the seventh edition:

Jami L. Anderson, *University of Michigan, Flint*
Brian Barnes, *University of Louisville*
Stephan Blatti, *University of Memphis*
Russell DiSilvestro, *California State University, Sacramento*
John Huss, *The University of Akron*
Court Lewis, *University of Alabama at Birmingham*
Bertha Manninen, *Arizona State University*
David Paul, *Western Michigan University*
Elisa Rapaport, *Molloy College*
John Ryan, *Community College of Vermont*
Michael Stanfield, *University of South Florida, Tampa*
Sandra Woien, *Arizona State University*

# Brief Contents

Chapter 1 Ethical Reasoning, Moral Theories, Principles, and Bioethics
Chapter 2 Requests to Die: Non-Terminal Patients
Chapter 3 Requests to Die: Terminal Patients
Chapter 4 Comas: Karen Quinlan, Nancy Cruzan, and Terri Schiavo
Chapter 5 Abortion: The Trial of Kenneth Edelin
Chapter 6 Assisted Reproduction, Multiple Births, and Elderly Parents
Chapter 7 Embryos, Stem Cells, and Cloning
Chapter 8 The Ethics of Treating Impaired Babies
Chapter 9 Medical Research on Animals
Chapter 10 Medical Research on Vulnerable Human Subjects
Chapter 11 Surgeons' Desire for Fame: Ethics of the First Transplants
Chapter 12 Just Distribution of Organs: God Committee and Personal Responsibility
Chapter 13 Using One Baby for Another: Babies Fae, Gabriel, and Theresa and Conjoined Twins
Chapter 14 Ethical Issues of Intersex and Transgender Persons
Chapter 15 Involuntary Psychiatric Commitment: The Case of Joyce Brown
Chapter 16 Ethical Issues in Testing for Genetic Disease
Chapter 17 Ethical Issues in Stopping the Global Spread of AIDS
Chapter 18 Ethical Issues with the Affordable Care Act
Chapter 19 Ethical Issues in Medical Enhancement

# Contents

*PREFACE*    iii

1.  Ethical Reasoning, Moral Theories, Principles, and Bioethics          1
    *Good Reasoning in Bioethics*      1
        Giving Reasons      1
        Universalization      2
        Impartiality      3
        Reasonableness      3
        Civility      4
    *Mistakes in Ethical Reasoning*      4
        Slippery Slope      4
        *Ad hominem* ("To the man")      5
        *Tu quoque*      5
        Straw Man/Red Herring      5
        *Post Hoc, Ergo Propter Hoc*      6
        Appeal to Authority      6
        Appeals to Feelings and Upbringing      7
        *Ad populum*      7
        False Dichotomy      7
        Equivocation      7
        Begging the Question      8
    *Ethical Theories, Principles, and Bioethics*      8
        Moral Relativism      8
        Utilitarianism      9
        Problems of Utilitarianism      10
        Kantian Ethics      11
        Problems of Kantian Ethics      12
        The Ethics of Care      12
        Virtue Ethics      13
        Natural Law      13
    *Theories of Justice*      15
        Libertarianism      15

Rawls' Theory of Justice     15
Marxism     16
Four Principles of Bioethics     16

2. Requests to Die: Non-Terminal Patients     19
*The Case of Elizabeth Bouvia*     19
    The Legal Battle: Refusing Sustenance     20
*The Case of Larry McAfee*     25
*The Case of Dax Cowart*     27
*Background: Perspectives on Suicide*     27
    Greece and Rome     27
    Philosophers on Voluntary Death     28
    The Concept of Assisted Suicide     31
*Ethical Issues: For and Against Assisted Suicide*     31
    Easy to Kill Oneself?     31
    Rationality and Competence     32
    Autonomy     33
    Treating Depression, Pain, and Symptoms Well     34
    Social Prejudice and Physical Disabilities     34
    Structural Discrimination Against the Disabled     35
    Disability Culture     36
*Further Reading and Resources*     37
*Discussion Questions*     37

3. Requests to Die: Terminal Patients     38
*Holland*     38
*Jack Kevorkian*     39
*Dr. Quill: Another Approach to Dying*     41
*Dr. Pou's Case, Continued*     41
*Oregon's Legalization*     42
*Background: Ancient Greece and the Hippocratic Oath*     43
*Dr. Pou's Case, continued*     44
*The Nazis and "Euthanasia"*     44
*Modern Developments*     46
    Recent Legal Decisions     46
*Ethical Issues*     47
*Direct Arguments—Physician-Assisted Dying*     47
    Killing Is Always Wrong     47
    Killing Is Not Always Wrong     48
    Killing vs. Letting Die     48
    Relief of Suffering     49
    Patient Autonomy     50
*Indirect Arguments About Physician-Assisted Dying*     51
    The Slippery Slope     51
    Inefficient Means     53
    A Financial Empirical Slope?     54

*The Roles of Physicians*     54
*Mistakes and Abuses*     55
*Cries for Help*     55
*Anna Pou, Again: Hero or Villain?*     56
*Further Reading*     57
*Discussion Questions*     58

4.  Comas: Karen Quinlan, Nancy Cruzan, and Terri Schiavo                              59
    *The Quinlan Case*     59
        Pulling the Plug or Weaning from a Ventilator?     62
        Substituted Judgment and Kinds of Cases     63
    *The Cruzan Case*     63
    *The Terri Schiavo Case*     66
        Enter Lawyers and Politicians     67
        What Schiavo's Autopsy Showed     70
    *Ethical Issues*     71
        Standards of Brain Death     71
        Chances of Regaining Consciousness from Coma and PVS     72
        Terri's Chances of Re-Awakening     75
        Compassion and Its Interpretation     75
        Religious Issues     76
        Nagging Questions     76
        Disability Issues     77
        Some Distinctions     77
        Advance Directives     80
        The Schiavo Case, Bioethics and Politics     80
    *Further Reading and Resources*     81
    *Discussion Questions*     81

5.  Abortion: The Trial of Kenneth Edelin                                              83
    *Kenneth Edelin's Controversial Abortion*     83
    *Background: Perspectives on Abortion*     87
        The Language of Abortion     87
        Abortion and the Bible     87
        The Experience of Illegal Abortions     89
        1962: Sherri Finkbine     90
        1968: Humanae Vitae     90
        1973: *Roe v. Wade*     90
        Abortion Statistics     91
    *Ethical Issues*     91
        Edelin's Actions     91
        Personhood     91
        Personhood as a Gradient     92
        The Deprivation Argument: Marquis and Quinn on Potentiality     93
        Viability     94
        The Argument from Marginal Cases     95

Thomson: A Limited Pro-Choice View    96
Feminist Views    96
Genetic Defects    97
A Culture of Life or a Culture of Death?    97
Abortion and Gender Selection    98
Abortion as a Three-Sided Issue    99
Anti-abortion Protests and Violence    99
Live Birth Abortions and How Abortions Are Done    100
Fetal Tissue Research    100
Emergency Contraception    101
Maternal versus Fetal Rights    101
Viability    102
The Supreme Court Fine-Tunes *Roe v. Wade*    103
Partial Birth Abortions    104
States Restrict Abortion Clinics    104
*Further Reading*    104
*Discussion Questions*    105

6. Assisted Reproduction, Multiple Births, and Elderly Parents    106
*The Octamom and the Gosselins*    106
*Background: Louise Brown, The First Test Tube Baby*    107
*Harm to Research from Alarmist Media*    108
*Later Developments in Assisted Reproduction*    109
    Sperm and Egg Transfer    109
*Freezing Gamete Material*    111
*Payment for Assisted Reproduction: Egg Donors*    112
*Payment for Assisted Reproduction: Adoption*    112
    Paid Surrogacy: The Baby M and Jaycee Cases    113
*Multiple Births: Before the Octamom and Gosselins*    114
*Older Parents*    115
*Gender Selection*    116
*Ethical Issues*    116
    Unnatural    116
*Physical Harm to Babies Created in New Ways*    118
*Psychological Harm to Babies Created in New Ways*    119
*Paradoxes About Harm and Reproduction*    119
*Wronging versus Harming*    120
*Harm by Not Knowing One's Biological Parents?*    121
*Is Commercialization of Assisted Reproduction Wrong?*    122
*Screening for Genetic Disease: A New Eugenics?*    122
*Designer Babies?*    123
*Assisted Reproduction Worldwide*    124
*Time to Regulate Fertility Clinics?*    125
*Conclusions*    126
*Further Reading*    126
*Discussion Questions*    126

7. Embryos, Stem Cells, and Cloning      128

*Historical Background of Embryonic Research*    128

   Two Important Cases    129

   History: Embryo Research, Cloning, and Stem Cells    130

*Ethical Issues Involving Embryos in Research*    135

   Valuable from Conception    136

   Potential for Personhood    136

   Slippery Slopes    136

   *Reductio ad Absurdum*    137

   The Interest View    137

   Embryos and Respect    138

   The Opportunity Cost of Missed Research    139

   My Tissue    139

   Moot?    140

*Reproductive Cloning*    140

   Reproductive Cloning: Myths about Cloned Persons    140

   Against the Will of God?    141

   The Right to a Unique Genetic Identity    141

   Unnatural and Perverse    142

   The Right to an Open Future    142

   Abnormalities    143

   Inequality    144

   Good of the Child    144

   Only Way to Have One's Own Baby    146

   Stronger Genetic Connection    146

   Liberty    147

   A Rawlsian Argument for Cloning and Choice    148

   Links Between Embryonic and Reproductive Cloning    148

*Further Readings*    149

*Discussion Questions*    149

8. The Ethics of Treating Impaired Babies      150

*1971: The Johns Hopkins Cases*    150

*1970s: Pediatric Intensivists Go Public*    151

*Ancient History*    152

*1981: The Mueller Case: Conjoined Twins*    152

*1982: The Infant Doe Case*    153

*1982–1986: The Baby Doe Rules*    154

*1983–1984: The Baby Jane Doe Case*    155

*1983–1986: Baby Jane's Case in the Courts*    156

*Follow-up on Baby Jane Doe*    157

*Media Ethics and Bias*    159

*Ethical Issues*    160

   Selfishness    160

   Personal versus Public Cases    160

*Abortion versus Infanticide*    161

   Killing versus Letting Die with Newborns    162

*Personhood of Impaired Neonates* 162
*Kinds of Euthanasia* 163
*Degrees of Defect* 163
*Wrongful Birth versus Wrongful Life* 165
*1984: Legislation* 166
*1992: The Americans with Disabilities Act (ADA)* 166
*The Strength of Disability Advocates* 167
*Conceptual Dilemma: Supporting Both Choice and Respect* 168
*Further Reading* 168
*Discussion Questions* 169

9. Medical Research on Animals 170
*The Animal Liberation Front and Gennarelli's Research* 170
*Evaluating the Philadelphia Study* 172
*PETA and Edward Taub's Research on Monkeys* 173
*The Law and Animal Research* 174
*Numbers and Kinds of Animals in Research* 175
*Descartes on Animal Pain* 176
*C. S. Lewis on Animal Pain* 177
    Philosophy of Mind and Ethics 177
*Peter Singer on Speciesism* 178
*Tom Regan on Animal Rights* 179
*Why We Need Animals in Research: The Official View* 181
*Critiquing the Official View* 182
*Chimpanzees and Research* 183
*Further Reading* 184
*Discussion Questions* 184

10. Medical Research on Vulnerable Human Subjects 186
*Infamous Medical Experiments* 186
    William Beaumont 186
    Nazi Medical Research 186
    Josef Mengele 187
*The Nuremberg Code* 188
    Questionable American Research 188
*The Tuskegee Study (or "Study")* 190
    Nature and History of Syphilis 190
    The Racial Environment 191
*Development of the Tuskegee Study* 192
    A Study in Nature Begins 192
    The Middle Phase: Poor Design 193
    Spinal Taps and Deception 193
    Revelation of the Study to the World 194
*Ethical Issues of the Tuskegee Study* 196
    Informed Consent and Deception 196
    Racism 196
    Media Coverage 197

Harm to Subjects     197
Effects on Subjects' Families     198
Kant and Motives of Researchers     199
*HIV Prevention in Africa: Another Tuskegee Study?*     199
The Krieger Lead Paint Study     201
1946–1948: The Guatemalan Syphilis Study     202
Financial Conflicts and Twenty-First-Century Research     202
*Toward International Standards of Research Ethics*     203
The Collaborative Model     204
The Death of Jesse Gelsinger     205
*Further Reading*     207
*Discussion Questions*     207

11. Surgeons' Desire for Fame: Ethics of the First Transplants     208
*The First Heart Transplant*     208
Fame Cometh     211
The Post-Transplant Era: "Surgery Went Nuts"     211
*Barney Clark's Artificial Heart*     212
The Implant     213
Post-Clark Implants     215
*Limb Transplants*     217
*Face Transplants*     217
*Ethical Issues*     219
The Desire to Be First and Famous     219
Concerns about Criteria of Death     221
Quality of Life     222
Defending Surgery     224
Cosmetic versus Therapeutic Surgery     224
Expensive Rescue versus Cheap Prevention     224
Real Informed Consent?     225
*Conclusion*     226
*Further Reading*     226
*Discussion Questions*     227

12. Just Distribution of Organs: The God Committee
and Personal Responsibility     228
*The God Committee and Artificial Kidneys*     228
*Shana Alexander Publicizes the God Committee; Starts Bioethics*     230
*The End-Stage Renal Disease Act (ESRD)*     231
*The Birth of Bioethics*     232
*Supply and Demand of Donated Organs*     232
*Ethical Issues*     233
Social Worth     233
*Personal Responsibility for Illness and Expensive Resources*     234
*Kant and Rescher on Just Allocation*     235
*Wealth, Celebrities, Justice, and Waiting Lists for Organs*     236

*Retransplants* 238
*The Rule of Rescue* 239
*Sickest First, UNOS, and the Rule of Rescue* 240
*Living Donors* 241
*Costs and the Medical Commons* 243
*Non-Heart-Beating Organ Transplantation* 244
*The God Committee, Again* 246
*Further Reading* 247
*Discussion Questions* 247

13. Using One Baby for Another: Babies Fae, Gabriel, and
    Theresa and Conjoined Twins 249
*1984: Baby Fae* 249
*1987: Baby Gabriel and Paul Holc* 251
*1992: Baby Theresa* 253
*1993: The Lakeberg Case: Separating Conjoined Twins* 254
*Ethical Issues* 255
    Use of Animals as Resources for Humans 255
*Alternative Treatments?* 256
*Babies as Subjects of Research* 257
*Informed Consent* 258
*The Media* 259
*Therapy or Research?* 260
*Ethics and Terminology: Infants as "Donors"* 262
*Anencephalics and Brain Death* 263
*Saving Other Children* 265
*Costs and Opportunity Costs* 265
*Conclusions* 266
*Further Reading* 266
*Discussion Questions* 266

14. Ethical Issues of Intersex and Transgender Persons 267
*David Reimer* 267
*Intersex People* 270
*Congenital Adrenal Hyperplasia* 271
*Fetal Dex* 272
*Ethical Issues* 273
    What Is Normal and Who Defines It? 273
*Secrecy in the Child's Best Interest* 274
*Ending the Shame and Secrecy* 274
*Transgender/Intersex and Civil Rights* 275
*Nature or Nurture, or Both?* 276
    An Alternative, Conservative View 276
    Ken Kipnis' Proposals 277
*Medical Exceptions* 277
*The Dutch Approach: Delaying Puberty* 278

*Conclusions*    278
*Further Reading*    278
*Discussion Questions*    279

15. Involuntary Psychiatric Commitment: The Case of
    Joyce Brown                                                                                       280
    *The Case of Joyce Brown*    280
        The Legal Conflict    281
    *Ideology and Insanity*    284
    *Patients' Rights*    285
    *Legal Victories for Psychiatric Patients*    286
    *Deinstitutionalization*    287
    *Violence and the Mentally Ill Homeless in the Cities*    288
    *Ethical Issues*    289
        Paternalism, Autonomy, and Diminished Competence    289
    *Homelessness and Commitment*    290
    *Psychiatry and Commitment*    291
    *Suffering and Commitment: Benefit and Harm*    292
    *Housing for the Mentally Ill as an Ethical Issue*    293
    *Mass Shootings and the Mentally Ill*    294
    *Further Reading*    295
    *Discussion Questions*    295

16. Ethical Issues in Testing for Genetic Disease                                296
    *Case 1: Angelina Jolie and Genetic Testing for Cancer*    296
    *Background: Basic Genetics*    297
    *Case 2: Nancy Wexler and Huntington's Disease*    297
    *The Eugenics Movement*    299
    *Case 3: Testing for Diabetes*    300
    *Case 4: Testing for Alzheimer's Disease*    302
    *Ethical Issues*    303
        Preventing Disease    303
    *Testing as Self-Interest*    303
    *Testing Only to Hear Good News*    304
    *Testing as a Duty to One's Family*    305
    *Testing One's Family by Testing Oneself*    306
    *Personal Responsibility for Disease*    307
    *Testing and Sick Identities*    308
    *Preventing Suicide by Not Knowing*    308
    *Testing Only with Good Counseling*    309
    *Genetic Testing and Insurance*    310
    *Premature Announcements and Over Simplifications*    310
    *Caveat Emptor: Making Money from Genetic Testing*    311
    *Preventing Genetic Disease: Final Thoughts*    312
    *Further Reading*    313
    *Discussion Questions*    314

*17.* Ethical Issues in Stopping the Global Spread of AIDS        315
  *Background: Epidemics, Plagues, and AIDS*    315
  *A Brief History of AIDS*    316
  *AIDS and Ideology*    317
  *Transmission of HIV and Testing for HIV*    319
  *Kimberly Bergalis's Case*    320
  *Three Ethical Issues in Stopping the Spread of AIDS*    321
    Homosexuality    321
  *HIV Exceptionalism*    322
  *Stopping the Worldwide Spread of HIV: Five Views*    322
    Educational Prevention    324
    Feminism    325
    Triage    326
    Structuralism    327
    Replies and Rebuttals    328
  *Conclusion*    331
  *Further Reading*    332
  *Discussion Questions*    332

*18.* Ethical Issues of the Affordable Care Act        333
  *Rosalyn Schwartz*    333
  *Universal Medical Coverage*    334
    1962 to Present: Canada    334
    The National Health Service in England    335
  *The American Medical System: 1962–2012*    335
    1965: Medicare Begins    336
    1965: Medicaid Begins    336
    1997: CHIP    337
    Tricare and VA Hospitals    337
    1985: COBRA    338
    1986: EMTALA    338
    1993–1994: Clinton's Health Care Security Bill    338
    1996: HIPPA    339
    1962–2012: Coverage at Work through Private Plans    339
  *Blue Cross/Blue Shield and Kinds of Ratings*    340
  *Oregon, Vermont, and Massachusetts Cover Everyone*    341
  *2010: The Patient Protection and Affordable Care Act*    342
  *For and Against The ACA*    343
    Opposing the ACA #1: Illegal Immigrants    343
    Favoring the ACA #1: Illegal Immigrants    344
    Favoring the ACA #2: Greater Efficiency    345
    Opposing the ACA #2: Federal Bureaucracy Is Inefficient    345
    Favoring the ACA #3: Making Medicine Rational    346
    Opposing the ACA #3: Government Cannot Make Medical Finance
    Rational    346
    Opposing the ACA #4: Health Care Is Not a Right    347

Favoring the ACA #4: Minimal Health Care Is a Right   348
Opposing the ACA #5: Health Care Is Not a Right   350
Favoring the ACA #5: Costs Can Be Controlled   352
Opposing the ACA #6: Intergenerational Injustice   353
Favoring the ACA #6: No Intergenerational Injustice   354
*Further Reading*   354
*Discussion Questions*   354

*19.* Ethical Issues in Medical Enhancement   356
*Ethical Issues of Medical Enhancement*   357
What Counts as an Enhancement?   357
Positional Advantage   358
An Arms Race   358
End Secrecy; Legalize Enhancements   359
Inauthentic   359
Cheating   360
Not Dangerous   362
Bad Effects of Legalization   363
*The Role of Physicians*   363
*Conclusions*   364
*Further Reading*   364
*Discussion Questions*   365

*NOTES*   *N–1*

*NAME INDEX*   *I–1*

*SUBJECT INDEX*   *I–6*

# CHAPTER 1

# Ethical Reasoning, Moral Theories, Principles, and Bioethics

## GOOD REASONING IN BIOETHICS

### Giving Reasons

*I*t is important to give *good reasons* for a position in ethics. More globally, giving reasons is part of what it means to *justify* a position in ethics. Justification is a complex affair, but for now we can state that it is more than saying "I feel this" or "I was raised that way" or "Most people think so."

First, the reason given must be *relevant* to the position. For example, in discussing whether humans should ever be created by cloning, someone might argue that such a way of originating people would not create zombies but be just another way of creating identical twins. In arguing this way, the proponent has done two things: first, attacked a common, relevant misconception about human cloning, and second, offered an insight, comparing creation of a new person by cloning from the cells of an existing person to the process that occurs when human embryos twin. In this second reason, the proponent is saying that cloning is really not unnatural but natural. Because the unnaturalness or naturalness of human cloning is highly relevant to whether it is ethical, this is a good reason.

Besides relevance, a good reason often provides *evidence* for a position. Suppose Martha favors in vitro fertilization and someone objects that such methods produce defective babies. Martha then replies that the rate of gene-linked defects in such babies is only a bit higher than the rate in the general population. (Chapter 6 discusses this claim.) That fact is good evidence, and hence, a good reason.

In arguing about abortion, an anti-abortionist might claim as a premise that a 12-week-old embryo feels pain, and therefore aborting such an embryo is wrong. Then someone pro-choice might counter that the neural system is undeveloped at 12 weeks, so no one exists who can feel pain. The anti-abortionist counters that "pain is pain," whether the being is a shrimp, rat, or human embryo. At this point, claims will continue to be exchanged back-and-forth, but notice that all these claims are *evidence* for and against the premise that the embryo feels pain at 12 weeks, and so, constitute good reasons.

Ideally, good reasons support a conclusion as an *argument*, that is, not a dispute, but a justified conclusion. Sometimes in an argument, a key premise is missing or assumed, but it needs to be made explicit. This missing premise is called an *enthymeme*. In the preceding argument, this premise is, "We should not cause pain to embryos." Without this premise, the argument doesn't work.

*Logic* is the study of the formal properties of arguments. It distinguishes between *truth* and falsehood, which governs how premises correspond or not to the world, and *validity*, which concerns the formal relations between premises and conclusion. In logic, an argument with true premises and a valid structure is called *sound*.

Another kind of good reason in bioethics appeals not to evidence, but to a *principle.* In the case where not everyone can get a scarce life-saving machine, questions arise about how to choose who is saved. In 1962, distributing dialysis machines raised just such a problem. One proposal was that, "Everyone should have an equal chance to get a machine," and to effect this, some advocated a lottery to select recipients. Here, the principle of equal consideration counted as a good reason.

Consider also the debate in bioethics as to whether alcoholics should be given a liver transplant, a practice that some critics believe wastes a good organ. (This is discussed in detail in Chapter 12.) A proponent of including alcoholics as recipients could argue from the principle of equal consideration that everyone should be able to get a new liver, so past behavior should not matter. An opponent might cite different principles such as, "Good organs should not be wasted" and "People must be held responsible for their bad behavior." In debating whether alcoholics get livers, these principles function as good reasons for and against the inclusion of alcoholics.

Finally, good reasons should not contradict each other but should be logically *consistent*. For example, if someone favors not making human cloning illegal by federal law, he might argue that it is not the business of federal government to tell citizens how to produce new humans. He might cite Huxley's novel *Brave New World* as an example of what could go wrong when government controls reproduction. To be consistent, he should favor keeping government out of all human reproductive decisions, including those about assisted reproduction, birth control, abortion, adoption, and whether to have children.

Consistency in ethics also entails not making exceptions for one's own case. For example, with brain death and organ transplants, one would not endorse bending the traditional criteria of brain death to generate more organs unless one would be willing to oneself be declared brain-dead by bending these rules. Or more commonly, we cannot consistently urge, "Everyone should volunteer to help the sick and needy, but I don't have the time to do so."

## Universalization

Most of us have been ethically challenged at some point in our lives by someone who asked us, "What if everyone did that?" Such a challenge assumes that the rules of ethics must be for everyone.

The idea of universalization often comes up in moral decisions. In bioethics, a controversy exists as to whether normal people with two kidneys should be encouraged to altruistically donate one so that someone on life-long dialysis could receive a kidney and live a normal life. Here the question, "What if everyone did that?" has a good answer: Because most people will need only one kidney for their life, if everyone agreed to donate a kidney (if they matched, were in good health, etc.), then all kinds of good things would occur. In short, the practice seems morally justified. Another way of putting this is that good reasons exist for altruistic donation of kidneys.

The twentieth-century ethicist R. M. Hare states this idea about universalization nicely,

> Universalizability means that, by saying "I ought," he commits himself to agreeing that *anybody* ought who is in just those circumstances. If I say "I ought, but there is someone else in exactly the same circumstances, doing it to someone who is just like the person I should be doing it to, but he ought not to do it," then logically eyebrows will be raised; it is *logically inconsistent* to say, of two exactly similar people in exactly similar situations, that the first ought to do something and the second ought not.[1]

## Impartiality

One of the most important ideas in ethics is that we should not make special rules for our own case, in other words, that we should not be *partial* to our own interests. Similarly, we should not be partial to those in our own gender, ethnicity, or age group. Instead we should be *impartial*, treating everyone the same.

Just how impartial we should be is an important question in ethical theory. Is it permissible to put the boundary of impartiality at our national borders, or should ethics be universal? For example, in research bioethics, should there be one standard for informed consent in developed countries and another in developing countries?

Over time, the tendency in ethics has been to widen the scope of impartiality. Thus in research bioethics today, there has been a movement to not have a double standard for developed and developing countries, but to treat both the same. (This is discussed in Chapter 9.)

One important idea here in reasoning concerns *onus of proof*. Suppose someone wants to apply a rule only to his own group, say, by arguing that cancer specialists, to encourage hope, should not always tell patients the truth about their diagnosis. Because it is now a norm in medicine to tell the truth and because most people want to know the truth, the "onus" or burden of truth for non-disclosure should be on cancer specialists. What this means is that this specialist needs especially good reasons for his actions and if he cannot present such good reasons, his position is unjustified.

## Reasonableness

It is hard to exactly characterize what is meant by being reasonable in ethics, but it is certainly composed of being open to other points of view. It is unlikely that the way any of us was raised—in, say, a Southern culture as a Baptist—is the only path to the truth about the universe. People raised in Jewish, Hindu, or Muslim cultures might also have insights into the universe, as might people raised in non-religious, secular households. Being open to other viewpoints is good for everyone, at least for people who share an interest in truth.

The same holds for other viewpoints on positions in bioethics. Most of us bring to these issues a general orientation that predisposes us to a certain position. For example, we might come from a culture that frowns on drinking alcohol and thus condemns rewarding alcoholics with liver transplants. But it is important to consider other points of view, for example, the theory that alcoholism is a disease over which drinkers have no control. If that theory is correct, then alcoholics should be blamed no more than people who get endocarditis from a virus.

Another quality of reasonableness is being fair-minded. This quality of intellectual life differs from being open-minded because it goes further and includes a willingness to try to see the best in the reasoning of other people. The opposite of this is the *fallacy of attacking a straw man*, where the attacker is not fair, does not attack the best version of his opponent's argument, but instead attacks a weak "straw man" who is easy to knock down.

Being unfair tends to generate hostility rather than goodwill. Being fair-minded includes a willingness to admit problems with one's own position, to admit good objections to it, and to admit that—given enough good reasons—one could even change one's mind. Most important, being fair-minded in discussing issues means trying to consider the best argument on the opposing side. Sometimes this can be expressed by the trial balloon, "If I understand what you are saying, you mean that ..." Such a tactic gives the opponent a chance to refine or modulate his or her position and engenders a spirit of mutual work toward discovering the best answer.

## Civility

In the United States in the past decades, a tone of incivility has permeated debates in public policy, including those in bioethics. This is unfortunate. Because of adamant divisions between political parties, between social conservatives and social liberals, and between liberal and conservative bioethicists, the tone of debate has sometimes descended to scoring cheap points, to demagoguery, to painting one's opponents as spawn of the Devil, and in general, to being nasty.

Being civil in discussions in bioethics improves everyone. Being uncivil degrades us all, both in class, as citizens, and as future professionals. This is juvenile, unprofessional behavior, and it is sad to see so many talk shows on cable television promoting it (seeing people argue badly seems to promote good ratings). It is important to realize that one can argue fairly and rationally without being mean and without attacking opponents personally. Some of the fallacies described in the following section involve cheap tricks in such mean-spirited attacks.

## MISTAKES IN ETHICAL REASONING

### Slippery Slope

Often in bioethics, champions of the status quo argue that a small change in a ~ent medical practice will lead to terrible results. Although the small change ~ not so bad, because there is no logical place to draw the line or because ~ horrible is unleashed in human nature, soon bad things will occur.

This is basically the idea of the *slippery slope*, which is one of the most famous ideas in ethics. It also called the "thin edge of the wedge"— or simply the "wedge"— argument. Claims about it in bioethics figure prominently in debates about physician-assisted dying, cloning, abortion, standards of brain death, and assisted reproduction.

Slippery slope arguments metaphorically see society as teetering like a ball perched atop a steep, greased slope and leaning downward, braced only by wedges on the ground, preventing it from descending. Our basic moral principles are the wedges.

For example, someone might invoke the slippery slope by claiming, "If we do not ban students taking the MCAT from using Adderall or Ritalin, soon there will be an arms race of mental enhancements by test-takers."

The counterargument to the slippery slope is multi-faceted: First, we can make a small change without going all the way down the slope. If we see that a change in a medical practice is bad, we can undo it. Also, not all change is bad; how else would progress occur? Finally, one's person's "slope" is another's "ascent." Integration and equal voting rights may have seemed like the pit to white male supremacists, but not to everyone else.

### *Ad hominem* ("To the man")

Generally, it's a mistake to make a personal attack on someone else, in part because you may not know an opponent well. Suppose Gina argues for the moral superiority of suicide for terminally ill patients because it gives patients control over their lives, because it is justified by the principle of autonomy, and because, after all, "it's the patient's body, not the doctor's." Her reasons are not affected by whether she is terminally ill. An *ad hominen* fallacy would be committed if someone said, "I'll bet you would change your mind if you were dying." This puts the focus incorrectly on her personal life and not on the reasons she gave for her position.

### *Tu quoque* (pronounced "tew-kwoh-kway")

Literally, "You, too." The mistaken idea here is that two wrongs make a right. First pharmacist: "You made an exception last week and let a 12-year-old girl buy emergency contraception when the law says she must be 14." Second pharmacist: "You made a similar exception for your 13-year-old niece."

"You, too!" resonates in ethics because when someone confronts us with wrongdoing, we feel less ashamed if the other person has also done it. But saying someone else also acted wrongly doesn't *justify* the first wrong.

### Straw Man/Red Herring

This occurs when someone brings up irrelevant issues. The fallacy is committed when someone focuses on a different issue than the one originally advocated, because the different issue is easier to refute. Example: "We should reject

Obamacare because it will lead to death panels where people are forced to have advance directives before they know they are dying or know what their options are."

Getting universal coverage for medical care does not entail death panels, but death panels sound scary and are easier to attack than universal medical coverage.

It is also not fair-minded to attack a position that one's opponent does not hold. Doing so is destructive, not constructive, to rational debate in bioethics.

The red herring fallacy is a bit different from straw man and consists of distracting an opponent from the real argument by raising an irrelevant, but associated, issue. (In hunting with dogs, the red herring across the trail of the tracked animal put the dogs on the wrong path.) So in discussing abortion and whether a fetus is a person, someone might object, "More African Americans have abortions as a percentage than white Americans." Obviously, raising race as an issue is always potentially controversial and, here, potentially distracting. The most important point is that the statement bears no relevance on whether the fetus is a person. Both, therefore, are fallacies of relevance.

### *Post hoc, ergo propter hoc* ("After this, therefore, because of this")

The mistake in reasoning here confuses temporal priority with causality. An example: "In the 1960s, women started working outside the home, and a few years later, rates of divorce soared. Therefore, if we want to preserve the family, we should prevent women from working outside the home."

Just because one event occurred before another does not mean the first caused the second. Why? Because when you think about it, *everything* in history came before X. Consider an example from the best-selling *Freakonomics*: "Abortion was legalized in 1973, and 15 years later, the crime rates went down. So if you want to lower rates of crime in the future, encourage abortions."

The problem here is the supposed causal links between abortion and crime rates. What might be true is that with more abortions in certain neighborhoods, there are fewer people 15 years later, or fewer people between ages 15 and 25 who could commit crimes. But more birth control pills might have had the same effect. Also, it may be that better education and counseling started at the same time and made a big difference.

### Appeal to Authority

Reasons and arguments justify a position, not just any authority. Moreover, when an authority is cited, it must be *relevant* to the topic in question.

Harvard Professor E. O. Wilson is probably the world's foremost authority on ants. When Wilson wrote *Sociobiology*, he claimed that, in certain aspects, organizations of ants and humans resembled each other. Quoting Wilson about Sociobiology is not erroneous but appropriate.

On the other hand, Wilson may have opinions about rock bands, but quoting these opinions is irrelevant to whether a band is good. Wilson's authority on ants is not relevant to rock bands.

## Appeals to Feelings and Upbringing

How you feel about something or what you were brought up to believe doesn't count as a reason for it. Example: "I was brought up to believe that men were the hunters and women were the hunted, so a woman should wait until a man finds her and asks her out."

Here is another example: "I was brought up to think being gay was repulsive, so I've got to feel that way." In this claim, we could substitute for "being gay" any number of other qualities, such as religion, race, ethnicity, or looks.

Obviously, you can be brought up in the wrong way, and as a result, or for other reasons, have irrational feelings as an adult. Again, *reasons justify a position in ethics*, not feelings or upbringing.

## *Ad populum*

"Everybody does it." Just because everyone does something does not justify it or make it ethical. Most physicians may take free gifts from drug reps who push expensive, brand name drugs over generics, but that doesn't mean it's right to take such gifts. The self-serving claim, "All the other physicians do it. Why shouldn't I take such gifts, too?" commits this fallacy.

## False Dichotomy ("Either-Or" Fallacy)

This fallacy is a version of simplistic thinking. "Either you're a liar or a completely honest man." The opponent presents an issue as if there are only two extreme, opposed alternatives, with nothing in between—black or white, no gray. "Either we ban cell phones, or people will use them while driving." Consider also: "Either we're all nuts, or we're all lucid."

Another example: "Either God exists, or everything is permitted." Counter-argument: Even if there's no God, good people will still act virtuously. If there is a God and people only act virtuously to please him, maybe they aren't virtuous anyway because only people who do the right thing *because it is right* are really virtuous.

## Equivocation

We should be careful to define key terms and not let key words contain many meanings. So we should clarify equivocal or ambiguous words with more than one meaning. Example: "Sex offenders should only be allowed to live in certain areas, so Alan Jones should not live here."

But who is a "sex offender"? It turns out that as an 18-year-old Atlanta teenager, Alan had consenting sex with a girl who was one month shy of 18, so technically he committed sodomy and was legally a sex offender in Georgia. But more commonly, the phrase is reserved for people who have non-consensual sex with a minor with a far greater age difference.

In bioethics, one of the most important terms is "person," where this evaluative term contrasts with "human," or mere biological membership in the human species. Some people consider 8 day-old human embryos to be persons and hence, that IUDs, which prevent embryos from implanting, are instruments of murder. Some people believe that victims of late-stage Alzheimer's disease are no longer persons, especially when they cannot recognize their children or remember how to take a shower. On the expansionist side of personhood, some bioethicists such as Peter Singer would include chimpanzees and great apes.

What is important in good reasoning is to define key terms such as "person." Sometimes, achieving clarity about such a definition is the major task at hand. Certainly in bioethics, philosophers, bioethicists, and theologians have penned untold volumes in trying to clarify the concept of personhood.

## Begging the Question

Begging the question occurs when a conclusion that requires good reasons is assumed without argument, so "begging" here means "assuming without proof." The end of the discussion in the previous section mentioned that Peter Singer considers adult chimpanzees to be persons. Someone might retort, "No. Only humans can be persons." Singer would reply that such a stance begs the question at hand, namely, whether only humans can be persons. That crucial point cannot just be assumed at the start, but must be backed up with good reasons. Indeed, that is the whole purpose of justification here.

Question-begging mistakes are not always obvious because synonyms may disguise the mistake. "I think everyone from the South is a racist." Why? "Because everyone who lives in states below the Mason-Dixon line is racist." The person has just said the same thing twice, both times assuming what should be argued for.

In bioethics and the abortion debate, an example of begging the question would be if an anti-abortionist began a debate by stating, "Abortion is murder." This statement begs at least two questions: that killing a fetus or embryo is the same as killing a full person and that the kind of killing in abortion is, like murder, an *unjustified* killing. (These claims are discussed in Chapter 5.)

## ETHICAL THEORIES, PRINCIPLES, AND BIOETHICS

In this section, some classic ethical theories are surveyed with emphasis on bioethics.

## Moral Relativism

Moral relativism is the theory that no universal truths exist across cultures but instead, what is right or wrong must be defined in each society. Inside a particular culture, some things are right, others wrong, but nothing is wrong across all.

This theory, popular in anthropology, initially seems attractive when students study various peoples around the world and different times in history. But it also has flaws, and medicine is one place where such flaws can be exhibited.

Consider that medicine under the Nazi regime in Germany was anti-Semitic, racist, and contemptuous of people with disabilities. As a result, physicians led the movement to "cleanse" the Aryan race of undesirable, "useless eaters," leading to the Holocaust and deaths of 6 million people. As described in Chapter 10, Nazi physicians also conducted horrible medical experiments on captives.

A moral relativist must accept the view that we cannot condemn Nazi physicians for such actions. The trials at Nuremberg were a farce. Inside Nazi culture, the Holocaust was not wrong but right. Only from an external, objective standard of morality can such actions be condemned.

## Utilitarianism

Utilitarianism was developed by philosopher-activists Jeremy Bentham and John Stuart Mill in late-eighteenth-century England. It holds that right acts produce the greatest amount of good for the greatest number of beings, which it called "utility." Its teachings can be summed up in four basic tenets:

1. *Consequentialism:* Consequences count, not motives or intentions.
2. *Maximization:* The number of beings affected by a consequence matters; the more beings affected, the more important the result.
3. *A theory of value* (or of "good"): A definition of what counts as *good* consequences.
4. *A scope-of-morality premise:* Each being's happiness is to count as one unit of happiness up to a certain boundary.

For utilitarians, right acts then contain four aspects, the greatest amount of good consequences for the greatest number of beings of a certain kind.

One distinctive aspect of utilitarianism is that it is wholly secular and posits no God or gods as the sources of morality. In this sense, it is naturalistic. In emphasizing consequences, it contrasts with deontology, such as Kantian ethics, which emphasizes motives, and virtue ethics, which emphasizes traits of character.

Each of the four tenets can be controversial. In reverse order, consider tenet 4, the scope of morality or who has "standing" in moral considerations. Bentham emphasized that the meaning of tenet 4, was whether a being could suffer, not whether it was human or animal. As such, many utilitarians include animals in their calculations of the "greatest number." This makes a big difference to research by psychologists and physiologists on animals. If an ape is 90 percent a human in interests and value, and utilitarianism calculates utility this way, then very few experiments on primates will be morally justified.

Some utilitarian thinkers such as Peter Singer take a large view of moral standing and hold that every being's happiness on the planet matters, not just citizens of America and not just humans. As such, they are more likely in bioethics to emphasize what benefits the poor people of the world.

Virtue ethicists and Kantians (discussed later) regard a physician's motives as a sign of his character. The poor patient without medical coverage doesn't care whether the physician volunteering to treat him without payment is doing it from a sense of duty or from guilt or to make others think him good. What matters is that the physician is there for him. Utilitarians think motives count only insofar as they tend to produce the greatest good.

In medicine, does it matter whether a physician listens because she really cares about patients or because she's found that having satisfied patients is an effective way to maximize income? A utilitarian might argue that if she is talented, whether she really cares about her patients matters little; in either case, her behavior produces good consequences to real people. For a larger view, she may do more good bringing clean water to a village than being a cameo medical missionary.

On the other hand, for virtue ethicists and Kantians, character and motives, not results, are everything, Good people sometimes fail to achieve good results, but if their motives are pure, they can't be faulted for such failures. Do we really want a physician who is faking compassion?

Utilitarianism also contains a theory of value (tenet 3), that is, a theory of harmful and good consequences. Utilitarianism is associated with, but not the same as, the Harm Reduction Movement in medicine, which focuses not on changing "immoral" behaviors such as IV-drug usage, prostitution, and gambling, but on the harmful results associated with them.

The most important claim of utilitarianism is that consequences matter to determining morality (tenet 1). Medicine can certainly live with that. When sick people see a physician, they want results, not just good intentions. And even other ethical theories, such as Kantian ethics and virtue theory, seem always to be indirectly appealing to consequences in calculating right actions.

## Problems of Utilitarianism

Maximization in utilitarianism has its benefits. It's an organizing principle; it sets a direction, and it provides guidance. In medicine, isn't it always better to save more lives than fewer?

Consider the famous *Trolley problem*. In its classical version, a streetcar loses its brakes and rolls uncontrollably down a steep mountain. At the bottom, the track divides into two parts: on the left side is one person and on the right, six. Shouldn't the conductor go left? Isn't he obligated to do so?

Similarly, suppose a surgeon can take liver, kidneys, heart, skin, eyes, and bone marrow from a brain-dead cadaver and save either the life of one patient, who gets everything, or save six separate patients. Again, it seems obvious that saving six is better than saving one.

In medicine, maximization and utilitarianism are often applied in public health ethics and situations of *triage*. Triage allocates scarce resources during emergencies when not all will live. Because consequences count, utilitarian physicians should *not* treat each patient equally, but should focus on those who can be benefited. Rigorous application of this principle gives utilitarianism its famous hard edge: Physicians should abandon those who will *die* anyway and, just as ruthlessly, abandon those who will *live* anyway. Physicians at the scene should help only those who waver between life and death and for whom intervention can tilt the balance toward life. The goal is always to save the maximal number of lives.

In these catastrophic situations, such as after a terrorist attack or tsunami, what other theory could help? Similarly in medical research, such as that focused on curing cancer, researchers need to focus on the big picture, which that is removing the scourge of cancer from tens of millions of lives. Yes, individual cancer patients may suffer in experimental trials of new drugs, but the goal is to help the huge numbers of cancer victims of the future.

Maximization tenet 2 can get utilitarians into trouble. Wouldn't utilitarianism be willing to violate the traditional sanctity-of-life principle to save many people? Wouldn't utilitarianism permit the sacrifice of an innocent, healthy person to transfer his organs to four patients who needed them to live?[2] Aren't four people alive better than one? If consequences and numbers define morality, what's wrong with doing so? Yet it's wrong to chop up a patient like this.

## Kantian Ethics

Immanuel Kant (1724–1804) lived during the Enlightenment, and he believed in the power of reason to solve human problems. The distinctive elements of Kantian ethics are these:

1. *Ethics is not a matter of consequences but of duty.* Why an act is done is more important than its results. Specifically, an act must be done from the right motive, and the right motive is the desire to do one's duty. Indeed, there is only one correct motive in Kantian ethics and that is the desire to be a good person, to do what is right, to have a "pure will."

   Kant's ethics celebrate duty (and are therefore called *deontological*, from *deontos*, duty) because they emphasize not having the right desires or feelings, but acting from obligation. We should praise only medical acts done from duty, not from compassion. For Kant, the correct motive for treating a patient well is not because a physician feels like doing so, but because it is the right thing to do. When we act morally, Kant says, reason must tell feelings what to do, not the other way around, as in popular culture.

   Kant says the only thing valuable in the world is a good will, the trait of character indicating a willingness to choose the right act simply because it's right. But how do we know what is right? What is our duty? Kant gives two formulations.

2. *A right act has a maxim that is universalizable.* An act is right if one can will its maxim or rule to be acted on by all others. "Lying to get out of keeping a promise" cannot be so willed because if everyone acted this way, promise-keeping would mean nothing.

3. *A right act always treats other humans as "ends-in-themselves," never as a "mere means."* To treat another person as an "end in himself" is to treat him as having absolute, infinite moral worth, not relative worth. His welfare cannot be sacrificed to the good of others or to one's own desires. So parents cannot create one child to help another, as with *savior siblings*.

   Consider the nurse who discovers a physician failed to tell patient Ruth an important fact years ago. Now it is too late for the truth to help Ruth. A consequentialist might argue that the nurse should not tell because Ruth won't benefit. But for Kant, Ruth must be told the truth. The only universalizable rule is, "Always tell patients the truth." Such a rule is the basis of trust and of treating patients as "ends in themselves." If the nurse were the patient, she would want to know. The nurse may *feel* that she shouldn't reveal the truth but reason will reveal her real duty.

4. *People are free only when they act rationally.* Kant would agree that much of how we act is governed by our emotions, as well as our biology. But controversially, Kant denies that we act morally when we do the right thing because we are accustomed to it, because it feels right, or because our society favors the act. We act morally only when we understand why certain rules are right and then freely choose to bind our actions to them. Kant calls the capacity to act this way *autonomy*. For him, it gives humans higher worth and dignity than animals.

It follows for Kant that one should not treat one's own person as a thing. That means one cannot think of oneself as a mechanical machine, subject only to the laws of chemistry and physics. So people are more than their bodies. Hence for Kant, alcoholism is not a disease of a body but a pattern of free choices.

## Problems of Kantian Ethics

Kantian ethics has several problems. First, it fails to tell us how to resolve conflicts between competing maxims. Because most cases in bioethics involve many competing interests of different people, there will be competing, universalizable maxims. In the preceding case about failing to tell a patient the truth, one maxim is, "Always tell the truth" but another is, "Be kind and don't inflict useless pain."

Second, the ideal of treating each person as if he has infinite value is not always practical: It does not tell us how to deliberate about tradeoffs when some humans will die in triage situations. Nor does it make sense in medicine when spending $5 million on one patient may mean spending little on the next 10 patients.

Third, some of Kant's ideas appear out of date. Why shouldn't Kantians accept an altruistic kidney donation? Why isn't everyone better off under such a maxim, and why isn't such a choice evidence of our best, free, rational natures?

Nevertheless, Kant provides useful insights to medical ethics. He would favor using a lottery to distribute a life-saving, but scarce new drug. His emphasis on people as "ends in themselves" explains the outrage that people have felt when learning of research done by Nazi physicians. Finally, Kantian autonomy explains why informed consent grounds participation in medical experiments. Also, when combined with the political autonomy of citizens of democracies, Kantian autonomy sets the stage for modern medical ethics.

## The Ethics of Care

During the 1980s, feminist psychologists and philosophers questioned whether traditional ethical theories were too male-oriented, too abstract, too intellectual, and too false to the experience of women, who valued trust, cooperation, nurturing, and bonding.

Carol Gilligan claimed that women analyze ethical dilemmas differently than men. Subsequent feminist theorists, who created the often-called *ethics of care theory*, explored family relationships by promoting "female" virtues of caring, nurturing, trust, intimate friendship, and love. Rather than focusing on atomistic individuals, the theory emphasized the family, which too often drops out of bioethical analysis. Overall, the ethics of care may be a useful corrective to abstract, semi-legalistic concepts, such as rights.

In criticism, the ethics of care does not tell us how to treat people we do not know or, worse, people we do not care about. This is important because physicians today often meet patients as strangers. Nor does it tell us how to resolve conflicts among people we care about, such as when a physician is torn between checking on a patient and being with his own daughter at childbirth.

Other feminists believe that only traditional gender roles make these virtues female and that the ethics of care reinforces stereotypes. As one wit said, "The ethics of care screams, 'Mommy!'" It should also be emphasized that female bioethicists often address concerns far beyond the family or their personal network of caring, such as the plight of HIV-infected women around the world.

## Virtue Ethics

In ancient Greek medicine, to know what made a good physician, we needed to know the physician's *role*. If that role was to heal the sick, then it required virtues of compassion, knowledge of healing, and skill in human relations. Virtues, then, were skills in performing a role well.

Socrates transcended role-defined ethics and asked about the virtues of a good person. Ancient Greek philosophers believed that the four great human excellences were human courage, temperance, wisdom, and justice, known as *the cardinal virtues*.

So we should not only ask, "What virtues should a good physician possess?" but also, "What virtues should a good person possess who happens to work as a physician?"

Role-based ethics suffer problems when roles conflict or the wider society calls into question whether the role has been properly defined. Greek virtues celebrated Hellenistic culture, but this culture was blind to being built on slavery. Role-based ethics still underlies the apprentice system in medical education, where medical students gradually assume more responsibility.

## Natural Law

When Rome conquered Greece, Greek culture in turn captured Rome. Rome's Stoic philosophers elevated one aspect of the Greek worldview to a higher level. Rules for human beings, they argued, were so embedded in the texture of the world that they were *law* for humans. These laws came to be known as "natural laws." They were apprehended by unaided reason, without Scripture or divine revelation.

The notion of a law-giver lies behind natural law. In the eleventh century, Thomas Aquinas synthesized Aristotelianism with Christian ideas to create his

*Thomistic* worldview. Aquinas then made explicit the connection between God and natural laws: A rational God made the world work rationally and gave humans reason to discover these laws. So studying Thomistic ethics is a rational process of discovering those rules. Correct *descriptions* of the world would yield correct *prescriptions* about how to act. To act rationally is to act morally, which in turn is to act in accordance with natural law.

These rules commanded humans to resist their feelings. St. Augustine taught in the fourth century C.E. that sin contaminated human feeling: as such, lust, sloth, avarice, and pride infected humans. This was in stunning contrast to modern times, for Aquinas ethics was *not* about examining one's feelings but about following the natural rules laid down by God.

Natural law condemns homosexuality. Aquinas believed that God made two sexes for procreation and that it was natural and rational for a man and woman to mate to have children. On the other hand, for two people of the same gender to have sex was contrary to natural law, and hence, immoral.

One problem with natural law theory is that what is considered against natural law may vary over the centuries. Many today do not consider homosexuality to be unnatural, especially because it has been practiced since the beginning of human history and because some great cultures, such as the ancient Greeks, celebrated it as ideal.

For natural law theory, consider marriage and children. Natural law regards loving, sexual relations between married man and wife as natural and good, and the natural product of such sex is children. But many forms of assisted reproduction today—in vitro fertilization, egg transfer, surrogate mothers, and artificial insemination of donor sperm—violate natural law because they don't involve sex between husbands and wives..

Natural law in bioethics tends to conflate "natural" with "primitive" or "traditional," and hence, it has no way to accommodate change or progress, for example, in helping infertile couples with assisted reproduction.

Natural law theory bequeathed to bioethics the famous *doctrine of double effect*. This doctrine holds that if an action had two effects, one good and the other evil, the evil effect was morally permitted: (1) if the action was good in itself or not evil, (2) if the good followed as immediately from the cause as did the evil effect, (3) if only the good effect was intended, and (4) if there was as important a reason for performing the action as for allowing the evil effect.

This doctrine justifies an exception to abortions with an ectopic pregnancy (an embryo growing in a Fallopian tube). This doctrine allows abortions only if the direct intention was to save the life of the mother and if the other conditions listed are followed.

This doctrine forbids physicians from assisting in executions, since it forbids an intention to kill. On the other hand, it allows increasing dosages of morphine for terminal patients, so long as the intention is to relieve suffering, not to kill the patient. (This idea entered the case of Ana Pou, the New Orleans physician caught by Hurricane Katrina—see Chapter 2).

The *principle of totality* also derives from natural law. It says that the human body may be changed only to ensure the proper functioning of that body. The underlying idea is that one's body is not something that one owns, but that one holds in trust for God: "The body is the temple of the Lord." So a gangrenous leg may be amputated or a cancerous breast removed, because these diseases threaten the body's overall health.

According to this principle, we are given our bodies as they are for a reason and we should not change our bodies for frivolous reasons. God wisely created human bodies as they are, and humans shouldn't meddle with these results.

## THEORIES OF JUSTICE

Many theories of justice exist. Most divide into *retributive* (about punishment) and *distributive* (about how to allocate benefits and burdens). Here, three main theories of justice are discussed.

### Libertarianism

Libertarians favor government for defense and for limited public works, perhaps not even including national parks or a public interstate road system (we could have private toll roads). They disfavor government programs such as Medicare, Medicaid, disability insurance, food stamps, and welfare. Libertarians oppose forced taxation by the government, especially when it redistributes property and income from rich to poor. They champion the property rights of the status quo, but tend to be silent about how those enjoying the status quo acquired their property. Harvard philosopher Robert Nozick saw forced taxation as equivalent to forced labor.

Accordingly, Libertarians oppose mandatory FICA taxes on workers' pay and taxes for Medicare and for the Hospital Insurance Trust Fund. Even though federal programs such as Medicare have made American physicians rich, libertarian physicians would rather have no government control over their business. In a libertarian society, physicians would be reimbursed only in cash.

Critics say that in such a system, fewer hospitals would be built, elderly patients would frequently forego procedures for lack of money, and physicians would earn far less income. In such a system, physicians would be controlled by few federal regulations.

### Rawls's Theory of Justice

John Rawls, a philosopher of the twentieth century, believed that moral constraints should be imposed on the social contract. He called his most important constraint "the veil of ignorance"—in the hypothetical social contract, no one should know his or her age, gender, race, health, number of children, income, wealth, or other arbitrary personal information. *Rawlsian contractarianism* assumes that people are self-interested and choose the basic institutions of their society in a social contract; it is Kantian in imposing impartiality or fairness on the choosers by ruling out arbitrary information on them.

Rawls argues that the only rational way to choose under his veil of ignorance is as if, when the veil lifts, one might be the least well-off person in society. Because you don't know anything personal under the veil, you don't know what place in society you will occupy. This justifies the choice of his famous *difference principle*: Choosers should opt for institutions creating equality unless a difference favors the least well-off group.

So *everyone* should be trained in medicine unless training only a few is better for the least well-off. Mandating the difference principle imposes the Golden Rule on the structure of society.

Rawlsian justice entails that every citizen should have equal access to medical care unless unequal access favors the poor. It reduces the inequalities of fate; hence, children and those with genetic disease must get good medical care *as a matter of justice*.

Advocates of free markets favor private medical insurance plans in which the healthy do not subsidize the unhealthy. Rawlsians see "healthy" and "unhealthy" as arbitrary distinctions, due more to genetics than individual merit. Libertarians would allow for-profit companies to practice experience rating, whereby citizens with preexisting illness may be excluded. Rawlsians favor community rating, whereby risk and premium rates are spread over all members of a large community, such as a state or nation.

### Marxism

Although both more and less than a theory of justice, Marxism is still an important tool for understanding the world and bioethics. Marx saw history as a struggle between the owners of the means of production (the rich) and the workers (the poor). He thought the rich got richer by not paying workers their true labor (theory of) value. Workers are exploited and create "surplus value"(i.e., unjustified value) for owners.

In bioethics, Marx's most important insight may be to always understand how money influences decisions in medicine. Although how people get reimbursed is certainly not the only issue that should be considered in bioethical analysis, it is also naïve to ignore how people get paid. For example, most services of physicians in assisted reproduction or enhancement medicine are not covered by traditional insurance plans, so these kinds of medicine are advertised aggressively in far different ways than, say, cancer surgery.

Marxist analysis may be more important than ever today, when the gap between income/wealth over the first years of the 2000s has grown considerably in North America and Europe. Moreover, a whole generation of young people may lack the upward economic mobility of past generations and be trapped into paying exorbitant taxes for medical care for seniors.

## FOUR PRINCIPLES OF BIOETHICS

One modern method of analysis is to dissect a medical case in terms of four principles. These principles are (patient) autonomy, beneficence, nonmaleficence, and justice.

*Autonomy* refers to the right to make decisions about one's own life and body without coercion by others. It honors the value that democracies place on allowing individuals to make their own decisions about whom to marry, whether to have children, how many children to have, what kind of career to pursue, and what kind of life they want to live. Insofar as is possible and to the extent that their decisions do not harm others, individuals should be left alone to make fundamental medical decisions that affect their own bodies and lives.

John Stuart Mill was a political theorist as well as an ethical theorist. In his most famous work of politics, *On Liberty* (1859), he defended this ideal of autonomy against the growing powers of government. He there defends "one simple principle," his so-called *harm principle*: "that the only purpose for which power can rightfully be exercised over any member of a civilized community, against his will, is to prevent harm to others. His own good, either physical or moral, is not a sufficient warrant. Over himself, over his own body and mind, the individual is sovereign."

Autonomy rejects paternalistic ethics. During the patient's rights movement in the early 1960s in America, feminists scorned paternalistic physicians as sexist octogenarians who imposed their rigid ideas on a more enlightened, freethinking, younger generation.

*Beneficence,* or helping others, grounds compassion. It grounds the moral difference between therapeutic and nontherapuetic experiments. If physicians intend to help diabetics, beneficence justifies experiments on diabetics, but if they have no such intent, the experiment may be unjustified.

Beneficence can be seen both as a principle and as a virtue for physicians. Physicians receive special powers, income, and prestige from society and, in return, are asked to help patients. Medical training requires this trait, as demands on a student increase on a slope between premedical years and residency. Self-sacrifice is part of medicine. Ideally, physicians should want to help others, but if the internal desire is lacking, they should act this way out of duty. The principle of beneficence spells out this duty.

Beneficence may conflict with autonomy (as any of these principles may conflict with each other). Consider the involuntary psychiatric commitment of schizophrenic, homeless people. Is it better to let such people wander the cold streets of a big city or to incarcerate and medicate them against their will? Should we let them "die with their rights on" or inject them with sedatives and antipsychotic drugs "for their own good"? Maybe we should do nothing at all and not risk making them worse off. After all, who are we to say that it is beneficent to do so? Maybe homeless schizophrenics want to stay as they are.

How beneficence and autonomy are balanced in particular cases is not easy to understand. Indeed, when John Stuart Mill advocated both utilitarianism and personal autonomy, critics wondered whether he contradicted himself.

*Nonmaleficence,* not harming others, echoes an ancient maxim of professional medical ethics, "First, do not harm." Above all, this maxim implies that physicians not technically competent to do something shouldn't do it. So medical students should not harm patients by practicing on them without consent: Patients are there to be helped, not to help students learn.

Patients should not leave encounters with physicians worse off than they were before. This crucial principle of medical ethics prohibits corruption, incompetence, and dangerous, nontherapuetic experiments. It explains why the 80,000 deaths per year in American hospitals from mistakes horrify critics.

The principle of nonmaleficence also accords with Mill's harm principle: The state and society should not attempt to shape all citizens for the better. In a fundamental sense, the first obligation we have is to leave each other alone, especially those who don't want our help. That means that physicians should not harm patients by unsolicited intrusions.

The last principle, *justice*, has both a social and a political meaning. Socially, it means treating similar kinds of people similarly (this is the so-called formal element of the larger principle). A just physician treats each patient the same, regardless of his or her insurance coverage.

Politically, the principle refers to distributive justice and, in medicine, to the allocation of scarce medical resources. Because there are many theories of justice, this principle is not self-evident. For example, Rawls's theory of justice demands that medicine serve the poorest people.

But another view equates justice with simple egalitarianism: Medicine is just if it treats each patient equally. Of course, that goal would not be easy to achieve either, and doing so would go a long way toward realizing Rawls's ideal. At the least, it would mean a guarantee of equal access to medical care for every citizen, such that insurance coverage would not be a factor in selection of which patient receives a liver transplant.

In the most minimal sense, justice requires physicians to treat patients impartially, without bias on account of gender, race, sexuality, or wealth. Even in such a minimal sense, justice requires a high standard of behavior among physicians.

# CHAPTER 2

# Requests to Die: Non-Terminal Patients

*T*his chapter presents Elizabeth Bouvia and Larry McAfee, two people with non-terminal physical disabilities who tried to die, won important cases in court, and whose outcomes surprised people. It discusses depression, autonomy, disability culture, philosophers on suicide, and whether physicians should assist non-terminal, disabled adults who want to die.

## THE CASE OF ELIZABETH BOUVIA

In 1983, Elizabeth Bouvia's father drove her from Oregon to Riverside General Hospital in California, where psychiatrists admitted her as a voluntary suicidal patient. Wanting "just to be left alone and not bothered by friends or family or anyone else and to ultimately starve to death," she had already attempted suicide once.[1] "Death is letting go of all burdens," she claimed. "It is being able to be free of my physical disability and mental struggle to live."

Almost totally paralyzed from cerebral palsy, Elizabeth, then 25 years old, never had the use of her legs, although her right hand could control a battery-powered wheelchair and smoke cigarettes. She could use her facial muscles to chew, swallow, and speak. She also had painful, severe degenerative arthritis. As a California resident, her medical care was paid for by Medi-Cal, a state–federal program.

She had a hard life. At age 5, her parents divorced. Afterward, her mother raised her for five years, but then abandoned her to a children's home. The following account comes from two physicians:

> For their 18th birthday, some children receive cars and gifts. When [Elizabeth] turned 18, her father, a postal inspector, told her that he would no longer be able to care for her because of her disabilities. The chief of psychiatry at Riverside says that what she did next showed great drive and promise. She gathered her requisite amount of state aid and lived on her own in an apartment with a live-in nurse. Although she earlier had dropped out of high school, she completed her general equivalency degree and went on to graduate from San Diego State University with a bachelor's degree in 1981. She even entered a master's program at the

university's School of Social Work, but left in 1982 over a disagreement about her field work placement.

For eight months, she worked as a volunteer in the San Diego placement program, but she has never been employed for salary or wages.

During the last year, Ms. Bouvia faced a series of devastating events. In August 1982, she married an ex-convict, Richard Bouvia, with whom she had been corresponding by mail. Together they conceived a child, but a few months later she suffered a miscarriage.

Her husband's part-time job did not provide enough income for the two to live decently, so they called her father to ask for help. He declined to aid them, Richard Bouvia said. They next went to Richard Bouvia's sister in Iowa to ask for help. That did not work out for long, and soon they ended up back in Oregon, where Richard Bouvia still could not find work. At that point, he abandoned her, stating—according to pleadings in the case—that he "could not accept her disabilities, a miscarriage, and rejection by her parents."

A few days later, Elizabeth Bouvia got a ride to Riverside General and wheeled herself into the emergency room, complaining that she wanted to commit suicide.[2]

During her first four months at Riverside Hospital, the chief of psychiatry, Donald Fisher, supervised her treatment. When he refused to let her starve, Elizabeth contacted the American Civil Liberties Union (ACLU) and telephoned a reporter. Richard Scott of Beverly Hills, both a physician and a lawyer, represented her free of charge.

## The Legal Battle: Refusing Sustenance

In a hearing before California probate judge John Hews, Fisher testified that because Elizabeth might change her mind, he would not let her starve and would force-feed her: "The court cannot order me to be a murderer nor to conspire with my staff and employees to murder Elizabeth."[3] Elizabeth Bouvia asked the judge to block her force-feeding.

Habeeb Bacchus, associate chief of medicine at Riverside Hospital and Bouvia's second physician, argued that "being allowed to die when there's no need for her to die—this is a dangerous precedent. Patients might wonder, `Am I next slated to be allowed to die?'"[4]

Advocates for the disabled feared that if Elizabeth died, other disabled people might follow. A lawyer at the Law Institute for the Disabled asserted that Bouvia symbolized a "social problem" of disabled people who are told they cannot be productive and said, "She needs to learn to live with dignity."[5]

At this point, the case escalated into a public debate:

Disabled individuals held vigils at the hospital to convince her to change her mind. Bouvia's estranged husband hitchhiked to Riverside from Iowa, retained lawyers, and asked to be named her legal guardian. He charged the ACLU with using his wife as a "guinea pig." She filed for divorce. Columnist Jack Anderson's offer to raise funds for Bouvia's treatment was rebuffed. Richard Nixon sent a letter to Bouvia to "keep fighting." A meeting with President Reagan was discussed. Two neurosurgeons offered free surgery to help her gain the use of her arms. A convicted felon volunteered to shoot her.[6]

Judge Hews allowed the force-feeding. Admitting Elizabeth's rationality, sincerity, and competence, he decided based on the "profound effect on the medical staff, nurses, and administration of the hospital," as well as the "devastating effect on other . . . physically handicapped persons."[7] Bouvia's lawyer said Hews accepted "the Chicken Little defense that the sky would fall if Ms. Bouvia wasn't force-fed."[8] Judge Hews held that since the patient was not terminally ill and could live for decades, "there is no other reasonable option."

Columnist Arthur Hoppe thought otherwise:

> I had the feeling that the judge, the doctor, and the hospital had found Elizabeth Bouvia guilty—guilty of not playing the game. It was as though the Easter Seal Child had looked into the camera and said being crippled was a lousy deal and certainly nothing to smile about.[9]

Boston University law professor George Annas blasted Hews:

> The judge's decision begs the question: Is there a reasonable option? In the adversary proceeding played out in California, no one seemed to search for reasonable options. The county, in fact, consistently took the most extreme position. It continually threatened to eject Ms. Bouvia from the hospital by force, and leave her out on the front sidewalk, hoping someone would pick her up and take her away. Almost from the beginning, the county and hospital made it clear that they did not care whether she lived or died but, because of their own fear of potential legal liability, would not let her die at Riverside Hospital.[10]

Elizabeth appealed, but continued to be force-fed. When aides pushed plastic tubing in her mouth, she bit through it. Thereafter, three attendants held her down while another inserted tubing through her nose into her stomach, pumping in a liquid diet. Annas commented on this gruesome scene:

> I do not believe competent adults should ever be force-fed; but efforts at persuading the individual to change his or her mind, and offering oral nutrition should continue. If a court determines, however, that invasive force-feeding is required, . . . then to [prevent] hospitals from becoming the most hideous torture chambers, some reasonable limit must be placed on this "treatment."[11]

Elizabeth Bouvia lost her first appeal and left Riverside Hospital in 1984. Individual commentators interpreted differently what happened next. Two physicians wrote in a medical journal:

> The standoff continued until April 7, when Ms. Bouvia unexpectedly checked herself out of the hospital. The hospital bill for the 217 days, excluding physicians' fees, was more than $56,000, paid by Riverside County and by the State of California. Ms. Bouvia went to the Hospital del Mar at Playease de Tijuana, Mexico, known for amygdalin (Laetrile) treatments for cancer. She believed the staff would help her die. Her new physicians, however, became convinced that she wanted to live. Two weeks later, Ms. Bouvia left the hospital, hired nurses, and moved to a motel. Three days later, with friends, a reporter, and an intern from Hospital del Mar at her side, she gave up her plan to starve herself to death and took solid food. Ms. Bouvia said that she wanted treatment, including surgery to reduce muscle spasms. . . . Her case was complicated further by the revelation that the newspaper reporter who covered the case most closely had a contract with Ms. Bouvia for a book, television, and movie rights to her story.[12]

This account emphasizes Elizabeth Bouvia's unexpected departure from the hospital, her costly hospital bills at public expense, the agreement of Mexican with American physicians in refusing to allow her to die, her seemingly arbitrary decision to give up starving herself, and a contract for book and film rights to her story.

In contrast, lawyer George Annas writes:

> Two years ago this column dealt with Elizabeth Bouvia's unequal and doomed struggle. . . . After losing both in the hospital and in the courtroom, Ms. Bouvia fled to Mexico on April 7, 1984, to seek her death. She was soon persuaded that Mexican physicians and nurses would be no more sympathetic to her plan than those at Riverside, and so returned to California. Because of the brutal force-feeding she had endured at Riverside, she was afraid to return there. Since no other facility would admit her unless she agreed to eat, she resigned herself to eating and entered a "private care" location. There she remained, without incident, for more than a year.[13]

An advocate for dignified dying, the Hemlock Society's Derek Humphrey, wrote even more sympathetically:

> Her troubles multiplied. The graduate school where she had been studying refused to readmit her, and her brother was drowned in a boating accident. Not long after, Elizabeth had a miscarriage, and she learned her mother was dying of cancer. . . . Determined once again to be in charge of her fate, she asked her father to take her to the county hospital in Riverside, near Los Angeles (an area where she had friends), for an examination. She checked herself into the psychiatric ward and told physicians she wanted to die by starvation. Elizabeth specifically asked that, until she died, she be looked after normally and given painkillers when her arthritis was troublesome.[14]

Disability advocate Paul Longmore offered a very different perspective on Bouvia's case, arguing that it reflected rank prejudice against the disabled. He wrote:

> The very agencies supposedly designed to enable severely physically handicapped adults like her to achieve independence . . . become yet another massive hurdle they must surmount, an enemy they must repeatedly battle but can never finally defeat. . . .
>
> [When she tried to go on internship,] the SDSU [San Diego State University] School of Social Work refused to back her up. They wanted to place her at a center where she would only work with disabled people. She refused. Reportedly, one of her employers told her she was unemployable, and that, if they had known just how disabled she was, they would never have admitted her to the program. . . .
>
> The attorneys brought in three psychiatric professionals to provide an independent evaluation. None of them had experience or expertise in dealing with persons with disabilities. In fact, Elizabeth Bouvia had never been examined by a psychiatric or medical professional qualified to understand her life experience. . . .
>
> Her examiners prejudicially concluded that because of her physical condition she would never be able to achieve her life goals, that her [physical] disability was the reason she wanted to die, and that her decision for death was reasonable. . . . [Judge Hews] too declared that Ms. Bouvia's physical disability was the sole reason she wished to die.[15]

Each account appeared in scholarly journals, implying objectivity, yet the physicians portray her as irresponsible; Annas and Humphrey portray her as a heroine fighting a cold bureaucracy; and Longmore portrays her as a victim of a prejudiced system and of misguided, do-gooder lawyers. Physicians refer to her as "Bouvia," Humphrey calls her "Elizabeth," and Longmore uses "Elizabeth Bouvia" or "Ms. Bouvia." The physicians say that, "she got a ride" to Riverside, as if she had hitchhiked to some arbitrary location; Humphrey says that her father took her to a place "where she had friends." Longmore emphasizes her desire to be independent; Humphrey emphasizes her physical pain and social trauma. Longmore suggests that society is prejudiced against disabled people and thus that Elizabeth Bouvia's disability is not so much her problem as society's problem. Humphrey writes from a point of view inside Elizabeth Bouvia; the physicians write from the viewpoint of hospital staff members who deal with problematic patients. Longmore critiques an inadequate system that forces terrible, desperate decisions.

In 1985, Elizabeth entered Los Angeles County–USC Medical Center, where physicians installed a morphine pump to control pain caused by her worsening arthritis. She promised to eat, so she was not force-fed.

After two months, physicians transferred her to nearby High Desert Hospital, another public hospital. Although she ate there, her physicians decided that she wasn't eating *enough* and again force-fed her. They reasoned that, "since she is occupying our space, she must accede to the same care which we afford every other patient admitted here, care designed to improve and not detract from chances of recovery and rehabilitation."[16] Critics objected: must all patients who occupy High Desert hospital's space do as they are told? Would the hospital want to market this theme "Enter High Desert Hospital and Do As: We Say."?

Elizabeth petitioned courts to stop her forced feeding. At this time, she weighed only 70 pounds. A consultant on nutrition noted that a weight of 75 or 85 pounds "might be desirable." Her physicians wanted her to weigh about 110 pounds.

At a hearing, Judge Warren Deering interpreted her low weight as "not motivated by a bona fide right to privacy but by a desire to terminate her life."[17] He said the right to privacy did not cover suicide by starvation and ordered force-feeding because, "Saving her life is paramount."

Elizabeth appealed and the California Court of Appeal ruled in her favor: "A desire to terminate one's life is probably the ultimate exercise of one's right to privacy."[18] This Court found "no substantive evidence to support the [lower] court's decision."

Judge Deering had been concerned that Elizabeth could live for decades, but the Court dismissed that concern: "This trial court mistakenly attached undue importance to the amount of time possibly available to her, and failed to give equal weight and consideration for the quality of that life; an equal, if not more significant, consideration."

The appeals court concluded:

This matter constitutes a perfect paradigm of the axiom: "Justice delayed is justice denied." Her mental and emotional feelings are equally entitled to respect. She has been subjected to the forced intrusion of an artificial mechanism into her body against her will. She has a right to refuse the increased dehumanizing aspect of her condition. . . . The right to refuse medical treatment is basic and fundamental. It is recognized as part of the right of privacy protected by both the state and federal constitutions. Its exercise requires no one's approval. It is not merely one vote subject to being overridden by medical opinion. . . .

[A precedent has been established that when] a doctor performs treatment in the absence of informed consent, there is an actionable battery. The obvious corollary to this principle is that a competent adult patient has the legal right to refuse medical treatment. [Moreover,] if the right of the patient to self-determination as to his own medical treatment is to have any meaning at all, it must be paramount to the interests of the patient's hospital and doctors. . . . The right of a competent adult patient to refuse medical treatment is a constitutionally guaranteed right which must not be abridged. . . .

In Elizabeth Bouvia's view, the quality of her life has been diminished to the point of hopelessness, uselessness, unenjoyability, and frustration. She, as the patient, lying helplessly in bed, unable to care for herself, may consider her existence meaningless. She is not to be faulted for so concluding. . . . As in all matters, lines must be drawn at some point, somewhere, but that decision must ultimately belong to the one whose life is in issue.

The state appellate court held that competent adults could refuse medical treatment: Building on prior decisions in other states,[19] this state court said that a competent adult patient had a constitutionally guaranteed right to refuse medical treatment that must not be abridged. This court also had strong words about force-feeding:

We do not believe it is the policy of this State that all and every life must be preserved against the will of the sufferer. It is incongruous, if not monstrous, for medical practitioners to assert their right to preserve a life that someone else must live, or more accurately, endure, for "15 or 20 years." We cannot conceive it to be the policy of this State to inflict such an ordeal upon anyone.

The court concluded that, "no criminal or civil liability attaches to honoring a competent, informed patient's refusal for medical service."

If nothing else, Elizabeth Bouvia, frail, small, alone, and barely able to move, won a remarkable victory. Preceding the U.S. Supreme Court's *Cruzan* decision by five years, she wrested from the courts a victory about the right to die for competent patients.

Yet after her victory, Elizabeth did not kill herself. When some caring people offered to help her die, she changed her mind. Most important, by giving her control over her life, they gave her a reason to live.

A decade after her victory in court, she described her body as "gnarled and useless."[20] In 1994, she lived in California on Medi-Cal, in a private hospital room with 24-hour-day care at a cost of $300 a day. A morphine pump controlled her pain, and she weighed 100 pounds. She said her life was "a lot of needles and bags," and she spent her time watching television. "I wouldn't say I'm happy, but I'm physically comfortable, more comfortable than before. There is nothing really to do. I just kind of lay here."

In 1992, Richard Scott, the physician and lawyer who represented Elizabeth Bouvia, and who battled depression most of his life committed suicide. When he did, Elizabeth Bouvia said, "Jesus, I wish he could have come in and taken me with him."

In 1996, Elizabeth, appeared on *60 Minutes* on the tenth anniversary of a previous *60 Minutes* story about her. Then she lived in Riverside County Hospital, but in 1997, a new pro bono attorney Griffith Thomas, M.D., got her disability payments put into a trust fund that allowed her to live in her own apartment with 24-hour-a-day, in-home assistants. Even though this cost far less than her hospital room, it took a decade to accomplish.

Elizabeth in 1996 still had pain each day and still needed morphine. She did not intend to be alive for another story by *60 Minutes* in 2006 and felt ambivalent about her life. An obituary for a disability rights advocate in 2008 mentioned that Elizabeth was still alive.[21] In 2013, she seemed to be still alive, but no one had heard anything about her.

## THE CASE OF LARRY MCAFEE

In 1985, an accident left 29-year-old Larry McAfee almost completely paralyzed (a C-2 quadriplegic). While studying mechanical engineering at Georgia State University, he fell forward over his motorcycle on a dirt road, snapped his head, and crushed his two top vertebrae. Left with use only of his eyes, mouth, and head, he could not clear his throat and sometimes choked. He needed a ventilator to breathe and could not control his bladder and bowels. He was unmarried and could feel no pleasure from sexual activity.

McAfee had a $1 million health insurance policy, and using it, remained for over a year at the expensive Shepherd Spinal Center in Atlanta, where the average stay for C-1 to C-4 patients is 19 weeks. He then moved to an apartment in Atlanta, where he insisted on certified nurses who were three times more expensive than home health aides. After 16 months of such living, he exhausted his insurance. Not wanting to be a burden, he refused his family's offer of care.

With no resources, he became eligible for Medicaid, the fund in each state that pays for medical care for the indigent. McAfee wanted Georgia Medicaid to pay for his care in an apartment and refused to enter a state nursing home. Only a small number of nursing homes in America admit ventilator-dependent patients such as Larry. Even fewer take Medicaid patients because Medicaid's reimbursement doesn't pay for the staffing needed for such patients. Georgia officials eventually transferred him to a Medicaid nursing home in Ohio that could care for respirator-dependent C-1 patients. This facility accepted McAfee on a temporary basis until Georgia could find a bed for him.

In Ohio, Larry wouldn't make appointments for vocational rehabilitation. The administrator there said, "Larry was very demanding, wanted things precisely the way he wanted them. . . . I had nurses toward the end who just couldn't work with him anymore because they were just extremely, extremely frustrated."[22] He noted that McAfee's family and friends all lived in Georgia.

McAfee claimed that he had been housed in Ohio with demented, senile, and brain-damaged patients who were being cheaply warehoused with only one or two staff for as many as 40 patients. The easiest way to warehouse such patients is to keep them heavily sedated. McAfee said that he experienced intense loneliness and received inadequate personal care. "You're just a sack of potatoes," he said.[23]

After two long years it became clear to Ohioans that McAfee had been dumped on them, so officials angrily hustled him onto a plane and left him in the emergency room at Grady Memorial Hospital in Atlanta.

There, Larry spent several miserable months in the intensive care unit. In 1989, Briarcliff Nursing Home, in a suburb of Birmingham, Alabama, accepted him as a patient, and he transferred there.

Larry one day called the radio talk show of Russ Fine, a disability advocate and director of the Injury Control Research Center at the University of Alabama at Birmingham. According to Fine, McAfee's treatment represented "everything that's wrong about the system that serves disabled people."[24]

On first meeting Larry, Fine found him lying in bed staring at the ceiling, with no voice-activated telephone and no television. All he could do was stare "at whatever happened to be in front of his face. From a quality of life standpoint, it was a devastating commentary on a society with a very advanced health-care system."[25]

A reporter once arrived to find McAfee's urinary catheter not connected to a container and spilling urine on the floor. Fine says, "These facilities were not equipped to take care of a patient such as Larry, with labor-intensive health-care requirements."[26]

In 1989, four years after Elizabeth Bouvia's victory, Larry filed suit in federal court to exercise his right to die. After a heart-wrenching 45-minute hearing in Fulton County Superior Court, Judge Edward Johnson found in McAfee's favor. Because his ventilator had once dislodged accidentally, causing him to suffocate, Larry did not want to experience such feelings again, so he asked to be sedated before disconnection. Judge Johnson granted this, declaring that no civil or criminal penalty would attach to any doctor who helped.

Everyone assumed that with his legal victory, McAfee would kill himself within days. Like Elizabeth Bouvia, he did not. Behind the scenes, Russ Fine had convinced McAfee to stay alive. But then Larry's financial problems began.

Social Security, besides financing income for Americans over 62, provides financial assistance to disabled people as Supplemental Security Income (SSI). In 2011, SSI payments averaged $700 a month and were paid to 10.6 million disabled Americans.[27] Larry qualified for SSI assistance.

In 1989, Russ Fine persuaded Birmingham's United Cerebral Palsy to let Larry live temporarily in its nine-person group home. Larry stayed there on-and-off until late 1990, but because he required expensive nurses, he then had to find somewhere else to live.

Federal regulations affecting Medicaid block using it to pay for disabled people to live in group homes. This structural discrimination forces such people to live either in public hospitals or be warehoused in huge public nursing homes. When President George Bush refused a waiver of Medicaid to help Larry, the Georgia legislature created an independent-living facility for him and for five other patients as an exception to Georgia's disability law and Medicaid plan. Larry then lived in Augusta, near its medical school.

In 1993, his accident and fight were portrayed in *The Switch*, a CBS movie. To keep his disability payments, McAfee could not accept any money from the movie.

A few months later, Georgia "forgot" to fund McAfee's group home in its state budget. Once again, Russ Fine held Georgia's feet to the fire for Larry, pointing out that the cost per person in the group home was only $52 a day. Georgia found funds to continue the home for another year.

In 1993, a kink in Larry's urinary catheter caused urine to back up. Being paralyzed, Larry could not feel what was happening; the backup caused toxicity and high blood pressure. This caused two devastating strokes.[28] Larry survived, but the strokes injured his brain and he was left with just a small amount of short-term memory.

He had planned to leave the group home for his own apartment but instead was transferred to a long-term nursing home. This was just the kind of place Larry had wanted to avoid. Ten years after his accident, Larry died in 1995. He died not by his own decision, but after being comatose for many months.

## THE CASE OF DAX COWART

Another famous case in bioethics concerned 29-year-old bachelor Dax (Donald) Cowart, who suffered burns over two-thirds of his body in 1973. Physicians treated him against his will for 14 months in a burn unit in Parkland Hospital in Dallas. He was left blind, disfigured, and with only partial use of his fingers.[29]

Afterward, Dax won a million dollars from an out-of-court settlement with a gas company. He then hired a plane, flew to Mexico, and spent several hours on a landing strip with a gun in his hand, debating whether to kill himself. Like Bouvia and McAfee, once he had the power to kill himself, he changed his mind.

Instead, he graduated from law school in 1986 and later married a nurse he had known previously when both of them were students in high school. He became interested in ham radio and raising golden retrievers. Since then, he has been an active trial lawyer, winning several lawsuits.

In retrospect, Dax rejects the decision of his physicians to keep him alive. He frequently tells his story in public, emphasizing the cruelty of the physicians who made him endure 14 months of terrible pain. He argues that even though he is glad to be alive today, his physicians wrongly treated him against his wishes. As he once said to this author, "If I should be so unlucky as to be burned that way again, and if I knew what was waiting at the end, I wouldn't go through that pain to get there."[30] In 2013, Dax was still alive, although living in some pain.[31]

## BACKGROUND: PERSPECTIVES ON SUICIDE

### Greece and Rome

Ancient Greek aristocrats strove not simply to live, but to lead lives of nobility, honor, excellence, and beauty. Believing that "the unexamined life is not worth living," they thought the "important thing is not to live but to live well." They thought that study of philosophy would provide wisdom to approach death (*philosophy* means "love of wisdom"). Plato records Socrates as saying, "True philosophers make dying their profession, and . . . to them of all men, death is least alarming. . . . So if you see one distressed at the prospect of dying, it will be proof that he is a lover not of wisdom but of the body."[32]

Socrates died famously. Sentenced to die for his political beliefs, he could have fled Athens, but chose instead to drink hemlock, a poison. At his end, he discussed death with a friend.

The friend argues that if one is convinced of life after death, it is easy not to fear death, but what if the soul is "dispersed and destroyed on the very day that the man himself dies [and] may be dissipated like breath or smoke, and vanish away, so that nothing is left of it anywhere. . . . No one but a fool is entitled to face death with confidence, unless he can prove that the soul is absolutely immortal and indestructible."

Socrates replies that the soul may be immortal, but if it is not, then death is like a sleep from which one never awakes. If so, we should not fear it, because no one will exist to feel pain or to miss life.

Hemlock acts as a poison by decreasing circulation at the extremities, creating distal numbness, and eventually stopping the heart. Hemlock began to work during Socrates' abstract discussion about death, moving up from his toes to his ankles. As the discussion ends, the state poisoner finds that Socrates' thighs are numb and says that, when the poison reaches the heart in minutes, Socrates will die.

As his friends begin to cry, Socrates says, "Calm yourselves and try to be brave!" He dies moments later. His admiring follower, Plato writes, "Such . . . was the end of our comrade, who was, we may fairly say, of all those whom we knew in our time, the bravest and also the wisest and most upright man."

Centuries later in Rome, emperor Marcus Aurelius wrote that suicide surpassed undignified dying. These Roman Stoics defended the argument for the open door: "If the room is smoky, if only moderately, I will stay; if there is too much smoke, I will go. Remember this, keep a firm hand on it, the door is always open."[33]

Another Stoic, Seneca, wrote about old age: "If it begins to shake my mind, if it destroys my faculties one by one, if it leaves me not life but breath, I will depart the putrid or the tottering edifice."[34]

In the twentieth century, existentialist philosopher Jean-Paul Sartre revived the argument for the open door.[35] He emphasized that choice—even the choice of staying alive each day—is inescapable. He famously wrote, "Not to choose is always still a choice."

## Philosophers on Voluntary Death

The Bible does not explicitly prohibit suicide, and seems to condone the suicides of Saul and Judas. During the fourth century, Augustine condemned suicide, basing his condemnation on the sixth commandment, "Thou shalt not kill" (Exodus 20:13).

Augustine distinguished between private killing and killing endorsed by divine authority. Killing on one's own authority is never right, but when God commands it, humans should obey. So Abraham had to obey when God commanded him to kill his son, Isaac. Individuals who so kill are instruments of God.

This reasoning underlies killing in capital punishment and just wars. The worldly Ambrose had already said that Christians could kill in war, and Augustine went further by condoning war against heretics. Frederick Russell in *The Just War in the Middle Ages* says that through Augustine's interpretation, "the New Testament doctrines of love and purity were accommodated to the savagery of the Old Testament and pacifism was defeated."[36]

The thirteenth-century philosopher Thomas Aquinas held that suicide is sinful because it leaves no time for repentance; repudiates a gift from God; deprives the community of talented people; deprives children of their parents; and is unnatural, going against the instinct of self-preservation.

Michel de Montaigne in the sixteenth century concluded in "To Philosophize Is to Learn How to Die" by saying, "If we have learned how to live properly and calmly, we will know how to die in the same manner."[37] The Dutch philosopher Baruch Spinoza wrote, "A free man, that is to say, a man who lives according to the dictates of reason alone, is not led by the fear of death."[38] The English poet John Donne in the seventeenth century wrote, "When the [terminal] disease would not reduce us, [God] sent a second and worse affliction, ignorant and torturing physicians."[39]

**Hume**    In the eighteenth century, Scottish philosopher David Hume argued that suicide "is no transgression of our duty to God." Hume hated vanity and observed, "The life of a man is of no greater importance to the universe than that of an oyster."[40]

In his "Essay on Suicide," Hume disagreed with Augustine and Aquinas. For dying patients, he argued, voluntary death is not a sin: "A house which falls by its own weight is not brought to ruin by [God's] providence."[41] Hume argued that if God made the natural world through the laws of causality—the laws of biology, medicine, and physics—then disease belonged to that world.

While Immanuel Kant argued that we have a station in life assigned to us by God that we must not give up, Hume replied, "It is a kind of blasphemy to imagine that any created being can [by taking his own life] disturb the order of the world. Any suicide is insignificant to the workings of the universe and it is blasphemy to think otherwise."

Hume disputed Aquinas's argument that suicide harms the community,

> A man who retires from life does no harm to society; he only ceases to do good; which, if it is an injury, is of the lowest kind. All our obligations to do good to society seem to imply something reciprocal. I receive benefits of society, and therefore ought to promote its interests; but when I withdraw myself altogether from society, can I be bound any longer? But [even] allowing that our obligations to do good were perpetual, they have certainly some bounds; I am not obliged to do a small good to society at the expense of a great harm to myself: when then should I prolong a miserable existence, because of some frivolous advantage which the public may perhaps receive from me?

**Kant**    Hume's contemporary, German philosopher Immanuel Kant, opposed suicide. For Kant, an act is right if it derives from a rule that can be universalized, that is, a rule we would want everyone to act on. Everyone cannot commit suicide or humanity would end.

Suicide also cannot be universalized because its motive is self-interest (for instance, escaping pain). For Kant, self-interest can never justify moral decisions, only respect for the moral law.

Second, a person "who does not respect his life even in principle cannot be restrained from the most dreadful vices." If I do not respect my own life, I will not respect anything else. To respect the sacred value of the lives of others, I must respect the sacred value of my own.

Third, Kant wrote, "Human beings are sentinels on earth and may not leave their posts until relieved by another beneficent hand. God is our owner; we are His property."[42]

Finally, suicide is immoral because people should always be treated as ends in themselves, never as mere means. This entails recognizing one's free will as an absolute, rather than as a relative, value, but destroying oneself entails destroying that freedom of will. "Man's freedom cannot subsist except on a condition which is immutable. This condition is that man not use his freedom against himself to his own destruction."[43]

In other words, Kant believed that each person must treat *his body* as an "end in itself." "To deprive oneself of an integral part of organ (to mutilate oneself), for example, to give away or sell a tooth so that it can be implanted in another person, or to submit oneself to castration in order to gain an easier living as a singer, and so on, belongs to partial self-murder."[44] (For this reason, Kant seems to reject giving another person a kidney.)

**John Stuart Mill**   In his 1859 essay, *On Liberty*, John Stuart Mill famously wrote that,

> One very simple principle [is] entitled to govern absolutely the dealings of society with the individual in the way of compulsion and control, whether the means used is physical force in the form of legal penalties, or the moral coercion of public opinion. That principle is, that the sole end for which mankind are warranted, individually or collectively, in interfering with the liberty of action of any of their number, is self-protection. That the only purpose for which power can be rightfully exercised over any member of a civilized community, against his will, is to prevent harm to others. His own good, either physical or moral, is not a sufficient warrant. . . . The only part of the conduct of any one, for which he is amenable to society, is that which concerns others. In the part which merely concerns himself, his independence is, of right, absolute. Over himself, over his own body and mind, the individual is sovereign.[45]

According to this principle, so long as others are not harmed, we can do whatever we want with our own lives and bodies.

Mill distinguished between *self-regarding* and *other-regarding* acts, arguing that we may censure others only for other-regarding acts. Paradoxically, Mill's analysis can both support and condemn suicide. On one hand, taking one's own life is clearly self-regarding; suicide is often described as the ultimate personal issue. On the other, suicide can affect others, especially when they believe they should have prevented it. If a suicidal person desired to make others feel bad, then Mill's principle condemns the suicide.

**The Modern Era**   American feminist Charlotte Perkins Gillman killed herself in 1935, writing that she preferred "chloroform to cancer" and that, "The record of a previously noble life is precisely what makes it sheer insult to allow death in pitiful degradation. We may not wish to 'die with our boots on,' but we may well prefer to 'die with our brains on.' "[46]

A century ago, only poor people without families went to hospitals to die. Before the Harrison Act of 1914, Americans could purchase heroin and opiates to lessen the pain of terminal cancer and to die at home. Today, physicians control such drugs, death has been medicalized, and most people die in hospitals.

The nature of deadly diseases has also changed. Before World War II, most people died of sudden-onset, acute diseases such as pneumonia and cholera. Today, people live longer and die slowly from chronic diseases such as emphysema, diabetes, dementia, cancer, and coronary artery disease. Such diseases slowly erode the quality of life, and many people want to die before such quality becomes too bad.

## The Concept of Assisted Suicide

One question raised by the cases of Elizabeth Bouvia and Larry McAfee is what to call their intended action: suicide, rational suicide, assisted suicide, euthanasia, voluntary death, or self-deliverance? Let us clarify some terms here.

First, *euthanasia* usually means the killing of one person by another for merciful reasons. The preceding cases do not involve euthanasia because in each case death would be initiated by the person herself.

Second, a terminally ill patient who forgoes medical treatment doesn't really "commit suicide." We should distinguish between (1) cases where an underlying disease is incrementally leading to death, and by choosing not to do everything possible, the patient accepts death; and (2) cases where a competent adult without a terminal illness causes his own death. The second kind of case is appropriately called "suicide." The Bouvia and McAfee cases are therefore best called cases of *assisted suicide*. Neither Elizabeth Bouvia nor Larry McAfee had a terminal disease, but they also could not easily kill themselves, hence they needed *assistance*.

One reason to make this distinction is that life insurance companies do not pay benefits for suicides. Another reason is that in all states it is illegal to assist in suicides.

## ETHICAL ISSUES: FOR AND AGAINST ASSISTED SUICIDE

### Easy to Kill Oneself?

Why didn't Elizabeth Bouvia and Larry McAfee simply kill themselves? Surprisingly, the answer is that it's difficult to kill yourself painlessly, aesthetically, and with certainty. When you're disabled, it's almost impossible to do so by yourself.

Whenever a suicide is botched, people infer ambivalence, but this is often mistaken. Emergency medicine contains many stories of bizarre survivals.[47] The hand holding the gun wobbles a fraction of an inch and leaves the would-be suicide a drooling zombie. Because drugs taken for courage also relax muscles and thus soften impact, some jumpers survive falls from the Golden Gate Bridge. One jumper hit a parked car, did not die, and did not lose consciousness.[48]

Although suicide attempts by teenagers increased 300 percent between 1967 and 1982, only one in 50 succeeded.[49] The elderly succeed one in three times. Women attempt suicide more than men, but succeed less. Men use violent means (such as guns); women use drugs.

Attempted suicides present a grim picture. People take lorazepam and benzo-diazepines in insufficient quantities to cause death, often ending up merely comatose. In 1987, National Security Advisor Robert McFarlane took 35–45 10-mg tablets of Valium. When he didn't die, people inferred he didn't want to die. An equally plausible explanation is that he didn't know how to kill himself. Even physicians don't. In 1985, physician Robert Rosier didn't know how much mor-phine to give his terminally ill wife to help her die.[50]

People using other methods may not die but awake in the ER. Carbon monoxide (CO) poisoning may not work because the car can stall or run out of gas; the CO may not concentrate enough to produce death, so that the person ends up with half his former intelligence.

Slitting wrists in a warm tub is not easy: the cuts are painful and must be made deep and in the right place. Nor is this method certain: in the time between unconsciousness and death, the arm may move out of the water and the blood may coagulate. One ER physician observes, "Most slashers just get a trophy: a claw hand."

Some people who don't kill themselves wake up with a nasogastric tube down their throat, into which syrup of ipecac is pumped to induce vomiting. ER physicians then inject saline solution and start gastric lavage—alternate flooding and suctioning of the stomach—and then pump granulated charcoal to absorb remaining toxins.

If they want to spare the feelings of others or be found in a dignified state, suicides should avoid certain methods. A drug overdose not only decreases respi-ration, but also relaxes bowels and bladders. Jumping off a building or shooting oneself in the head leaves a crushed body. Hanging is difficult to do correctly because the neck may not break and the victim, kicking in agony as he partially asphyxiates, may not die. Men who do die this way are found with an erection and may have lost control of their bladder and bowels.

## Rationality and Competence

In the movie *Whose Life Is It, Anyway?*, the quadriplegic hero, Ken Harrison, wants to die and offers rational arguments for suicide to his psychiatrist. Harrison makes a convincing case for suicide, but his psychiatrist decides he's too depressed to make the decision to die. A judge decides that Harrison is of sound mind and his psychiatrist allows him to discontinue dialysis and tells Harrison no attempt to revive him will be made if he slips into a coma.

In Elizabeth Bouvia's case, psychiatrist Nancy Mullen testified that because Elizabeth was suicidal, she could not rationally make decisions about her life. Mullen said that she could conceive of no situation where people could make competent decisions to take their own lives.[51] Carol Gill, a clinical assistant professor of occupational therapy who used a wheelchair, criticized the ACLU for backing "a handful of medical experts" who found that Bouvia was competent.[52]

Mullen and Gill may have begged the question of rational suicide. A question is begged when the answer is assumed to be true rather than proved. In these cases, the question or point is whether a decision to die is irrational: whether it indicates misinformation or faulty reasoning. Just assuming that a decision to die is always irrational begs that question.

This is not to say that a decision to die is always rational. Elizabeth Bouvia may have been depressed, and psychological tests might have shown this. But Mullen and Gill did not base their arguments on such tests. They were not Elizabeth's therapists and were not treating her. Mullen and Gill reacted to the content of Elizabeth's decision rather than to psychological tests. Indeed, three psychiatric professionals who actually tested Elizabeth found her competent.[53]

In America a patient is legally competent until proven otherwise and proven so in a legal hearing. No patient can be held in a hospital against her will without having been proven legally incompetent. In practice, hospitals sometimes break such laws. Although physicians never legally declared Dax Cowart incompetent, they treated him against his will for 14 months in a burn unit.

## Autonomy

At the start of bioethics in the 1970s, autonomy fueled the patient rights movement. Applied to the right to die, an autonomous person who has not been proved incompetent and who is terminally ill always has a right to end his life.

But not everyone glorifies autonomy in bioethics. Critics argued that Bouvia and McAfee did not want to die because they made dramatic demands on public institutions, "acting out" and pleading for attention. In such cases, critics argue, physicians must not accede to wishes of unstable patients. Only fools would assist every distraught patient who came to an ER wishing to die.

The Roman Catholic Church opposes autonomous suicide. In 1990, Father Kevin O'Rourke argued that humans are not in control of their lives.[54] O'Rourke argued that God has a plan for each person and it never includes suicide.

One problem with uncritical acceptance of autonomy is the famous SUPPORT study (Study to Understand Prognoses and Preferences for Outcomes and Risks of Treatments). It discovered that competent people do not accurately predict what they will later find unacceptable as quality of life.[55] People who predicted that they would rather die than go on a ventilator most often did *not* choose to die but chose life on a ventilator. It's one thing to say abstractly that one would "rather be dead than live like that," but when actually faced with death, most people decide to live.

Moreover, in rehabilitation medicine there is the equally famous *adaptation effect*, in which after six months or so, patients like Larry McAfee or Dax Cowart, who were disabled in accidents, adapt their views about acceptable quality of life. What they once considered unacceptable then becomes acceptable. For most patients, it may take six months or more for this effect to occur.

Supporters of assisted suicide argued that providing such assistance continues good medical care, even if a patient is not terminally ill. When qualify of life diminishes, the fact that a patient does not have a terminal disease is irrelevant. The real issue is whether a quality of life is acceptable to the person who must endure it, and that is an evaluative judgment that can be made only by that person.

If physicians ignore autonomy, patients can be flogged to death with unnecessary tubes, surgery, and radiation. Such barbaric end-of-life treatment differs little from involuntary commitment of competent people in psychiatric wards.

So the key question was not whether Elizabeth Bouvia was demonstrably competent or incompetent, but where the onus of proof should lie. For rugged individualists and Libertarians who abhor the growing powers of government and physicians, this onus should be on those who would take away autonomy.

As we shall see in Chapter 4, in 1990, the United States Supreme Court decided in its *Cruzan* decision that no state may pass a law limiting the right of competent patients to decline medical treatment, even if declining treatment would hasten death. *Cruzan* built on the *Bouvia* and *McAfee* decisions, and was a victory for the right of competent adults to control how they died.

## Treating Depression, Pain, and Symptoms Well

Although every decision to die is not irrational, some suicidal people suffer from treatable depression.

This is especially true of the three patients of this chapter, who were young, non-terminal, competent adults. Although it is understandable to want to die after being horribly burned or after losing physical abilities, people in the throes of depression do not understand how much better they can later feel. Anti-depressants can lift mood and should be given to all non-terminal patients who wish to die.

A different clinical issue concerns relief of symptoms. One physician in palliative care always asks his patients, "What is the chief symptom that makes you want to die now?"[56] That answer is often not what outsiders predict. One patient suffered obviously from air hunger but most missed going to a public park in his trailer, so volunteers quickly arranged such visits. With good coverage, almost any symptom can be controlled, including pain, air hunger, itchiness, fatigue, and boredom.

End-of-life care varies considerably across developed countries. A survey by a charity ranked Britain best for such care, followed by Australia and New Zealand, then the United States.[57]

## Social Prejudice and Physical Disabilities

Disability advocate Paul Longmore, whose commentary was quoted earlier and who was a ventilator-dependent person with quadriplegia, opposes voluntary death for people with disabilities. For him, Bouvia's case shows how a prejudiced system destroys the independence of disabled people.

By creating intolerable conditions, society paints people with disabilities into a corner, leaving them with only one autonomous decision consistent with their former selves: to decide to die. Professionals who keep them passive and dependent make every other decision for them. In Longmore's words:

Given the lumping together of people with disabilities with those who are terminally ill, the blurring of voluntary assisted suicide and forced "mercy" killing, and the oppressive conditions of social devaluation and isolation, blocked opportunities, economic deprivation, and enforced social powerlessness, talk of their "rational" or "voluntary" suicide is simply Orwellian newspeak. The advocates of assisted suicide assume a nonexistent autonomy. They offer an illusory self-determination.[58]

To see Bouvia or McAfee or Cowart simply as cases of a right to die is to miss a much bigger issue. Elizabeth Bouvia wanted to die because of centuries of prejudice against people who are physically disabled—prejudice that society expresses daily—prejudice that idealizes youth, beauty, sex, athleticism, fitness, and wealth. Other values also can make life valuable, such as caring for others, erudition, creativity, and community, but our culture does not idealize them.

Longmore despises films that encourage disabled people to view killing themselves as a rational response to their miserable conditions. He cites *Annie Hall*, *Elephant Man*, and especially *Whose Life Is It, Anyway?* He claims that watching the latter depressed Elizabeth Bouvia. He could have also cited the 2004 film *Million Dollar Baby*.

Longmore sees Bouvia as one who slipped through the cracks of an impersonal system. She was tragic not because of her physical situation, but because of her *social* situation. Even as a hospitalized patient, she remained sadly alone. It was this aloneness that underlay her fierce desire to tear herself away from life.

## Structural Discrimination Against the Disabled

In 1990, the Americans with Disabilities Act (ADA) became federal law. This legislation represents one of the most sweeping changes in American life and was intended to integrate Americans with disabilities into normal life. Despite it being passed over two decades ago, some institutions still do not comply with it because of lack of financial resources.

Raising the issue of inadequate resources puts physicians in an awkward place. On the one hand, they do not want to torture disabled people who want to die. On the other hand, they do not want to kill disabled people because a prejudiced society is too cheap to help such people.

The catch is that to provide such great care, the patient must be rich or have great insurance, or society must be generous. If the true measure of a society's humanity is how it treats its least well-off members, then our society is not humane toward the disabled.[59]

As a result of childhood polio, Professor Longmore's arms were paralyzed, his spine was curved, and he used a ventilator as much as 18 hours a day. As a professor of history at San Francisco State University, his success would have been impossible without his ability to live on his own, which required home health care aides. Fortunately, California's generous Medicaid program paid for his domestic aides ($15,000 a year) and Medicare disability paid for his ventilator ($12,000 a year). Had he lived in Georgia, Longmore, too, might have wanted to die, where he would not have been able to find a group home and where, as he said, he "probably would have found my life unendurable."

Longmore maintained that Elizabeth Bouvia's problems resulted in part because she did not receive her maximum payments and because her county is notorious for its stingy benefits to disabled people.

When a disabled person takes a job or marries, officials reduce her benefits. California's In-Home Supportive Services program allowed Elizabeth to manage her own life at home only while she was single; when she married, however, her husband was expected to care for her. Given these circumstances, it is no wonder that Bouvia later divorced or that she did not complete her training for a job. Longmore concludes:

> This is a woman who aimed at something more significant than mere self-sufficiency. She struggled to attain self-determination, but she was repeatedly thwarted in her efforts by discriminatory actions on the part of the government, her teachers, her employers, her parents, and her society. Contrary to the highly prejudiced view of the appeals court, what makes life with a major physical disability ignominious, embarrassing, humiliating, and dehumanizing is not the need for extensive physical assistance, but the dehumanizing social contempt toward those who require such aid.

Russ Fine believes that McAfee's desire to die also resulted from his inadequate care. Public officials control costs by requiring patients to live in the most cost-effective facilities, but McAfee said that if he couldn't live in his own apartment he would rather die. According to Fine, McAfee "was very vocal about inferior nursing care, which was the rule, not the exception, in these marginal health-care facilities that had accepted these contracts."[60]

Once, Fine had brought McAfee a Thanksgiving dinner and the two were watching a televised football game while waiting for McAfee's family to arrive. Fine was drowsing in an armchair when he suddenly realized that McAfee had stopped breathing. Aides soon got Larry breathing and Fine then saw tears streaming out of his eyes. "He didn't really want to die," Fine concluded. "He was just terrified."[61]

It should be noted that McAfee, like Bouvia, wanted to work, but getting paid for working would have made him ineligible for publicly funded assistance in housing or for Medicaid.

Cases such as Bouvia's and McAfee's suggest that we often give severely disabled people three grim choices: to become a burden on their families, to live miserably in a large public institution, or to kill themselves.

## Disability Culture

During the last decades, people with disabilities increasingly resisted discrimination, asserting their right to 24-hour-a-day attendants, public transportation, and good housing.[62] They asserted that they had a condition, not an illness. For them, "Disability Culture" is not bad, but a source of identity.

Indeed, the disabled community is the only minority that one may join at any time. James Meredith had to sue in 1962 to become the first black person admitted to the University of Mississippi, and so also quadriplegic Edward V. Roberts had to sue to be admitted to the University of California. But has society more successfully integrated the races than the disabled?

People with disabilities despise Mattel's "Share-a-Smile Becky" in a wheel-chair (sold in some hospitals' gift shops) and demonstrate outside of classes of Princeton bioethicist Peter Singer, whose views on quality of life, they fear, will allow society to easily kill the disabled or deny them adequate resources. They hectored the Hemlock Society (now called Compassion and Choices) for being too sympathetic to the assisted death of non-terminal patients. They cite psychologist Faye Girsh, this society's executive director, who testified on behalf of Bouvia, on behalf of Jack Kevorkian, on behalf of George DeLury who in 1996 in Manhattan killed his wife in the late stages of multiple sclerosis, and on behalf of Canadian Robert Latimer, who in 1993 killed his 12-year-old daughter with cerebral palsy. Disability groups accused Girsh of siding with rich, well-insured, autonomous elites, not of securing better conditions for the disabled.

## FURTHER READING AND RESOURCES

"A Man of Endurance," *20/20* television show on March 22, 1999, on Donald Cowart's case. Call 1-800-CALL-ABC to order tape.
"Elizabeth Bouvia: 10 Years Later," *60 Minutes* Special, www.cbs.com.
Pat MilmoreMcCarrick, "Active Euthanasia and Assisted Suicide," Scope Note 18, *Kennedy Institute of Ethics Journal* no. 1 (March 1992).
James Rachels, *The End of Life*, Oxford, UK: Oxford University Press, 1986.
Lonnie Kliever, *Dax's Case: Essays in Medical Ethics and Human Meaning*, Dallas, TX: Southern Methodist University Press, 1989.

## DISCUSSION QUESTIONS

1. Can decisions be justified by their outcomes? What if, when they had the opportunity, Bouvia or Cowart had killed themselves? Would that mean the physicians who prevented their earlier deaths were wrong?
2. How do you know when you've really properly treated depression and "debilitating symptoms" when a patient has sustained a terrible accident or is dying? Isn't that a Catch-22, where you only know you've successfully treated it when the patient decides to live?
3. Is the right to die glamorized in movies? What if the paralyzed fighter, portrayed by actress Hillary Swank in *Million Dollar Baby*, had to suffocate slowly for 20 minutes in dying? What if her reflexes kicked in and her body resisted? She lost bowel and bladder control? It didn't work and she was left comatose or brain-damaged?
4. Right now, society seems to exalt young bodies, sexiness, athleticism, and wealth. Do these images set young people up for failure? As most people can't have these traits, what message do these images send to people who are the opposite? Is this a good set of values to live by?
5. How do diversity and autonomy go together, or not? Will some ethnic groups be more interested in autonomy in medicine than others? Is autonomy more meaningful to some than others? Should autonomy be defined as a check or balance against the power of the medical establishment over the individual?

# CHAPTER 3

# Requests to Die: Terminal Patients

$I$n a dark, humid hospital that had been damaged when Hurricane Katrina struck New Orleans in 2005, physician Anna Pou stood her post, caring for dozens of critically ill patients who had been abandoned by other physicians. With overflowing toilets, no fresh water, no electric power, a flooded first floor preventing delivery of supplies, and temperatures above 100 degrees Fahrenheit, Dr. Pou allegedly killed four patients who could not be evacuated. Was she a hero or a villain?

In 1971, a Dutch physician killed her terminally ill mother, making Holland an ethics laboratory for physician-assisted dying. In 1998, a decades-long battle ended when a physician legally assisted a terminally ill Oregonian to die. During the same decade, Dr. Jack Kevorkian assisted more than 100 patients to die before being jailed in 1999. In 2009, physicians legally helped five terminally ill residents of Washington to die. In 2009, the Montana Supreme Court also legalized physician-assisted dying and in 2013, the Vermont legislature did too.

Critics saw these physician-assisted deaths as accelerating a growing culture of death. They claimed that this culture began in 1973 with legalization of abortion.

## HOLLAND

In 1973, the Dutch formed guidelines for physician-assisted death: (1) Only competent patients can request death; (2) requests must be repeated, non-ambivalent, unpressured, and documented; (3) physicians must consult another physician; (4) patients must be in unbearable pain or suffering, without likelihood of improvement.[1]

Holland has universal medical coverage, including long-term nursing home care. Dutch patients see physicians who have known them for years.

So did Holland's mercy killings create a slippery slope into barbarism? In 1990, its Remmelink Commission reported that between 1973 and 1990, Dutch physicians had killed a thousand *incompetent* patients, a direct violation of the guidelines.[2] All patients were terminally ill. Most had cancer or AIDS, and when competent, had asked to have physicians help them die. So voluntary euthanasia did spread to the killing of incompetent patients. Nevertheless, some limits exist. Without prior discussion with a physician or an advance directive, comatose patients like Terri Schiavo could not be legally assisted to die in Holland.

Some cases pushed the limits, such as when a physician killed a woman in her 20s who had suffered a decade of severe anorexia. In 1993, a physician killed a woman after the death of her two children and the failure of her marriage left her depressed.

In 2001, after 30 years of agreements and semi-legalization, physician-assisted dying became completely legal in Holland. By then it had the support of 90 percent of Dutch citizens. Dutch law now includes the right of patients in the early stages of dementia or amyotrophic lateral sclerosis to sign advance directives to be killed at a later date.

In early years, Dutch physicians rebuffed 66 percent of patients who requested death. By 2005, and in a pattern also seen in the American Northwest, the number of patients rejected had dropped to 12 percent, with another 13 percent changing their minds and another 13 percent dying before the physician could assist.[3]

In 2002, the Dutch Parliament extended its previous euthanasia legislation to competent adolescents aged 16 to 18 and, with consent of parents, teenagers aged 12 to 16. The *Groningen protocol* began in March 2006 where children under age 12, and especially babies, could be killed with parental consent. Two physicians had to agree that the child was terminally ill with no prospect of recovery and suffering great pain.[4] This protocol legalized previously secret euthanasia in babies in Dutch hospitals, especially for babies with spina bifida.

In 2002, Belgium legalized physician-assisted dying for adults, Luxembourg did so in 2011, and also in 2011, Switzerland legalized some kinds of physician-assisted dying.

## JACK KEVORKIAN

In the 1990s, retired pathologist Jack Kevorkian created an ethical firestorm by helping more than 100 American patients to die.

The son of Armenian immigrants, he grew up in Michigan and graduated from medical school in 1953. After residency, he worked from 1969 to 1978 in Detroit at Sarasota Hospital as director of laboratories. Later, he worked at hospitals in Southern California.

In the mid-1980s, he retired and lived on his savings and Social Security, $550 a month. He lived simply in a tiny, two-room apartment near his two sisters.

Compassion did not originally motivate Kevorkian. Instead, he wanted to increase organs available for transplantation. This failed because most terminal patients are unsuitable donors.

Always a loner, he scorned membership in medical societies. "Instinctively, as a student, I thought they were corrupt," he says. "I've been independent all my life."

Afraid to fly and hating to drive far, his patients had to come to him. He also accepted no money from the patients whom he helped to die.

In 1990, he helped 54-year-old Oregonian Janet Adkins to die, setting off a national debate. In 1988, Adkins had become frustrated by her inability to remember. She had early Alzheimer's disease, the fourth-largest killer of Americans. She tried the experimental drug Tacrine, but it didn't work.

Characterized by progressive loss of memory, Alzheimer's results from irreversible degeneration of neural cells. After the onset of symptoms and with excellent care, its victims on average live 8 to 10 years. In the disease's final phase, patients will not recognize their own children.

At the time, assisted suicide was not illegal in Michigan. Adkins flew there with her husband and her three sons. Her family disliked her intention to die and hoped she would change her mind, but in the end, they supported her.

When Adkins arrived in Michigan, Kevorkian and his sister interviewed her for two hours. Nobody thought she was depressed or that she could be helped by medicine. She signed documents and made videotapes to prove she knew what she was doing.

The next day, June 4, 1990, Adkins met Kevorkian alone and the two drove away in his rusty Volkswagen van. He had asked several clinics, churches, and funeral homes, but none would let him use their facilities. So he drove to a park in Oakland County. Inside his van, he had Janet, a cot, and a device.

The simple device consisted of three intravenous (IV) bottles hung from an aluminum frame; Kevorkian called it the *Mercitron*. At the park, he connected an IV line to Janet Adkins and started a saline solution for fluid volume. Then she pushed a switch that stopped the saline and released thiopental, a powerful sedative. The switch started a six-second timer that activated a drip of potassium chloride. Thiopental rendered Janet Adkins unconscious, and about a minute later, potassium chloride killed her. Kevorkian said that Janet had in effect "a painless heart attack while in deep sleep." The whole process took less than six minutes.

Neither the Adkins family nor Kevorkian anticipated the resulting publicity. The local district attorney prosecuted Kevorkian for murder. Because no law prohibited assisted suicide in Michigan, a local judge dismissed the case but ordered Kevorkian not to use his Mercitron again (although the judge had no legal basis for his order).

In 1991, Kevorkian assisted in the death of a woman with chronic vaginal-pelvic pain. An autopsy showed no physical cause of her pain. With Kevorkian again indicted for murder, a judge dismissed the charges because of the absence of a Michigan law. However, authorities suspended Kevorkian's medical license.

Without a license, Kevorkian couldn't obtain sodium pentothal or potassium chloride, so he began using carbon monoxide (CO). He claimed the gas "has no color, taste, or smell; and it's toxic enough to cause rapid unconsciousness in relatively low concentration. Furthermore, in light complexioned people it often produces a rosy color that makes the victim look better as a corpse." He taught patients to attach one end of a plastic tube to a canister of CO and the other to the kind of small plastic mask used in hospitals for oxygen therapy. When he turned on the gas and the patient breathed, death occurred within five minutes. In 1992, he helped another victim of multiple sclerosis, who donned a mask to breathe CO.

Most bioethicists and physicians denounced him. Kevorkian responded, "Why should I care what brainwashed ethicists and non-thinking physicians say?"[5]

Nor did he worry about violating the Hippocratic Oath; he called physicians who followed it "hypocritic oafs." He regarded himself as a Socratic gadfly and saw his struggle in heroic terms, comparing himself to Mahatma Gandhi and Martin Luther King, Jr.

In 1995, he opened a suicide clinic in Michigan, but the building's owner evicted him. By 1998, he had assisted 100 patients in committing suicide and had been acquitted in three trials involving five of those deaths.

In 1998, the Michigan legislature passed a law making physician-assisted dying illegal. Kevorkian then assisted in the videotaped death of ALS patient Thomas Youk. The videotape offered irrefutable evidence at Kevorkian's trial that he had deliberately broken the law.

The then-70-year-old Kevorkian received a 10–25 year sentence and later entered jail in Jackson, Michigan. After Kevorkian promised to help no more terminal patients to die, authorities paroled him eight years later in 2007 at age 79. He died in 2011 at age 83.

## DR. QUILL: ANOTHER APPROACH TO DYING

In 1990, Timothy Quill, an internist in Rochester, New York, helped his patient Diane to die. She had terminal, acute myelomonocytic leukemia, and had experienced three tumultuous months, during which her son stayed nearby.

When Dr. Quill knew that her end had come, he gave her the drugs she needed to commit suicide. He wrote:

> When we met, it was clear that she [Diane] knew what she was doing, that she was sad and frightened to be leaving, but that she would be even more terrified to stay and suffer. In our tearful goodbye, she promised a reunion in the future at her favorite spot on the edge of Lake Geneva, with dragons swimming in the sunset.[6]

Quill wrote of Diane's death in a medical journal and his district attorney then prosecuted him for murder; however, the grand jury refused to indict him.

Quill's case contrasted with those of Jack Kevorkian: Quill knew his patient well and had treated her for a long time; he first offered her a course of treatment that might allow her to survive; he helped her die privately and without publicity; he presented his account in an established medical forum; and he did not specialize in assisted dying but in primary care medicine.

## DR. POU'S CASE, CONTINUED

The 7th floor of Memorial Hospital had been leased privately to LifeCare as a long-term care facility for senior citizens with multiple medical problems. Anna Pou, then 51 years old and a native of New Orleans, worked as a Ear-Nose-and-Throat doctor there, supervising residents at Louisiana State University School of Medicine.[7]

Memorial Hospital lies three miles southwest of the French Quarter in New Orleans, a city that is essentially a big bowl around which, high above, mighty waters flow behind levees. Historically during hurricanes, local residents had fled to Memorial Hospital for shelter. When a nearby levee broke, water surrounded the hospital, trapping everyone inside.

After Hurricane Katrina made the hospital unlivable, most physicians fled. Calling her a hero for remaining, Dr. Pou's fellow physicians described her as hardworking, dedicated, and exerting a "huge presence."[8]

Helicopters on Tuesday began to evacuate the sickest patients at the hospital. On Thursday, an important date to remember, someone informed Dr. Pou that further evacuations might not happen. Meanwhile, thousands of survivors in New Orleans had fled into the Super Dome, begging for rescue from the appalling conditions.

According to Dr. Pou, at that point, "When we realized that help was not imminent . . . the standard of rescue changed to that of reverse triage. It was recognized that some patients might not survive, and priority was given to those who had the best chance of survival. On Thursday morning, only category 3 patients [the most gravely ill] remained on the LifeCare unit." That left nine patients there, all of whom eventually died.

## OREGON'S LEGALIZATION

After intense battles, Oregonians in 1994 by referendum approved the Oregon Death with Dignity Act, but its legislature refused to go along. Another referendum in 1997 approved the measure 60 to 40 percent, forcing the act into law beginning in 1998.

The act had draconian restrictions: Patients had to be (1) clearly competent, (2) have less than six months to live, and (3) wait 15 days before filling prescriptions to avoid impulsive decisions. Physicians could not administer the fatal dosage, only prescribe it.

Most Oregonians prefer to die at home. Oregon has the lowest in-hospital mortality rate, suggesting many referrals for home health care and respect for advance directives.[9] Under its groundbreaking Oregon Health Plan, all its previously uninsured, terminally ill citizens could utilize hospice programs.[10]

What about managed care organizations subtly pushing early death to save money? One misperception is that hospice and palliative care are cheap. A 1998 study showed that physician-assisted death might make a difference in only one-half of 1 percent of costs at the end of life.[11] Nevertheless, critics charge that state-run plans will encourage early death. In 2009, some Americans feared that mandatory "death counseling" under one Obama plan for public medicine might be a screen for saving money.

Doctors cannot be forced to participate in such deaths. They also cannot *abandon* patients. As in the case of abortion, those who object to participating in the death "must transfer care so that the needs of the patient can be met" and "must not hinder the transfer."[12]

In the 13 years that assisted death has been legal in Oregon, about 60 to 90 terminal patients a year requested prescriptions, and about 30 to 50 used such prescriptions to die.[13]

As these data make clear, about a third of patients who use this act do not kill themselves. Why? They either die before the waiting period is over or die without using the pills. Most seem to like the control that having the pills gives them. Over 10 years, only 670 of about 100,000 dying Oregonians requested terminal drugs.[14] The most frequent diseases were ALS, AIDS, and cancer. Physicians most commonly prescribed the barbiturates secobarbital and phenobarbital.

The guidebook for Oregonian physicians encourages them to obtain the drugs, keep them until the time of death, and be there with the patient in his home as he takes them.[15] A "Do Not Resuscitate" (DNR) order should be signed for emergency-response personnel, and the physician should counsel the family that death may take hours and have complications. Physicians should also be ready to administer antiemetics and analgesics, counsel and support the family during and after the death, sign the death certificate, and arrange transfer to a funeral home.

Finally, here is a tip for all of us who want to avoid undignified dying and loss of control in an impersonal hospital. When patients really are dying, the urge to eat disappears. In such a state, fasting becomes easy. Although patients must be determined, such dying can be a peaceful alternative to intravenous lines and the sleep of barbiturates. Before succumbing, one dying patient went 11 days without fluids and 51 days without food. One study in 2003 discovered that more Oregonians died by ceasing food and water than by asking physicians to give them drugs, and as said, most died at home.[16]

## BACKGROUND: ANCIENT GREECE AND THE HIPPOCRATIC OATH

The Hippocratic Oath, considered the origin of medical ethics, forbids physicians to kill patients. It originated in ancient Greece at the time of Socrates in fifth century B.C.E. But did Hippocratic doctors represent most ancient Greek physicians?

Hippocrates followed the mathematician Pythagoras, who developed the famous theorem, worshipped numbers as divine, and held that all life was sacred. But as a Pythagorean, Hippocrates did not represent his fellow physicians.

The Hippocratic corpus, or body of writings, does not represent the work of one man named "Hippocrates," but a number of his followers. These practitioners "possessed no legally recognized professional qualifications" and competed with gymnastic instructors, drugsellers, herbalists, midwives, and exorcists.[17]

Many people today misunderstand the content of the original Hippocratic oath, which makes physicians promise:

> I swear by Apollo Physician and Asclepius and Hygeia and Panaceia and all the gods and goddesses, making them my witnesses, that I will fulfill according to my ability and judgment this oath and this covenant:
>
> To hold him who has taught me this art as equal to my parents and to live my life in partnership with him, and if he is in need of money, to give him a share of mine, and to regard his offspring as equal to my brothers in male lineage, and to teach his art—if they desire to learn it—without fee and covenant; to give a share of precepts and oral instruction and all the other learning to my sons and to the sons of him who has instructed me and the pupils who have signed the covenant and have taken this oath according to the medical law, but to no one else.
>
> I will apply dietetic measures for the benefit of the sick according to my ability and judgment; I will keep them from harm and injustice.

I will neither give a deadly drug to anybody if asked for it, nor will I make a suggestion to this effect. Similarly I will not give to a woman an abortive remedy. In purity and holiness I will guard my life and my art. I will not use the knife, not even on sufferers of stone, but will withdraw in favor of such men as are engaged in this work.

Whatever houses I visit, I will come for the benefit of the sick, remaining free of all intentional injustice, of all mischief and in particular of sexual relations with both female and male persons, be they free or slaves.

What I may see or hear in the course of the treatment or even outside of the treatment in regard to the life of men, which on no account one must spread abroad, I will keep to myself holding such things shameful to be spoken about.

If I fulfill this oath and do not violate it, may it be granted to me to enjoy life and art, being honored with fame among all men for all time to come; if I transgress it and swear falsely, may the opposite of all this be my lot.[18]

With this oath, Hippocratic physicians solidified their membership against competing healers, such as surgeons or sophistic physicians who charged for teaching. Note that the oath refers only to teaching males and forbids those who swear by it from performing surgery, abortions, or giving deadly drugs.

Ordinary Greek physicians thought that life had natural limitations, beyond which only fools extended life. The concept of a natural limit infused Greek culture, especially in architecture and theater. To attempt to go beyond such limits was *hubris* and invited the gods to strike one down. So most ancient Greek physicians helped their patients die.

## DR. POU'S CASE, CONTINUED

Shocking conditions prevailed at Memorial Hospital after Hurricane Katrina. More than 2,000 people had sought shelter there—neighbors, family members, family of staff, and previous outpatients—crowding the hallways and draining the hospital of food, water, and clean toilets. Staff rushed by people sprawled on the floor, crying out for water and help.

On the top floor, conditions for the last nine patients worsened each day. One paralyzed 61-year-old person weighed 380 pounds, but seemed alert, oriented, and interactive. Others could breathe only on ventilators; some had chronic, non-healing wounds that required intensive nursing. All sweltered in rooms as hot as 105 degrees. Another aspirated food and suffered a heart attack but was resuscitated.

## THE NAZIS AND "EUTHANASIA"

Debates about physician-assisted dying frequently refer to German physicians during the Nazi era, who in the name of "euthanasia" killed 90,000 patients because of mental or physical inferiority. This so-called Nazi argument bears some scrutiny.

First, Nazi physicians administered the *Final Solution* to the "problem" of how to cleanse Germany of racially inferior non-Aryan peoples. Physicians kept this program secret, and under it, killed 6 million Jews, 600,000 Poles, thousands of Gypsies, and hundreds of gay men and lesbians.

Leo Alexander, a New York psychiatrist who observed the Nuremberg trials, famously argued in 1949 that the killing programs began with their belief that some people are better off dead than alive because their quality of life is poor.[19]

In 1986, another New York psychiatrist, Robert Jay Lifton, argued similarly, although his "first step" differed from Alexander's:

> The Nazis justified direct medical killing by use of the . . . concept of "life unworthy of life," *lebensunwertes Leben*. While this concept predated the Nazis, it was carried to its ultimate racial and "therapeutic" extreme by them.
>
> . . . Of the five identifiable steps by which the Nazis carried out the destruction of "life unworthy of life," coercive sterilization was the first. There followed the killing of "impaired" children in hospitals, and then the killing of "impaired" adults—mostly collected from mental hospitals—in centers especially equipped with carbon monoxide. The same killing centers were then used for the murders of "impaired" inmates of concentration camps. The final step was mass killing, mostly of Jews, in the extermination camps themselves.[20]

People opposed to physician-assisted dying often cite Alexander's and Lifton's work. They emphasize that fact that in Nazi Germany medical professors in elite medical schools took the first dangerous step down the slope.

J. C. Wilkes argued differently that the first steps down the Nazi slope came when physicians mercy-killed a few severely handicapped infants.[21] Starting in 1937, a father who killed his mentally challenged child, received only a mild rebuke. Two years later, Dr. Karl Brandt examined an infant named Knauer, born blind and missing an arm and a leg. Hitler cleared him to kill Knauer and all similar infants. Wilkes claims these two test cases led to the first phase of deaths in Germany where physicians killed as many as 6,000 disabled children.

These cases differ from the so-called Baby Doe cases (discussed in Chapter 8) in that most German parents did *not* consent to these killings. Officials took the babies and children out of the home and parents never heard from them again.

What about claims by Alexander, Lifton, and Wilkes about the first step that led down the slippery slope? In rebuttal, many history professors say this is just bad history. They emphasize that Germany had been blatantly anti-Semitic since the time of the Crusades. Instead of a subtle first step propelling them downward, Nazi physicians rode a tsunami that had been building for centuries.

The Nazi "euthanasia" program also misleads people in at least three ways: it had nothing in common with *competent* patients who are *dying* and who *voluntarily* request assistance in dying from physicians. Nazi "euthanasia" was not "good deaths" but despicable murders.

A little analysis also helps. The Nazi argument contains many different claims, including:

1. Involuntary killings of people *for medical reasons* led to the Holocaust.

2. Involuntary killings of people *by physicians* led to the Holocaust.

3. Justifying medical killings of people *for reasons of quality of life* led to the Holocaust.

4. *Involuntary sterilization* of retarded, psychotic, and demented people led to the Holocaust.
5. The *killing of impaired children* led to the Holocaust.
6. *Eugenics*, the desire of Nazis to create a Master Race, led to the Holocaust.
7. Deep *cultural racism and anti-Semitism* led to the Holocaust.
8. Acceptance by physicians of a *new role as killers* led to the Holocaust.

Because all its victims died *involuntarily*, and because no terminal patients died voluntarily by Nazi physicians, "playing the Nazi card" does not illustrate good reasoning. (Nevertheless, in any long discussion in bioethics, the possibility—especially on talk radio or in letters to the editor—that someone will bring up the Nazis or Hitler approaches 100 percent, a fact often referred to as "Godwin's Law").

## MODERN DEVELOPMENTS

Founded in the United States in 1980 by Derek Humphrey, the Hemlock Society helped people with terminal illness die with dignity. After merging with other organizations, in 2005 it became Compassion & Choices, which advocates legalizing physician-assisted dying.

In the 1960s, two physicians—one working in America and the other in England—changed medicine to help dying patients. Elisabeth Kübler-Ross, working in Chicago, and Cicely Saunders, in Britain, emphasized making terminal patients comfortable.

Their programs began the *hospice movement*. Hospice tries to give dying patients dignity and maximal control over the final months of their lives. Originally, hospices were independent facilities, often residences, but the concept evolved to visiting nurses treating patients at home.

Because of the work of these two women, physicians today better relieve pain and better attend psychologically to dying patients than 40 years ago. In the United States, Medicare now pays for six months of hospice.

Around 1986, *palliative care* began in medicine, which does not mean giving up on patients but does forego experimental treatments. Palliative care strives for maximal relief of nausea, boredom, itching, feelings of suffocation, immobility, depression, and especially pain.

### Recent Legal Decisions

In 1994, a federal judge struck down a law in Washington state banning assisted suicide, holding that the equal protection of liberty guaranteed in the Fourteenth Amendment covered not only a woman's right to end a pregnancy but also a terminal patient's right to physician-assisted dying.[22] The liberty guaranteed to Americans by the Constitution included the right to die with assistance by physicians, she said.

Over the next three years and in two important decisions, the U.S. Supreme Court disagreed. Although a state such as Oregon *could* legalize physician-assisted dying, no fundamental liberty existed in the Constitution to this assistance—such that state laws banning this assistance might be unconstitutional.

One appeal alleged discrimination against dying patients because only some patients could decide to die by removal of a ventilator or feeding tube. If physicians could legally kill by withdrawing treatment, it argued, why not by more direct means? The highest Court answered that "the distinction between assisting suicide and withdrawing life-sustaining treatment, a distinction widely recognized and endorsed in the medical profession and in our legal traditions, is both important and logical; it is certainly rational. . . . "[23]

In the second appeal, the same Court accepted the AMA's claim that legalization of physician-assisted dying threatened the medical profession's integrity, as well as claims that physician-assisted dying would hurt the disabled and poor. It also found "ample concern" for a slippery slope from increased acceptance of physician killings.

These decisions only said that a fundamental right to die did not already exist in the Constitution, such that state laws banning assisted suicide would violate it. They left the door open for states such as Oregon to legalize physician-assisted dying. In this way, these decisions mirrored what *Cruzan* said about laws about incompetent patients, i.e., states *could*, but *need not*, pass this kind of law.

## ETHICAL ISSUES

Two different kinds of arguments occur in ethics. One focuses directly on the morality of acts and argues that they are intrinsically wrong or wrong without regard to consequences. The other grants that in a few cases, such acts may be justified, but opposes them based on their bad indirect effects. These are *direct* and *indirect* arguments.

The main direct argument against physician-assisted dying is that it is always wrong to kill. Most other arguments against it are indirect and predict slippery slopes.

## DIRECT ARGUMENTS—PHYSICIAN-ASSISTED DYING

### Killing Is Always Wrong

The best direct argument against physician-assisted dying is that such actions wrongly kill vulnerable humans. It is always wrong to kill humans under all circumstances, and just because a human is dying, no exceptions can be made. Evil occurs when one human ends the life of another.

This argument does not claim that what is wrong about killing is that it can become uncontrollable after a few justified cases, for that would be appealing to a slippery slope. Instead, it claims that all killing is *intrinsically wrong*, no matter what the circumstances.

Whether or not an afterlife or God exists, once a person is dead, he's not coming back. Without an afterlife, this life is all a person has, and to take it away is to take away all values because the valu*er* is gone.

For many decisions, such as transplanting a kidney, if mistakes occur, there is backup, for example, hemodialysis. But mistakes in killing have no backup. Once a person is dead, that's it.

For this reason, killing must not be taken lightly. Life must not be cheapened. The ultimate power on earth is to take away life. All life should be valued, not just some in the right circumstances. Life is precious, not matter how low in quality. Of all values in medicine, this one must reign supreme.

## Killing Is Not Always Wrong

The most ancient justification of the direct argument is based on religious metaphysics: that God exists, that Scripture correctly reveals his laws for humans, and that one such law is for humans never to kill another human. Based on this view, some Christians and some orthodox Jews prefer death to self-defense, refuse war and the draft, and will never kill.

One should note that Scripture really bans "unjustified" killings, and hence, allows just wars and the death penalty for murderers. The question here concerns whether helping terminally ill patients die is "unjustified killing." After all, God presumably allows us to get terminal illnesses and to die, so in one sense, dying for each of us is His Will.

More important, the background conditions need to be examined about the rule against killing. In the past, most people have wanted to live as long as possible, but that fact is less true today. Why? Because medicine has cured the acute diseases, and left us with chronic diseases. In previous centuries, people tried to live as long as possible because most never experienced the disability and dysfunction that come with chronic diseases.

Now consider the rule against killing and physician-assisted dying. When you help me accomplish what I want to do, you do a good thing, and morality encourages you to help me. When you prevent me from doing what I want to do, you hurt my interests, and your actions may be immoral. Whether or not dying assisted by physicians is good or bad may depend, not on what has been traditionally been judged moral or immoral, but on the wishes of the patient.

Of course, critics can object that helping me do what I want to do is not always a good thing, such as if I want to steal my neighbor's car. And, they say, helping people die is immoral.

But why should we allow this objection? Why should we accept the underlying premise that "helping dying people die is immoral" unless some further reason is given? To simply assert this as an objection is to beg the question. It is not an argument against a position to assume that it is wrong.

## Killing vs. Letting Die

For several decades, bioethicists have debated whether killing differs from letting die. A 1997 survey by the American Hospital Association found that 70 percent of deaths in hospitals involve some decision by a physician or relative to cease treatment.[24] However, intentional termination of a dying patient's life is still illegal in most states.

A leading physician in medical ethics once admitted, "I have had occasion to give a patient pain medication we both knew would shorten her life."[25] Does this differ from killing her?

In palliative care, physicians practice *terminal sedation*, which stands on the doctrine of double effect where the physician must not intend death but merely the relief of pain (see Index and Chapter 5 for discussion of this doctrine). Does such sedation differ from killing the patient? Is the difference only semantic?

In 1975, philosopher James Rachels attacked the distinction between active and passive euthanasia in a famous article in the *New England Journal of Medicine*.[26] Rachels argued that this distinction, though still dominant in modern medicine and law, has no inherent moral value and, when it is taken for anything more than a pragmatic rule, leads to decisions about death based on irrelevant factors.

Rachels' logic cuts two ways: first, letting a vegetative patient die is just as bad (or good) as killing her; second, killing a vegetative patient is just as good (or bad) as allowing her to die. There is nothing moral or immoral in the act of passive or active euthanasia itself; instead, morality or immorality is determined by motives and results in the context of that act. Focusing on whether an act is active or passive, he argued, may confuse our judgments, leading us to think that passively allowing people to die slowly and horribly is morally superior to actively bringing about a quick, painless death.

Rachels caused controversy. Is intending death by removing a respirator equivalent to suffocating a patient with a pillow? If a patient is allowed to die, isn't that patient killed by the disease? But if someone acts directly to bring about dying, isn't that human agent the cause of death? One critic argued:

> What is the difference between merely letting a patient die and killing that patient? Does it depend upon activity or passivity? Does it depend on an agent's intentions? I think that neither of these factors is relevant. What is relevant is the cause of death. When the cause of death is the underlying disease process, the patient is simply allowed to die.[27]

So after Hurricane Katrina, diseases didn't kill Ana Pou's patients, Ana Pou did.

Philosopher Bonnie Steinbock argues that Rachels confuses ceasing treatment with killing or "intentionally letting die."[28] The former may stem from rights of protection against unwanted interference and medical standards of appropriate treatment. The latter connotes a different motive, wanting a life to end *soon*.

In support of Rachels, it can be argued that in practice the line between active and passive is hard to draw. In some cases, not acting can be considered active, e.g., omitting antibiotics to Karen Quinlan to treat the pneumonia she developed in her final weeks.

This does not entail that killing and assisted dying do not differ; as Jean Davies argued, just as "rape and making love are different, so are killing and assisted suicide."[29]

## Relief of Suffering

One of the most persuasive arguments for physician-assisted dying is the appeal to mercy. Ana Pou probably saw panicked patients suffering in terrible heat, dehydration, and discomfort. Observing another human being in untreatable pain howling like a wounded animal should move us to tears and we should end such suffering. We do this for our pets; why can't we do so for humans? Moreover, the suffering of terminal patients is not confined to physical pain, as bad as that is; it also involves helplessness, stress, exhaustion, terror, loss, and other experiences that are difficult even to imagine.

A big issue here has to do with relief of pain. Is it possible to relieve all pain and make dying patients completely comfortable? Cicely Saunders, who founded St. Christopher's Hospice in London, said her dying patients never needed to suffer pain. She gave them Brompton cocktails, a powerful brew of morphine, heroin, alcohol, and cocaine.

On the other hand, Derek Humphrey of the Hemlock Society argued that, "it is generally agreed that 10 percent of pain cannot be controlled. That is a lot of people."[30] Margaret Battin and Timothy Quill acknowledge that even with excellent palliative care, 2 to 5 percent of terminal patients experience pain that is incontrollable.[31] It is also true that not everyone experiences pain in the same way, and a condition that would be acceptable to some might be intolerable to others.

A second question concerns what the cost of relief might be, and what costs are acceptable. In this context, we are not talking about financial costs: the issue is the cost to the patient's well-being. Powerful narcotics such as Brompton cocktails numb consciousness and make patients mostly unconscious.

Dying patients must make a tradeoff between consciousness and relief of pain, and not every patient considers that tradeoff acceptable. For some patients, being conscious and able to talk to relatives and friends is more important than avoiding pain. Here again, autonomy becomes relevant. What counts as a benefit or a harm must be defined within each patient's own value system, and who else but patients can make such judgments?

Ethics and medicine commonly distinguish between pain and suffering. *Pain* is physical; *suffering* is a broader and more personal matter. Pain covers one aspect of suffering, but relieving pain does not necessarily relieve suffering

Peter Admiraal, a physician and one of the leaders of assisted dying in the Netherlands, agrees that uncontrollable pain is rarely the only reason for death:

> There is severe dehydration, uncontrolled itching and fatigue. These patients are completely exhausted. Some of them can't turn around in their beds. They become incontinent. All these factors make a kind of suffering from which they only want to escape. . . .
>
> And of course you are suffering because you have a mind. You are thinking about what is happening to you. You have fears and anxiety and sorrow. In the end, it gives a complete loss of human dignity. You cannot stop that feeling with medical treatment.[32]

In Dr. Pou's case, one could argue that her nine patients were suffering badly and it was unlikely that they would be saved. Gravely ill with many medical problems, lying in hot, humid rooms with no fresh water—it is hard to imagine a more uncomfortable place to be.

## Patient Autonomy

Let's be frank: people believe different things about the sanctity of life and the wrongness of killing, but what if you're not religious? Or don't see religion as against helping people die? What are we to do? Fight about it? Kill each other over who's right about killing?

One way to say that each person should decide things himself is to say that the *autonomy* of patients should count most. "Autonomy" means the ability to be self-governing and self-directed. Its opposite is to be treated paternalistically, like an incompetent child.

Autonomy mattered to John Stuart Mill, who argued in his *On Liberty* that, "over his own body and mind, the individual is sovereign." Mill's view implies that government should not impose its view of when and how people should die.

Autonomy raises some questions about risks: Who is best qualified to assess the danger of dying too soon? What degree of risk is acceptable? Who should determine acceptability? How does the risk of dying too soon compare with the risks entailed by alternatives?

Physicians usually believe that they are best qualified to assess risk, and they're right as far as statistical risk is concerned. But *acceptable* risk is evaluative as well as statistical, and many patients want the right to make their own judgments about what is acceptable risk.

When terminal patients make such evaluations, their concern is more than just fear of pain. Derek Humphrey of the Hemlock Society has written, "It isn't just a question of pain. It is a question of dignity, self-control, and distress. If you can't eat, sleep, or read, and the quality of life is so bad, and there is a certainty that you are dying, it is a matter of dignity" to be able to end your life.[33]

In order to evaluate acceptable risk, patients need information. Margaret Battin holds that physicians rarely discuss options with dying patients.[34] She believes that patients' informed consent should be sought not only for medical research but also for ways of dying. Especially when experimental drugs and surgery are involved, terminal patients should be informed about different outcomes and different ways of dying so that they can choose the *least worst death*. Alas, few patients get such information and are allowed to make such choices.

Ana Pou's patients did not seem to ask to die. At least one of them seems to have been oriented and alert, and could have been asked. Maybe she thought asking was moot, as no rescue was coming and conditions were worsening. Nevertheless, this lack of consent seems to be the most serious charge against Dr. Pou.

## INDIRECT ARGUMENTS ABOUT
## PHYSICIAN-ASSISTED DYING

### The Slippery Slope

One of the most famous ideas in ethics is the *slippery slope*, also called the "thin edge of the wedge argument," and already introduced in Chapter 1. Claims about it figure prominently in debates about physician-assisted dying, as we saw in decisions by the U.S. Supreme Court.

There are two general kinds of claims about slippery slopes: *empirical* and *conceptual*.[35] Claims about *empirical slopes* assert that once you take the first step, something bad in human nature is unleashed. Leo Alexander refers to an empirical slope: "The destructive principle, once unleashed, is bound to engulf the whole personality and to occupy all its relationships."[36]

A *conceptual* slippery slope asserts that once a small change is made in a moral rule, other changes will soon follow. Why? Because of the demands of reason for consistency in treating similar cases similarly. Alexander also assumes this kind of slope:

> The beginnings at first were merely a subtle shift in emphasis in the basic attitude of the physicians. It started with the acceptance of the attitude, basic in the euthanasia movement, that there is such a thing as life not worthy to be lived. This attitude in its early stages concerned itself merely with the severely and chronically sick. Gradually the sphere of those to be included in this category was enlarged to encompass the socially unproductive, the ideologically unwanted, the racially unwanted and finally all non-Germans. But it is important to realize that the infinitely small wedged-in lever from which this entire trend of mind received its impetus was the attitude of the nonrehabilitable sick.[37]

According to a conceptual slippery slope, once physicians kill one kind of patient because quality of life is so low as to make "life not worthy to be lived," they not only can, but *will*, use the same reasoning to kill in similar cases.

An *empirical* slope prediction says that once society changes a rule about protecting one class of patient, powerful forces will be unleashed that cannot be restrained and kept contained to the original class. Something like this was unleashed in Michael Swango: Charged and convicted in 2000 with killing three patients in New York State, Dr. Swango was found to have killed at least 60 patients, possibly hundreds, starting in Zimbabwe in the early 1980s and moving around the world. His diary revealed that he killed for the thrill of the power to kill and "the sweet, husky, close smell of an indoor homicide."

It is just such malice in human nature that could be unleashed with legal, physician-assisted deaths. Law professor Yale Kamisar observes that, "not all people are kind, understanding, and loving.[38]

After four patients under her care died suspiciously, Anna Pou was charged with second-degree murder.[39] The Louisiana Attorney General alleged that they died of overdoses of morphine and midazolam. Although the grand jury declined to indict Dr. Pou, it may have done so in part because other physicians abandoned the hospital while she heroically stayed, because the four patients might well have died anyway, and because she seemed compassionate. But it still may be true that, given the changing ethical climate about physician-assisted killing in America, she felt more free to do this than she would have decades ago. To that degree, and under those circumstances, perhaps some slippage has occurred.

Consider another example of a conceptual slope: first we will allow abortion of a fetus because of Down syndrome, and then we will let a newborn with Down syndrome die. In this kind of slope, as opposed to empirical slopes, *it is always the demand of reason to treat similar cases similarly that expands the initial change.*

This kind of reasoning is seen in the following claims: At the time of the Karen Quinlan case in 1976, disability advocate James Bopp said that if you "accept quality of life as the standard," then "first you withdraw the respirators, then the food and then you actively kill people. It's a straight line from one place to the others."[40] Bioethicist Daniel Callahan then said that the logic of the case for euthanasia would inevitably lead to its extension far beyond terminally ill competent adults. If relief of suffering is critical, Callahan said, "[W]hy should that relief be denied to the demented or the incompetent?"[41]

Contrasts may be made among the two kinds of slope claims. The empirical claim is a prediction about consequences if some moral change occurs, whereas the conceptual claim refers to a linkage in reasoning once particular premises are accepted. Where the empirical slope says one small change will create many others because of something bad in humans, the conceptual slope says the same kind of change can occur because of something higher—reason's need to treat similar cases similarly.

Claims about slippery slopes are difficult to evaluate because the predicted, final bad event often lies so far away. However, critics predicted that slippery slopes would occur during the Karen Quinlan case, with Holland's changes, and with Oregon's legalization, so we can evaluate such predictions.

In 1975, columnist Nat Hentoff predicted that the *Quinlan* decision would bring on an empirical slippery slope. In 1992, he felt vindicated in describing Jack Kevorkian's actions and the decriminalization of physician-assisted dying in the Netherlands, all of which he called a "reckless cheapening of life."[42]

What can we say about these claims? First, if the danger of an empirical slippery slope was real, we would have expected the precedent of the Quinlan case to first, make it easy for competent patients to die, and second, generalize to other kinds of incompetent patients, such as senile, demented patients in nursing homes. Yet neither happened. It took 22 years after the *Quinlan* decision before the first terminal patient legally died with the help of a physician in Oregon in 1998, and the Schiavo case (see next chapter) showed us how far we are from readily accepting the deaths of incompetent, comatose patients.

In Oregon, physician-assisted deaths over the first eight years averaged 35–40 per year. In Holland, a real expansion of cases occurred. Teenagers, psychiatric patients, and newborns who were suffering and terminal were killed with their parents' consent but against the initial guidelines.

Adequate screening for depression in patients with terminal cancer continues to be a concern. One review of patients requesting assistance in dying in Oregon questioned whether such patients had received such screening.[43]

Callahan's prediction has come true, but the Dutch regard it not as a descent but as a moral elevation: The Dutch agree that if it's justified to kill a consenting 64-year-old with terminal cancer, why isn't it also justified to kill a consenting 16-year-old with terminal cancer?

## Inefficient Means

Opponents of legalization claim that physician-assisted deaths botch 25 percent of cases in Holland and therefore it should be illegal.[44] This is a strange argument because it complains about the "how to" part of the legalization. In other words, physicians at present aren't good enough to guarantee death.

Of course, death for some patients will not be easy. Some AIDS patients who were intravenous drug users and who attempted suicide at dosages recommended by the Hemlock Society had high tolerances to central nervous system depressants. Instead of dying, they sometimes became comatose.

To avoid this possibility, the patient needed to ask a friend to be present to possibly help at the end by attaching a large plastic bag over the patient's head and securing it with duct tape, such that the patient could suffocate to death. (Called the "Exit Bag" by critic Nat Hentoff, this refers to the efficient, self-administered form of it with Velcro straps that once could be ordered from the Hemlock Society.[45]) The use of Exit Bags subjects friends to charges of murder. It leaves dying patients faced with the dilemma of dying alone and botching the attempt or asking a friend to be present, assist, and risk prosecution for assisting in suicide.

This is why Oregonian physicians may attend the deaths of terminal patients. If something goes wrong, they can adjust medications or deal with unexpected complications. In short, this argument is not an argument for no physician-assisted dying, but for *more* of it.

## A Financial Empirical Slope?

Will the greed of families and the avarice of physicians conspire to speed sick patients to an early grave? The honest answer is that we don't know. Hard times have not tested American physicians this way. They are used to aggressively treating patients and being well paid to do so, especially in oncology, cardiac surgery, and cancer surgery.

One nagging worry is that some historians think that the ultimate reason for the rise of Nazi Germany was economic. After losing World War I, the Germans were made to pay huge war reparations, which caused great harm to the German economy and created much ill will. Since World War II, and especially in the last decades, North America has experienced an unparalleled economic boom. What will happen when times turn bad and families must choose between grandma's care and a child's college tuition?

Most patients and families are shielded from the true costs of long-term coverage at the end of life. What might be truly dangerous is to give physicians incentives to curtail care at the end of life while ethical bulwarks against physician-assisted dying were weakened. That could easily become not just a wave but a tsunami, especially during a major depression and intergenerational war over who should pay the medical costs of an aging population.

> The financial and emotional burdens of lingering deaths [slow deterioration from chronic diseases] are discussed in an excerpt from Gregory Pence's *Elements of Bioethics*. To read this material, go to Chapter 3 in the Online Learning Center (OLC) at www.mhhe.com/pence7e where you will find "A Duty to Die?"

## THE ROLES OF PHYSICIANS

Some physicians argue that "physicians should not kill" and should always be healers. This statement assumes incorrectly that physicians can always heal. That is false. Everyone will eventually die. No human has ever been "healed" of death.

Second, to simplistically assert that, "Physicians should not kill" begs the key question of this chapter. It is like saying that, "Physicians should do not what is wrong," while assuming without argument that such-and-such is wrong.

More than one way exists to be a compassionate physician to dying patients: Quill vs. Kevorkian. A good physician makes sure his patient isn't depressed and doesn't choose death because of treatable symptoms. The short interviews by Dr. Kevorkian and his layperson sister, of his patients who arrived in town the day before they were killed, did not meet the highest standards of humanism in medicine.

As for Ana Pou, her role drew mixed reactions. On one hand, if it was a triage situation, she acted mercifully. But what if it wasn't a true situation of triage, because unknown to her, help was on the way? What if the definition of a "triage situation" is more subjective than it first appears?

## MISTAKES AND ABUSES

Physicians make mistakes. Surgeon Christiaan Barnard recalled a young woman with ovarian cancer who repeatedly begged him to kill her painlessly with morphine.[46] Aware that she was terminal—and hearing her screams at night—Barnard decided to help her. When he came into her room with a syringe loaded with morphine, she was quiet, and he thought that she was in too much pain even to scream. Then he realized that she was semiconscious, beyond pain, and changed his mind. The next morning, she felt better; soon was in remission, and lived another few months. Stories like this abound in medicine.

What if Ana Pou had hesitated? Waited one more day? As we shall see, rescue would have come and some of her patients would have lived.

In Holland, critics claim that physicians often misdiagnose "intractable and unbearable" suffering. In Janet Adkins's case, some critics said that physicians aren't infallible diagnosticians and that patients sometimes defy a dire prognosis.

Let us put this point differently. In bioethics, many discussions begin with a phrase like, "If a patient has a terminal illness. . . ." Notice the word "if." In presumably terminal illnesses, few claims are absolute until the patient's last days. Before then, how "terminal"—how close to death—the patient is may depend on many factors that are not easy to assess: the patient's attitude, the family's attitude, the attitude of staff members, the quality and level of care, and so on. Some terminal patients were misdiagnosed and recovered. Physician-assisted dying allows a mistaken diagnosis to become a death sentence.

Israeli physician Seymour Glick once revealed a dirty little secret of medicine: every physician has some patients whom he dislikes. Some illnesses are messy, some families are intolerable, and some physicians make mistakes and harm patients. In such cases, physicians want the patients to "go away." They "go away" most easily if the patients immediately die. But patients should only die for the right reason, not reasons like these.

## CRIES FOR HELP

Joanne Lynn, a physician who has cared for over 1,000 hospice patients, believes that most terminal patients who request physician-assisted death seek attention, control, dignity, relief of symptoms, or relief from depression. Sometimes a request to die is a plea to see "if anyone really cares whether he or she lives.[47]

It is especially important with terminal patients not just to deal with physical symptoms. Terminal patients are often bored and depressed: people avoid them. People who once did important work now have nothing to do. People who never watched television now watch it all day long. Good psychiatrists know how to help.

Dying at home cures some problems. It is empowering to be dying in your own home rather than a hospital, which has its own routine and hierarchy. But allowing physician-assisted dying would be the easy way out on several fronts. First, physicians don't need to aggressively treat symptoms. Second, the system doesn't need to change or to train more people in hospice and palliative care.

In a review of the literature, bioethicist Margaret Pabst Battin and Timothy Quill conclude that physician-assisted dying should be an option of last resort after all resources are exhausted of excellent palliative care.[48] Even though they defend legalizing physician-assisted dying, they stress that it must be no substitute for lack of great palliative care.

## ANNA POU, AGAIN: HERO OR VILLAIN?

**Hero.**    According to statements Dr. Pou made to *Newsweek*, the remaining staff met on Thursday and believed that no further evacuation or help was coming to them. They then decided to euthanize the remaining nine patients by sedation and that Dr. Pou would administer the drugs.

Unknown to her, the parent organization of LifeCare, which leased a floor that housed these nine patients, had hired private contractors to remove the patients. In addition, all other critically ill patients had been successfully removed from Memorial Hospital, including two 300-pound men who could not walk, patients from intensive care units, and tiny, premature babies.

Bioethicist Alto Charo notes, "From her perspective, these patients are now terminal . . . and they're terminal under particularly terrifying conditions: extreme discomfort, [probably] panic, and the prospect of being abandoned while helpless. [If Pou could not save them] her next obligation would seem to be . . . to give them enough medicine that they're not in any pain and they're not in any panic and it may or may not hasten their deaths."[49]

Dr. Timothy Quill said the drugs Dr. Pou gave are typically used to relieve pain and anxiety, not for euthanasia. For the latter, she would have used drugs such as barbituates and paralytics, but instead she used morphine, which both eases pain and decreases respiration, and midazolam, a powerful sedative.

At her trial, like Kevorkian, Dr. Pou insisted she did not intended to kill her patients but only to relieve their pain. The grand jury concluded that not enough evidence existed to conclude otherwise.

**Villain.**    In 2009, investigative reporter and M.D./Ph.D. Sheri Fink won a Pulitzer Prize for her story on what happened at Memorial Hospital after Hurricane Katrina.[50] Based on four years of research, Dr. Fink discovered several things. First, patients who had signed DNR orders were judged to be the last to be evacuated because they were judged by Dr. Pou to have the least to lose. Second, some patients on the LifeCare floor were DNR and some were not. Third, all were patients in rehabilitation on electricity-dependent ventilators, but they were not terminally ill patients in any ordinary sense but patients who, with excellent care, might reasonably be expected to leave the hospital.

When electricity failed, nurses and Dr. Pou at first kept some patients breathing by manually pumping airbags, but by Thursday, they became physically exhausted and stopped, so these patients died.

Among the 41 dead bodies analyzed by forensic pathologists, Pou was charged with killing nine patients. The cadavers of these nine contained high levels of morphine and midazolam, drugs not justified by any previous symptoms. A coroner testified that all nine patients died within three-and-a-half hours of each other, timing that could not have occurred naturally.

In case-based bioethics, details matter a lot, and in new interviews, Dr. Fink discovered that two of Life-Care's patients on the 7th floor died on Wednesday, but that the other nine made it through the night to Thursday. On Thursday morning, Dr. Pou told some staff that the nine patients were not going to make it and would not be evacuated. Other physicians agreed and thought that when everyone left Memorial, these nine patients might be subject to degradation at the hands of vandals looking for drugs inside the evacuated hospital.

Emmett Everett was one of the nine remaining patients. He was a 380-pound Honduran hospitalized for a colostomy to relieve his bowel obstruction. He was not terminal, had no DNR order, and had pleaded, "Please don't leave me behind." According to one staff member, Dr. Pou and others concluded that Everett weighed too much to be carried down five flights of stairs to where helicopters were airlifting the last patients away. This is despite the fact that Rodney Scott, weighing more than 300 pounds, had been taken to the helipad and evacuated on Thursday.

In new interviews years afterward, Fink heard descriptions from staff of Ana Pou and John Theile, a pulmonary physician, administering large dosages of morphine and midazolam to the nine remaining patients, including Alice Hutzler, a 90-year old woman with bedsores and pneumonia and to Emmett Everett, as well as to Wilda McCanus, who had a blood infection, and 90-year-old Rose Savoie, who suffered from bronchitis and kidney problems. These last two women were described late Thursday morning as alert and stable, but both died that day.

Emmett Everett did not die immediately from the injection of drugs, but required staff to cover his face with a towel for a minute to stop his breathing. By the time Dr. Pou, Dr. Theile, and two nurses left, all nine patients on the 7th floor of Memorial Hospital were dead.

## FURTHER READING

Gerald Dworkin, Ray Frey, and Sissela Bok, eds., *Euthanasia and Physician-Assisted Suicide: For and Against,* New York: Cambridge University Press, 1998.

Kathleen M. Foley and Herbert Hendin, eds., *The Case Against Assisted Suicide: For the Right to End-Of-Life Care* Johns Hopkins University Press, 2002.

Tom Beauchamp, ed., *Intending Death: The Ethics of Assisted Suicide and Euthanasia,* Upper Saddle River, NJ: Prentice-Hall, 1996.

Timothy Quill and Margaret Pabst Battin, eds. *Physician-Assisted Dying: The Case for Palliative Care and Patient Choice*, Baltimore, MD: Johns Hopkins Press, 2004.

R. Steinbrook, "Physician-Assisted Death—From Oregon to Washington State," *New England Journal of Medicine* 359:24, 11 December 2008, pp. 2513–2515.

Sheri Fink, "Deadly Decisions at Memorial," *New York Times Magazine*, August 27, 2009.

## DISCUSSION QUESTIONS

1. If you were Ana Pou and believed no rescue was coming for your nine patients, would you have done the same as she did?

2. Almost all the patients who died in Oregon and Washington were white and educated. Why do you think other kinds of people didn't use the law?

3. If physicians were on salary rather than being paid per procedures, would more terminal patients be killed more quickly?

4. Do views about physician-assisted killing depend on whether you think humans are basically selfish and sinful or good and compassionate?

5. Does the doctrine of terminal sedation (double effect) make sense? Can anyone really know what is in someone else's mind?

# CHAPTER 4

# Comas: Karen Quinlan, Nancy Cruzan, and Terri Schiavo

*Inco mpetent*

$B$uilt on previous cases of Nancy Cruzan and Karen Quinlan, the famous case of Terri Schiavo exploded in 2005. All three cases involved incompetent adults and whether their medical treatment could be stopped. The Quinlan case started in 1975 in New Jersey courts. Fifteen years later in 1990, the U.S. Supreme Court decided the landmark case of Nancy Cruzan. The Schiavo case started then and lasted another 15 years, until 2005.

## THE QUINLAN CASE

In April 1975, just after turning 21, perky, independent Karen Quinlan became comatose from drinking alcohol after taking either barbiturates or benzodiazepines, or both.[1] Karen had also been dieting, and at hospital admission, weighed only 115 pounds.

Benzodiazepines—anti-anxiety drugs such as Valium, Librium, Ativan, and Xanax—act on specific nerve receptors in the brain and are considered safer than barbiturates. The latter have been around since 1912, when physicians first used phenobarbital.

Both benzodiazepines and barbiturates intensify with alcohol, an effect called *synergism*. Alcohol *potentiates* (intensifies) the effects of these drugs, and an empty stomach also increases the effects. Actor River Phoenix unintentionally killed himself in 1993 by mixing barbiturates, alcohol, and benzodiazepines.

Karen lost her brain from a synergistic reaction of barbiturates, benzodiazepines, and alcohol taken on an empty stomach. These drugs suppressed her breathing, caused loss of oxygen to her brain, and after 30 minutes, destroyed her higher brain.

At St. Clare's Hospital, a Catholic institution in New Jersey, a small ventilator, also called a respirator, kept Karen breathing. It also prevented aspiration of vomit, which could cause pneumonia.

Ventilators began to be used in medicine during the 1960s and by 1975 had become common in cases of emergency and trauma. The ventilator's use in this case showed that the *criteria of death* needed clarification. Because the brain must have a fresh supply of oxygenated blood to function, lack of such oxygenated blood (anoxia) quickly damages the brain and over time, destroys it. The traditional definition of death—where the body stops breathing and the person is declared dead—indirectly *assumed* brain death to be inevitable, but now a ventilator prevented this.

Karen's appearance shocked her sister, who said:

> Whenever I thought of a person in a coma, I thought they would just lie there very quietly, almost as though they were sleeping. Karen's head was moving around, as if she was trying to pull away from that tube in her throat, and she made little noises, like moans. I don't know if she was in pain, but it seemed as though she was. And I thought—if Karen could ever see herself like this, it would be the worst thing in the world for her.[2]

Sometimes Karen would choke, sit bolt upright with her arms flung out and her eyes wide open, appearing to be in intense pain. Eventually her breathing stabilized, but even then she didn't breathe deeply enough to sigh. Without such breathing, the lower sacs of her lungs risked infection. Hence she was put on a larger ventilator for a "sigh volume." This larger ventilator required a tracheotomy (a hole cut surgically in the throat or trachea) to which her mother, Julia Quinlan, reluctantly agreed.

This more powerful ventilator altered her appearance. At a later hearing in September 1975, her lawyer testified about Karen that:

> Her eyes are open and move in a circular manner as she breathes; her eyes blink approximately three or four times per minute; her forehead evidences every noticeable perspiration; her mouth is open while the ventilator expands to ingest oxygen, and while her mouth is open, her tongue appears to be moving in a rather random manner; her mouth closes as the oxygen is ingested into her body through the tracheotomy and she appears to be slightly convulsing or gasping as the oxygen enters the windpipe; her hands are visible in an emaciated form, facing in a praying position away from her body. Her present weight would seem to be in vicinity of 70–80 pounds.[3]

Karen Quinlan was in a coma, of course, but what does that mean? The word "coma" is vague. Despite popular belief in 1975, under New Jersey law Karen was not brain-dead, which required *all* of her brain not to be functioning.

Karen Quinlan lay in a serious form of coma called *persistent vegetative state* (PVS). PVS is a generic term covering a type of deep unconsciousness that, if it persists for a few months, is almost always irreversible. In this case, her eyes were *disconjugate,* i.e., they moved in different, random directions at the same time. Despite eye movements, she was also thought to be *decorticate;* Karen's brain could not receive input from her eyes. She had slow-wave—not isoelectric or "flat"—electroencephalograms (EEGs).

At one time, a patient in such a condition would simply starve to death; but in the late 1960s, crude intravenous and nasogastric feeding tubes began to be used. Initially, an intravenous tube fed Karen, but as her condition persisted, the rigidity of her muscles made it difficult to insert and reinsert such a tube into her veins. Five months after her admission, in September 1975, she required a nasogastric feeding tube.

The Quinlans never allowed a picture to be taken of Karen in PVS. So the public never saw a realistic picture of her with a shaved head and on a ventilator and feeding tube.

In October 1975, deciding that Karen would never regain consciousness, the Quinlans decided to remove the ventilator and let her body die. They had no idea that their decision would be the easy part.

The Quinlans averred that Karen had twice said that if anything terrible happened to her, she did not want to be kept alive as a vegetable on machines. But was she really a "vegetable"? We now know that a rare patient may recover from PVS.

The Quinlans asked the physicians of record, Robert Morse, a resident in internal medicine, and Arshad Javed, a fellow in pulmonary medicine, to disconnect Karen's ventilator. These physicians balked. Why?

First, in 1975 the American Medical Association (AMA) seemed to equate withdrawing a ventilator for death to occur with euthanasia, and then equated that with murder. Back then, no federal or state court had clarified the rights of *competent* dying patients, much less the rights of *incompetent* patients.

Second, the physicians feared that the Quinlans might later change their minds and sue them for malpractice. One common definition of malpractice is "departure from normal standards of medical practice in a community," and in 1975—when most physicians continued treatment until the last moments of life—assisting in the deaths of comatose patients would have been such a departure.

At a legal hearing, Dr. Morse testified that no medical precedent allowed him to disconnect Karen's ventilator. Neurologist Julius Korein described Karen as having no mental age at all and as being like "an anencephalic monster."[4] Neurologist Fred Plum described Karen as "lying in bed, emaciated, curled up in what is known as flexion contracture. Every joint was bent in a flexion position and making one tight sort of fetal position. It's too grotesque, really, to describe in human terms like fetal."[5]

Because Karen had never written down her wishes in an advance directive, the judge did not know what she would have wanted, so he decided that her ventilator must continue. He ruled that her parents' testimony about her wishes would not be final, because it entailed her death. He also ruled that he could not find a right to die in the U.S. Constitution.

Several weeks later, the New Jersey State Supreme Court heard the case on direct review. Physicians testifying there surprised these justices by distinguishing between disconnecting a ventilator and not starting it. They argued that once they accepted patients, they had an absolute duty to pursue patients' welfare, such that they could never cause death. But neurologist Julius Korein counter-testified that physicians privately used "judicious neglect" to let terminal patients die.

The justices pressed the hospital's lawyers about the physician–patient relationship. Why couldn't Morse and Javed allow Karen to be transferred to another hospital, where other physicians could disconnect her? St. Clare's lawyers hemmed and hawed, but finally said it would be immoral. The justices found this reasoning "rather flimsy."

In 1965, the U.S. Supreme Court cited a right to privacy in *Griswold v. Connecticut*, when it found state laws unconstitutional that banned physicians from giving contraceptives to married couples. *Griswold* found this kind of right in *Oklahoma vs. Skinner* in 1942, which noted a fundamental right to reproduction and control of one's body to block a law allowing involuntary sterilization of habitual criminals. *Griswold* said that banning contraception violated a couple's *fundamental liberty to lead their personal life as they saw fit*, which the U.S. Constitution assumed throughout.

In 1973, the U.S. Supreme Court strengthened the right to privacy in *Roe vs. Wade* (see Chapter 5), deciding that this same right included the right of a woman to decide whether she would remain pregnant or abort her fetus.

In January 1976, the New Jersey Supreme Court ruled unanimously for the Quinlans. The right to privacy allowed the family of a dying incompetent patient to let her die by disconnecting her ventilator. The Supreme Court of the United States had not yet made a comparable decision about the end of life, so the New Jersey Supreme Court's decision helped define a family's right to let an incompetent patient die based on the right to privacy (liberty). the right to privacy.

The New Jersey court allowed Joseph Quinlan to become Karen's guardian, gave legal immunity to Morse and Javed for disconnecting Karen's life support, and suggested (though it did not require) ethics committees of laypeople in hospitals to help in future cases.

## Pulling the Plug or Weaning from a Ventilator?

In April 1976, four months after the higher-court decision, a ventilator helped Karen Quinlan's body breathe. By then, decubitus ulcers had eaten through her flesh, exposing her hip bones.

But why was Karen still alive four months later? This is the least understood and most controversial aspect of this case.

According to the Quinlans, Morse resisted implementing the decision of the New Jersey Supreme Court, because "this is something I will have to live with for the rest of my life."[6] The head nun at St. Clare's lectured Mrs. Quinlan more bluntly: "You have to understand our position, Mrs. Quinlan. In this hospital we don't kill people."[7] To this, Julia Quinlan replied, "Why didn't you tell me ten months ago? I would have taken Karen out of this hospital immediately."

The nuns saw the *Quinlan* decision as another step down a slippery slope that had started three years earlier with *Roe vs. Wade*. During the trial, a Vatican theologian criticized the Quinlans: "A right to death does not exist. Love for life, even a life reduced to ruin, drives one to protect life with every possible care."[8] A pulmonologist in Rome said removal of the ventilator "would be an extremely dangerous move by her doctors, and represents an indirect form of euthanasia."[9]

Instead of simply disconnecting Karen's ventilator, Morse and Javed weaned her from it. "Weaned" means that, by building up different muscles, they gradually trained her body to breathe without the ventilator. The tired, confused Quinlans did not understand what this meant and its real implications would become painfully clear over the next 10 years. Eventually, Javed had Karen off the ventilator for four hours; then, after intensive work over many weeks, for 12 hours. By late May of 1976, Karen was off the ventilator altogether.

This weaning confused the public: Some people took it to mean that Karen had gotten better. Others thought that Karen's physicians had "pulled the plug," but a miracle had prevented her death. Both impressions were false.

St. Clare's Hospital now wanted Karen transferred and in June 1976, New Jersey's Medicaid office forced a nursing home to accept her. At this point, Karen had been in PVS for 14 months.

After more than 10 years in the nursing home, Karen Quinlan's body expired in June 1986. For several months before that, Karen had had pneumonia and the Quinlans at the time declined antibiotics to reverse it.

## Substituted Judgment and Kinds of Cases

The *Quinlan* decision used the standard of *substituted judgment* according to which relatives or friends could say what they believed to be the wishes of the incompetent patient.

But this standard has two major problems. First, substituted judgment is notoriously subjective.[10] It presumes that decisions made by a patient's family will reflect what the patient herself would have wanted. In the Quinlan case, like the later Cruzan and Schiavo cases, it was unclear whether these women had really expressed a wish not to have their lives prolonged or whether the families just wished it so.

Second, how did a family's right to exercise substituted judgment derive from *Griswold*? Critics felt that the New Jersey court had jumped too quickly from married people's right to control their own reproduction to the parents' right to decide that an adult, comatose incompetent child wanted to die—especially because few intervening decisions had been made about whether competent, terminal adults could refuse medical treatment. Given that quick, big jump, critics wondered what was next? Given parents the right to make life-or-death decisions for never-competent patients? For brain-damaged babies?

*Quinlan* also ran two different kinds of cases together.[11] As noted, the Court based its decision partly on the right to privacy, a right that in medical contexts would presumably apply only to competent patients. But the right to privacy most obviously applies to competent patients and their rights to determine their own medical destinies. Ideally, the U.S. Supreme Court would have first laid out these rights and then tackled incompetent patients. But life is messy and it didn't happen that way, so the *Quinlan* decision tackled incompetent patients first. It took 15 more years before things were straightened out, when the U.S. Supreme Court finally decided in *Cruzan*.

## THE CRUZAN CASE

The Cruzan case led to a landmark decision by the United States Supreme Court in June 1990.[12] Before this decision, 20 states had recognized the right of competent patients to refuse medical life-support, and all these states (with the exception of New York and Missouri) had recognized the right of surrogates to make decisions for incompetent patients.[13] Although other decisions by lower courts had come to similar conclusions, this was the first U.S. Supreme Court declaration that a competent patient could decline all medical treatment to die as his definitive Constitutional right.

On January 11, 1983, 24-year-old Nancy Cruzan lost control of her car at night on a lonely, icy country road in Missouri.[14] Thrown 35 feet from the car, she landed face down in a water-filled ditch. Paramedics found that her heart had stopped. Injecting a stimulant into her heart, they restarted it, but because her brain had been anoxic for 15 minutes, Nancy did not regain consciousness.[15]

Over seven years, Nancy's body became rigid, her hands curled tightly, and her fingernails became claw-like. Like Karen Quinlan, Nancy could take nothing by mouth and somebody turned her every two hours to prevent ulcers. She drooled much of the time, wetting her hair, pillow and sheets. Her care cost the state of Missouri $130,000 a year.

Where the Quinlan case focused on withdrawal of a ventilator, the Cruzan case, like the Schiavo case 15 years later, focused on withdrawal of a feeding tube. Because she could not swallow, Nancy could not be fed by mouth. Loss of ability to swallow signals a key decision in the care of incapacitated patients, especially those with dementia or neurological damage. As mentioned, before feeding tubes began to be used in the 1960s, such patients naturally died by starvation.

Artificial feeding can now done in three basic ways: (1) by a temporary nasogastric tube run up the nostrils and down into the gastrointestinal tract; (2) by a permanent intravenous feeding line, surgically attached to one of the major veins of the chest; and (3) by a surgically implanted gastrostomy (PEG) tube. All feeding tubes carry the risk of infection; with many, such a large volume of fluid is needed to supply the nutrients that other problems are caused.

Morally, the question arose in the Cruzan case of whether a PVS patient is *owed* food and water forever. Karen Quinlan's parents thought so; they never withdrew the nutrition that kept her body alive. Nancy's parents, Joe and Joyce Cruzan, thought otherwise: they sought permission in court to disconnect her feeding tube.

In discussing the Cruzan case, it is necessary to understand different standards of legal evidence. The minimum standard is *preponderance of evidence;* a more rigorous standard is *clear and convincing evidence;* the most rigorous standard—the standard used for serious felonies—is *beyond a reasonable doubt.*

*Preponderance of evidence* simply means that there is more evidence one way than another; in some cases, this simply means there is a bit of evidence rather than none. *Clear and convincing* denotes something more rigorous and with dying, requires an advance directive (living will) or durable power of attorney. Finally, *beyond a reasonable doubt* requires the most evidence and is used in trials of homicide to establish guilt and where the accused is presumed innocent.

The Cruzans won their case in lower (probate) court, but upon direct review, the Missouri Supreme Court reversed, and its reversal had to do with the standard of clear and convincing evidence. Because Nancy had no advance directive and because only her parents and a sister testified about her alleged wishes, the Cruzans did not provide "clear and convincing" evidence about Nancy's wishes.

Missouri felt it had a duty to protect an incompetent adult child against parents who might be merely seeking financial and emotional closure. The Missouri Supreme Court agreed and concluded that the state had an interest in preserving life, regardless of quality of life, and no matter how strongly the family felt otherwise, that before medical support could be withdrawn from an incompetent patient, the family had to meet the higher standard of clear and convincing evidence.

In this case, the United States Supreme Court declared three things. First, it recognized a right of *competent* patients to decline medical treatment, even if such refusal led directly to their death.

Second, the Supreme Court found that withdrawing a feeding tube did not differ from withdrawing any other kind of life-sustaining medical support. Some state laws, which permitted forgoing or withdrawing ventilators but not artificial nutrition, were hence unconstitutional.

Third, with regard to *incompetent* patients, the Supreme Court held in Cruzan that a state *could, but need not,* pass a statute requiring the clear and convincing standard of evidence about what a formerly competent patient would have wanted done. Because Missouri had such a standard, its law was constitutional. Because the Cruzan family had not met that standard, Nancy's feeding tube could not be removed.

*Cruzan* said nothing about never-competent patients, such as people with profound mental retardation. Because of past abuses, it is reasonable to expect that in these cases only state laws with the most rigorous standards of proof would pass the Supreme Court's review. For such cases, the Supreme Court could require the standard of beyond a reasonable doubt.

Legal commentators agreed that the previous legal standard of *substituted judgment* was a mockery "[leading] us to pretend that we are merely complying (however reluctantly) with the wishes of the patient. The result in most states is mere lip service to substituted judgment. Almost any evidence is deemed sufficient to establish a preference for death over PVS and/or families are empowered to express patient preferences for death-with few questions asked."

The case of Nancy Cruzan illustrates this problem. Nancy' father, Joe, said that because Nancy was strong-willed and a fighter, she wouldn't want to exist in PVS. But others might infer a different conclusion: that she might have wanted to fight for any chance to return to normalcy.

In contrast, another standard used in such cases was that of *best interests of the patient.* So in the Cruzan case, would the best interests of Nancy be to live on in such a state? Some people would say no, although this judgment is not open-and-shut, especially as Missouri argued that Nancy's best interests entailed continued feeding, as activists argued in the later Schiavo case.

A different kind of reaction came from physicians who worked with families of vegetative patients. Neurologist and bioethicist Ronald Cranford of Minnesota, who would later testify in the Schiavo case, predicted that, "many families will experience the utter helplessness of the Cruzans." Allowing the standard of clear-and-convincing evidence would "place an enormous burden on society, which will spend hundreds of millions of dollars each year for a condition that no one in their right mind would ever want to be in."[16]

Hospice physician Joanne Lynn emphasized that in Missouri and New York, "the suffering of the patient and family, the costs, the kind of life that can be gained, are all to count for nothing. If life can be prolonged, then it will have to be."[17]

Nancy had been divorced just before her accident, and some of her old friends knew her only by her married name, Davis. When her case first became widely known, these friends had not realized who she was. After the major decision, the case was reheard in a lower court and Nancy's old friends testified. In that hearing, the lower court decided that Nancy Cruzan's parents had now met the clear-and-convincing standard.[18] So five months after the Supreme Court decided *Cruzan*, on December 14, 1990, physicians legally removed Nancy Cruzan's feeding tube, and her body died.

## THE TERRI SCHIAVO CASE

While the U.S. Supreme Court Justices deliberated *Cruzan*, another coma case began on February 25, 1990. Terri Schiavo, a 27-year-old woman, went into a coma probably because of anoxia, a lack of oxygen to her brain, perhaps from a heart arrhythmia caused by extreme hypoalkemia (an imbalance of potassium in her body), causing severe hypoxic ischemic encephalopathy (brain damage).[19]

Before her heart attack, Terri Schiavo seemed anorexic. People with anorexia may suffer from an imbalance of potassium. According to documents filed in a malpractice suit by her family, a three-stage imbalance of potassium led to Terri's heart attack, which led to anoxia and subsequent brain damage.

To keep her alive, physicians inserted a PEG (percutaneous endoscopic gastronomy) feeding tube. When a patient lacks the reflex to swallow, surgeons place PEG tubes through the abdominal wall into the stomach, through which flows a nutritious, slushy mixture. Doctors sometimes insert PEG tubes after an emergency to buy time, with the understanding that they may be temporary and removed later.

Once attached, feeding tubes can be difficult to remove. Years later, removal of her feeding tube became the legal focus of Terri's case.

In April 1990, husband Michael Schiavo transferred Terri from the hospital to a rehabilitation center. In May, and with no objection from her parents, Robert and Mary Schindler, Michael became Terri legal guardian. Later, her parents took her to their home for care but, overwhelmed by the task, they returned her to the center. Michael also flew Terri once to California for a two-month experiment with a "thalamic stimulator implant" in her brain. After that experiment failed, Terri returned to the Mediplex Rehabilitation Center in Brandon, Florida, and for months 13–18 into her coma, three shifts of workers worked 24 hours a day trying to rehabilitate her.

In July 1991, Terri went to Sable Palms, a skilled care facility, where neurologists continued to test her and where speech, occupational, and physical therapists worked on her for three more years, until 1994. At this point, Terri had received nearly five years of intensive efforts to return her to consciousness.

Michael Schiavo and Terri's parents stopped living together in May 1992. That August, Michael received a settlement from the malpractice case against Terri's obstetrician for failing to diagnose a potassium imbalance. He got $750,000 from the hospital for a trust fund specifically set up for Terri's care and $300,000 for loss of her companionship.

The three adults allegedly then fought over money. The Schindlers believed they were entitled to part of the $300,000 for loss of spousal companionship, but Michael disagreed. After this dispute, their relationship soured.

Based on what several physicians told Michael, at this point Terri had no chance of meaningful recovery. Michael agreed to a "Do Not Resuscitate" order for Terri, but her parents violently disagreed and he later rescinded the order.

The Schindlers then tried to remove Michael as Terri's guardian, but a court-appointed special guardian investigated and determined that Michael had acted appropriately toward Terri, which the court accepted.

Three years passed, during which Terri's condition did not improve. During this time and in order to help care for Terri, Michael became certified as a licensed respiratory therapist.[20]

In May 1998, eight years after Terri's heart attack, Michael asked a court to allow removal of the PEG tube so that Terri could die. Michael testified that, while watching television many years before, Terri had once remarked that she wouldn't want to live in a vegetative state. The Schindlers retorted that their daughter wanted to live.

Nearly two years after Michael Schiavo's request to have Terri's feeding tube removed, Judge George Greer in 2000 approved the request. He ruled that clear and convincing evidence existed that Terri would not have chosen to live under such circumstances. Legally, this ruling seemed wanting, because Terri's parents disputed the claim and because Terri had no advance directive.

The Schindlers appealed, which took a year, but they lost. They appealed again, this time to the Florida Supreme Court, which in 2001 denied their appeal.

Over the next few years, the Schindlers began to allege that Michael caused Terri's condition, perhaps because of domestic abuse. An autopsy after her death proved that no such abuse occurred. Moreover, if Terri had arrived at an emergency room with this kind of trauma, Michael would have been reported—as required by law—to authorities for domestic violence, battery, or possible manslaughter. Also, if such evidence had existed, the hospital and its physicians would have been unlikely to settle a malpractice case or to allow Michael to become Terri's guardian.

The Schindlers testified that, even if Terri had asked them to do so, they would not remove Terri's feeding tube under any circumstances. They said that even if she developed gangrene and all her limbs had to be amputated, they would still keep her alive.[21]

A year later in the fall of 2003, having exhausted all appeals in Florida, the Schindlers appealed in federal court to prevent removal of Terri's feeding tube. The Schindlers also appealed to the public through the media, and several physicians publicly joined their side, including a pathologist and a physician who hoped to try exotic "coma stimulation" therapies.

## Enter Lawyers and Politicians

Governor Jeb Bush, a Catholic, filed a brief on the side of the Schindlers; he praised the parents in the media for defending their daughter's right to life. President George W. Bush praised his brother's stand. The Advocacy Center for Persons with Disabilities filed a lawsuit claiming that removal of Terri's feeding tube would abuse a person with disabilities. The anti-abortion group, Life Legal Defense Fund, helped the Schindlers hire lawyers, eventually paying bills of $300,000.

Three neurologists, including the late, distinguished neurologist Ronald Cranford, testified that Terri was in PVS (Cranford substituted "permanent" for "persistent" to emphasize the irreversibility of her condition). The Schindlers cited Terri's ability to swallow saliva as evidence that she was not in PVS; Cranford rebutted and testified that primitive functions in her brain stem controlled such swallowing.

Physicians William Mayfield and William Hammesfahr, champions of hyperbaric oxygenation therapy (HBOT), claimed HBOT would benefit Terri.[22] Neurologist Ronald Cranford retorted, "Increase the blood flood to dead tissue, and what do you get? Dead tissue."[23] Others found Hammesfahr unprofessional and noted that he required cash in advance for his treatments and had never documented any success.

These physicians disagreed about what Terri's movements meant. Ability to respond to a squeeze or pinch is consistent with PVS. In the Cruzan case, when neurologist Cranford examined Nancy, her lawyer William Colby described what happened:

> Cranford next grabbed hold of Nancy's stiff right leg and tried to bend it straight. Nancy grimaced. Then he reached for the soft skin on the inside of the upper part of her right arm, and held the pinch. Slowly, as if she were a robot, Nancy's head lifted off the bed and turned. Her face locked on her father's for about ten seconds, before she lowered just as slowly to the pillow.[24]

Despite being there and witnessing this phenomenon in this case, Dr. Cranford insisted that Nancy Cruzan's biography was over, that no one was conscious within the reflexes of her body, and that further treatment was futile.

In the fall of 2003, the Florida legislature passed a special bill, *Terri's Law*, which allowed the governor to issue a one-time stay of a judge's order to remove a feeding tube in certain cases where a patient is in PVS. After its passage, Governor Bush immediately issued the stay.

Michael and the American Civil Liberties Union appealed in state court and won, but Governor Bush appealed to a mid-level appellate court, lost, and appealed again to the Florida Supreme Court.

On September 23, 2004, Florida's Supreme Court ruled 7–0 that Terri's Law was unconstitutional. It based its decision upon two constitutional canons: the separation of powers and the unlawful delegation of authority. "It is without question an invasion of the authority of the judicial branch for the Legislature to pass a law that allows the executive branch to interfere with the final judicial determination in a case," wrote Chief Justice Barbara Pariente.[25]

About two months later, the top U.S. Court let stand without comment the decision by the Florida Supreme Court against Terri's Law.[26] Activists predicted Terri's imminent "brutal murder" and claimed that she was a "purposefully interactive, alert, curious, lovely young woman who lives with a very serious disability."[27]

Much of these claims came from an edited video, clips of which cable television often showed (because such stories need visual background). These pro-Schindler clips can be easily seen on YouTube or by searching for videos on Terri Schiavo.

At the end of February 2005, 15 years after the case began, the Schindlers filed a variety of desperate motions in Judge Greer's court, but he still ordered the feeding tube removed. The Schindlers appealed, but a Florida appellate court again rebuffed them.

Extraordinary events ensued, of a kind never before seen in the history of modern bioethics. As the Schindlers lost in court, they became desperate; they turned to the media for their cause, encouraging their other son and daughter to appear on television. Catholic priests dressed in robes of monastic orders appeared with them. People flooded Florida legislators with e-mail and phone calls.

Activists and the Schindlers then turned to the U.S. Congress. First, House leaders tried to compel Terri to appear before a House committee as a witness, and fall under protection of the federal program that protects witnesses. Judge Greer ignored this subpoena.

Senator Bill Frist was a physician who was planning to run for president in 2008 and may have wanted to align himself with the same culture-of-life constituency that had helped George W. Bush narrowly win. So they worked to get Congress to pass a federal version of Terri's Law, having President Bush fly back during a congressional recess to sign a bill passed at midnight.[28]

Some critics said that Senator Frist crossed a dangerous line and committed virtual malpractice by declaring—merely by watching the edited video clip and never actually visiting or examining Terri—that Terri "did not seem to be" in a persistent vegetative state. As one critic fumed, "It's quackery. It'd be hilarious if it weren't so grotesque, how his presidential ambition and pandering to the right wing is clashing with his life's work."[29] Congressman Dave Weldon, a physician and also a pro-life Republican, agreed with Frist. These high-ranking politician-physicians publicly contradicted the fellow physicians who had actually examined Terri and whose area of expertise covered PVS and comas.

Congressmen Frist and Weldon had one problem here: the federal government cannot order a physician to insert a feeding tube. The only thing it could do is order a federal judge to review the case again, which it did. Judge James Whittemore reviewed the whole case over two days and concluded, like two dozen appellate judges before him, that nothing was amiss, that Terri had no chance of recovery, that Michael was properly motivated, and that previous courts had made no errors. An appeal to the U. S. Court of Appeals for the 11th Circuit in Atlanta, a conservative group, produced the same conclusions.

During March 2005, media exposure escalated, producing what *Newsweek* later called "a public spectacle airing nonstop on cable and playing on front pages around the world."[30] Terri's supporters traveled to Pinellas Park, Florida, to hold prayer vigils, while others threatened to kill Michael and his lawyer, George Felos. Various members and friends of both sides went on cable television shows and endlessly discussed the family's problems.

A juggernaut for Terri ensued: soon four Schindlers, plus recovered coma patients, shady physicians, activist monks, Patrick Mahoney, director of the Christian Defense Coalition, and anti-abortion activist Randall Terry campaigned on television, radio, and the Internet against Michael Schiavo, who was media shy and had only his brother, Scott, and lawyer, George Felos, to help him.

Barbara Weller, an attorney working for the Schindlers, went from lawyer to witness, swearing that she had seen Terri trying to talk. Protestors called Judge Greer a "judicial murderer" and Republicans blasted the "imperial judiciary." The Reverend James Kennedy urged Governor Jeb Bush to ignore the federal judges the way Alabama's Governor George Wallace did in defying federal orders to integrate the University of Alabama.[31] The FBI arrested a man offering $250,000 to kill Michael Schiavo and $50,000 to do the same to Judge Greer. Police arrested two others trying to break into the hospice.

Terri was said to be "suffering terribly" by starving, even though physicians in palliative care repeatedly denied that when feeding tubes are removed, terminal patients suffer, and that in this case, any person still existed to suffer.[32]

The case showed the limitations of television and the Internet because what made great visuals (people praying and screaming outside Terri's hospice), great drama (the Schindlers crying on television), and great tension (various people claiming that Michael was evil), distorted the facts. What had been a private family dispute became a take-no-prisoners war on national television.

On March 18, the last appeal failed to the U.S. Supreme Court (which had already twice refused to the review) and physicians removed Terri's feeding tube. Palliative care physicians predicted it would take two weeks for the body to die and emphasized that it would not be painful. Opponents outside decried "murder by starvation." After 13 days, while protestors prayed and rallied outside, Terri's body expired on March 31, 2005.

## What Schiavo's Autopsy Showed

Chief Medical Examiner for Pinellas County, Florida, Jon Thogmartin, M.D., released Terri's autopsy on June 13, 2005. It answered some questions and left others as mysteries.

The big surprise of the autopsy was that, "Mrs. Schiavo's heart was anatomically normal without any areas of recent or remote myocardial infarction. Her heart (including the cardiac valves, conduction system and myocardium) was essentially unremarkable. . . . " That was a surprise because, although people debated the cause of her heart attack, few doubted that she had had one.

We will never know exactly what happened to Terri's heart. Two crucial pieces of evidence are that she may have consumed as much as one gram of caffeine a day and that she had hypoalkemia. Perhaps this combination, after the extreme weight loss, stressed her heart too much.

The night of her original collapse, no other drugs were found in her system.

Another surprise was that the autopsy showed no clinical evidence of bulimia, especially the kind of wear on the enamel of the back teeth that is often caused by this condition. Despite the fact that the malpractice suit was settled on the assertion that Terri had an undiagnosed eating disorder, the coroner's report showed no physical evidence of it.

However, it still was true that 15 years before, she had seemed anorexic. Certainly her low potassium level, the fact that her weight dropped more than

100 pounds in a few months, combined with her drinking gallons of iced tea, give evidence to this hypothesis.

The autopsy by the coroner also implied that Terri Schiavo was not in (what later would be called) "a minimally conscious state." It said that she had massive brain damage. "Mrs. Schiavo's brain showed global anoxic-ischemic encephalopathy resulting in massive cerebral atrophy. Her brain weight was approximately half of the expected weight. Of particular importance was the hypoxic damage and neuronal loss in her occipital lobes, which indicates cortical blindness. Her remaining brain regions show severe hypoxic injury and neuronal atrophy/loss. No areas of recent or remote traumatic injury were found."[33]

Finally, without the PEG feeding tube, she would have died. "Oral feedings in quantities sufficient to sustain life would have certainly resulted in aspiration." Aspiration of food in such patients is a serious, even lethal, complication, causing infection, choking, and possible suffocation.

## ETHICAL ISSUES

### Standards of Brain Death

People have always feared being declared dead prematurely and buried alive. In the eighteenth century, gruesome stories circulated about exhumations discovering scratches on the inside lids of coffins. In the nineteenth century, some legislatures required delays before burial, and in 1882, an undertaker named Kirchbaum attached periscopes to coffins and put cowbells inside, so people waking up inside could signal for help.[34]

This whole-body standard became inappropriate when ventilators allowed respiration of brain-damaged patients. Before them, heart-lung machines could maintain immobilized patients. In 1967, when Christiaan Barnard transplanted Denise Darvall's heart into a dying patient named Louis Washkansky (discussed in Chapter 10), the question arose whether Denise Darvall had really been dead before Barnard removed her heart. Because Barnard needed a healthy heart for transplantation, Denise obviously hadn't been declared dead by the whole-body standard. So medicine needed a new standard of death, specifically of *brain death,* to determine when organs could be removed.

Shortly after that event, an ad hoc committee at Harvard Medical School developed the Harvard criteria of brain death.[35] The Harvard criteria operationally defined brain death as behavior that indicated unawareness of external stimuli, lack of bodily movements, no spontaneous breathing, lack of reflexes, and two isoelectric (nearly flat) electroencephalogram (EEG) readings 24 hours apart. These criteria required loss of virtually all brain activity (including the brain stem, and hence breathing).

The Harvard criteria personify caution: no one declared dead by them has ever regained consciousness. (One could say, "If you're Harvard dead, you're really dead.") Its extreme conservatism disappoints people waiting for organ transplants: during the last half-century, it has covered relatively few patients.

Another standard of brain death is the *cognitive criterion.* This criterion identifies a philosophical core of properties of persons and assumes that without such a core, a human body is no longer a person; the core properties commonly include reason, memory, agency, and self-awareness. For example, neurological disorders such as Alzheimer's or Lewy body dementia destroy brain cells at a high rate, so that over a decade, none of the higher person remains.

The cognitive criterion has the greatest potential to generate organs for transplantation. So far, however, it has been too controversial and too vague to be adopted by any state, although countless families use it to cease treatment to speed a body's death.[36]

A third standard of brain death is *irreversibility* and it falls between the Harvard and cognitive criteria. According to it, death occurs simply when unconsciousness is irreversible. Operationally, this judgment would be made by a neurologist and another physician. The irreversibility standard would allow PVS patients to be declared dead after several years (perhaps, in some cases of anoxia, after several months).

In popular culture, some people believe that a metaphysical event with physical manifestations marks death, perhaps the counterpart of a similar event at the beginning of life. Some people would describe this event as the entrance and departure of a soul. But the occurrence of such metaphysical events cannot be proven, and even if they are, seem to have no physical manifestations.

So in medical reality, the definition of death is often not so much a *discovery* as a *decision* that families and physicians make—not an event—but a process.[37] Unfortunately, many families lack preparation to make such decisions and find it easier to believe that physicians "discover" that a patient has died.

As it turns out, the phrase "brain death" misleads in various ways. Newspapers commonly refer to someone as being "brain dead" for months until "life-support" is removed, after which the patient is said to "expire." Reformers such as North Carolina medical ethicist Lance Stell believe that such terms incorrectly imply that a patient could be dead in two different ways and that there are degrees of being dead. Such equivocation creates confusion about the epistemological criteria for declaring death, implying that someone might die more than once. Stell thinks a more accurate phrase would be "death by neurological criteria." A being that meets these criteria, he says, "is not a patient but a cadaver."[38]

Proposals to redefine brain death create controversy. On the one hand, reformers want to end public uncertainty over brain death, expand the number of organs available for transplantation, save the medical system money by not maintaining comatose patients, and help families move on after the death by having a universally accepted practical definition. On the other hand, advocates for vulnerable patients want to give them every chance of recovery.

## Chances of Regaining Consciousness from Coma and PVS

The question of whether the movements of PVS patients are intentional behavior or merely reflexes raises philosophical as well as medical issues. *Intentional* behavior indicates an organism seeking a goal, such as freedom from pain, and might indicate awareness. As the seventeenth-century philosopher Rene Descartes noted, consciousness in others is always an inference from outward behavior and cannot be directly observed.

Permanent lack of consciousness is also an inference. Some people claim that shrimp aren't conscious; they infer that from the behavior of shrimp and by comparing the anatomy of shrimp and humans.

Consider four surprising cases of long-term unconsciousness. First, after an automobile wreck in Arkansas, Terry Wallis emerged from a coma after 19 years, and three years later, continued to improve.[39] In 1996, police officer Gary Dockery of Tennessee emerged out of his coma of eight years to talk for a few hours to his family, after which he lapsed back into a coma and died a year later in April.[40] Third, Patricia White Bull became comatose while giving birth to her fourth child and could not speak, swallow, or move much, but suddenly awoke 16 years later to full consciousness on Christmas Eve, 1999. Fourth, after a car accident, Sarah Scantlin of Kansas went into a coma and emerged 19 years later.[41] Comas in all four cases were caused by trauma, not anoxia.

Ethically, the fact that anyone at all comes out of a long-term coma is crucial because it changes the prognosis from certainty to probability. Families who want emotional closure prefer to hear physicians say that the patient has "no" chance of recovery. The emotional weight changes when a patient has a "tiny" chance.

A review of these cases reveals an interesting conceptual disagreement among neurologists. Some claim that any patient who emerges from PVS was not really in PVS. But this is a non-falsifiable, circular argument: if you awaken, you weren't in PVS. If you never awaken, you were in PVS.

In 1994, in a then-definitive study in the *New England Journal of Medicine* by the Multi-Task Force on PVS, 7 of 434 adults with traumatic head injuries who were in PVS for more than a year made good recoveries and regained consciousness, some with normal quality of life.[42] Should traumatic PVS befall some people, they might want this 7/434th chance of recovery. Several other studies have shown that, although few patients ever emerge from PVS, some people do within the first year, and once in a thousand times, after three years.[43] Again, all these patients suffered *traumatic* injuries, not anoxia.

In a 1995 study of 19 patients with severe head injuries and persisting post-traumatic unawareness, 58 percent (11 patients) recovered within the first year and 5 percent (1 patient) within the second.[44] In a 1996 study of 34 patients with *anoxic* coma, 2 patients with "malignant EEGs" (the worst classification, where patients were expected to die based on lack of brain wave activity), eventually made a "good recovery."[45]

Some patients emerge, especially in the first few months, after coma caused by trauma, but rarely in coma caused by anoxia. "It's the difference between taking a blow to the brain, which affects a local area—and taking this global, whole-brain hit," asserted New York bioethicist Joseph Fins in explaining the difference.[46]

In 2005, some neurologists proposed a new category of *minimally conscious state* (MCS) for patients in long-term coma-like states, a category between the previous ways of classifying them as either *comatose* or *vegetative*.[47] After working with brain-damaged patients at several facilities around New York City, neurologists Nicholas Schiff, Joy Hirsch, and Joseph Giacino, along with seven other co-authors, proposed this new category.[48]

These claims generate some passion in neurology. Alan Shewmon, a famous pediatric neurologist, calls the new category "an inaccurate name for an invalid concept." Shewmon argues that there is no scientific way to distinguish between minimal consciousness and full consciousness, implying that consciousness is something one either has or does not have, like saying you can't be a little bit pregnant.

But maybe that's the wrong analogy. Why can't a light bulb be, not on or off, but bright or dim? Why can't consciousness be a *gradient*? Terri's defenders retort that people are minimally conscious all the time—in sleep, or after injury—and what is important is the potential for recovery of consciousness. If it's impossible to prove any difference between minimal consciousness and consciousness, it also must be impossible to *disprove* a difference. So if Terri was in MCS, she might at times feel something. After all, the brain does not get injured in neat taxonomic lines.

By 2007, the claims centered not so much on ability to recover from anoxia-caused PVS as on patients classified as in PVS but *misdiagnosed*. In a 1996 study in England, one researcher estimated that 17 of 40 patients in PVS had been so misdiagnosed. Another study in 2010 claimed that 40 percent of disorders of consciousness are misdiagnosed.[49] Could Terri Schiavo have been misdiagnosed?

An important study in 2007 by Owen et al. noted that,

> The assessment of patients with disorders of consciousness, including the vegetative state, is difficult and frequently depends on subjective interpretations of the observed spontaneous and volitional behavior. . . . However, it is becoming increasingly apparent that in some patients damage to the peripheral motor system may prevent overt responses to command although the cognitive ability to perceive and understand such commands may remain intact. Recent advances in functional neuroimaging suggest a novel solution to this problem: in several cases, so-called activation studies have been used to identify residual cognitive function and conscious awareness in patients who are assumed to be in a vegetative state yet retain cognitive abilities that have evaded detection using standard clinical methods.[50]

In this study, a PVS patient was asked to imagine playing tennis and walking through a house, and every time she was asked about playing tennis, a key part of her brain lit up, whereas it did not when she was asked about walking through rooms.

The latest claims focus on MCS, fMRI scans, and deep-brain stimulation of supposed PVS patients. Through an intense program with probes that stimulated the thalamus, a deep part of the brain, they enabled one or two patients to return to MCS. Using fMRI scans of blood flow to the brain, physicians have identified dozens of patients with this potential, and improved one or two remarkably.[51]

In 2009, Belgian researcher Steven Laureys awoke Rom Houben, who for 23 years had been conscious and falsely diagnosed as in a vegetative state, but unable to move. "Once someone is labeled as being without consciousness, it is very hard to get rid of that," Laureys said.[52]

In conclusion, patients who are stimulated during the first six months after injury and who became comatose through trauma rather than anoxia or global ischemia are most likely to recover. Also, the potential for recovery diminishes as the years increase, but—as the cases show at the beginning of this section—is rarely zero.

## Terri's Chances of Re-Awakening

No case exists of anyone emerging from PVS of three years' duration. Toward the end of Terri Schiavo's life, when activists shouted the contrary at cameras, she had been in PVS for *15 years*, and hence, according to clinical evidence, had no chance of returning to normal consciousness. Physicians who have seen her CT scan said that her brain, instead of being filled with normal brain tissue, then contained only cerebrospinal fluid, an indication of gross neurological damage and vegetative status.[53]

Terri's electoencephalogram (EEG) was flat and her CT scan showed severe atrophy in her cerebral hemispheres. Schindler-friendly physicians suggested vasodilators, but the autopsy showed what professional neurologists claimed: nothing would have helped her regain consciousness.

Dartmouth neurologist James Bernat agreed, but understood why laypeople rallied behind Terri. "Just looking at a videotape of someone propped up in bed, with their eyes blinking and so on, it look's like they're aware," he said.[54] They are awake, he said, but not aware. With an intact brain stem, their eyes can still follow things, but only slightly to the left or right.

## Compassion and Its Interpretation

In cases like Karen Quinlan's or Nancy Cruzan's, the Golden Rule might imply that,

> If I ended up in a condition like Karen's or Nancy's, I would want to die, and I hope that those around me would be merciful enough to let me die. If I could somehow possibly be "conscious" in such a state, I wouldn't want to go on. I wouldn't want to be imprisoned in such a body for months or years, which would be worse than being buried alive. Mercy requires us to make dying humane, not an endless torture.

Such a thought illustrates how the Golden Rule can be interpreted in different ways. Some people might want a chance to recover, even if it is very slight. "Doing whatever someone else wants" must take into account that people differ in their personalities and wants.

The Quinlans and the Cruzans did argue that allowing Karen and Nancy to die would be merciful. The issue of mercy is relevant in these and similar cases because we can't know for certain that such patients do not feel—we cannot be certain that they do not experience sensations such as pain and discomfort; we may not even be certain that they do not experience distress, fear, frustration, loss, or other tormenting emotions.

Eventually, the cases of Karen Quinlan and Nancy Cruzan came to symbolize mercy as an issue for both patients and families. These cases seemed to represent an inversion of values in medicine: instead of doing what families wanted, medicine did what bureaucracies required; instead of a dignified death, breathing machines and feeding tubes maintained existence; instead of a quick death, there was slow withering of an emaciated body over a decade. On top of all that, the chance that a shell of a person might still exist in pain was too much for most people. For many people, the long dying of these two patients lacked mercy.

Would not most people abhor such a life? Abhor the thought of inhabiting a body for 15 years in which they could not scratch an itch, express a wish, or perform any human act? No one knows what might be going on in such a mental remnant. Whatever destroyed the original mind might have left it in disarray, such that Terri's mental life had become an endless nightmare.

If Terri Schiavo could have awakened for 15 minutes and could have understood her condition, what she looked like, and what the case was doing to her family, can anyone think that this shy, weight-conscious woman would have wanted her brain-damaged, disfigured body exhibited to the world this way? If emotional revulsion is going to count in ethics, what about *her* revulsion?

Her parents saw this differently. They felt she would have wanted to live, even in such diminished circumstances. This shows the problem with simplistic interpretations of the Golden Rule or substituted judgment.

## Religious Issues

As we saw, in 1976 the Catholic Church opposed withdrawal of a ventilator for Karen Quinlan. Over the next 40 years, Catholic hospitals softened their opposition to such withdrawals, and indeed, became models of compassionate dying, routinely removing feeding tubes from comatose patients.

But in 2004 during the Schiavo case, Pope John Paul II said that removal of feeding tubes from patients in PVS was "euthanasia by omission."[55] Although not delivered *ex cathedra*, the Pope's remark cast doubt on that practice.

In contrast, Father Kevin O'Rourke, one of the leading Catholic medical ethicists in North America, argued that feeding tubes were extraordinary care and should not be used to prolong the life of PVS patients. He noted that both Catholic ethicists working in hospitals, as well as doctors and nurses there, routinely allowed removal of life-support from patients in PVS. Father John Paris, a leading Jesuit bioethicist and professor of ethics at Boston College, noted that the Pope's remarks targeted a specific audience and predicted they would have little impact in America. "I think the best thing to do is ignore it, and it will go away," Paris said. "It's not an authoritative teaching statement."[56]

After the Schiavo case, Catholic hospitals could remove life-sustaining care under very few conditions.[57] The case also had other effects. In 2013, in Washington State, as Catholic hospitals merged with other hospitals, big political issues emerged whether the new Catholic-controlled entity would perform abortions, allow assisted reproduction or removal of ventilators and feeding tubes, or recognize rights of same-sex couples.[58]

## Nagging Questions

Not everything in the Schiavo case adds up. First, as the attorney general for Missouri said about the case of Nancy Cruzan, "We generally don't allow a life to be ended on hearsay." He was referring to statements by Nancy's father and sister that they thought they remembered her saying she wouldn't want to live on a feeding tube.

Michael Schiavo's very late recollection of a comment by Terri years before to the same effect seems ad hoc, that is, remembered for the purpose at hand. Regardless of its veracity, it simply does not meet the standard of clear and convincing evidence, especially when directly contradicted by both Schindler parents and her brother, Bobby. Three-to-one *against* doesn't add up to clear-and-convincing evidence *for*.

Second, why not relinquish guardianship to the Schindlers? Michael's position was that, first, he had long ago exhausted all the money on her care, and second, she had died long before. But if that were so, why not let her parents care for her body? After a few years, they would probably come to agree, as Karen Quinlan's mother did, but why not let them get closure that way? If Terri was already dead, she couldn't be harmed anymore.

Third, although the coroner's report closed some questions, it opened others: how did she lose so much weight so fast? Just by drinking ice tea? That doesn't add up. Why did she suddenly stop breathing? If not a heart attack, then what?

## Disability Issues

As interest grew in the Schiavo case, advocates for disabled people began to take notice. While the Quinlan and Cruzan cases had never been conceptualized as involving discrimination against disabled persons, the last decades have witnessed the growing influence of disability culture.

Advocates for Terri Schiavo claimed that this severely, cognitively impaired person was *a victim of discrimination against the disabled*. Since passage of the Americans with Disabilities Act (ADA) in 1990, denial of medical resources to a disabled person because he is disabled violates federal law. However, the ADA has never specified end-of-life cognitive deterioration (which also would include Alzheimer's disease) as a covered disability.

Groups such as Not Dead Yet, the World Association of Persons with Disabilities, the National Spinal Cord Injury Association, and Joni and Friends opposed removal of Terri's feeding tube. Of course, to claim that Terri Schiavo is a victim of discrimination against disabled persons assumes that she is still a person. That is exactly what disability advocates claimed. Given the increasing acceptance that a patient in PVS for a decade cannot revert back to consciousness, Terri's advocates thus increasingly *claimed that she is not in PVS but in a minimal consciousness state*.

Charleston disability rights lawyer Harriet McBryde Johnson charged that, "Ms. Schiavo has a statutory right under the Americans with Disabilities Act not to be treated differently because of her disability. Obviously, Florida law would not allow a husband to kill a non-disabled wife by denying her nourishment. Because the state is overtly drawing lines based on disability, it has the burden under the ADA of justifying those lines."[59]

## Some Distinctions

**Futile vs. Non-Futile Care.**  In December 1991, Helga Wanglie, age 87, had been in PVS for eight months, sustained by a ventilator and a feeding tube, at Hennepin County Hospital in Minneapolis, Minnesota.[60] At the hospital the physicians (who included Ronald Cranford) decided to withdraw treatment. Helga's husband refused permission for discontinuation of her ventilator and feeding tube, and he went to court.

The Wanglie case surprised for two reasons. First, since Helga's insurance covered her hospitalization, the hospital lost money by withdrawing artificial life-support. Second, the case involved a philosophical dispute about whether a relative could force the medical team to continue care it regarded as futile. When Helga died unexpectedly, the legal case ended.[61]

In 1989 in Massachusetts, physicians were sued for removing medical support that they unanimously believed to be futile. Even though the jury agreed that Caroline Gilgunn would have wanted to remain on life-support, the physicians won because the jury agreed that patients could not force physicians to render futile treatment.

In the 1990s, some physicians believed that medical futility was a descriptive concept that could help physicians and families easily make decisions about treatment at the end of life. Today, most bioethicists believe that medical futility is not entirely descriptive and contains the evaluative assumption that continued treatment is "not worth it."[62]

The Schiavo case is a good example: competent neurologists unanimously agreed that, after three years, further treatment was futile for Terri, yet some staff, her parents, and rogue neurologists disagreed, claiming it could be worthwhile.

Most American patients and their families now decline treatment when their physicians advise them that further treatment is futile. A study in 1994 that followed over 4,000 patients whose condition was diagnosed as life threatening or terminal found that only 14 percent of them were resuscitated after being near death. This figure was far less than most physicians predicted and far less than it would have been a decade earlier, when most of those patients would have been resuscitated.[63]

**Extraordinary versus Ordinary Treatment.** In 1957, a group of anesthesiologists asked Pope Pius XII what they owed dying patients. The Pope said that they need not take heroic steps to keep such patients alive: patients were owed merely ordinary, but not extraordinary, treatments. However, "extraordinary" is equivocal and has meaning across the end points of a continuum that shifts with medical progress. In 1967, when Christiaan Barnard first transplanted a human heart, his heart-lung bypass machine was extraordinary. That machine was the forerunner of the large, bulky ventilator that kept Karen Quinlan breathing. Today, miniaturized ventilators—some small enough to be used with premature babies—are used everywhere in medicine. Yesterday's extraordinary treatment becomes today's ordinary treatment, rendering the distinction less helpful than it was a half-century ago.

**Artificial Nutrition and Hydration.** In the 1980s, some people believed that whatever might be said about extraordinary and ordinary care in the future, providing food and water would always be considered ordinary and humane medical care. They felt that such basic care was morally owed to PVS patients. This issue arose in the Schiavo case.

The reality of feeding a chronically vegetative patient is not like spooning chicken soup into the mouths of patients who are simply weak. Most vegetative patients have no swallowing reflexes, so they cannot be fed by mouth. Therefore, an artificial liquid diet must be mechanically pumped into their bodies.

The chicken-soup image can distort people's impression of a PVS case. Karen Quinlan's sister, for example, thought that her comatose sister would look like Sleeping Beauty and was shocked by the emaciated figure she saw. By the time of Nancy Cruzan's case in 1990, improvements in artificial feeding would create the opposite effect: because of retention of fluids, PVS patients now had the rotund "Porky Pig" face seen in Terri Schiavo. Moreover, with many kinds of feeding tubes, patients must be tied down to avoid dislodging the line. A restrained, bald woman with a "porky" face is not how most people visualize PVS patients.

As said, neither dehydration nor starvation distresses semiconscious, dying patients. Patients near death *not* on nutritional support seem more comfortable than patients on whom such support is forced. One important national commission noted in 1983 that loss of appetite is "almost the norm in the latter stages of terminal illness" and concluded, "Only rarely should a dying patient be fed by tube or intravenously."[64] Indeed, such feeding may actually make the patient suffer and thus harm her.

Shaky arguments abounded in the 1980s against withdrawing nutrition and hydration. Some states allowed removal of ventilators but not of feeding tubes, and champions of a sanctity-of-life worldview saw removal of feeding and hydration tubes as the immediate cause of death and hence as mercy killing. One philosopher argued in 1983 that providing food and water to PVS patients is the ordinary care "that all human beings owe each other"; another argued at about the same time that such feeding involves "the most fundamental of all human relationships," and that "to tamper with, or adulterate, so enduring and central a moral emotion" is "a most dangerous business."[65]

By the 1990s, most physicians had come to feel that artificial IV feeding lines for PVS patients compared to ventilators: both were advanced medical technology. The *Cruzan* decision in 1990 agreed.

**Withdrawing and Forgoing Treatment**    During the last forty years, a central moral debate has concerned the degree to which a physician may hasten deaths of dying patients. One cause of this debate was a declaration by the AMA in 1973 (two years before Quinlan):

> The intentional termination of the life of one human being by another—mercy killing—is contrary to that for which the medical profession stands and is contrary to the policy of the American Medical Association.
>     . . . The cessation of the employment of extraordinary means to prolong the life of the body when there is irrefutable evidence that biological death is imminent is the decision of the patient and/or immediate family.[66]

In this statement, the word "extraordinary" is ambiguous, and AMA policy did not clarify it. Are all patients on ventilators receiving extraordinary care? Is a physician who withdraws a dying patient's ventilator or feeding tube guilty of mercy killing?

Concern about mercy killing led some physicians to forgo the use of ventilators and artificial feeding. Since withdrawal of such care might be seen as mercy killing, it was far easier to just forgo support. This reasoning created an odd situation, in which physicians would forgo the same treatment that they would not otherwise withdraw.

Others believed that because outcomes are never certain, patients were owed treatment on a trial period—perhaps both a ventilator and artificial feeding—to see if they could recover.

In 1975, Karen Quinlan's physicians, Morse and Javed, upheld the official position of AMA: that withdrawing medical support from a patient was "active euthanasia." In 1986, the AMA decided that an ethical physician, after consulting with the family, could withdraw ventilators and feeding tubes from irreversibly comatose patients.

This new AMA policy did not say that being irreversibly comatose meant being brain dead. Criteria for ethical removal of medical support differ from criteria of brain death.

## Advance Directives

The Quinlan case caused written advance directives to become popular in various forms. A *living will* informs physicians about conditions under which a person would not want medical support. A *values inventory* specifies what a person values in life and may be useful to a patient's family and physicians if they must make decisions for that person. A *durable power of attorney* assigns to someone else the right to make financial and life-and-death medical decisions if the signee becomes incompetent.

*Cruzan* emphasized that such a document would be crucial in meeting the "clear and convincing" standard required by New York and Missouri. After the Schiavo case, many Americans rushed to sign such directives (which may be downloaded at the Caring Connections website). In 1991, the Health Care Financing Administration required all American hospitals to ask incoming patients if they wanted to create an advance directive.

Advance directives contain two major problems. First, as the SUPPORT study showed, most people do not accurately predict their own future preferences.[67] Second, evidence has grown that spouses designated as legal proxies do not accurately predict the wishes of previously competent but now incompetent spouses.[68] As frequently as they wrongly predict a desire for mere palliative care, they just as frequently wrongly predict desires for aggressive treatment.[69]

Advance directives often do not cover non-terminal, though permanently comatose, patients. As such, advance directives should specify whether food and water is included under unwanted medical treatment or name a specific person to be a proxy for an incompetent patient. Because such directives are requested of patients only upon admission to hospitals, most people under 30 do not have one.

## The Schiavo Case, Bioethics and Politics

Outsiders made things worse in the Schiavo case. Not understanding the history of the false report of abuse and trauma on the 1991 bone scan, outside experts guessed that something malevolent had happened to Terri, making her advocates suspect a cover-up by Terri's husband and the courts. Outside physicians, push-ing their own exotic, for-profit schemes, exploited gullible parents and friends. Outlier neurologists, pushing a new category of consciousness not in journals of neurology but on the front pages of the *New York Times* and the *Hastings Center Report*, a bioethics journal, also didn't help.

When Terri's parents went to national media, especially in an age of fierce competition among cable news stations for sensational topics, the floodgates opened. And because politicians on the national scene love media attention, and as Florida Senator Mel Martinez predicted, U.S. senators, congressmen, and even the president got involved.

Since 1997 when scientists announced the cloning of the lamb Dolly (see Chapter 7), bioethics has become increasingly politicized, with social conserva-tives extolling the personhood of human embryos and opposing all forms of clon-ing. The Schiavo case landed on this pedigree and exploded. Whether it's good for bioethics to be covered all evening on cable news outlets remains to be seen.

## FURTHER READING AND RESOURCES

Margaret Battin, *The Least Worst Death: Essays in Bioethics at the End of Life*, New York: Oxford University Press, New York, 1993.
Joanne Lynn, ed., *By No Extraordinary Means: The Choice to Forgo Life-Sustaining Food and Water*, expanded ed., Bloomington, IN: Indiana University Press, 1989.
Joseph and Julia Quinlan with Phyllis Battelle, *Karen Ann: The Quinlans Tell Their Story*, New York, NY: Doubleday, 1977.
William Colby, *The Long Goodbye: The Deaths of Nancy Cruzan*, Carlsbad, CA: Hay House, 2002.
Robert and Mary Schindler, with Suzanne Schindler Vitadamo and Bobby Schindler, *A Life that Matters: The Legacy of Terri Schiavo*, New York, NY: Time Warner Books, 2006.
Michael Schiavo, and Michael Hirsh, *Terri: The Truth*, New York: Dutton Adult Books, 2006.
Mark Fuhrman, *Silent Witness: The Untold Story of Terri Schiavo's Death*, New York: William Morrow, 2005.

*Between Life and Death: The Terri Schiavo Story*, A&E films. This excellent 45-minute sum-mary of the case, made by CBS News, has good pictures of Terri in various stages of her life and pictures of Patricia White Bull and Terry Wallace (coma patients who awakened after many years).

## DISCUSSION QUESTIONS

1. If you had only a 1 percent chance of coming out of a long-term coma or PVS, would you want physicians to keep treating you, or would you rather they let you die?

2. In the above case, what burdens or benefits would continued treatment place on your family and loved ones?

3. Many elderly people will succumb to coma-like states in their final years as they decline into neurological conditions such as Alzheimer's disease. Can society afford long-term care for millions of such people? Is there a

morally relevant difference between such care for a 90-year-old with dementia and a 25-year-old in PVS?

4. If families won't or can't make decisions about death, is it permissible for physicians to act as if they've discovered that death has occurred in a relative, to help out the family? Is this a white lie? Would Kant approve?

5. Are worries about a slippery slope legitimate in the coma cases of this chapter? If society starts triaging such marginal people, will it lead to a "culture of death" rather than a "culture of life"? What will happen if society faces a great financial crisis over paying for medical care for cognitively impaired patients and we don't have a strong culture of life? Will society fail this new test?

6. James Rachels argues that it's morally irrelevant whether physicians withdraw or forgo ventilators and feeding tubes, but the two actions certainly feel different to families and physicians. Are these feelings relevant to accessing the morality of letting die?

7. How do expanded definitions of death by neurological criteria depend on great trust in the integrity of the transplant community not to abuse such definitions?

8. What is the proper role of state and federal government in cases like Nancy Cruzan and Terri Schiavo? Should it protect vulnerable patients and assume the worst of families or should it assume the best of families and give them wide latitude to decide?

9. Given the SUPPORT study, would it help to avoid family disputes if most people had an advance directive? What are the limitations of such directives and hospital ethics committees to resolve these cases?

10. Is it fair to conceptualize the cases in this chapter as "disabled people" needing protection under the Americans with Disabilities Act? If we do so, what problems arise?

11. In the Schiavo case, did Michael Schiavo meet the standard of clear and convincing evidence for removal of Terri's feeding tube? Why didn't he turn the case over to her parents and let them take care of her, as they volunteered to do?

# CHAPTER 5

# Abortion: The Trial of Kenneth Edelin

*T*his chapter discusses abortion and its history prior to its legalization by the U.S. Supreme Court in 1973 in *Roe v. Wade*. It also discusses the controversial case of Kenneth Edelin, who aborted a late-term fetus; experiments on fetuses, fetal and fetal-tissue research; and emergency contraception (Plan B).

## KENNETH EDELIN'S CONTROVERSIAL ABORTION

In January 1973, just nine months before Kenneth Edelin aborted a fetus in Boston in October, the U.S. Supreme Court had legalized abortion. Edelin served as chief resident in obstetrics at Boston City Hospital.

Over those nine months, researchers at this hospital had performed experiments on to-be-aborted fetuses and reasoned this way: Since the aborted fetuses were going to die anyway, why not use them in experiments to help other fetuses?

What about this reasoning? If unclaimed, runaway pets will be killed after three days in the pound, why not use them in medical experiments to help other dogs? If terminal patients will die anyway, why not test new drugs or procedures on them? If Jews are going to die anyway in concentration camps, why not use them—as Nazi physicians reasoned—in medical experiments? (These claims illustrate *reductio ad absurdum* reasoning.)

The research at this hospital studied which drugs crossed the placenta and, hence, which might harm the fetus. Physicians gave women undergoing abortions the antibiotics clindamycin and erythromycin, later examined the aborted fetuses, and found that these drugs concentrated in livers of fetuses.

In another study in 1973, researchers tried to develop an artificial placenta. Eight fetuses, weighing between 300 and 1,000 grams, were obtained by hysterotomy. A hysterotomy is abortion by caesarean surgery that involves cutting through the lower abdominal wall. When researchers placed the largest of them in a warm saline solution that mimicked the amniotic sac, it gasped frantically and moved its limbs as it died.[1] In another experiment on the effect of lack of glucose to the brain, researchers severed heads of 12 nonviable fetuses after stopping their hearts but before anoxia damaged their brains. The researchers successfully maintained the fetal brains with artificial replacements for glucose.[2]

An article describing the first experiment appeared in June 1973 in the *New England Journal of Medicine*, a publication edited in Boston.[3] Someone mailed a copy to several Boston Catholics.

Protestant theologian Paul Ramsey called such experimentation "unconsented-to research on unborn babies" and exploitation of a "tragical case of dying" babies.[4] These experiments outraged Americans. After publicity about them in 1975, Congress banned all federally funded research involving fetuses. Because it did not know where to draw a line, it also banned funding of research involving human embryos.

A councilman held a hearing in September 1973 to investigate the experiments on fetuses. Anti-abortionists packed the auditorium and heard Mildred Jefferson, an African-American assistant professor of surgery at Boston University, speak of her opposition to abortion.

At Edelin's trial, Jefferson testified that some women undergoing abortion in studies at Boston City Hospital were too young to consent legally and had not consented in writing. If this were true, researchers could be charged with "grave robbing," i.e., illegally procuring bodies for medical experimentation.

As a result of these hearings, nothing happened to the researchers or to Boston City Hospital, which continued to experiment. But Catholic Bostonians festered about legalized abortion. In this milieu in October 1973, Edelin performed a controversial abortion.

In 1973, Kenneth Edelin was 35 years old. The son of a postman, he grew up poor in Washington, D.C. Graduating with a B.S. from Columbia University, he received his M.D. from Meharry Medical College, interned in Ohio, and then served three years as a U.S. Air Force physician. In 1971, he began his residency at Boston City Hospital, known as the public hospital for poor people and the model for the television show *St. Elsewhere*. When the case occurred, Edelin was the first African-American chief resident in OB/GYN in the hospital's history.

"Alice Roe" is a pseudonym for a 17-year-old African-American student from Roxbury, a poor suburb of Boston, whom Edelin (decades later) called "Evonne." Edelin's faculty supervisor, Hugh Holtrop, examined Evonne, estimating her to be 22 weeks pregnant. Enrique Giminez, a first-year resident from Mexico, estimated her to be 24 weeks pregnant (Giminez later testified against Edelin); a third-year medical student, Steve Teich, who assisted during the abortion, agreed with Giminez's estimate. At the time, the under-funded hospital had no ultrasound machine and couldn't make a more precise estimate.

Even though Holtrop had admitted Evonne, and even though the fetus to be aborted was late-second trimester, Holtrop delegated third-year resident Edelin to perform the abortion. Like most attending physicians, Holtrop had a private practice and spent little time at this hospital, so third-year residents normally did such operations.

To complicate matters, Holtrop had obtained Evonne's and her mother's permission for another fetal experiment, this time to see if aminoglutethamide increased the hormone output of the placenta. Accordingly, Holtrop gave Evonne aminoglutethamide intravenously and analyzed her urine over the next 24 hours. His study took place on October 1–2, 1973.

Edelin planned to abort the fetus by injecting saline solution into the amniotic sac, but the next day, when he inserted a needle to sample her amniotic fluid, he drew blood. This indicated that Evonne had an anterior placenta, attached to her uterine front wall, with the fetus behind it (the placenta normally develops near the spine with the fetus near the abdomen). Saline injected into the placenta could travel into her bloodstream, where it could be lethal to Evonne.

So Edelin rescheduled Evonne for a hysterotomy the next day. Instead of Giminez, Edelin chose Teich, the third-year medical student, as his assistant. Uninvited, Giminez watched the hysterotomy from a distance.

What happened next is controversial. Giminez later testified that Edelin made the Cesarean section, reached in, cut the placenta from the abdominal wall, waited three minutes, and then removed a dead fetus. If such a wait took place, it is important because a baby cannot breathe on its own inside the uterus: it begins breathing only when brought outside. Edelin would soon be charged with manslaughter for not immediately removing the baby, causing it to suffocate.

Afterward, someone took the fetus to the morgue, and—as required by hospital policy for aborted fetuses weighing more than 600 grams—preserved it in formalin. This meant that the district attorney had a body for the crime and photographs to show a jury.

A grand jury indicted Edelin. Newman Flanagan, a competent, tough, and showy district attorney, prosecuted Edelin. William Perkins Homans, Jr., a wealthy Boston lawyer who often defended unpopular causes, defended Edelin; Judge James McGuire presided

Flanagan charged Edelin with manslaughter, defined in Massachusetts as "wanton, reckless" omission or commission of an act which causes death; Massachusetts law further defined "wanton, reckless" conduct as "the legal equivalent of intentional conduct" and as "disregard of the probable consequences to the rights of others." Judge McGuire told the jury: "The essence of wanton or reckless conduct is the doing of an act or the omission to act where there is a duty to act, which commission or omission involves a high degree of likelihood that substantial harm will result to another."[5]

Massachusetts did not pass an abortion law until August 1974 (19 months after *Roe v. Wade*), and in the absence of a specific state law, Judge McGuire instructed the jury that *Roe v. Wade* was "absolutely controlling." Since *Roe v. Wade* equated personhood with viability, the jury thought it had to determine whether Evonne's fetus had been viable.

The Supreme Court had said only that viability is "usually" placed at 24 to 28 weeks, not that viability necessarily falls within that range. It had not specified how to determine the viability of a late-term fetus. If Evonne's fetus wasn't viable, no person had been killed; and if no person had been killed, no manslaughter charge could be brought.

Edelin testified that his operation on Evonne had seemed long to Giminez because her thick abdominal wall had not yet stretched enough to sever easily. Considered safer than vertical incisions and to leave less scarring, Edelin made a Pfannenstiel ("bikini") incision. Surgeon William Nolen wrote that making such an incision could not take three minutes.[6] Edelin testified that Giminez confused his initial abdominal incision with his second incision to detach the placenta.

Flanagan showed the jury a picture of the fetus. Homans objected angrily, arguing it would inflame the jury and prove nothing about viability. Judge McGuire allowed it, but charged the jury with not viewing it "from any emotional point of view."[7]

Flanagan concluded that when Edelin cut the placenta, the fetus had been viable and hence was a person; Edelin had waited three minutes and this delay constituted "wanton, reckless conduct"; finally, the goal of legal abortion was not to produce a dead fetus but merely to end a pregnancy, so Edelin should have saved the viable fetus before cutting its placenta.

Judge McGuire instructed the jury that an unborn fetus was not a person and could not be the subject of a manslaughter indictment. Such an indictment could refer only to a person, defined by Massachusetts law as *a baby*—a fetus that has been born. Because birth was critical, Judge McGuire instructed the jury: "You must be satisfied beyond a reasonable doubt . . . that the defendant caused the death of a person who had been alive outside the body of his or her mother."

So the jury had to decide: (1) Had Evonne's fetus been alive outside Evonne's body? (2) If so, did the baby die as a result of "wanton, reckless conduct" by Edelin? The jurors said "yes" to both points and convicted Edelin of manslaughter.

Judge McGuire sentenced Edelin to a year of probation. If this conviction had stuck, Edelin would have lost his medical license. While Edelin appealed, Boston City Hospital immediately offered him a permanent position.

In 1976, three years after Evonne's surgery, the Massachusetts Supreme Court overturned Edelin's conviction, declaring that the district attorney had presented no evidence of criminal negligence and writing, "In the comparative calm of appellate review, the essential proposition emerges that the defendant had no evil frame of mind, was actuated by no criminal purpose, and committed no wanton or reckless act in carrying out the medical procedures on Oct. 3, 1973."[8] The Court did not require a new trial but simply acquitted Edelin.

Upon hearing of his acquittal, Edelin was "jubilant." He said, "It's great to be able to smile again after two-and-a-half years."[9] Television anchor Walter Cronkite that evening triumphantly announced that Edelin had been acquitted of "manslaughter by abortion."[10]

William Nolen, a surgeon who examined the case in his book *The Baby in the Bottle*, concluded that the fetus had not been outside the womb, so it had not been born and thus no manslaughter charge had been warranted.[11] Nolen's conclusion was made not only as a surgeon but also as someone who opposed abortion.

For the ethics of abortion, Nolen believed that Edelin had intended to abort a late fetus and once he had opened Evonne, he was surprised to find her fetus viable. Nolen doesn't say that Edelin suffocated the fetus, but he does say that whether a newborn has a will to live can be known only if the physician takes it out of the womb, slaps it, and helps it to breathe:

> What is disturbing in the Roe case is that, by his own admission, Edelin made no attempt to see if the child had that spark. As [Jeffrey] Gould [another physician who testified] said, the will to live isn't always immediately apparent; it becomes

obvious only if "the physician will try to stimulate, will try to give a little bit of oxygen, and look for a favorable response." . . .

The Roe baby wasn't given this bit of provocation that might—just might—have shown it had the will to live. Why? The answer is distressingly simple. No one wanted the Roe baby to live.[12]

For the next three decades, both Newman Flanagan and Edelin worked in Boston: Newman, as one of the longest serving district attorneys in America; Edelin, as chair of OB/GYN at Boston City Hospital and associate dean at Boston University School of Medicine. He later became Chairman of the Board of Planned Parenthood Federation of America. (A 2008 tribute to him by Planned Parenthood can be seen on YouTube, as well as the famous anti-abortion video, "The Silent Scream").

In 2013, another African-American physician, Kermit Gosnell was sentenced to life in prison for the death of a patient under his care and the deaths of seven newborns said to have been born alive after attempted abortions.[13]

## BACKGROUND: PERSPECTIVES ON ABORTION

### The Language of Abortion

This book will use medically accepted terms for the stages of a human life. When sperm meets egg, conception starts an *embryo*; after nine weeks and until birth, this being is a *fetus*, and at birth is a *baby*.

Definitions of these terms have legal and ethical consequences. For example, a baby can be the subject of a homicide charge, but not a fetus. Critics of abortion object to the connotation of "fetus" as a being containing less value than a baby and refer to the growing fetus as a "baby."

### Abortion and the Bible

Without interpretation, the Bible or the Torah do not explicitly forbid abortion. In this regard, Paul Badham, a British professor of church history, writes:

> The Bible certainly teaches the value of human life, and forbids the murder of any human being (Psalm 8). But life, in biblical terms, commences only when the breath enters the nostrils and the man or woman becomes a "living being" (Genesis 2:7). . . . Consequently in biblical terms the fetus is not a person. This is brought out clearly in the laws relating to murder. . . . For whereas "whoever hits a man and kills him shall be put to death" (Exodus 21; 12), " . . . if some men are fighting and hurt a woman so that she loses her child, but is not injured in any other way, the one who hurt her is to be fined." . . . And this absence of concern for the fetus is also implied by the imposition of the death penalty on women who conceive out of wedlock, without any consideration being given to the fact that this killed both the fetus and the woman (Deuteronomy 22:21, Leviticus 21:9, Genesis 38:24).[14]

Jesus never explicitly speaks about abortion anywhere in the Gospels.[15] If the Old Testament or the Gospels do not explicitly condemn abortion, why do so many conservative Christians condemn abortion today? An answer comes from the development of Church doctrine.

The Old Testament took its final form during the fifth century Before the Common Era (B.C.E.) and the New Testament was finalized around the year 200 of the Common Era (C.E.)—when Christianity began as an organized religion. As an organized religion, Christianity always opposed abortion, but its view of abortion has changed over 1,800 years.

By the fourth century C.E., Christian teaching about sex was in crisis. Christianity idealized celibacy, but if too many Christians were celibate, Christianity would die out (as the Shakers did). Practically, most people could not practice perfect celibacy. Consequently, Augustine revised Christian teaching in the fourth century to allow sexual intercourse in marriage, *but only if the couple intended to have children.*[16] It follows for Augustine that abortion is sinful because it thwarts the only justification for having sex: to produce a child.

In the twelfth century, Christian doctrine began to separate abortion from homicide by distinguishing between "formed" and "unformed" embryos. The concept had to do with the soul rather than with physical development.

In the thirteenth century, St. Thomas Aquinas held that God ensouled male embryos at day 40 of gestation;, female embryos, at day 90. Aborting a male embryo after day 40 was punished more severely than aborting a female embryo at the same age, since the male was formed but the female was not. Although abortion at any time was sinful, penalties increased when the fetus was formed.[17]

During the nineteenth century, scientific evidence discredited the Thomistic concept of ensoulment. Microscopes revealed life at tiny stages, including human life. Around 1850, popes began denouncing abortion in increasingly absolutistic terms. During this time, Catholicism came close to teaching that personhood began at conception, a view called immediate animation. (Over the last 30 years, the Church has moved closer to immediate animation, especially with its emphasis on the value of the human embryo.)

In 1870, Pope Pius IX resisted the growing power of science by convening the First Vatican Council. It declared that his edicts and those of future popes would be infallible.[18] From 1869 to 1900, the Church encouraged veneration of Mary (which had been neglected), supported Creationism against geological explanations of the origins of the Earth, emphasized miracles (Fatima was recognized shortly afterward), and vigorously attacked Darwinism.

In Catholic ethics, the *doctrine of double effect* allowed abortions for two cases: ectopic pregnancy and uterine cancer (in which the uterus and fetus must be removed together). According to this doctrine, an action having two effects, one good and the other evil, is morally permissible under four conditions: (1) if the action is good in itself or not evil, (2) if the good follows as immediately from the cause as from the evil effect, (3) if only the good effect is intended, and (4) if there is a proportionately grave cause for performing the action as for allowing the evil effect.

Historical Catholic doctrine was stricter than the law. During the seventeenth century, European common law did not indict women for aborting even a quickened fetus. Finally, in 1803, an English statute made abortion of a quickened fetus a capital crime.

From the seventeenth through the nineteenth centuries, American law followed English common law: Abortion before quickening was only a misdemeanor.

In 1973 in its *Roe v. Wade* decision, the United States Supreme Court reviewed the legal background of abortion and concluded:

> It is thus apparent that at common law, at the time of the adopting of our Constitution, and throughout the major portion of the nineteenth century, . . . a woman enjoyed a substantially broader right to terminate a pregnancy than she does in most States today. At least with respect to the early stage of pregnancy, and very possibly without such a limitation, the opportunity to make this choice was present in this country well into the 19th century.[19]

In America, this leniency changed after the Civil War, when most states criminalized abortion. From 1870 to 1970, the American medical profession opposed abortion.

Historians argue that this opposition stemmed from paternalism, misogyny, and protection of professional turf by male physicians and men: "Anti-abortion legislation was part of an anti-feminist backlash to the growing movement for suffrage, voluntary motherhood, and other women's rights in the nineteenth century."[20]

Before the Civil War, midwives delivered most babies, and in doing so, competed with physicians over births. After this war, physicians took over deliveries, and most physicians were men. So bans on abortions both drove out midwives and helped medicalize birth.

## The Experience of Illegal Abortions

Before the Supreme Court legalized abortion in 1973, women undergoing abortions often had horrible experiences. Physicians performing abortions usually did so only for money; some demanded sex. Others lectured women on their promiscuity.

Though abortion is painful, abortionists didn't use anesthesia. Abortionists didn't explain to women beforehand what would happen or why. If damage occurred, women had no legal recourse. Women usually didn't know the names of abortionists, who forbade further contact. Illegal abortions cost a lot, condemning poor women to unwanted children. (And still may be costly: a legal abortion at 10 weeks of gestation costs between $300 and $900, depending on location and not including costs of getting there; 26 states require a woman to wait 24 hours between being informed of risks about the abortion and the procedure itself thus increasing costs for women traveling from other areas.[21])

Despite these conditions, during the 1950s and 1960s, hundreds of thousands of American women had illegal abortions. Some died as a result: 193 died in 1965 alone, and during the 1960s, over 1,000.[22] In contrast and in 2007, the most recent year for the Centers for Disease Control reporting data, abortion clinics reported that only six women died from consequences of legal abortions.[23]

Because what they had done was illegal, victims of botched abortions entered emergency rooms only at the last moment. Some died of widespread abdominal infections, and those who recovered often were sterile. Poor women of color ran the greatest risks; in 1965, 55 percent of abortion-related deaths were among them.

## 1962: Sherri Finkbine

In 1962, Sherri Finkbine, living with her husband and their four children in Phoenix, Arizona, became pregnant with a fifth child.[24] During her second month of pregnancy, she took thalidomide, an anti-nausea drug (also marketed in Germany as a sedative). It was just becoming apparent then that thalidomide is a teratogen ("monster former") that produces babies with missing arms or legs. (Thalidomide had been tested on animals, but not on *pregnant* animals. The tragedies it caused made the FDA test all future drugs on pregnant animals.)

Sherri Finkbine requested an abortion at a local hospital, ostensibly for her health, but really to abort a fetus likely to be born without arms or legs. However, the district attorney threatened to prosecute the abortion, so she flew to Sweden, where therapeutic abortion had been legal since 1940. Swedish physicians then aborted her fetus, which was severely deformed.

The case caused many people to demand legalized abortion. In the years preceding *Roe v. Wade*, 18 states liberalized laws about abortion. Hawaii began in 1970, followed by Colorado, North Carolina, and California. Governor of California, Ronald Reagan, signed its bill into law.

## 1968: Humanae Vitae

In 1968, five years before *Roe v. Wade*, Pope Paul VI issued his encyclical *Humanae Vitae* that declared use of birth control to be a sin. The edict startled liberal Catholics and drove them to defy church teachings. A quarter of a century later in 1993, Pope John Paul II vigorously defended *Humanae Vitae* and its ban on birth control.[25]

The 1968 encyclical had an unintended effect: when they were not allowed to teach about contraception at Catholic University in Washington, D.C., Catholic priests Warren Reich, Albert Jonsen, William Curren, and Paul Tong left the priesthood and Catholic universities. These apostates became founders of bioethics, a field that tries to teach both sides of moral issues.

## 1973: *Roe v. Wade*

The decision of the United States Supreme Court in *Roe v. Wade* (1973) concerned "Jane Roe" (Norma McCorvey) from Dallas, Texas. Wade was Henry Wade, district attorney of Dallas County. When this case began in 1970, Norma wanted a safe, legal abortion and could not get one in Dallas County, so she challenged the Texas law. (She later recanted, becoming anti-abortion.)

The Supreme Court had already decided in *Griswold v. Connecticut* (1965) that the Constitution's implied right to privacy or liberty allowed couples to receive birth control pills. The Court also saw this entitlement in 1942 in *Oklahoma vs. Skinner,* which noted a fundamental right to reproduction and control of one's body in blocking a law allowing involuntary sterilization of habitual criminals.

In *Roe v. Wade*, it decided that the same liberty included the right of a woman to decide whether she wanted to stay pregnant or to abort her fetus, or put differently, whether a state could pass a law prohibiting such abortions, which most had previously done.

This new right was not unqualified. A woman's right to abort her fetus was balanced against the rights of the fetus to live, which expanded as its gestational age increased. The Court decided that the State's interest in protecting unborn life becomes compelling at viability, such that after that point, their interest in protecting unborn life allows states to pass laws banning most abortions.

In 1973 in *Roe v. Wade*, the Court used a trimester system to mark viability, where viability divided the second from the third trimester of fetal development. The Court defined viability as the point when a fetus is able to live outside the mother's womb. It placed viability between 24 and 28 weeks. A later decision by this Court ignored the trimester system but retained viability as the key marker.

Note two things: first, a state *may* forbid abortion during the third trimester, but need not. Second, even if states pass laws forbidding abortions in that trimester, exceptions must be allowed to preserve the *life* or *health* of the mother.

Anti-abortionists argue that this permission constitutes a loophole justifying any abortion. Two physicians can often be found who will say that continuing the pregnancy would endanger the mother's health.

## Abortion Statistics

After abortion became legal, American women had about 1.5 million abortions per year, a figure that remained steady for a decade.[26] During the last decades, the number has steadily dropped. The exact number of abortions per year is controversial. The Centers for Disease Control are required by federal law to track this number, but they rely on voluntary reporting by clinics, some of which don't cooperate. The Alan Guttmacher Institute, which calls abortion providers, has the most accurate figures. It says that in 2009, this figure dropped to 750,000.

## ETHICAL ISSUES

### Edelin's Actions

Edelin waited a long time before he removed Evonne's fetus. Even if he was innocent of any legal charge, were his actions ethical? As Nolen said, all he had to do was remove it, slap it on the bottom, and it would have lived. If it had trouble breathing, he could have given it oxygen or technical assistance.

The baby may have been healthy and someone may have adopted it. If Evonne had wanted the baby and the baby had been born premature at this time, Edelin certainly would have done everything to keep it alive. Should a life be so precariously valued merely because a teenage mother doesn't want it? Because a physician won't take it out of the womb and slap its bottom?

### Personhood

What is a person? With abortion, some philosophers draw a distinction between a person and a human being. They argue that although a fetus is human, it does not meet certain criteria of personhood; and that since a fetus is not a person, it does not have a right to life. In this sense, *human* is a factual term, whereas *person* is an evaluative term.

The late Mary Ann Warren famously defends *a cognitive criterion of personhood* and holds that a fetus does not meet this criterion.[27] According to her, to be a person is to be able to think, to be capable of cognition. What separates a person from a rat is certain capacities—for advanced reasoning, reflective self-awareness, use of language, agency, and consciousness of the external world. Warren does not think that any one of these capacities alone is sufficient for cognition; rather, these capacities define as a group the core criterion. A being lacking *all* of these capacities fails to meet the cognitive criterion and cannot be a person. So a first trimester fetus (when most abortions are done) for her is not a person.

The cognitive criterion may be both too broad and too narrow. It seems to admit some beings that we don't traditionally regard as persons: some chimpanzees communicate, are conscious, may reason and may be self-aware, yet we don't ordinarily consider them persons. (Perhaps, though, we are prejudiced against chimpanzees and the cognitive criterion should make us reconsider our views?)

The cognitive criterion may also be too broad if it implies that society should not protect human beings in the late stages of Alzheimer's disease, permanently comatose patients, or anencephalic babies. Philosophers such as Peter Singer argue that such beings are not persons and do not deserve special protection.[28]

## Personhood as a Gradient

Why does personhood have to be all-or-nothing? In practical reasoning, the all-or-nothing fallacy consists of treating complex issues as if they have only two simplistic, extreme answers when in fact there are many compromises in between. Often, practical solutions reside not on black or white poles but in gray areas in the middle.

Biologically, we know that the human embryo develops by degrees during the first trimester into a fetus, and then over the next trimester, the fetus grows into viability, and finally, during the last trimester, into a baby. No single event or day along this nine-month journey marks *the* day of personhood. The most accurate view is that personhood accumulates by degrees over time.

On this view, a 2-year-old is more of a person than a newborn baby, and a 26-year-old at the height of his powers and health is more of a person than a 2-year-old. If personhood depends on capacities, then a human at maximal capacities is more of a person than a human with few capacities.

At the end of life, people lose personhood by degrees, especially with diseases that rob them of their minds. A 90-year-old man who once had an I.Q. of 140 is only "half the man he once was" at age 90 with initial Alzheimer's and an I.Q. of 70.

We think of personhood as all-or-nothing for two reasons. First, some people believe that a metaphysical event occurs in which human bodies get ensouled or where a soul departs. Before that event, there is no personhood and no moral value, and after that event, there is.

Second, people confuse personhood with moral concern. If granddad with Alzheimer's at 90 is only half the person he once was, that does not mean we owe him only half our previous concern. Indeed, humans who have lost their former capacities may need *more* concern than those at maximal capacity. Who is a full person differs from whom we care about.

That's also true for non-human animals. Some of them may function in families as only semi-persons, but they may be as high on our scale of concern as are our own children.

In biology, humans evolved on a gradient by degrees from other primates, and primates in turn from lesser organisms. In biology, all life is an evolving continuum, connected by common ancestors and by degrees, not huge leaps.

Nevertheless, the gradient may raise as many problems as it solves. If end-stage Alzheimer's patients have lost 99 percent of their cognition, should they be killed? If baboons share 99 percent of their genes with humans, should they be protected as persons?

## The Deprivation Argument: Marquis and Quinn on Potentiality

If we accept the cognitive criterion, a problem arises. If cognition makes people valuable, is it wrong to deprive beings of potential cognition?

Philosophers Don Marquis and Warren Quinn argue this way. They start with two premises: first, what is wrong about killing a person—such as a college student—is depriving him of future cognitive experiences; second, what is wrong about killing an adult matches what is wrong about killing fetuses.[29]

*This deprivation argument* is an interesting one, and many people accept their first premise. Other explanations of why it is wrong to kill persons—that killing violates peoples' rights, for instance, or that killing is against God's will—beg the question: phrases such as "violation of rights" and "against the will of God" are simply other ways of saying that killing is wrong.

As for the second premise, it does seem that what is wrong with killing a competent, adult human is that such an adult strongly desires to go on living, and his family strongly desires this too. When he is killed, all these people have their desires thwarted. Moreover, because almost everyone in society wants to continue living, the murder of anyone threatens us all and makes us skeptical of society's ability to protect us.

Back to the first premise: can a being like an early fetus, without an already existing self or identity, have a personal future of which to be deprived? Marquis's and Quinn's second premise may be vulnerable here to attack.

Consider an analogy: Imagine an omnipotent deity—God—who creates a universe, considers creating a second parallel universe, but then decides against it. Now imagine a powerful evil force—Satan—who wants to destroy the existing universe. It seems that destruction of the existing world by Satan would be wrong; but it does not seem wrong for God to refrain from creating a second world. Although God has disallowed a vast amount of cognitive experiences in the parallel universe, he has neither done any wrong nor wronged any person in not creating it. In the same way, failing to allow the potential cognition of a human fetus to come into existence wrongs no existing person.

Could you imagine yourself as a fetus and feel sad because you have had been aborted and not come into existence? No, that is not fair. It puts one's self erroneously into the picture when, by definition, that self will never exist.

What about contraception or masturbation? This objection is intended as a *reductio ad absurdum* of the idea that we should bring into existence beings with future cognitive experiences. As either of these prevents potential persons from coming into existence, are they wrong? Probably not. They seem to be a straw man—a false opponent, too easily refuted. No anti-abortionist wants to produce billions of extra people and once conception occurs, things do seem different as a distinct human life has started.

Indeed, pro-life champions see each particular person as valuable from conception. Federal Judge John Noonan advocates *a genetic criterion of personhood* and argues that when sperm and egg meet and merge genes, a genetically unique individual is created. The resulting embryo has all the potential in its DNA to be a full person, provided that it finds a nurturing uterus.[30] This seems to be the root idea behind the objection to using human embryos in medical research, or using them as little factories to make embryonic stem cells.

But is *potential* to become a person the same as being a person? What about the thousands of frozen embryos stored around the world? If some woman doesn't adopt them and implant them in her uterus, they will eventually deteriorate and die. Are we thus allowing thousands of "persons" to die by lack of adoption?

Another problem with the genetic criterion is that it collapses the distinction between being human and being a person—as we realize when we consider that a brain-dead human has a unique set of genes. Moreover, through human cloning, 99.9 percent of his genes could be replicated one day, and would that imply that he has been 99.9 percent resurrected? That's unlikely, because what most of us want by immortality is not for our genes to continue but for ourselves to do so, i.e., our memories and our present desires that exist in that bundle of perceptions we call "ourselves." So these implications seem to be a *reductio ad absurdum* of the genetic criterion.

A third possible criterion for personhood might be called the *neurological criterion*. This minimal version of the cognitive criterion defines a person as a human being with a detectable brain wave. This simple standard applies to many issues of medical ethics; it recognizes as persons both quasi-anencephalic babies and adults in persistent vegetative states. With regard to abortion, the neurological criterion would consider a fetus a person when it develops brain waves at about 25 weeks, but not before.

## Viability

The concept of viability is vague. A vague concept is one with no sharp boundaries, for example, baldness. When does viability begin? In *Roe v. Wade*, the Supreme Court said only that viability is "usually placed" at about 28 weeks, but "may occur earlier, even at 24 weeks."

In Edelin's trial, district attorney Newman Flanagan seized on this vagueness and tried to establish that Evonne's fetus had been viable. One anti-abortion physician testified that a 12-week-old fetus could live outside the womb. But for how long? Only a few minutes, the physician answered.

The defense attorney, William Homans, countered by asking the physician how he defined viability; the witness replied, [viability is the] "capacity to survive [outside the womb] even for a second after birth." Homans got several obstetricians to admit that they had never known a fetus to survive for even a few days outside the womb before 24 weeks of gestation.

Remember that legally, viability didn't matter in this case. Even if Evonne's fetus was viable, if it didn't exist outside the womb, no charge of manslaughter could be brought.

On the other hand, legality isn't ethics. Viability matters a lot to ethics. It's one thing to abort a tiny fetus at 13 weeks with no chance of living on its own; it's quite another at 24 or 26 weeks when continued life is possible. That's one reason why many physicians refuse to perform late-stage abortions.

Edelin's critics knew exactly what was meant by viability: the ability to survive independently of the mother. In reality, some fetuses that are born early are not viable: They will die no matter how hard physicians try to keep them alive. Others will survive, and will do so only if given the chance.

To Edelin's opponents, the point was that he had never tried to determine viability. His supporters replied that of course he had not tried because *the whole point* of abortion is to kill a fetus. The point is not to look inside the uterus, see if the fetus is viable, and if it is, rescue it. No, the goal of abortion is to produce a dead fetus.

## The Argument from Marginal Cases

In the Edelin case, one question that arose was, "Where do you draw the line?"— that is, the line between fetuses which may and may not be aborted. Reasoning based on this kind of question is called the *argument from marginal cases*, and it is one of the most widely used ideas in ethics.

With abortion, the argument from marginal cases is as follows: Beings at the margins of personhood cannot be nonarbitrarily distinguished from those at the core. If it's wrong to kill a newborn baby, it's wrong to kill it the day before it's born, and so on, being wrong to kill the growing being anytime after conception.

This argument can be used against the gradient of personhood. Where prochoice advocates say an embryo is not a baby, anti-abortionists point to the smooth continuum and say there is no place to draw the line. No matter what week of gestation we consider, it is arbitrary to make that week the marker of personhood, because the fetus of a week earlier has almost the same qualities. Whatever time or marker is chosen, someone can always ask: Why not choose the week before or after?

Is the argument from marginal cases a good one? Consider an analogy with the color spectrum: although each shade in the spectrum resembles the shades next to it, we can distinguish widely separated colors. Similarly, a full-grown oak tree differs from an acorn, even though an acorn becomes an oak by continuous growth. Similarly, we can distinguish an 8-cell human embryo from a newborn baby. Marginal cases do not make distinctions impossible.

In *Roe v. Wade*, the Court said that in the first two trimesters, the interests of competent adults to control their bodies outweighs the growing interests of fetuses to live. But it could have equally stressed a continuum of development from embryo to birth, such that fetuses have some rights in the second trimester, such that only very strong reasons justify abortions then. Especially with abortions available now in the first trimester, and with genetic screening available then for many common conditions, second semester abortions seem less justified, especially as the fetus has more of those qualities that make it a person.

## Thomson: A Limited Pro-Choice View

Suppose we admit that the fetus in the Edelin case was a person. Does it follow that killing it was immoral? Philosopher Judith Jarvis Thomson says "No."[31]

Imagine you have been admitted to a hospital for an operation, and awaken to find yourself hooked up to a famous violinist. His kidneys have failed and his blood is entering and leaving your body through tubes. Without your permission, your kidneys have been used to keep the violinist alive.

Thomson argues that it is immoral for the hospital to force you to keep the violinist alive. Although it would be saintly of you to agree to stay, you are not *obligated* to do so. Why? Because you did not consent to have your body burdened this way and no one else has a right to make you use your body to keep another person alive.

Just as the violinist cannot demand as a right that you keep him alive by allowing your kidneys to be used, so a fetus has no right that a woman keep it alive. For Thomson, the most telling case is rape, because a rape victim has not consented to sexual intercourse or conceiving a child. She thinks a similar argument applies when a woman has used contraception responsibly but it fails.

Thomson's argument is an example of reasoning by analogy. The violinist's dependence on the other patient is analogous to the fetus's dependence on the mother. In analogical reasoning, the closer the fit between the two things compared, the stronger the inferred conclusion is supported.

Philosopher Francis Kamm objects to Thomson's analogy. Kamm argues that the dialysis patient can simply detach herself, and that such detachment is not like killing a fetus. Since something active must be done to end a fetus's life, for a proper analogy, Kamm says, imagine the violinist blocking the patient's way out of the room, so that the patient could escape only by cutting up the violinist.[32]

The above arguments suggest abortion as self-defense. In the sixteenth century, theologian Thomas Sanchez used Augustine's doctrine of just war to identify an unwanted embryo growing in a fallopian tube as an unjust aggressor against the mother's life. So Sanchez maintained that a mother could kill such a lethal embryo in self-defense.[33]

## Feminist Views

One feminist writer argues that the key question about abortion is whether women should be forced to bear children in a way in which men are not. If an embryo is a person who has a right to life at the mother's expense, then women will always be potential slaves of biological reproduction:

> With all the imperfections of our present-day attitudes, I'm still a lot better off in terms of the sexual choices I have than women of my mother's generation. I was a lot better off after the sixties than I was before then. What sexual freedom I now have has been very hard-won. I wouldn't give it up for anything. . . . There

is a larger crisis, one that has to do with the tensions between feminism and the backlash against it. On the one hand, society is encouraging sexual freedom; on the other hand, it's punishing people for indulging in it and not emotionally preparing them for it. Both women in general and teenagers in particular are caught in the middle.[34]

## Genetic Defects

Genetic testing of embryos and fetuses can reveal worrisome future genetic conditions in babies, such as cystic fibrosis, Tay Sachs disease, sickle cell anemia, Down syndrome, and spina bifida. Medicine now allows testing in the first semester of fetal development, allowing abortions at the usual time after a positive result.

Some people regard such a result the most legitimate reason for abortion; others fear that such results will create a stealth eugenics movement. God Must Want Be to Be Pregnant, or Else I Wouldn't Be (section heading)Some people believe that each human pregnancy happens for a reason. Each human embryo that has been conceived and survived to implant itself in the uterine wall was meant by God to have been created at this place and time. Any interference with the growth of that embryo would thwart God's plans. As one sometimes hears, "God must mean for me to be pregnant, or else I wouldn't be."

Abortion done after genetic tests have revealed undesirable conditions in the fetus is discussed in an excerpt from Gregory Pence's *Elements of Bioethics* book. To read *"Are Genetic Abortions Eugenic?"* go to Chapter 5 in the Online Learning Center (OLC) at www.mhhe.com/pence7e.

Two replies can be made to this view. First, how does a woman know God's will about a particular pregnancy? Unless God speaks to her directly, how can she just assume that *planning* when to have children is not God's will for her? How does she know that God does not want her to do what she believes will be best for her, now and in the future?

Second, such a view is fatalistic in one's personal relation to God. It seems reasonable to ask, "Why must I accept everything that happens? If everything comes from God, doesn't the choice to have an abortion also come from Him? Why make the fatalistic assumption that one can follow God's will only by accepting pregnancy? Why can't a reasoned choice to have an abortion also reflect God's will?"

## A Culture of Life or a Culture of Death?

By 2013, after 40 years of legalized abortion, and with at least a million abortions on average a year, American women had aborted at least 40 million human fetuses. Worldwide, the figure is probably hundreds of millions. Pro-life champions argue that such a tsunami of abortions has created a "culture of death," one that has increased with the legalization of assisted suicide for terminally ill patients in several states.

As noted in earlier chapters, it is easy to push a false autonomy that masks underlying scarcities for the disabled or lack of treatment of symptoms for the dying. Too often, death seems the easy way out. Is this true, too, with abortion?

Take the Edelin case. The doctor did not have to produce a dead baby. He could have saved the viable fetus and Evonne could have given it up for adoption. She had a right to end her pregnancy, not to a dead fetus.

Since World War II, America has had no great crisis such as a world war or a great depression, but that may change in the future. Is our culture ready? If millions of Baby Boomers need long-term care, will the culture help them or urge them to take an early Final Exit? Has society's pendulum swung too much toward death?

Suppose, for the last 40 years, no opposition to abortion had existed. What might have happened? Abortion would be much more easily available, with perhaps every small city having a clinic and competition bringing down prices. Instead of 40 million abortions, we might have had 400 million. Would that have been a good thing?

Catholicism, conservative Protestantism, Islam, and Orthodox Judaism oppose the easy availability of abortion. Are they not right to say, "This involves who we are and we must oppose this?" Aren't hospitals affiliated with such religions within their rights not to provide abortions? As such, shouldn't they oppose abortion as good citizens? Just as Jews are horrified that so many stood by passively when 6 million Jews went to death in concentration camps, shouldn't others be horrified that 40 million fetuses never got a chance to live?

On the other hand, perhaps all this should be seen in a wider context. The world is overpopulated. Extra people pressure the environment with more mouths to feed, more cars emitting noxious gases, and more consumption of scarce water. Suppose contraception was still banned. Then one or two billion more people might exist. Would that be a good thing? All unchosen, unwanted? Yes, contraception and abortion prevented many people from coming into existence—prevented, as Marquis and Quinn would say—many future cognitive experiences from existing, but is that really all bad?

## Abortion and Gender Selection

Gender selection-plus-abortion has been a problem in countries such as China, the Republic of Korea, and India. For centuries, parents there have seen females as less desirable than male children. Using sonograms, many families aborted female fetuses to try again for a male child.

Because X chromosomes weigh more than Y chromosomes, a flow cytometer can separate heavier from lighter sperm, producing accurate results 90 percent of the time. Although intended for use in pre-implantation genetic diagnosis, this technology may be used to select male babies, making gender selection cheap and easy.

Despite laws that ban testing for sex in India and China, at least 160 million females there are missing. After decades of such practices and in China in 2012, never-married men outnumber their female counterparts 124 to 100.[35] By 2020, 1 million excess Chinese males will seek to marry. Both Northern India and China contain large bands of young men who will never marry, leading to social discontent in a society where marriage, family, and children are highly valued.

Sex selection is sexist and leads to imbalances of the sexes in the population, the way it happened in China. Perhaps it, too, should be banned.

## Abortion as a Three-Sided Issue

Many people living in a tolerant democracy, where individual liberties are respected, fail to understand how they got where they are or to understand the larger, worldwide picture. In the United States, they forget that our modern policy of individual rights and personal liberty represents a hard-won victory that citizens of many other countries never achieved.

For instance in China, if they become pregnant before their mid-20s or after they already have a child, beginning in 1979—when the government imposed a limit of one child per family—thousands of women underwent forced abortions—a practice that continues today in rural areas. In Romania, the dictator Nicolae Ceaucescau (in office from 1965-89) denied millions of women contraception or abortions because he wanted a larger population.

Perhaps this ignorance explains why the media frame abortion as an issue with only two sides: anti-abortion versus pro-choice. In fact, the global picture of abortion is three-sided, with two extremes and a compromise: *forced birth* versus *forced abortion,* with individual choice as the middle ground.

## Anti-abortion Protests and Violence

During the 1980s, two Texans attacked several abortion clinics in Florida. In 1984, protestors bombed or burned 24 abortion clinics, including one in Pensacola that took place on Christmas morning and was described by one conspirator as a "birthday present to Jesus."[36]

By 1990, public opinion had turned against anti-abortion violence. As a result, the anti-abortion movement turned to *Operation Rescue,* an organization founded by Randall Terry in 1988. Modeling themselves on the nonviolent demonstrations in the South during the Civil Rights Movement, protesters practiced civil disobedience in front of abortion clinics. During the 1990s, they picketed the homes of physicians who performed abortions.

Some also killed in the name of stopping abortions. They killed physician David Gunn in 1993 as he left an abortion clinic in Pensacola. In 1994, anti-abortionist Paul Hill, a former minister, killed physician John Britton and his security escort as they left another abortion clinic in Pensacola. In 2003, Florida executed Hill for the murder.

In January 1998, an explosion rocked the campus at the University of Alabama at Birmingham. Across the street at Ronald McDonald House and a block away from a dorm, windows shook from the blast. When touched, a package outside the small abortion clinic exploded, the dynamite inside causing hundreds of nails to ricochet off a steel plate inside into the face, torso, and legs of Emily Lyons, a nurse at the clinic, and killing Robert Sanderson, an off-duty Birmingham policeman. Due to intense efforts a few blocks away at UAB hospital, Lyons survived.

An alert UAB student spotted Eric Rudolph leaving the scene and copied the license number of his truck. Police searched for Rudolph for five years in the hills of North Carolina. Arrested in 2003, he confessed in 2005 to bombing abortion clinics in Birmingham and Atlanta, to bombing gay/lesbian nightclubs, and to bombing the Centennial Olympic Park during the 1996 Olympics, where he killed three people and injured 111 others.

In 1998, anti-abortionist James Koop crouched behind the backyard fence with a high-powered rifle and shot Dr. Barnett Slepian through his kitchen window. During the previous four years, snipers shot and wounded three Canadian physicians. In 2009, physician George Tiller was killed in his church in Wichita, Kansas. Both Slepian and Tiller had been targeted by anti-abortion groups for decades and had vowed not to stop providing abortions.

## Live Birth Abortions and How Abortions Are Done

Attempts to abort late-term fetuses have sometimes resulted in live births. In 1977, physician Ronald Cornelson testified in a California criminal court that after a botched saline abortion resulted in a live-born 2.5-pound baby, his colleague William Waddill had choked the infant and suggested injecting it with potassium chloride to kill it.[37] Tried twice for murder, both juries deadlocked on convicting Waddill. In 1979, at the University of Nebraska Medical Center, after an attempted abortion, another 2.5-pound baby was born alive; purposefully left unattended, it died after a few hours.

Because of such cases, physicians today rarely abort a fetus after 23 weeks. They also rarely use prostaglandins to induce abortion because, although safer than suction or surgical techniques, they result in 30 times more live births.

For first-trimester abortions, the most typical technique was formerly injection of saline or urea, followed by dilatation and curettage (scraping, a technique called D&C), but D&C has been replaced by suction curettage or uterine aspiration. Physicians do most abortions in the first trimester.

For late-term abortions, dilatation and evacuation (D&E) is used: The fetus is cut into parts and removed piecewise. To ensure that all the pieces have been removed—since any fragments left behind would produce infection in the mother—the dismembered fetus must be reassembled outside the womb. Late second-trimester or third-trimester abortions use hysterotomy, as in the Edelin case.

Because abortion is controversial, residency programs in obstetrics sometimes offer no training in performing abortion. Some residents in obstetrics have demanded such training.[38]

In 2005, a review of several hundred scientific papers concluded that nerve connections in the fetal brain are not developed enough before 29 weeks for the fetus to feel pain.[39] As such, the authors concluded, aborting a fetus before this point caused it no pain and no anesthesia need be used to spare the fetus pain.

## Fetal Tissue Research

Tissue from aborted fetuses may help patients with neurological disorders such as Parkinson's disease. The tissue required for such neurological research must be adrenal tissue producing dopamine, and it must be obtained from fetuses whose gestational age is 8 to 11 weeks, since after 12 weeks the tissue begins to differentiate into the normal cells of the brain and loses its elasticity. Treatment consists of dopamine delivered as fetal cells: In the operation, a small hole is drilled through the patient's skull and fetal cells are dripped directly into the devastated area of the brain.

A panel of the National Institutes of Health studied this issue and concluded that even if abortion were immoral, fetal tissue obtained from abortions could be used for research if the woman's decision to donate tissue was separated from, and came after, her decision to abort.[40] In 1993, President Clinton lifted the four-year ban on fetal tissue research.

## Emergency Contraception

In America, the traditional approach to preventing pregnancy has been either abstinence or contraception, with abortion as a backup for failures. A middle ground exists between these extremes.

Emergency contraception has been used without publicity for 40 years in America. It consists of taking a double dose of birth-control pills within 72 hours after an act of unprotected sex, followed by a second dose 12 hours later.[41] When the first dose is taken within 72 hours after unprotected sex, emergency contraception reduces the risk of pregnancy by 75–90 percent.

Such pills contain estrogen and/or progesterone and block the release of the egg from the ovary, block the movement of the embryo down the fallopian tube, or prevent implantation of the embryo in the endometrium.

Emergency contraception requires a woman either to have birth control pills on hand, or to be able to obtain them 72 hours after unprotected sex. A woman cannot wait for a pregnancy test because her urine changes chemically only after embryonic implantation.

In 2006, the FDA approved Plan B, a progestin-only form of emergency contraception, for over-the-counter sales to women over 18. In 2009, a federal judge ordered the FDA to approve the same for 17-year-old women.

The American Medical Association defines pregnancy as beginning when the embryo implants on the uterine wall, but not all physicians accept that definition. Some believe that pregnancy begins with conception in the fallopian tubes, and as such, refuse to prescribe IUDs, which interfere with implantation.

In 2005, pharmacists at a Walgreens in Illinois refused to fill prescriptions for Plan B, as did some at WalMart pharmacies. Since Plan B blocks implantation of a fertilized embryo, these pharmacists considered Plan B to be an abortion agent.

Women physicians successfully sued Walgreens and WalMart to make Plan B available by prescription at all its pharmacies. Walgreens then fired pharmacists who refused to fill prescriptions for Plan B, igniting a debate about conscientious refusal of pharmacists to fill prescriptions. This debate became moot in 2013 when the FDA-approved sale of Plan B *without prescription* for any woman regardless of age.

## Maternal versus Fetal Rights

In her 20s in 1989, Nancy Klein went into a coma at an early stage of her pregnancy. Her physicians wanted to abort her fetus to increase her cerebral blood volume and to awaken her. They were also reluctant to give Nancy certain drugs that might injure a fetus brought to term. Anti-abortionists went to court to block the abortion, while Nancy Klein's husband, Martin, pressed for it. Martin prevailed and physicians aborted her fetus while protestors chanted outside. After 11 months, Nancy emerged from the coma and now lives a normal life.

In 1985, Angela Carder in Washington, D.C., dying of a rare form of cancer, requested chemotherapy and resisted a Cesarean section to save her 26-week-old fetus. The baby was delivered alive anyway, but died two hours later. Angela died two days later.[42]

Both cases raised the issue of who was the patient, the mother or the fetus. Legally, the answer is clear. A fetus inside the womb is not a baby and not a person, but the mother is a person, so her wishes rule. But ethically, things become murky *if* either the mother is going to die or *if* the fetus is going to be born. But these "ifs" are difficult to know in advance.

A flashpoint for maternal–child conflict concerns pregnant mothers using alcohol or illegal drugs. Fetal alcohol syndrome causes the most mental retardation in children.[43] Between 1987 and 1992, 160 women in 24 states were charged with injuring a fetus during pregnancy by taking drugs such as cocaine.[44]

In 1993, the law tried to force Comelia Whitner to stop using cocaine for the good of her fetus, forcing her to choose between mandatory drug rehabilitation and jail. The South Carolina Supreme Court upheld the law in *Whitner v. South Carolina (1997)*.

Critics said the law prosecuted pregnant African-American women using cocaine, but not pregnant white women drinking alcohol, and claimed that prosecutors exaggerated harm to the fetus during gestation from cocaine. Defenders of the law estimated that 70,000 American women used cocaine while pregnant and agreed that pregnant women abusing alcohol, whether Caucasian or African-American, should also be prosecuted. Some wanted to prosecute smoking during pregnancy.

## Viability

In 1983, Justice Sandra Day O'Connor predicted that medicine would push viability "further back toward conception" and that the trimester system established in *Roe v. Wade* would be on a collision course with itself. Her prediction has not come true.

Although medicine has made intense efforts to treat premature babies more effectively, the consensus in neonatology is that "before 23 or 24 weeks, [the fetus] simply cannot survive. And nothing that medical science can do will budge that boundary in the foreseeable future."[45] The unsolvable problem is that even with a respirator, the lungs are too immature to function earlier than at 23 or 24 weeks of gestation, and certain essential organs, such as the kidneys, do not develop early in pregnancy.

This recently acknowledged fact weakens one argument against abortion. Clearly, the argument from marginal cases must lose some of its force, since lung viability has served for over 30 years as a practical indicator of viability and as a mark of when a state can outlaw abortion.

In 1979, in *Colautti v. Franklin*, the Supreme Court made its major decision about viability. It said that "the determination of whether a particular fetus is viable is, and must be, a matter for the judgment of the responsible attending physician," thus precluding another case like Kenneth Edelin's.

## The Supreme Court Fine-Tunes *Roe v. Wade*

In the decades since *Roe v. Wade*, abortion-rights advocates have pressed for broader protection and anti-abortion forces have mounted legal challenges to the original decision. All of this came to a head in 1992 with the Supreme Court's decision in *Planned Parenthood v. Casey*. The Court reaffirmed the "essential holding" of *Roe v. Wade*, including "the right of a woman to choose to have an abortion before viability and to obtain it without undue interference from the State."[46] This decision appeared to say, "Here we stand on abortion, and we will hear no more cases challenging it." Since then, the Court turned down cases aimed at challenging *Roe v. Wade*. However, over the last decades, it has fine-tuned *Roe v. Wade*.

In 1976, in *Planned Parenthood v. Danforth*, the Court invalidated state laws requiring a woman to get consent for an abortion from either a matrimonial or a biological father. The Court held that such consent amounted to giving these men a veto over the woman's decision.

The *Danforth* decision also said that a state couldn't pass a law giving parents of teenage girls an absolute veto over a decision to have an abortion. Two later decisions allowed a state, before a teenager's abortion, to require the minor to obtain the *consent* of one or both parents, or required the clinic to *notify* one or both parents. By 2006, 44 states had laws requiring a parent's consent or notification when minors sought abortions, although nine of those states did not enforce their laws.[47] Such laws had to have an escape clause where the minor could appeal to a judge for an exception to parental notification or consent.

In *Harris v. McRae* (1980), the Court held that, although a woman has a right to an abortion, she does not have a right to one at government expense. Congress passed laws banning use of public funds for abortions for women unable to afford them, and many states followed suit. *Webster* (1989) said that states may ban public employees or public hospitals from performing abortions.

In *Casey* in 1992, the Court ruled that informed consent and a 24-hour waiting period did not constitute an "undue burden" on women seeking abortions. Anti-abortionists said this change brought abortion into line with informed-consent requirements for other surgical procedures. Pro-choice advocates pointed out that many surgical procedures would not occur if hospitals enforced a similar 24-hour waiting period.

As said, *Casey* signaled a pivotal affirmation of "the essential holding" of *Roe v. Wade*, that the right to abortion is grounded in the Constitution and a majority of justices repeated what a previous Court had said in *Eisenstadt v. Baird*, "If the right of privacy means anything, it is the right of the individual, married or single, to be free from unwarranted governmental intrusion into matters so fundamentally affecting a person as the decision whether to bear or beget a child."

## Partial Birth Abortions

Critics define as a "partial birth abortion" one that is performed in the third tri-mester or especially, just before birth. The phrase connotes the advanced state of the fetus, and how, even on the gradient view, it is almost a person.

The rights of late-term fetuses arise in murders of pregnant mothers (for example, Lacy Peterson) and abortions in the late third trimester. Killing a preg-nant woman and her child is a heinous crime, and to inflict greater punishments, people advocate for a charge of double homicide. Similarly, few reasons justify killing a fetus after eight months of gestation, and the methods to do so are grim and surgical.

Opponents of abortion hope that everyone can agree to protect fetuses from such acts and push for changes in the law to do so. Pro-choice advocates oppose such legal changes, fearing a slippery slope to protecting the fetus from abortion at earlier stages.

State legislatures frequently have passed bills making such changes, but fed-eral courts have struck them down 18 out of 19 times.[48] Why? Because a long legal tradition has defined a baby as created at birth, not before, with only a criminal charge being capable of being made against a baby, and courts have been reluctant to overturn that tradition. To do so would be to go into territory where there is no logical stopping point until before viability.

## States Restrict Abortion Clinics

Faced with 35 years of defeats in federal courts, anti-abortion activists focused on state courts and state legislatures in closing abortion clinics. Activists pres-sured for physicians performing abortions to have admitting privileges at a local hospital, an almost impossible condition for clinics to fulfill because the physi-cian performing the abortions almost always does not live in the area (to avoid people picketing his house or trying to shoot him). Nor were hospitals likely to give admitting privileges to a physician who did not practice regularly in their area and moreover, most hospitals did not want to get involved with the politics of abortion. Many clinics closed in Alabama, Mississippi, North Carolina, Penn-sylvania, and especially in politically conservative "red" states, forcing pregnant women to travel long distances to get an abortion, to wait 24 hours and stay over-night to watch movies of movements of second-trimester fetuses, and in general, to make it more costly and emotionally traumatic to get abortions.

### FURTHER READING

Kenneth Edelin, *Broken Justice*, Martha's Vineyard, Massachusetts, Pond View Press, 2007.

Francis M. Kamm, *Creation and Abortion*, New York: Oxford University Press, 1992.

Don Marquis, "Why Abortion Is Immoral," *Journal of Philosophy*, vol. 86, 1989, pp. 183–202.

Warren Quinn, "Abortion: Identity and Loss," *Philosophy and Public Affairs*, vol. 13, 1984, pp. 24–54.

Michael Tooley, *Abortion and Infanticide*, New York: Oxford University Press, 1983.

Mary Ann Warren, *Moral Status: Obligations to Persons and Other Living Things*, New York: Oxford University Press, 1997.

## DISCUSSION QUESTIONS

1. If the fetus had slipped out during the procedure and been outside the womb, even attached to an umbilical cord, would it have been illegal to kill it? Should that matter *ethically*?
2. How should "pregnancy" be defined? By formation of a unique embryo in the fallopian tubes or by implantation of an embryo in the uterus?
3. How can anyone ever truly know what's in the mind of another to judge someone by the doctrine of double effect? Someone may say he's trying to save the life (or health) of a pregnant mother, not desiring to end the life of fetus, but who can tell? Isn't this a fault of the doctrine?
4. Fetal sonograms are now being used to give pregnant women vivid pictures of their fetuses in the first and second trimesters. Some women viewing such pictures reverse their decisions to have abortions. Given that fact, should all women planning abortions be required to view such live images?
5. Some women regret having abortions. What weight should we give such regrets in public policy about abortion?
6. Is a fetus necessarily a person at birth? What's so magical about birth? Maybe, even on a gradient view, we should not declare personhood until much later, say, six months.
7. "God must want me to be pregnant or I wouldn't be." Is this a fair view?

# CHAPTER 6

# Assisted Reproduction, Multiple Births, and Elderly Parents

$B$etween 1978, which saw the world's first test tube baby, and 2008, which saw "Octamom" Nadya Suleman add to her brood of test-tube-produced kids, assisted reproduction raised many ethical issues. This chapter discusses Louise Brown's birth, surrogate mothers, buying eggs of younger women, the McCaughey septuplets, and older women having children (such as Carmen Bousada, who died at age 69 after giving birth at 66).

## THE OCTAMOM AND THE GOSSELINS

Nadya Suleman, 32 years old of Whittier, California, in 2008 had six embryos left over from previous in-vitro fertilization treatments with fertility physician Michael Kamrava. She did not want the remaining embryos destroyed and underwent another cycle of IVF to have all of them implanted. Two of the six embryos split into twins, resulting in a total of eight embryos. When sonograms in the first trimester revealed at least five fetuses, Suleman refused reduction and on January 26, physicians delivered eight babies.

Much criticism focused on Dr. Kamrava, who implanted Suleman not once but twice with six embryos. He certainly breached the guidelines of the American Society for Reproductive Medicine, which recommends implantation of ideally just one embryo and, permissibly, two. Because Nadya already had children from previous cycles of IVF, and because two of these children were disabled, for Kamrava to implant six more embryos was unethical and likely created even more disabled children.

The year 2009 also saw another bad situation involving Kate and Jon Gosselin in suburban Pennsylvania. A labor-and-delivery nurse and a network engineer, the two married in 2001. The Gosselins had a family of twin girls (born in 2001 from artificial insemination by husband or "AIH") when sextuplets (three girls and three boys) were born to them in 2004. Fertility doctors started the sextuplets by injecting Kate with drugs to stimulate her ovaries and afterward, introduced Jon's sperm. Informed of six pregnancies, the Gosselins chose not to reduce and all six babies were delivered by caesarean in 2004.

*Jon & Kate Plus 8* filmed the controlled chaos of this family of 10 and became a hit show in 2007 on cable television. Putting the kids on television also glamorized having multiple babies. Shortly after birth, a plastic surgeon did free plastic surgery to correct the distortion of Kate's stomach from gestating six babies.

In 2009, after both had extra-marital affairs, the Gosselins divorced. Thereafter, Jon seemed to abandon his responsibilities as a father. Both parents seemed immature and not focused on the best interests of their eight children. Kate went on television in 2010 on *Dancing with the Stars* and had the kids on new reality TV shows, *Twist of Kate* plus updates called *Kate Plus 8*, but in 2011, low ratings sank the shows and in subsequent years, Kate scrambled as a single mother to find the money to raise eight kids.

Meanwhile, Nadya Suleman wanted her own reality show, but it didn't happen. She began to work occasionally in the adult entertainment industry. In 2012, she filed for personal bankruptcy; authorities auctioned her $1 million home; her children lived on public assistance; and she spent a month in rehab for addiction to Xanax.

## BACKGROUND: LOUISE BROWN, THE FIRST TEST TUBE BABY

Test tube conception is the popular name for in vitro fertilization (IVF). ("In vitro" means "in glass.") It involves fertilization outside the womb, in a Petri dish.

Lesley Brown, the mother of the first child conceived in vitro, had damaged fallopian tubes from ectopic pregnancies. For her IVF, scientists removed one of her eggs and placed it in a Petri dish, where they mixed her husband John's sperm to form an embryo. With the embryo returned to her uterus, Lesley then carried it to normal gestation.

In such development, sperm move up the vagina, through the uterus, and into one of the narrow fallopian tubes. The two tubes, the size of the lead in a mechanical pencil, can each carry an egg from an ovary to the uterus.

A woman has all her eggs at birth, but only one egg is normally primed for conception each month. Drugs such as Clomid and Pergonal stimulate the ovaries to release more than one egg, a process called *superovulation*.

In at least 40 percent of pregnancies, and possibly as many as 70 percent, the embryo fails to implant on the wall of the uterus, often because of genetic irregularities. More commonly, the mix of hormones is not quite correct.

After one year of trying, about one married couple in 11 cannot conceive a child. Infertility stems from many factors, including a woman's age, damage from pelvic inflammatory disease, previous abortions, uterine abnormalities, and low sperm count or low sperm motility. Infertility is often blamed on the woman, but men account for 50 percent of it.

Two decades of research by Robert Edwards, a physiologist at Cambridge University, preceded the first IVF birth. Edwards' work with mice in the 1950s had taught him how to precisely balance hormones to induce ovulation.

In 1965, 13 years before the birth of Louise Brown, Edwards created a human embryo after adding his own semen to a ripe human egg in a Petri dish.[1] Edwards thereby fulfilled one of the great fears about scientists: lone scientist late at night in his lab artificially creates human life, stealing mystery from creation. Perhaps

Edwards realized people would be frightened by his feat, so he destroyed the embryo. Later, he tried to repeat it, but could not. Nor did he announce to others what he had done.

In his research, Edwards needed to create many embryos and returned only the healthiest to the uterus. To do so, he needed eggs from female volunteers. Enter Patrick Steptoe, a gynecologic surgeon practicing in a small hospital near Manchester, who became Edwards' partner. Steptoe used a newly created laparascope (a long thin tube containing a lens with a light) to remove the eggs.

Over the next decade, the duo attempted IVF many times. In the first phase, they implanted an embryo 41 times in a fallopian tube, but each time, it failed to go farther. In the next phase, they recruited a hundred infertile female volunteers and implanted an embryo directly into the uterus of each. Their 102nd attempt resulted in Louise Brown.

In 1977, Dr. Steptoe told Lesley she was pregnant. Before this, some women had had eggs successfully fertilized in vitro, but all had lost the embryo. Lesley made it to five months, and her amniocentesis showed a normal pregnancy (if it had been abnormal, Steptoe would have aborted it). She spent the last month of her pregnancy at Oldham Hospital under siege by the media.

Steptoe delivered the baby, a girl, by cesarean section on July 25, 1978. In order to avoid reporters, he operated around midnight with only a few people present.

The Browns called the normal, 5-pound, 12-ounce girl Louise Joy, who the father said was "beautiful, with a marvelous complexion, not red and wrinkly at all."[2] Immediately after the birth, John Brown said, "For a person who's been told he and his wife can never have children, the pregnancy was 'like a miracle.' I felt 12 feet high."

For Louise Brown's birth, London newspapers ran huge banner headlines, "IT'S A GIRL!" "THE LOVELY LOUISE!" "BABY OF THE CENTURY! JOY TO THE WORLD!"

One competitor who had hoped to be first to deliver an IVF infant dismissed Steptoe's achievement as a "cheap stunt." Another criticized Steptoe for not revealing how many failures had preceded his success and for giving "false hope to millions of women."[3] But they missed the point: Louise Brown mattered not because of her improbability, but because she proved that IVF could succeed.

Patrick Steptoe died at age 74 in 1988, a week before Queen Elizabeth II was to have knighted him at Buckingham Place. The same week, Robert Edwards became a Fellow of the Royal Society, a great honor in the English scientific community.

Louise Brown's mother chose to have a second child, Natalie, by IVF in 1982. In 1993, the three female Browns appeared on American television to support research in assisted reproduction. At age 15, Louise was a chubby girl whose friends teased, "How did you ever fit into a test tube?" In 2004, she married, with Edwards attending her wedding. Her naturally conceived son was born on December 20, 2006. Robert Edwards died at age 87 in 2013.

## HARM TO RESEARCH FROM ALARMIST MEDIA

New ways of making babies have always fascinated the media, whose approaches to this subject have ranged from alarmist to naively uncritical.

Warren Kornberg, editor of *Science News*, wrote in a 1969 op-ed in the *Los Angeles Times* that questions about assisted reproduction, cloning, and human genetics raised questions "more important" than those raised by nuclear weapons.[4]

In his early years, Edwards worked on infertility at the National Institute for Medical Research in London. A television show on IVF opened with pictures of an exploding atomic bomb and the institute then suspended his funding. Edwards claims that his scientific supervisor, who had also frozen sperm, flatly told him his work was "unethical"; when asked "Why?" she only replied, "Because it is."[5]

Edwards left for Cambridge University, where he worked on a Ford Foundation grant to study population control and fertility. Because his work offended some people, the Ford Foundation stopped funding him in 1974.

The press incorrectly called Louise Brown a "test tube baby." This term implied something bizarre—that a baby had been created without egg or sperm. When Lesley first took her baby outside, neighbors expected to see a little monster.

The press equated means of overcoming infertility with genetic manipulation and, as with cloning later, predicted creation of mindless slaves or dangerous superhumans. The *London Times* equated in vitro fertilization with state-controlled eugenics. In contrast, John Brown saw IVF as "helping nature along a bit."

Newspapers and television shows constantly compared IVF to Aldous Huxley's 1932 novel *Brave New World*. Yet most had not read the book: The controls that Huxley feared stemmed from psychological conditioning. *Brave New World* worries about behaviorism, a school of psychology then as poorly understood as IVF was in 1978. Although Huxley wrote *Brave New World* to dramatize the evil of taking away choice from citizens, people cited his novel as advocating taking away choice.

## LATER DEVELOPMENTS IN ASSISTED REPRODUCTION

The first IVF baby in America, Elizabeth Carr, was born in 1981. In 500 clinics, American fertility physicians now deliver about 58,000 babies a year from IVF and IVF has helped create about 4 million babies worldwide.[6]

Only 5 percent of babies today conceived by assisted reproductive technology (ART) result from IVF. Less dramatic techniques create most ART babies, such as egg stimulation and injection of concentrated sperm.

Unfortunately, for most of the last three decades, about 75 percent of couples who pay for cycles of IVF spend from $13,000 to $100,000 and go home without a baby. In 2002, fertility clinics claimed that about 23 percent of attempts at IVF allowed couples to have a baby, although the actual figure may be more like 20 percent.[7] Chances worsen for women over 40 and drop with each unsuccessful attempt, from 13 percent on the first to 4 percent on the fourth.[8] At age 43, chances drop to almost zero. We read a lot about successful IVF, but hardly anything about all the couples for whom it fails.[9]

### Sperm and Egg Transfer

**Sperm.** Around 1850, physician J. Marion Sims, while practicing in Montgomery, Alabama, artificially inseminated 55 infertile women with their husbands' sperm

(AIH).[10] He produced one pregnancy, though it later miscarried. Condemnation of his work by other physicians forced him to stop. In the 1890s in America, critics vilified Dr. Robert Latou Dickinson for practicing AIH, accusing him of abetting "adultery."[11]

It took another century for people to accept artificial insemination of sperm. Had Sims *paid* his first sperm donor, his critics would have been legion. The net result? Hundreds, maybe thousands, of couples in America and Europe remained infertile, blaming each other for being barren, going childless not by choice but by fate.

Today, most people accept insemination of sperm. Indeed, Americans have gone from accepting (1) artificial insemination (AI) of a husband's (AIH) sperm into the wife's womb, to (2) insemination of another donor's (AID) sperm into a woman's womb, to (3) paying a man for use of his sperm to create a pregnancy, to (4) insemination of anonymous donor sperm into unmarried women wishing to become pregnant, to (5) selection of sperm from a catalog of pictures of men listing their achievements. Today, couples and single women can select sperm from men at about 400 sperm banks, where sperm donors receive between $50 and $75 per visit or where they have donated their sperm free.

**Eggs**   Australia's Carl Woods in 1983 created the first human pregnancy from an egg transfer. In the next 15 years, 6,000 middle-aged women gave birth using eggs from young women.[12]

In the 1980s, scientists began *gamete intrafallopian transfer (GIFT)*, which unites sperm and egg not in a Petri dish but inside a fallopian tube, approximately where normal conception takes place. A Belgian group in 1993 succeeded in using a single sperm to fertilize an egg, a process called *intracytoplasmic sperm injection (ICSI)*, making it possible for one sperm to be used to achieve a pregnancy.[13]

The world's first IVF child conceived with a younger woman's egg occurred in California in 1984, but then eggs had to be removed cumbersomely under anesthesia. The end of that decade saw another technological breakthrough when a thin needle guided by ultrasound retrieved the eggs by going through a vaginal wall.[14] That 10-minute procedure under light anesthesia could be done in offices, not operating rooms of hospitals, and changed the industry. By 1990, with a new, steady supply of young eggs, fertility doctors showed that many older women could gestate embryos.[15]

Because of assisted conception of twins to celebrities such to Celine Dion at 42, Geena Davis at 48, Jane Seymour at 44, Holly Hunter at 47, and singletons in their 30s to Christie Brinkley and Angelina Jolie, today's young women too often believe they can wait to become mothers until their 30s. Most celebrities don't disclose their use of egg donors or how many failed IVF cycles they had (Celine Dion had five before her twins). Only 8 percent of women at age 43 will have children with their own eggs because 90 percent of their eggs will be abnormal.[16]

But a woman over 40 can gestate embryos created from eggs of younger women, giving the older woman a biological connection to the baby, creating a *bio-genetic child*, one connected biologically and genetically to two different females. About 10 percent of IVF attempts today use such eggs. This works for women who have severe genetic diseases in their families, who have eggs damaged by chemotherapy or poisoning, who have had several miscarriages, or who suffer from premature menopause.

Scientists once thought age of sperm or age of gestational mothers caused infertility, but these can be overcome. The absolute barrier to successful gestation is age of the egg, with rapid drop-offs as eggs deteriorate in women over age 31. As said, an even bigger drop-off occurs for women over age 43.

Young eggs in older surrogates make a big difference. Using egg transfer, the success rate for taking a baby home jumps to 60–80 percent, and more important, 30 percent *regardless of the age of the female gestator*, making egg donation the great hope for many infertile couples.

## FREEZING GAMETE MATERIAL

In 1997, the first birth using previously frozen human embryos occurred at an Atlanta clinic run by Bruce Tucker.[17] In 1990, two embryos were created from different eggs at a California clinic.[18] One was implanted and became a baby; the other remained frozen. Seven-and-a-half years later, doctors implanted the second embryo and it became a male fraternal twin to his 7-year-old brother. Emma Davis was an IVF baby born in Britain in 1989; her sister, Niamh, also created as an embryo in 1989, was born 16 years later in 2006.[19] The record for such siblings created together by IVF but born apart is 21 years.

In 2002, a California clinic began to freeze eggs of young women about to undergo hysterectomy but who wanted to later bear children.[20] In 2007, other clinics similarly froze ovarian tissue for women who wanted to preserve or delay childbearing.[21] Questions remain about how viable these eggs/tissue will be after thawing.

When scientists store embryos and sperm, mishaps can occur. In the 1990s, a white Dutch couple had non-identical twins, one of them black. In 2002, a white couple in London had black twins because scientists implanted the wrong embryos. (We'll never know how many embryos got mixed up between same-ethnicity couples.)

Keeping embryos frozen costs couples $200 a year and creates ethical dilemmas for originating couples.[22] Some couples do not want their embryos destroyed, but also do not want them donated to other couples or used for research.

On the criminal side, IVF pioneer physician Cecil Jacobsen of Fairfax, Virginia, used his own sperm instead of the intended fathers' to create as many as 75 embryos throughout the 1980s. In 1992, he went to jail for this. In the mid-1990s, Dr. Ricardo Asch at UC Irvine was caught switching donor eggs around without women's consent and fled the country to avoid prosecution.

In 2013, physicians pioneered the use of the EmbryoScope, which allows fertility doctors to use high-resolution photos to monitor the dynamic development of individual embryos day-by-day in real time, thus enabling them to pick the very best embryo for implantation and reducing the need for implanting more than one embryo. A study in Manchester, England, showed that the EmbryoScope could raise success rates by 50 percent.[23]

## PAYMENT FOR ASSISTED REPRODUCTION:
## EGG DONORS

Originally, young volunteers supplied eggs for older women, but altruism didn't meet the demand. Paying for eggs is euphemistically called "egg donation," and in America in 2006, egg donors earned on average $4,217.[24]

Egg retrieval is more complicated than obtaining sperm. A woman takes drugs daily for a month or more to induce superovulation, after which eggs are aspirated as previously explained. Some people claim that the drugs increase risk of some cancers over the life of the woman, but no long-term data support this claim.

In 1999, a famous ad ran in newspapers at Princeton and Yale universities stating that an anonymous couple would pay $50,000 for the eggs of a "woman over six feet tall and with SAT scores over 1450."[25] Payment also runs high for donors of Jewish or Asian background, because they donate less frequently.

Critics rarely complained when clinics paid males to donate sperm, even though genetically, sperm and eggs are both gametes and contain the same amount of genetic information. Critics condemn only payment of women for eggs.

## PAYMENT FOR ASSISTED REPRODUCTION:
## ADOPTION

Because roughly 1 out of 11 couples in North America is infertile after a year of trying to conceive, and because in vitro fertilization works for only 20 couples out of 100, infertile couples create high demand for healthy, adoptable babies. Because most such couples in North America are white and want a white child, demand for healthy, white babies has skyrocketed.

Because of this demand, the average couple in 2002 seeking to adopt a baby paid agencies $20,000. In their quest for a healthy toddler, some couples paid $100,000. Other couples paid on average $22,000 for a Vietnamese baby, $17,000 for a Chinese baby, and $8,000 or less for a black baby.[26]

Like transfer of eggs or organs, agencies do not technically sell babies, which is illegal. But a new industry has sprung up that connects couples to pregnant women who might put their babies up for adoption. According to one investigative journalist, "That has left only the thinnest line between buying a child and buying adoption services that lead to a child."[27] The doubling of licensed child placement has increased adoptions in North America in the last few years to nearly 2,000.

In 1993, Russia had no foreign adoptions, but in 2001, it placed more children in America than any other country (990). Because of alleged abuse of adoptees, including claims by an 18-year-old adopted teenager who returned after five years, Russia in 2013 banned adoption by Americans, creating a scarcity of adoptable babies. In 2011, the other top countries for adoption (and number adopted) were Ethiopia (448), South Korea (280), China (278), Taiwan (88), Congo (48), and Columbia (41).[28]

Although black critics have recently decried the lesser payments that seem to demean black babies, virtually no one has condemned payment itself. No one has criticized "pregnancy counseling centers" that encourage pregnant girls to give up their babies for adoption, while charging lucrative fees to couples who adopt those babies.

## Paid Surrogacy: The Baby M and Jaycee Cases

Fertilization of embryos outside the womb made it possible for another woman to gestate an embryo to birth, creating so-called surrogate mothers, either for pay or altruistically. For short, we'll call them surrogates.

By 1986, several hundred women had helped infertile women gestate babies when biochemist Bill Stern and pediatrician Elizabeth Stern hired Mary Beth Whitehead for $10,000 to gestate an embryo created by his sperm and White-head's egg through artificial insemination. Giving birth on March 27, 1986, in Monmouth County Medical Center in Long Branch, New Jersey, Mrs. Whitehead claimed to have bonded with the Baby M, aka Melissa Stern, and refused to give her to the Sterns. When Mr. Stern threatened legal action, Mrs. Whitehead fled to Florida with Melissa, but was discovered and returned to New Jersey.

At the lower court trial in 1987, Judge Harvey Sorkow upheld the contract, said it did not constitute baby selling, required Whitehead to hand over the baby, awarded her $10,000, and decided it would be best for the baby never to see Mrs. Whitehead again. The New Jersey Supreme Court in 1998 unanimously reversed his decision, declared Mrs. Whitehead the legal mother with full visiting rights, and invalidated surrogacy contracts. Mrs. Whitehead later became a well-known critic of surrogacy. Melissa graduated from George Washington University and then wrote a Master's thesis on children of surrogacy at King's College in London, where she now lives

Several states reacted to the Baby M case by criminalizing commercial surrogacy; some laws are still in effect in 2010. Arkansas, Florida, Ohio, Virginia, Nevada, and New Hampshire legally recognized paid surrogacy. At least 26 states have no law about surrogacy. California, which has many paid surrogates, recognizes a series of decisions in case law that regulate paid surrogacy.[29]

Jaycee Buzzanca, aka "the child with five parents," was born in March 1995 from a paid surrogate and became embroiled in a divorce between the parents who hired the surrogate. Jaycee was also conceived from sperm and egg other than from the parents who hired the surrogate. A California Appeals court ruled in 1998 that the parents who had hired the surrogate were legally responsible for him.

A common objection to paid surrogacy is that it's not best for the child. Paying for gestation creates a confused identity for a child who has at least three, and maybe five, parents. On the other hand, most cases of surrogacy do not involve so many parents.

In 2013, surrogate Crystal Kelley made national news when she refused to abort the fetus she carried because it had severe heart defects, a cleft palate, and a cyst in its brain.[30] After multiple surgeries after birth, surgeons told the donor parents that the baby would have only about a 25 percent chance of a normal life. The donors had contracted to pay Kelley $22,000 for the surrogacy and the contract contained a clause requiring abortion in case of gross defects of fetus.

They offered her $10,000 to abort, but Kelley refused. Then the donors sued to get their already-paid $8,000 back and refused to be the legal parents if a child was born. Kelley continued the pregnancy.

Baby S at birth had worse problems than previously imagined: *holoprosencephaly*, where the brain fails to completely divide into distinct hemispheres, and *heterotaxy*, in which many organs develop in the wrong places. A Michigan couple adopted Baby S, who has had multiple surgeries, paid for by Medicaid at the University of Michigan Medical Center.

## MULTIPLE BIRTHS: BEFORE THE OCTAMOM AND GOSSELINS

Although the Octamom and Gosselins made news in 2009, multiples and their problems have a sad history.

Births of multiples have been growing steadily since the birth of Louise Brown in 1978, For most couples without reimbursement for in vitro fertilization, the easiest way to overcome infertility is to take the drug Clomid, and if that doesn't work, Pergonal or Metrodin, to stimulate the ovaries to release many eggs at the same time. The problem then is that introduction of sperm can fertilize one, two, or eight eggs.

In vitro fertilization, in contrast, allows physicians to control how many embryos they implant.

In 1985, a Mormon couple, Patti and Sam Frustaci, conceived septuplets but refused to have such a reduction, so four of their seven babies died; the three survivors had severe disabilities, including cerebral palsy.

In 1987 and with the help of Pergonal, Ron and Roz Helms of Peoria, Illinois, had quintuplets. One child spent a year in a neonatal intensive care unit (NICU), another had seizures, and a third has cerebral palsy. The quints' medical bills for their first decade topped $3 million.

Multiple-birth babies are usually premature (each may weigh less than two pounds), three times as likely to be severely handicapped at birth, and often spend months in NICUs.

During gestation, nutrients and oxygenated blood in the womb are scarce (a uterine lifeboat, if you will); thus, not all seven fetuses will likely emerge healthy. To prevent disabilities resulting from uterine deprivation, physicians recommend selective reduction of all but one or two embryos.

In 1996 in England, after taking the fertility drugs Merton and Pregnyl for two days, Mandy Allwood released seven eggs, had sex, and all of her eggs were fertilized. Four months later, a London tabloid offered her a large payment for exclusive rights to her story if, and only if, all her embryos made it to term. This began a pattern of exploitation of mothers of multiples by the media. Mandy announced she would not reduce any embryos and would go for maximal births. As a result, she lost all seven.

In 1997, Denise Amen and her husband were offered the chance to reduce five growing embryos but refused. One of their quintuplets was born blind and others are "developmentally slow."[31]

In 1997, an Iowa couple, Bobbi and Kenny McCaughey, used Pergonal to superovulate Bobbi and introduced Kenny's sperm, conceiving seven embryos, refused to reduce any, and choose to risk having disabled babies. They said that the results were God's will.

At their fourth birthday in 2001, the McCaughey septuplets lagged in development and were not all potty trained. Joel suffered seizures; Nathan had spastic diplegia, a form of cerebral palsy requiring botox injections (to paralyze spastic muscles) and orthopedic braces. Alexis had hypotonic quadriplegia, a cerebral palsy that causes muscle weakness. After two major orthopedic surgeries, at age 7, Nathan still could not walk. For four years, Alexis had an indwelling feeding tube. Although they homeschooled, the McCaugheys in 2006 began to send Nathan and Alexis to a public school for developmentally challenged children.[32]

In 1997, Jacqueline Thompson had sextuplets in Washington, D.C. After the death of one child, the mother today struggles to raise five teenagers.[33] Unlike the McCaugheys', this single black mother's story drew scant media attention, no offers of television appearances or reality shows, and few donations by volunteers or companies.

In 1998, octuplets—six girls and two boys—were born to Nigeria-born American citizens Nkem Chukwu, age 27, and Iyke Louis Udobi, 41. In 2009, the Chukwus tried to tour the world with their eight 10-year-old children under their self-chosen theme, "Promote Healthy Families," but their tour did not garner fame and donations similar to those generated by the Gosselins, the Octamom, or the McCaugheys.

The probability of an impaired baby varies directly with the number of embryos allowed to gestate. In other words, if six are implanted, one is almost certain to be born with cerebral palsy or blindness. Unfortunately, the chance of having any baby at all also varies directly with the number of embryos implanted—hence, the ethical dilemma of how many embryos *should* be implanted.

## OLDER PARENTS

As said, by using eggs of younger women and ICSI, older people can create their own children. In 1980, Carl Woods accepted a 42-year-old woman as his first IVF candidate because of her increased chances of birth defects. She had a normal baby.

In 1993, a 59-year-old Englishwoman gestated twins from embryos fertilized by her husband's sperm and eggs donated by a young woman. In 1998 and at age 57, American Judy Cates did the same.[34]

In 1990, one-third of American Assisted Reproduction (AR) clinics excluded women over 40. By 1998, the practice of using eggs of younger women had moved such limits to age 55.

Several births pushed this debate into public consciousness. In 1997, after lying about her age, 63-year-old Arceh Keh gave birth to a healthy baby girl. In 2005, 66-year-old Adriana Iliescu gave birth to a healthy baby daughter in Romania. In 2004, two 57-year-old women, Aleta Saint James, unmarried, and Rosee Swain, a great-grandmother, gave birth to twins using IVF and eggs from younger women.

In 2007, at age 67 and after having lied about her age at a fertility clinic in Los Angeles, Maria Carmen del Bousada gave birth to twins in Barcelona, Spain. Two years later, she died of cancer, leaving two orphans.

Should society encourage seniors to have children when they may be dead before their children reach 18? In 1968, at age 66, Senator Strom Thurmond married a 22-year-old former Miss South Carolina and had four children with her (he died at age 100 in 2003). Actor Tony Randall fathered a daughter in 1997 at age 77 (he died at age 89 in 2005). Should fertility clinics place restrictions on women that they don't place on men?

One answer focuses on the best interests of the children. Regardless of whether it's a man or a woman, is it in a child's best interest to be a newborn of a parent approaching 70? How likely is it that the elderly parent will be around for the child's senior prom, let alone grade school graduation? Certainly being orphaned at age 2 is not ideal for the Bousada twins, and Adriana Iliescu will be unlikely to see her daughter's 18th birthday. Moreover, raising children takes energy and vigor, qualities that diminish rapidly in the senior years.

Given these facts, are 70-year-old seniors vain in having children? Or selfish, in wanting something to cherish, carry on one's name, or possibly, take care of one in old age? Shouldn't we make it illegal for them to have children so late?

## GENDER SELECTION

Because X chromosomes weigh more than Y chromosomes, a modified flow cytometer called Microsort can separate heavier from lighter sperm, producing accurate results 90 percent of the time.[35] Although intended for use in preimplantation genetic diagnosis, Microsort may be used to select male babies.

Gender selection has been an issue in countries such as China, the Republic of Korea, and India. For centuries there, parents have seen females as less desirable than males. Using sonograms, many families there aborted female fetuses to try again for a male child.

Despite laws that ban testing for sex in India and China, at least 60 million females there are missing. After decades of such practices in China, in 2001, 20- to 44-year-old never-married men outnumber two-to-one their female counterparts, who are sometimes kidnapped and sold into marriage. By 2020, one million excess Chinese males will seek to marry.[36]

Sex selection is sexist and leads to imbalances of the sexes in the population, as happened in China. Perhaps it, too, should be banned.

## ETHICAL ISSUES

### Unnatural

In 1978, the year of Louise Brown's birth, the Vatican condemned in vitro fertilization and has not changed its position since. Its *Instructions* of 1987 equated IVF with "domination" and "manipulation of nature."[37] In 2008, in "Dignity of the Person," it emphasized that children should be created only through sexual intercourse of a married couple.[38] The document bans IVF, freezing embryos, and screening them genetically.

Paul Ramsey, a famous, socially conservative Protestant theologian at Princeton University, in 1970 equated IVF with genetic manipulation and predicted societal horrors from it. He implied that if physicians could find a tiny egg and fertilize it, why couldn't they alter its genes?[39] He predicted that if they could, they would, and he held that if they did, it would be sinful.

Ramsey came up with some provocative phrases suggesting vague but disturbing harms to society: "test tube babies," "dial-a-baby," "playing God." He was especially good at creating neologisms for rhetorical effect: "mercenary gestation," "supermarket of embryos," "spare-parts man" (a hypothetical cloned twin grown for this purpose and kept unconscious), "celebrity seed" (sperm banks), "human species suicide" (eliminating genetic diseases).

When Lesley Brown was several months pregnant, Robert Edwards attended a symposium on the ethics of IVF at Washington's Kennedy Institute for Bioethics at the invitation of Sargeant Shriver. While senators, national columnists, and other scientists listened, Ramsey condemned IVF and Edwards. As Edwards described it:

> He had to be seen and heard to be believed. I had to endure a denunciation of our work as if from some nineteenth-century pulpit. It was delivered with a Gale 8 force, and written in a similar vein a year later in the *Journal of the American Medical Association*. He doubted that our patients had given their fully understanding consent. We ignored the sanctity of life. We carried out immoral experiments on the unborn. Our work was, he thundered, "unethical medical experimentation on possible future human beings and therefore it is subject to absolute moral prohibition." I was as much surprised as made wrathful by this impertinent scorching attack. He abused everything I stood for.[40]

Ramsey condemned IVF not based on its possible harmful consequences to the child, to the parents, or to society, but rather, and in a view that resurfaced twenty years later, from the idea of wronging the embryo-person. IVF is wrong in itself, Ramsey held, because it is "unconsented-to experimentation" on a person, the embryo."[41]

During the 1970s, then Episcopal priest Joseph Fletcher defended IVF against the claim that it was unnatural:

> It is depressing, not comforting, to realize that most people are accidents. Their conception was at best unintended, at worst unwanted. There are those who are so bemused and befuddled by a fatalist mystique about nature with a capital N (or "God's will") that they want us to accept passively whatever comes along. Talk of "not tinkering" and "not playing God" and snide remarks about "artificial" and "technological" policies is a vote against both humanness and humaneness.[42]

For Fletcher, each kind of case should be considered on its own merits to see if it would help or hurt humanity; society must not be locked into antiquated religious prohibitions that take no account of consequences. Religion is best when it is "pro people," not when it worships abstract "thou shall not's":

The real choice is between accidental or random reproduction and rationally willed or chosen reproduction. . . . Laboratory reproduction is radically human compared to conception by ordinary heterosexual intercourse. It is willed, chosen, purposed and controlled, and surely those are among the traits that distinguish Homo sapiens from others in the animal genus, from the primates down.[43]

In part because he disagreed so much with the views of conservative Christianity, Fletcher gave up the priesthood around 1980 and became a secular thinker, becoming one of the first secular bioethicists.

## PHYSICAL HARM TO BABIES CREATED IN NEW WAYS

Many people predicted that the first baby born from in vitro fertilization might be defective. This is understandable because in the 1940s, an Italian researcher named Petrucci had claimed to have fertilized a human egg in vitro, grown it for 29 days, and then destroyed it because it was "monstrous." Petrucci's story fueled fears about monsters, though he never gave evidence for his claims.[44]

At Louise Brown's birth, one obstetrician emphasized that severely defective babies could be created, and that "the potential is there for serious anomalies should an unqualified scientist mishandle an embryo."[45] Another obstetrician said, "What if we got a cyclops? Who is responsible? The parents? Is the government obligated to take care of it?"[46]

Leon Kass, later chair in 2002 of the George W. Bush Bioethics Commission, warned, "It doesn't matter how many times the baby is tested while in the mother's womb," he averred, "they will never be certain the baby won't be born without defect."[47] Without the certainty of a normal baby, Kass condemned all experimental conception.

Some Nobel Prize winners surprisingly condemned experimental methods of conception. James Watson feared that deformed babies would be born and that they would need to be raised in custodial homes or killed.[48] (Watson later recanted.) Max Perutz, who won a Nobel in chemistry, agreed:

I agree entirely with Dr. Watson that this is far too great a risk. Even if only a single abnormal baby is born and has to be kept alive as an invalid for the rest of its life, Dr. Edwards would have a terrible guilt upon his shoulders. The idea that this might happen on a larger scale—new thalidomide catastrophe—is horrifying.[49]

In 1977, in *Who Shall Play God?* alarmist Jeremy Rifkin began three decades of opposition to new reproductive techniques. Rifkin decried assisted reproduction as evil "genetic engineering," which he defined as "artificial manipulation of life."

Socially conservative, pioneering bioethicist Dan Callahan argued that the first case of IVF was "probably unethical" because no one could guarantee that Louise Brown would be normal, though scientists could ethically proceed after Louise's healthy birth. He added that many medical breakthroughs are "unethical" because we cannot guarantee that the first patients will not be harmed—implying an odd criterion of ethics for medical experiments.[50]

These general arguments do not seem compelling. What these critics overlooked was that no reasonable approach to life can avoid all risks. A highly unlikely result, even if that result is bad, still represents a small risk.

Over the last 35 years, we learned a few things about actual physical harm to IVF babies. Babies conceived through IVF have approximately twice the normal rate of birth defects, around 4 percent overall—instead of the norm of 2 percent.[51] IVF children are at greater risk for Beckwith-Wiedemann syndrome, which causes enlarged organs and cancer in children, and five to seven times more likely to develop retinoblastoma, a rare cancer of the eye.[52] Another study found that 9 percent of babies conceived through IVF or ICSI had birth defects versus 4.2 percent of those naturally conceived. Another American study found that babies conceived through IVF were three times more likely to be born underweight and premature than babies naturally conceived.

One possible cause of these defects may be subtle change in expression of genes caused by IVF that in turn may cause serious genetic damage.[53] Researchers have suggested an IVF registry to track such problems.[54]

A 2012 Australian study suggested that assisted reproduction itself might pose no extra risk and that the increase in defects associated with it were really caused by infertile women previously taking clomiphene citrate (Clomid), having previously conceived embryos with defects, or other factors associated with infertility.[55]

The concept of absolute versus relative risk matters here. Given that the *absolute risk* of an abnormal child overall is small, a slightly increased *relative risk* from IVF conception doesn't matter that much, as couples having IVF babies still have small risks of serious problems.

## PSYCHOLOGICAL HARM TO BABIES CREATED IN NEW WAYS

Jeremy Rifkin first raised the issue not of physical harm but of *psychological harm* by having a new kind of origin:

> What are the psychological implications of growing up as a specimen, sheltered not by a warm womb but by steel and glass, belonging to no one but the lab technician who joined together sperm and egg? In a world already populated with people with identity crises, what's the personal identity of a test-tube baby?[56]

*Psychological trauma* could also come from badly motivated or immature parents, an issue discussed below in connection with the children of Nadya Suleman and the Gosselins.

## PARADOXES ABOUT HARM AND REPRODUCTION

Can children be harmed by in vitro conception? Theologian Hans Tiefel wrote, "No one has the moral right to endanger a child while there is yet the option of whether the child shall come into existence."[57] But can a "being" be harmed when it may not exist?

Call this the *paradox of harm*, the seemingly self-contradictory idea that someone can be harmed by being born. This idea appears to be paradoxical because, first, it seems queer to say that we can harm a being by bringing it into existence; but second, it seems equally odd to say that a mother, who could have prevented harm to her child but did not, did no wrong.

A *paradox* results when two different meanings of a key term are used simultaneously. Paradoxical statements can be dissolved by carefully specifying the different meanings in each part of the statement and deciding which meaning applies to each. With the paradox of harm, any approach to dissolving it must distinguish between different meanings of "harm." Like "good," "harm" covers a broad range of meanings. In law school, such meanings are covered in one of the major courses, *torts*.

Let's distinguish two ways of thinking about harm. In the first, both a baseline and a temporal component are necessary, so that a change occurs that makes someone worse off. In this *baseline harm*, harm requires an adverse change in someone's condition. With the baseline concept, someone who doesn't yet exist cannot be harmed, because there is no baseline from which change can occur. (Consider the old Yiddish joke: 1st—"Life is so terrible! Better to have never existed." 2nd—"True, but who is so lucky? Not one in a thousand.")

In the second way of defining harm, harm involves comparing a present deficient condition with what normally would have been. In this *abnormal harm*, someone can be harmed by being brought into existence with some defect that could have been avoided by taking reasonable precautions. With abnormal harm, the event or omission that causes the defect is the cause of harm. The abnormality concept underlies the belief that women should do everything possible to have healthy, unimpaired babies: That anything less than the maximal effort is blameworthy, and that it is wrong for a woman to take risks with a future person's intelligence or health. To sum up these two concepts of harm:

> **Baseline Harm**. Requires a starting point (baseline) from which an adverse change is plotted; that is, it requires an existing being who is made worse off.
> **Abnormal Harm**. Requires a norm of development that is not met, for example, because of a doctor's actions or omissions while a woman is carrying a fetus.

In *wrongful life* cases in the courts, it is claimed that the lives of some children are so miserable that their very existence is a tort. In *wrongful birth* cases, the claim is not that the child's life is totally miserable, but simply that the child has been damaged by being born less than normal. Wrongful birth suits appeal to the normality concept. The courts have rejected wrongful life suits by assuming the baseline concept; that is, they have assumed that preventing a birth or killing a baby cannot possibly be a benefit, even to prevent or end a life of total harm.

These two concepts of harm can be applied to IVF. According to baseline harm, a person created by IVF cannot thereby be harmed because, otherwise, that person wouldn't have existed. According to abnormal harm, IVF could harm a baby if it caused some defect or deficiency that a normal baby would not have had.

## WRONGING VERSUS HARMING

For utilitarians or consequentialists, what matters about new kinds of human creation is that babies are not harmed. On the other hand, virtue theories or deontologists such as Kantians focus on the motives of prospective parents. Whether it is AID, IVF, surrogacy, or cloning, they ask, "What would a good mother do? What kinds of risk would she take?"

This deontological approach emphasizes that, even though a child might not be harmed by being brought into existence, a mother can still be wrong in bringing the child into existence. That's because "wrong" here is divorced from consequences to the child and instead married to the motives of the mother in conceiving a child. To take a mundane example, if a mother conceives a child not because she wants a child but to try to force a wealthy man to marry her, then—regardless of any later possible harm to the child—the mother is wrong to create it for this reason.

In a Scottish study in 2005 of women trying to conceive at an infertility clinic, most of the 81 women would, if given an either-or choice, rather have a child with cerebral palsy or partially blind than no child at all.[58] But is this the right motive for approaching childbearing? This issue intensifies with dilemmas raised by implanting multiple embryos, where couples face choices between risks of no child and risks of several children with disabilities.

Let us distinguish between the ideal and the permissible regarding traditional conception and assisted reproduction.

> **Best Interests.** What methods of conception are best for children brought into the world? What methods are permissible?
> **Best Motives.** What motives are best for parents to have in creating children? What motives are permissible?

Using this distinction, some motives might be allowable, e.g., the motive of having kids so "someone will take care of me in my old age," even though we acknowledge they are not ideal. Similarly, it is probably in the best interests of children to be created by traditional sex by a married couple.

## HARM BY NOT KNOWING ONE'S BIOLOGICAL PARENTS?

Can a child be harmed by not knowing his genetic ancestors? Yes, if he later needs to find out specific genetic information or to discover who his biological parents were. Even if a donor of sperm or egg wishes to be anonymous, there are ways of giving the child this information.

One compromise solves this problem by allowing gametic donors or surrogates to be *confidential* but not *anonymous*. In this practice, agencies keep from children the names and identities of donor gametes, but donors can update their files every few years, so that their biological children can know about their genetic diseases and lives. This practice protects the desire of some donors and some surrogates not to have contact with children created from their gametes, while also giving them the chance to change their minds.

It is mainly the adoptive parents who don't want their children to know such donors.[59] Surprisingly, many sperm and egg donors, or surrogates, do not mind maintaining such records and want to know about the lives of such children.[60]

Pediatrician/internist Matthew Neidner registered online in 2006 with the Donor Sibling Registry and discovered that his sperm over 10 years had helped create nine children, who can see his picture online and follow his career.[61]

Single women in San Diego selected his sperm from his profile at the Fertility Center of California.

## IS COMMERCIALIZATION OF ASSISTED REPRODUCTION WRONG?

Sale of gametes either could be intrinsically wrong—just wrong in itself—or indirectly wrong because of associated bad consequences. The first belief stems from religious or Kantian premises about the inherent value of humans being incompatible with aspects of their conception being priced in the market. Valuing human life is incompatible with paying someone a price for sperm, eggs, embryos, or gestation, making the resulting baby a commodity.

Someone looking at the larger structure of society may claim, emphasizing a view of justice, that reproductive relationships between people should not be subjected to money. They could also argue that such transactions violate natural law. In other words, reproduction should be natural and free, not something bought through a contract. So payment for sperm, eggs, and surrogacy is wrong, as is physicians working in fertility clinics where money is exchanged for these goods and services.

A large number of articles over the last decades sensationalized payment to young women for their eggs, predicting dire consequences such as the commodification of life, millions of women reduced to being egg sellers, and made-to-order embryos.[62]

Defenders of payment ask whether enough young women will go through egg donation for altruistic reasons. Altruism hasn't worked in other areas of medicine. Voluntary donation has failed to meet the need for blood for operations, organs for transplantation, or bone marrow for leukemia patients.

So if we don't permit compensation, we will not get enough eggs from young women, and hence, infertile couples will not get the babies they want. If we regulate compensation and ban a real market, other problems arise, such as trying to set the right fee for everyone. Finally, if payment for assisted reproduction is wrong, why isn't payment for adoption wrong? If payment for assisted reproduction is not for babies but merely for services, why isn't payment also banned for adoption?

Sometimes, objections about payment to women imply that men are exploiting women. From reading interviews with paid surrogates, this does not seem to true.[63] Paid surrogacy empowers many women who do it, making them special and contributing to their family's income. A surprisingly large number do it despite objections from husbands, or battle husbands who want to keep the gestated baby.

## SCREENING FOR GENETIC DISEASE: A NEW EUGENICS?

At some clinics and with permission, researchers store extra eggs or embryos for later use with infertile couples.[64] Other agencies store sperm. Prospective couples can screen for future traits of children in two ways: by scrutinizing the background of the egg or sperm donors, or by testing actual embryos for genetic conditions such as Down syndrome. Is such expanded choice good for couples and children or a new eugenics?

Some critics oppose any selection by prospective parents and argue that parents should be forced to accept the first available embryo or that embryos should be randomly assigned. Similar critics once argued that all adoptable babies should be adopted before couples could try IVF.

Some prospective couples, e.g, Japanese-American, want an embryo from parents who will be ethnically as close to them as possible. They also desire to maintain, as much as possible, the illusion that the child came from their gametes. For them, choice of skin color or ethnicity matters a lot.

Other couples want to avoid a child with disabilities, such as a Down child or a child with fragile X syndrome (a condition leading to retardation). If couples are allowed to do some screening for genetic diseases, will this lead to them wanting only perfect babies or to a new eugenics?

Perhaps not. One reason is the cost of screening: for a single disease, it can be as much as $20,000, which most insurance companies will not pay.[65] It is unlikely that a couple will screen out hundreds of embryos and implant only the perfect ones because few couples have the millions of dollars to pay for so many screening tests. Should a cheap screening test be available where a couple could cheaply screen an embryo for hundreds of genetic diseases, this objection might carry some moral weight.

Even if such a test becomes available, we need to ask, what's wrong with couples wanting as healthy a baby as possible at birth? Isn't this what properly motivated parents should desire? Isn't this why pregnant mothers should avoid alcohol, tobacco, or other harmful drugs during pregnancy?

> More ethical issues raised by new ways of creating babies by older women are discussed in an excerpt from Pence's *Elements of Bioethics*. To read "Emotivism and Banning Some Conceptions", go to Chapter 6 in the Online Learning Center (OLC) at www.mhhe.com/pence7e.

## DESIGNER BABIES?

This is a large question, connected in part to questions about eugenics and controls on biotechnology. Note that many people believe that it is permissible to use such techniques to let infertile couples choose *against* diseases that embryos might carry. Sensationalistic stories imply that pre-implantation diagnosis will lead to eugenics, but is this leap realistic?

When clinics pay young women for their eggs, they fertilize the eggs with a variety of different sperm, keeping records of each embryo created. Couples may then select an embryo from this woman's eggs (seeing a photo and description of her) that will be fertilized by sperm from a man whose photo they view and whose life they read about.

Critics worry that traits of men and women will be selected that the purchasing couple deem desirable. As one such critic put it in discussing a market for egg donors, "this approach is harmful not only because it serves to reinforce social prejudice but also because it fragments women as persons by commodifying their characteristics, which seems at least as harmful as commodifying their eggs."[66]

But critics who decry selection of traits in embryos always ignore adoption. Why is selection by ethnicity or race bad in one case but permissible in the other? Why is selection by ethnicity and race plus large payment permissible for adoption but not for eggs or embryos or surrogates?

In other areas of life, people decide what they value in others in joining fraternities, sororities, and country clubs, in hiring and firing, in dating, in choosing a person to marry and to create children with, in making friends, in deciding where to live, and in choosing whom to mentor. Many of these choices reinforce existing attitudes and the government does not ban them.

On the other hand, perhaps things are subtler. The media and advertising shape the way millions of young people dress and wear their clothes, and could easily sway them similarly about the kind of children they should want. Maybe we should be worried.

## ASSISTED REPRODUCTION WORLDWIDE

As one would expect, countries vary about their attitudes to assisted reproduction. The highest per capita users in the world are Israelis, where unlimited cycles of IVF are free for up to "two take-home babies" until a woman is 45.[67]

As one might also expect, global capitalism, the Internet, and outsourcing have combined to create what some dub "reproductive tourism." PlaneHospital .com LLC operates from California and brings together clients, gamete donors, and surrogates from around the globe.[68] Because many foreign countries such as China deny gay and lesbian couples the right to adopt, such couples often use global services to obtain children. Using one of the couple's sperm or eggs can create a genetic tie to a child gestated by a woman in, say, India.

Egg donors usually come from North America or Eastern European countries because clients prefer fair-skinned babies. Greece, Cyprus, Panama, and Gujarat, India are centers for reproductive services.

In the Gujarat State in southeast India, the Akanksha Infertility Clinic run by Dr. Nayna Patel offers many willing surrogates for foreign couples at $5,000–$7,000, instead of the $50,000 fee common in North America. The Oprah Winfrey Show has profiled the Akanksha Infertility Clinic in Anand. The Akanksha Clinic has been criticized for keeping its mothers in prison-like seclusion behind barbed-wire gates and for the death of a young surrogate named Easwari, who delivered her contracted-for baby but died afterward from uncontrolled bleeding.[69] As the second wife in a polygamous marriage, Easwari may have had little real choice about accepting the $5,000 for surrogacy, more than what she could have made at best in 10 years of working outside her home If a woman has twins, as surrogates often do after Dr. Patel implants several embryos, she can make $6,000–$7,000, equivalent to 12–14 years of work outside the home.

## TIME TO REGULATE FERTILITY CLINICS?

Perhaps it's time to ban implantation of sperm or embryos where more than two births are possible and ban implantation of embryos in women over age 55 (and with rigorous proof required of birth).

Given that the ART industry generates $1 billion in fees per year and given what critics call "the wild west of medicine," where almost anything goes, some minimal regulation of AR might be good for it, and especially for the children it creates.[70]

We know that being a multiple is not good for the resulting children, who run a high risk of having a life-long disability. Nor is it good to be born to a single, nearly 70-year-old woman, who will likely die and leave the child an orphan. Even if the woman is rich, the emotional health of the child will be severely compromised.

Governments could regulate fertility clinics in four ways: (1) No assisted reproduction for women over age 55, and real testing must be enforced (seriously, in America it's easier for the elderly to buy reproductive services than it is for teenagers to buy alcohol). (2) No implantation of more than two embryos and no introduction of sperm when ovaries mature more than two eggs. This will reduce the number of multiple births, and attendant disabled children, by 99 percent. (3) No selection of gender of embryos except for sex-linked genetic disorders. As explained, it violates the dignity of women and is sexist to allow people to use AR to get a first-born male child. (4) No selection of a child to match the disability of existing parents with a disability, e.g., deaf parents who want a deaf child. It is not in the best interests of any child to be born deaf, and parents who want such disabilities in their children are not properly motivated.

To insure the creation of a baby, especially when a couple lacks insurance to cover IVF, American physicians and infertile couples want to implant more than one embryo or multiples. In 2009, Missouri and Georgia proposed laws to limit such physicians to implanting two embryos. Such laws would limit multiples and resulting babies with disabilities.

On the other hand, some reasons exist *not* to regulate fertility clinics. During the 1970s, America banned use of federal funds for experimentation on embryos. This ban hoped to stop AR research, but fertility clinics subsidized their research from fees paid by clients. At the time, critics doubted that couples would pay much for AR, especially given such low chances of having a baby. But critics erred. Over a million American couples paid for some form of assistance in ART clinics.

An unintended but foreseeable by-product of the ban was that neither the National Institutes of Health (NIH) nor IRBs could regulate AR research in private clinics. That lack of regulation led to breakthroughs, fueled by competition between ART clinics. It created a billion-dollar industry, where patients fly to enlightened countries to get what they can't get in repressive countries.

So, if it's not broke, don't fix it. A few aberrant cases should not bring down the whole system. Physician Michael Kamrava can be sued on behalf of the disabled babies for breach of the standard of care, sending a message to other physicians in fertility medicine.

Another problem is that reproductive medicine, with its research on human embryos, fires passions in social conservatives, who believe such research attacks the dignity of humans. Once politics controls who can buy AR services, will a slippery slope occur? If we make it illegal for a physician to help a couple have a first-born male child, or a 60-year-old woman to gestate a child, what's next? Banning assisted reproduction altogether, the way the Vatican advocates?

Finally, given that assisted reproduction has gone global, how can we regulate services in Greece or India? Perhaps the only avenue for doing so involves citizenship and immigration, where children born to North American couples at non-sanctioned foreign clinics would be denied citizenship or entry to North America.

## CONCLUSIONS

Given that Nadya Suleman already had six children, Dr. Sharma's acceptance of her as a fertility patient certainly was "a huge ethical failure."[71] And for him then to implant all six of Suleman's remaining embryos moved the case from ethical failure to ethical tragedy—tragedy for the 14 kids to be parented by this immature, single woman.

Assisted reproduction is a special kind of medicine, wrapped in the joys of creating wanted babies, but also rife with controversies. As older women bear such babies, as more embryos are implanted creating more multiple births, we need to think more about harm to new children and less about the desires of infertile parents.

## FURTHER READING

Cynthia Cohen, ed., *New Ways of Making Babies: The Case of Egg Donation*, Bloomington, IN: Indiana University Press, 1996.

Joseph Fletcher, *Ethics of Genetic Control: Enduring Reproductive Roulette*, New York: Doubleday Anchor; reprinted by Prometheus, Buffalo, NY, 1984.

Marcia Inhorn and Frank Balen, *Infertility Around the Globe: New Thinking on Childlessness, Gender and Reproductive Technologies*, Berkeley, CA: University of California Press, 2002.

Scott Carney, *The Red Market: On the Trail of the World's Organ Brokers, Bone Thieves, Blood Farmers, and Child Traffickers*, New York: William Morrow, 2011.

Elaine Tyler, *Barren in the Promised Land: Childless Americans and the Pursuit of Happiness*, Cambridge, MA: Harvard University Press, 1995.

Paul Ramsey, *The Ethics of Fetal Experimentation*, New Haven, CT: Yale University Press, 1975.

Stephanie Coontz, *The Way We Never Were*, New York: Basic Books, 1992.

## DISCUSSION QUESTIONS

1. If fertility clinics are regulated, shouldn't adoption agencies also be regulated? Shouldn't there be age limits on who can adopt? Shouldn't couples also be banned from saying they want only a baby of a certain sex?

2. Is it better to be born with a 65-year-old single mother than not to exist at all? Is this a fair question? What's wrong, if anything, with the way this question is asked?

3. Why should there be any restrictions on choices of parents about babies with assisted reproduction? What's different about AR that gives governments the right to impose such restrictions? We don't impose any tests on who can have a baby and we let people who use tobacco and alcohol during pregnancy have babies. Given such low standards, isn't it contradictory to impose higher standards on AR?

4. Isn't selling one's eggs to the highest bidder like prostitution? Kant would object to both because they treat one's body as "a mere means." Is it wrong to so commodify one's body and be paid for doing so?

5. IVF may not be unnatural, but gestating eight fetuses is. There's perversity going on here and Nature extracts a terrible price on the resulting kids. The same thing when an elderly woman gestates a baby with artificial hormones. Aren't both processes thwarting nature, unnatural, and, hence, "just wrong"?

6. Is assisted reproduction "pro life?" Since 1 in 11 couples in America can't conceive after a year of trying, and if they want to have babies, what's wrong with their using AR? Even if some tiny embryos are lost in the process of trying to conceive—which also occurs for 50 percent of embryos conceived through normal sexual relations—what's wrong with couples wanting their own kids and using medical science to try to have them? How can such desires not be "pro life"?

# CHAPTER 7

# Embryos, Stem Cells, and Cloning

Over the last two decades, ethical controversies about embryos intricately mixed with controversies about cloning and stem cells. The announcement in 1997 of cloning the sheep Dolly created even more controversy about using human embryos in research and cloning anything human. This chapter discusses such controversies, including one of the greatest frauds in science. At its end, it discusses cloning to produce children, or *reproductive cloning*.

## HISTORICAL BACKGROUND OF EMBRYONIC RESEARCH

In 1973, *Roe v. Wade made* abortion legal in all states. As soon as laws permitted abortions, researchers *legally* experimented on 20 live-born fetuses, seemingly degrading nascent human life (see Chapter 5).[1]

Five years later, and without cultural agreement or approval of an ethics committee, Patrick Steptoe and Robert Edwards reversed infertility by creating "test tube" baby Louise Brown (see Chapter 6). In doing so, and using in vitro fertilization (IVF), they created and destroyed about a hundred human embryos. Then, as today, the creation of babies by IVF had the foreseen but unintended byproduct of sacrificing human embryos that did not implant.

In 1979, obstetricians Howard and Georgeanna Jones established the first American IVF clinic at Eastern Virginia Medical School. In 1981, they were responsible for the first American baby born via IVF, Elizabeth Carr. While the embryo that became Elizabeth Carr was being formed, opponents protested outside. Conservative Christians saw IVF as alien and suspect, and as violating principles of natural law because scientists were creating humans in artificial ways, outside of sexual intercourse and the womb.

So began the politics of the embryo, which have intensified over the last 35 years. In 1977, the Ethics Advisory Board concluded that some research with embryos should be permitted, but Congress never accepted its conclusions.

## Two Important Cases

**The Rios Case**   In 1981, Mario and Elsa Rios, a wealthy American couple, died childless. Their IVF-created embryos then existed in frozen limbo. Because neither the Rioses nor their infertility clinic in Australia had provided for the death of their embryos, the question arose whether they could be destroyed. If implanted in surrogates, the embryos could result in children who could later sue for support.

An ad hoc committee of the Australian government required scientists to preserve the embryos until they were adopted. They never were, and over the years, freezing made them deteriorate (as all frozen embryos will eventually deteriorate), making the issue moot.

**The Davis Case**   In 1990, Mary Sue and Junior Davis of Tennessee divorced and fought for custody of seven embryos frozen in an IVF clinic. Both remarried. After her remarriage, Mary Sue Davis wanted to donate their embryos to an infertile couple. In 1992, the Tennessee Supreme Court decided that Junior needn't become a father against his will. After that, a lower Tennessee court ruled that he could destroy the embryos, which he did.[2]

In 1994, the Human Embryo Research Panel concluded that federal funding of research with embryos would improve the success and safety of procedures to reduce infertility and that prohibiting federal funding would harm the quality of such research.

It called embryos created specifically for *research embryos*, and those leftover after successful IVF *spare embryos*. The panel rejected the compromise that research could be done only on spare embryos. As expected, leftover embryos from couples unsuccessfully attempting IVF had higher rates of genetic abnormalities, and research needed to be done on exactly such embryos.

Politically savvy members of the panel thought Congress would accept their modest recommendations, but, preoccupied with partial-birth abortions in 1995, Congress rejected them.

In 1996, Congress added the Dickey-Warner Amendment to NIH's appropriations bill: "None of the funds made available in this act may be used for . . . research in which a human embryo or embryos are destroyed, discarded, or knowingly subjected to risk of injury or death greater than allowed for research on fetuses in utero." English and Australian governments allowed public monies to fund research on embryos up to day 14 of life. As a result, companies based in these countries soon licensed breakthroughs to American researchers.

Geneticist Marl Hughes had once made *Science* magazine's list of top breakthroughs for his technique of taking DNA from a single cell of a human embryo and testing it for cystic fibrosis. Taking the cell did not damage healthy embryos, but such testing did mean that embryos with cystic fibrosis would be destroyed.

Although the ban on federal funds had stayed in effect, scientists such as Hughes could work on embryos that were *privately funded* i.e., from private charities such as Planned Parenthood or the March of Dimes. In 1997, Hughes had private funds to pursue embryonic screening and much larger federal funds to pursue other research that did not involve human embryos. Yet Hughes lost all federal funding because federal funds had paid for a small refrigerator mistakenly placed in his private lab.

## History: Embryo Research, Cloning and Stem Cells

**1997: Dolly Is Cloned**   On February 24, 1997, every newspaper in the world screamed that a lamb named Dolly had been created by cloning (she was actually born on the previous July 5, 1996, but patents on the techniques were finalized only in February). Cloning, a technique previously thought impossible to use to create mammals, conjured scary scenarios from science fiction. Dolly's birth galvanized interest in cloned human embryos, especially embryos that might be created, implanted in a woman, and gestated to a human baby.

Where they had felt ambushed by *Roe v. Wade* and the birth of Louise Brown, as well as the unanticipated success of IVF clinics, social conservatives vowed this time to resist. It is as if they said to scientists, "At cloning, we draw the line and beyond, 'You shall not pass!' "

**Cloning Science**   "Cloning" is ambiguous, even in science, and may refer to molecular cloning, cellular cloning, embryo twinning, or *somatic cell nuclear transfer* (SCNT). The latter is what occurred in Dolly and what most people care about. It takes the nucleus of an adult cell and implants it in an egg where the nucleus has been removed.

A variant of this process called *fusion* (which was actually done to produce Dolly) puts the donor cells next to an enucleated egg and fuses the two with a tiny electric current. Because the pulse that produces fusion also activates egg development, a blastocyst—an embryo of about 100 cells—starts to develop.

In cells, *mitochondria* are oragnelles that do many things, such as fueling the cell, signaling, and carrying genes implicated in serious human diseases. In fusion, mitochondria from both the donor and the egg recipient mix, whereas in strict transfer of a nucleus, mitochondria are present only in the enucleated egg.[3]

At a 1997 conference on mammalian cloning, Ian Wilmut, Dolly's originator, tissue stressed that his techniques were inefficient: he started with 277 sheep eggs and got only one live lamb. Nevertheless, his statement has been widely misunderstood, partly because he has emphasized how many eggs he started with and not how many fetuses resulted in live births. The actual statistics were 277 eggs fused with sperm in oviducts, 247 of 277 recovered from oviducts, 29 transferred at the stage of morula or blastocyst to create 13 pregnancies in lambs, three of which came to birth, and one of which was healthy and lived, Dolly.[4]

**1998: Immortalized Human Stem Cell Lines Created**   Found in embryos, bone marrow, and the umbilical cord, stem cells help the injured body grow new cells. If the body loses blood, it activates stem cells to make new blood. As primordial cells, stem cells can develop into any kind of differentiated cellular tissue: bone, muscle, nerve, etc. In theory, they could be directed to form new bones, neural cells, cardiac tissue, and cure diseases.

Physicians already knew that the human body had stem cells, but they had no easy way to grow them. Then John Gearhart of Johns Hopkins University and

James Thomson of the University of Wisconsin in 1998 discovered how to continually produce stem cells—to create an immortalized stem cell line—rather than tediously derive them from minute amounts of tissue from embryos or fetuses.

In effect, Gearhart and Thompson discovered how to make human embryos into tiny "stem cell factories." Such objectification of human bothered critics, who felt that using human embryos for such purposes demeaned tissues the dignity of human life and led down the slippery slope.

**1998: ACT Uses Cow Eggs to Grow Human Embryos**  In 1998, Advanced Cell Technology (ACT) of Massachusetts announced that it had made differentiated human cells revert to a primordial state by fusing them with cow eggs. Although the cow egg was just the medium for the nucleus of the human cell (the nucleus of the cow egg had been removed), the procedure sounded alarms. Once again, biotechnology seemed out of control. President Clinton and his National Bioethics Advisory Commission (NBAC) condemned any attempts to create children out of such hybrids (although no one wanted to try to create such beings or was suggesting doing so).

**2001: NBAC Backs Research on Embryonic Stem Cells**  Although it condemned reproductive cloning in 1998, the National Bioethics Advisory Commission (NBAC) concluded in 2001 that the government should fund research on stem cells created from human embryos. Congress never accepted this recommendation, in part because cloning embryos connected to the larger, controversial issue of reproductive cloning.

**Fraudulent Claims and Kooks**  Cloning soon took up more media time than any issue in the 35-year history of bioethics. With physicist Dick Seed wanting to clone himself, and with the bizarre cult called "the Raelians" and Pamayiotis Zavos and Severino Antinori falsely claiming to have cloned a human fetus, cloning created one sensational story after another, scaring people about identical babies being produced like immortalized stem cell lines.

**2001: Adult Stem Cells Discovered**  In 2001, scientists discovered stem cells not only in bone marrow but also throughout the human body. Researchers started using adult stem cells in research rather than using stem cells derived from human embryos.

In the next five years, researchers discovered that many organs and tissues contain precursor cells that act like stem cells. These adult stem cells became specific kinds of cells more quickly than embryonic stem cells, for which scientists do not know how to do the same. One director of an institute for regenerative medicine says, "Brain stem cells can make almost all cell types in the brain, and that may be all we need if we want to treat Parkinson's disease or ALS. Embryonic stem cells might not be necessary in those cases."[5] Similar, specific adult stem cells can be obtained from the intestine, skin, liver, and bone marrow. For heart disease (and many other organs or tissues), the director of Harvard's Stem Cell Institute says, "If you could find a progenitor cell in the adult heart that has the ability to replicate, it's likely easier to start with that than begin with an embryonic stem cell, which has too many options."[6]

But most adult organs contain few stem cells, not nearly enough to use medically, and adult stem cells are even harder to grow than embryonic stem cells. More fundamentally, "Unlocking the secrets of self-renewal will most likely involve studying embryonic stem cells," says Harvard's director.

**2001: President George W. Bush's First Press Conference**   On August 11, 2001, President George W. Bush, in the first press conference on bioethics by an American president, announced his policy on federally funded research on human embryos. He rejected using such funds to create embryos for research, but allowed them for research on 60 stem cell lines created from spare embryos. Carried live on television in prime time, his press conference signaled that bioethics had arrived in American politics.

A year after that press conference, the number of stem cell lines appeared to be small, about 15. Scientists then questioned whether President Bush's policy would get them the biological material they needed. Three years later, scientists regarded the 15 stem cell lines as inadequate.[7]

**Cloning and the Law**   Senator Sam Brownback (R, Kansas) introduced his Human Cloning Prohibition Act of 2001, which stated: "It shall be unlawful for any person or entity, public or private, in or affecting interstate commerce, knowingly (1) to perform or attempt to perform human cloning; (2) to participate in an attempt to perform human cloning; or (3) to ship or receive for any purpose an embryo produced by human cloning." Also, "It shall be unlawful for any person or entity, public or private, knowingly to import for any purpose an embryo produced by human cloning, or any product derived from such an embryo."

A similar proposal to ban all forms of cloning worldwide, backed by the administration of George W. Bush, stalemated in the United Nations. Hoping to excel in biotechnology, Asian countries such as Korea, Malaysia, and China aligned with European countries to resist the measure. Malaysia invested $26 million in BioValley, a cluster of 100 new biotech companies to work on stem cells and raise Malaysia to a world power in biotechnology.[8] China invested in cloning technology, hoping to succeed where the West had stumbled.[9]

With Congress stalemated, action about cloning fell to the states. Californians in 2002 passed Proposition 71, giving $3 billion for stem cell research from human embryos. State legislatures across the land then battled to fund or to criminalize embryonic cloning. Wisconsin, New Jersey, Connecticut, Illinois, Washington, Ohio, and Maryland funded similar research, whereas Massachusetts, Missouri, Arkansas, Indiana, Iowa, Michigan, and North and South Dakota voted to criminalize all cloning.[10]

By 2006, 13 states passed laws making attempts at reproductive cloning a crime, including Arkansas, California, Connecticut, Indiana, Iowa, Maryland, Massachusetts, Michigan, New Jersey, North Dakota, Rhode Island, South Dakota, and Virginia.[11]

**Animal Cloning**   In the years after Dolly's birth, scientists cloned animals important for food and research: two calves (1998), the lambs Molly and Polly to create Factor IX (1998), three generations of mice (1998), a Rhesus monkey (1999), five pigs, (2002), a goat (2002), a rat (2003), many champion dairy cows and bulls (1998–2004), a horse named "Prometea" (2003), a mule named "Idaho Gem" (2003), and a deer named "Dewey" (2003). Scientists also cloned ferrets, rabbits, frogs, fruit flies, a water buffalo, a wolf, and carp.

They also cloned animals of endangered species such as the banteng (2003), a bovine native to Indonesia; the mouflon (2001); and the African wildcat (2004). Critics feared that such cloning would lessen preservation of natural habitat for such species.

Scientists also cloned a cat named "Carbon Copy" or "CC" (2001). CC had a striped gray coat over a white base, unlike her ancestor, an orange calico. Critics claimed this showed that cloning didn't work, while CC's originator, Mark Westhusin, replied that of course CC's coat color differed, because random genetic re-programming controls coat coloring and patterns.

In March 2005, the South Korean team of Hwang Woo-suk announced it had cloned an Afghan hound that it named "Snuppy." Because of their complex reproductive system, dogs had previously eluded cloning scientists, but Hwang's team succeeded, an achievement that remains undisputed. Later, they produced five cloned "sniffer dogs" possessed of extraordinary ability to smell drugs at airports.

Efforts to clone primates, however, went nowhere. The most intense efforts occurred at the Oregon Health and Science University, where one researcher speculated in 2013 that the extra fragility of eggs of primates (compared to other species) makes cloning primates more difficult.[12]

**2004: Hwang Woo-suk's Fraud about Cloning Embryos**   In 2004, seemingly out of nowhere, South Korean researcher Hwang Woo-suk announced that he had not only successfully cloned viable human embryos but had also derived viable stem cells from these embryos.[13] Before this claim, biologists thought that creating a human stem cell in primates by cloning could not be done. His account emphasized the relaxed Buddhist attention and skills of his team. Importantly, he said these stem cell lines genetically matched cells of donors, opening doors to study cells of victims of diseases such as Alzheimer's or Lou Gehrig's disease.

His story, and a subsequent one the next year,[14] received almost as much publicity as Dolly's birth. Carefully planned, it was announced at a meeting in Seattle of the American Association of Science. Richard Doerflinger of the U.S. Conference of Catholic Bishops called the success a "clear and present danger" to the dignity of human life. Champions of victims of Parkinson's disease, such as the actor Michael J. Fox, hailed it as a major breakthrough. Handsome and wearing a business suit, Dr. Hwang seemed to symbolize progress in medicine, especially when condemning President George W. Bush's hostility to his research.

But questions soon arose about the photos of embryos published in *Nature* and *Science* of Hwang's research, which did not seem to be of different embryos but of the same ones.

In 2005, Hwang's university and the South Korean government investigated Hwang. Assistants testified that Hwang had forced them to fabricate results and to alter pictures of embryos. The investigation concluded that Hwang had not in fact produced any stem cell lines from human embryos, had not discovered easy techniques for doing so, and had not produced matching stem cell lines to cells of donors. Hwang went on trial in South Korea for misusing millions of dollars of funds specially given to him for his work and for violating Korean laws in bioethics. Like Enron's Ken Lay and Health South's Richard Scrushy, Hwang claimed that underlings had deceived him.

So one of the biggest medical breakthroughs of the decade had been faked. After an investigation by his university, *Science* magazine retracted both of his landmark papers of 2004 and 2005.

Why was it hard to expose this fraud? Simple: American researchers at the time using federal funds could not do any research on human embryos, so the Korean's research could not be easily falsified or verified in America, the leading center for biotechnology.

Like the Raelians, a fake cult, Hwang was a fake. Stories about both of them received saturation coverage by the media, and both damaged legitimate medical progress.

**2006: The Senate Vote and Presidential Veto**   On July 18, 2006, the U.S. Senate voted to expand federal funding of embryonic stem cell research, passing a bill that had passed the House the year before. The next day President Bush, as he had promised to do, vetoed the bill, the first of his administration. At a news conference at the White House explaining his veto, the president said the bill would be "crossing a moral line and would support the taking of innocent human life." He was surrounded by dozens of "Snowflake" children, who were born from an embryo-adoption program, and their parents. "These boys and girls are not spare parts," the president affirmed.[15]

Representative Nancy Pelosi of California, the House minority leader, retorted that Bush's veto was "saying 'no' to hope." And Senator Orrin Hatch agreed, saying the veto "sets back embryonic stem cell research another year or so." In truth, during the eight years of George W. Bush's presidency, very little research from federal funding occurred on stem cells from human embryos, a real setback to medical progress.

**2009: Obama Administration Reverses Bush Policies**   On July 7, 2009, federal regulators in the Obama administration set new rules for research with embryonic stem cells.[16] The president created a panel of scientists and ethicists to ensure that couples truly consented to using their embryos to create stem cells. Scientists and the American Medical Association liked the results.

**2007–2009: IPS Cells Discovered**   In 2007, researcher Shinya Yamanaka of Kyoto University discovered how to use four genes to tell skin cells to revert back to pluripotent cells, or *induced pluripotent stem (IPS) cells*. It took a while for the world to understand this Nobel Prize–worthy achievement.

In essence, Yamanaka learned how to use a few genes to tell a differentiated, somatic cell how to revert back to a primordial, undifferentiated stem cell, which then could turn into anything. These powerful cells eliminate the need for both embryonic stem cells derived from actual embryos and eggs from female donors to create embryos.

In July 2009, further progress occurred with induced stem cells.[17] Two Chinese teams created identical mice using embryonic stem cells created from IPS cells derived from the skin of the ancestral mice. This achievement seemed to prove that IPS cells are the equivalent of human embryonic cells in producing stem cells.

**2009: Controversies about Swapping Mitochondria in IPS Cells**   Although Yamanaka's achievement appeared to greatly diminish needs in research for human embryos, it started others.

In August 2009, a lab produced monkeys when researchers substituted the healthy mitochondrial DNA of mothers with DNA from mothers with terrible genetic diseases, then used the nucleus of the mother with the bad DNA to create the embryo that became the monkey.[18] In essence, because mitochondrial carry genes, this is gene therapy (discussed in Chapter 15).

Although mitochondrial DNA can carry terrible diseases such as Alzheimer's disease, blindness, and muscle degeneration diseases, changing the mitochondrial DNA in an embryo will not only affect the future adult, but also the grandchildren and future progeny of that adult. This involves germ-line, not somatic cell, gene therapy. Historically, such a change has been thought to be a momentous ethical bright line, one not to be crossed lightly, because if anything unexpected happens, it cannot be reversed and will affect many people.

Lastly, if IPS cells and gene transfer could be used safely (and that is a big "if"), then fears arise about both cloning and designer babies. As said Robert Lanza of ACT, "It raises many of the issues raised by reproductive cloning."[19] If the mice are normal, as they seem to be, then this is a gigantic step toward creating safe cloning of humans.[20]

**2010–2012: Setbacks to Stem Cell Research**   Many "gee whiz" predictions about stem cells did not come true. First, IPS cells derived from, say, skin cells seem to retain memory traces of being skin, such that they cannot easily be turned into functioning cardiac cells.[21] Second, IPS cells have been employed in clinical trials to help patients with heart disease, with damaged spinal cords, or needing bone marrow transplants, but results so far have not been hugely therapeutic.[22] Hence, we may need to create stem cells derived from cloned embryos created from a patient's own cells and then use those stem cells in new research to help people. This would put controversies back into play about using such human embryos in research.

## ETHICAL ISSUES INVOLVING EMBRYOS
## IN RESEARCH

Nevertheless, controversies about human embryos remain. As long as IVF clinics implant more than one embryo for maximal chances of taking home a baby, the moral status of the embryo will be debated. Some scientists also believe that stem cells derived from embryos may work better than IPS cells for certain purposes.

## Valuable from Conception

For Thomas Aquinas in the thirteenth century, ensoulment occurred at 40 and 90 days for male and female fetuses, respectively, and therefore nothing of value resided in the womb before those points. In 1869, Pius IX announced that abortion at any stage resulted in excommunication.[23] Since then, Catholic teaching has emphasized the value of human life from the moment of conception. So it was no surprise that in 1982, Pope John Paul II said to a group of scientists,

> I condemn, in the most explicit and formal way, experimental manipulations of the human embryo, since the human being, from conception to death, cannot be exploited for any purpose whatsoever.[24]

## Potential for Personhood

Many scientists say that before 14 days, the human embryo has no human form and cannot experience pain. Why then give it value? One reply is that, despite the fact that some zygotes become pathological tissue and some zygotes become twins, the embryo is, as Jesuit priest Richard McCormick says, "powerfully on its way" to development as a person. Even though it may later twin or not implant, conservative believers see it as already a member of the human family.

Why is that? As McCormick writes about the human embryo:

> . . . it remains [as having] potential for personhood and as such deserves profound respect. This is *a fortiori* weighty for the believer who sees the human person as a member of God's family and the temple of the spirit. Interference with such a potential future cannot be a light undertaking.

The fact that 400,000 embryos are frozen and deteriorating over time and may become non-viable has created a new kind of adoption. The Snowflake program to date arranges adoptions of embryos, of which about 20 became babies.[25] The program charges up to $20,000 for this service, as it considers itself arranging an adoption.

However, we now know that *any* cell of the body can become a person. The nucleus of a differentiated cell can be put into an enucleated human egg, a spark applied, and a new embryo can be formed that is a near-copy of the genetic ancestor. Whether we use SCNT, IPS cells, or fusion, the truth is that we can form human embryos in a variety of ways—and they all contain full potential for personhood.

The revolutionary aspect of recent advances in biology is that they do not make embryos, but *any human cell*, special. The dignity of the embryo begins to collapse into the dignity of the cell.

## Slippery Slopes

In addition to asserting the intrinsic value of the embryo, McCormick worries about what happens when human embryos are regarded as mere commodities for research (or as little factories to produce stem cells). (In the following passage, "preembryo" refers to the embryo before implantation on the uterine wall.)

> If we concluded that preembryos need not be treated as persons, would we little by little extend this to embryos? Would we gradually trivialize the reasons

justifying preembryo manipulation? . . . Furthermore, there is uncertainty about the effect of preembryo manipulation on personal and societal attitudes toward nascent human life in general. Will there be further erosion of our respect? I say "further" because of the widespread acceptance and practice of abortion.[26]

Here, we first have a conceptual slippery slope argument, asserting that if trivial reasons justify experimenting on embryos before 14 days, then similarly trivial reasons will justify experimenting on first-trimester fetuses and then on more developed fetuses. McCormick also has an empirical slippery slope argument here, predicting that acceptance of the deaths of embryos will generalize to acceptance of deaths of fetuses. (Chapter 2 discusses these two kinds of slippery slopes).

## Reductio ad Absurdum

Many commentators think that treating the embryo as valuable because it is a potential person can be refuted by a *reductio ad absurdum*: a line of reasoning that shows that implications of an idea are absurd and thus cast doubt on the idea itself. In this instance, if a woman starts procreating in her teens and continues throughout her fertile years, she can produce a dozen or more children. If each potential person is valuable, then she ought to conceive as many children as possible. Given the consequences of overpopulation, this conclusion hardly makes sense.

If embryos are persons, the following involve killing persons: creating embryos for in vitro fertilization and freezing them for later use, pre-implantation genetic diagnosis, or medical research. Similarly, if embryos are persons, then intrauterine devices (IUDs) and Plan B (the "day after pill"), both of which prevent implantation of embryos, also kill persons.

If these implications are false, then the premise that generated these claims is false, and that premise is that human embryos are persons.

Of course, it might be possible, thinking of Judith Jarvis Thomson, to accept the premise that embryos are persons, but to deny a further premise that persons can never be killed. Also, when no particular woman has a duty to gestate them, there is clearly a philosophical difficulty in claiming a right to life for frozen embryos.

## The Interest View

Philosopher Bonnie Steinbock argues that having moral status (i.e., being the kind of being who must be considered from the moral point of view) is limited to beings "who have interests." For her, a necessary condition of having an interest is being able to desire something. One of the most basic desires is to avoid pain. We don't think vegetables feel pain, so we don't think they have desires. We do think cats and dogs feel pain, so we think they have an interest in avoiding pain.

Courses in law school say a great deal about interests, conflicts among interests, and how to resolve conflicts of interest. As such, the concept of interest covers a lot of intellectual territory.

As for embryos, it is commonly accepted that before the emergence of the primitive streak at 14 days, there is no possibility of any neural development such that any being could "be there" to feel pain. The human embryo at this stage is more like a blackberry than a tadpole. To say this a different way, embryos cannot feel pain at 14 days.

As such for Steinbock, the embryo has no desires about what happens to it, so it has no interests and no moral status. So it does not matter whether an embryo fails to implant in the uterine wall, whether it is dislodged by an intrauterine device (IUD), or whether it is used in research. It only begins to matter when neurons form to create *sentience*, the ability to feel pain.

Steinbock distinguishes between moral status and moral value. Beings can have moral value, even if they lack moral status. For her, to say that something has moral value is to say that there are good reasons for protecting it or being concerned about it. So wilderness and works of art can have moral value, even if they lack interests and lack moral status.[27]

For Steinbock, embryos have moral value but no moral status, and as such, reasons exist for protecting their usage, for respecting them, and for not devaluing them as mere tissue.

But how much do people really value embryos? Two-thirds of the human embryos stored at two fertility clinics in England had to be destroyed because the owners did not respond to a letter asking about their wishes.[28] Given that these owners are the most affected by their destruction, such couples do not seem to put much value on these embryos—at least, in responding to a letter about consenting to keep them alive in public clinics.

England has allowed its scientists to create human embryos for research and to use them in such research for up to 14 days of development.[29] In the years in which that has been legal, no great changes in the fabric of English life seem to have occurred, nor has there been a massive slide down a slippery slope of loss of human dignity.

## Embryos and Respect

Bioethicist David Ozar once argued that although an embryo may not be a person, neither is it just a pebble or a tissue.[30] Embryos are not simply the property of an owner. They deserve respect in view of their potential as persons.

What does respecting an embryo mean? Well, for one thing, embryos should not be eaten, encased in plastic as earrings, or bred into mixed-species hybrids. Gene Outka claims that respecting embryos also means that human embryos should not be substituted for the eyes of rabbits in testing cosmetics.[31]

Another way to put this point is to emphasize that a large amount of bodily products, such as bone, cartilage, blood, and tissue, can be legally sold from cadavers. Some firms specialize in such sales and broker them to research institutions and medical schools. Respecting embryos would include banning them from being bought and sold this way.

It is possible to be a good scientist and treat human embryos with respect in medical research. One might make an analogy with animal experimentation. To test new forms of heart surgery or new kinds of lenses for human eyes, we harm animals. But in using animals for our benefit this way, we should minimize their pain and psychological terror, and not make fun of them in any way.

In the same way, researchers who have the privilege of using human embryos should be taught, required, and legally enjoined to treat them with the greatest respect. That respect prevents a slippery slope to devaluing other human lives.

To make another analogy: physicians and medical students should treat the newly dead with respect and not practice intubation or spinal taps or surgery on them without the family's permission, for to do so is to offer no respect to the life just expired or to those who loved the patient. In the same way, one could argue that human embryos should be treated carefully in view of the persons that—under different circumstances—they could have become.

**Indeterminacy**   Father Richard McCormick does not assert that human embryos are persons but thinks we should treat them as if they were. Why? Because we don't know exactly where personhood begins. To use his analogy, if the hunter is unsure whether something moving in the bushes is a deer or a human, he shouldn't shoot.

Similarly, at the other end of life, if we are unsure whether a patient will emerge from a coma, shouldn't we wait as long as possible before removing a feeding tube?

A subtler objection emphasizes the indeterminacy of the boundaries of sentience. When patients are under sedation for surgery, well-publicized stories have taught us that they can hear. Some patients have been declared dead and then awakened, recalling jokes made in their presence and procedures done on them (an important argument for not allowing medical students to train on the newly dead).

Similarly, we are not sure exactly when the embryo develops sentience. Perhaps the most rudimentary form is like phototropism when a plant bends toward light. Even so, when any doubt exists, we should be cautious and, under a general principle of respect, not subject embryos to any medical research, just as we would not subject patients in vegetative states to such research.

## The Opportunity Cost of Missed Research

In any decade, few really major breakthroughs occur in medical research. The creation of immortalized stem cell lines from human embryos was one such breakthrough. Not allowing this line of research to be federally funded was a major tragedy.

It is not enough to let private companies or other countries fund the research. America's National Institutes of Health (NIH) is the crown jewel of the world's scientific treasure, and it is a tragedy that its researchers could not pursue this new area. Moreover, by allowing federally funded studies, we ensure the highest level of peer-reviewed, objective research.

By banning use of embryos in federally funded projects, NIH deprives millions of people of new medicines that otherwise might not be discovered for another hundred years.

## My Tissue

One of the well-known problems of transplants of foreign organs, blood, and tissue into a patient's body is rejection of the foreign material when recognized by the immune system. Drugs that suppress the immune system to allow acceptance of foreign tissue may cause cancer after decades of use. It would be much better to grow bone, blood, organs, or particular masses of cells from one's own body for future use.

Creating embryos from one's own cells could be used to grow tissue for one's future medical needs. By using donor cells, embryos could be created by embryonic cloning that are nearly identical copies of one's genome.

Libertarians argue that what an individual does with his or her body should be up to him or her. A federal ban on storing self-made medicine from one's own embryos allows government to take away this personal liberty. By denying citizens such new medicines made from their own embryonic tissue, it takes away years from their lives.

## Moot?

The creation of IPS cells means that we can get the valuable stem cells we need for research without destroying human embryos. Whether you see this as a brilliant scientific discovery or a gift from God, or both, the fact is that the impasse of the last decade motivated scientists to seek a way around it, which they did.

Some researchers say we should keep all the tools on the table and that human embryonic stem cells may be better for some purposes that IPS cells cannot fulfill. Even so, with this new source of stem cells, some of the preceding arguments lose their punch.

## REPRODUCTIVE CLONING

Reproductive cloning alarms many people, perhaps because of the way it's portrayed in movies and science fiction. As such, we first need to address some misconceptions about it.

### Reproductive Cloning: Myths about Cloned Persons

**1. Cloning Does Not Reproduce an Existing Person**   Reproductive cloning re-creates the genes of the ancestor, not the ancestor himself. Cloning re-creates the genetic base of a person, but a person's identity partly stems from non-genetic sources, such as his experiences growing up.

This means that you can't reproduce yourself. Of course, any resulting child would not have the memories of the adult ancestor. Narcissistic people who want to clone themselves will be disappointed. Cloning reproduces about 99.8 percent of the ancestor's genes (the other 0.2 percent come from mitochondrial genes in the host-egg), but even 0.2 percent difference at conception can be significant. Identical twins have small differences in random inactivation of the X chromosome in embryonic development, and this results in their different personalities and traits as adults.

**2. Cloned Humans Would Not Be Drones but Persons**   A child created by reproductive cloning would, like any other fetus, need to be gestated by a woman for nine months. He would have no distinguishing marks on him to indicate his origins. He would feel, sense, think, and hurt like any other human child.

Would a cloned child's origins affect his status as a person? Critics once thought that IVF kids might suffer discrimination, but that never happened. Most likely, children created by cloning would be persons with all the rights of other persons.

Leon Kass implied that prejudiced people might treat cloned children as less-than-human. If this were so, it might not be in the best interest of them to be originated this way.

But notice that the same logic implies that it might not be best to be created as a child of an interracial couple because "other people" might be prejudiced against such marriages and their children. The effect of such reasoning is to strengthen prejudice, not to weaken it, and to give prejudice too much weight in what, after all, is supposed to be *moral* reasoning. For this reason, we must be careful when we speak of children originated by cloning. To call them "clones" may be prejudicial if this term implies bad things about such children. Similarly, to imply that children created by cloning would be raised in batches connotes all kinds of bad, silly things, such as seeing them as zombies, as sources of organs for genetic ancestors, and in general, as less than human.

In short, babies created by cloning would not be *zombies*, but—legally and morally—*persons*.

## Against the Will of God?

Many clergy believe that originating children by cloning is not God's will. God ordained in Genesis that humans should reproduce as did Adam and Eve, man and woman begetting children, and that is God's plan for humanity. To deviate from the plan is wrong. Just as gay men and lesbians were not meant in this plan to have children, so children were not meant to be created asexually.

Notice that this argument is an inference about God's will. Nowhere in any scripture does it say that medical science should not use reproductive cloning to produce children. Notice too that most advances in the history of medicine have overcome the argument that the change is against God's will.

## The Right to a Unique Genetic Identity

With Dolly's birth, the possibility emerged of cloning a human baby. Various people began to assert that what was wrong with cloning a human baby from a genetic ancestor's cells was that it would violate the right of each person to a "unique genetic identity." Some theologians at the Vatican made this claim (although they had never made it before Dolly's birth).

An initial problem about this argument concerned twins. Since so-called identical twins share 99.9 percent of their genes, is their right to a unique identity violated by being a twin? Certain techniques of assisted reproduction, such as implanting many embryos, drastically increase the likelihood of such twins. Are they wrong?

A bigger problem with this objection is the assumption that one's genes are one's identity. This reductionist line of thinking in modern genetics lies behind similar objections that a child created by cloning would not have a soul because it shared the same genes as the ancestor. Both objections assume that genes make the person, the self, the identity, and yet we know that is incorrect because environment also contributes to personhood (and possibly, so does free choice).

## Unnatural and Perverse

Many people also wonder about the motives behind cloning. They ask, Why would anyone want to create a child by cloning? Why not use the fun method of sex? If a couple is unable to have a child through sex, why not adopt?

Sexual reproduction is natural. Cloning, or asexual reproduction, is unnatural. What is good for plants or animals should not be used for humans.

Something is wrong with parents who want to clone a child. They are either narcissistic or so desperate—after all other methods of having children have failed—that they will subject their future child to a perverted experiment in which his personhood will be at risk when he later learns that he is "just a clone."

In reply, it should be noted that this objection begs a lot of questions. First, it assumes that what is primitive or natural is always best. That is certainly not true for a man and woman who are naturally infertile. Second, it assumes that the new way of making babies is perverse and therefore wrong, a charge that greeted many other new ways of making babies in the past. Finally, it assumes bad motives on the part of would-be parents.

## The Right to an Open Future

Critics claim that parents will choose to create a child with a certain genotype, say, that of an athlete, actor, or dad, with certain expectations. After their investment in in vitro fertilization, they would expect the resulting child to have qualities similar to the ancestor.

But the future should be open to every child. It is wrong for tennis mothers to impose their wills on their children in their hell-bent determination to make them into tennis stars, wrong for certain parents from an early age to push their children into medical careers, and wrong for soccer dads and Little League coaches to push their children into athleticism.

Why is this so? The heart of the objection about a closed future lies in explaining this answer. At bottom is the premise that parents should not have children to fulfill their own needs, desires, or fantasies, but for the good of the child. In this sense, parenting should be Kantian, not egotistic.

If parents create children expecting specific traits (basketball skills, acting talent), then children can be damaged psychologically when they cannot, or choose not to, fulfill such expectations.

This argument lies behind the widely heard objection about "designer babies," i.e., that it is wrong for parents to try to create children with blue eyes and blonde hair and with a strong interest in music and tennis. Instead, parents should accept whatever God gives them as a gift.

The most dangerous idea of all is that parents should be free to reject, or not love, babies who lack the qualities they want. Already a dangerous tendency has started among some parents to not aggressively treat impaired babies suffering from genetic diseases at birth, followed by equally dangerous practices of death-by-abortion after a sonogram has determined that it's a female fetus. If we add to this the possibility of using pre-implantation diagnosis during in vitro fertilization not to implant any embryo with cystic fibrosis or Down syndrome, we are already halfway to the bad place of parents rejecting children in the nursery when they emerge with the wrong genes.

Suppose a child is created from the genes of a girl who was an all-state champion in the breaststroke and who had ability in math, scoring in the top 1 percent of standardized tests and excelling in AP math classes in high school. What is often overlooked is the role of supportive parents in such achievements. Now suppose that the cloned child never learns to swim and is never exposed to math—and doesn't develop these abilities while she is young enough. In that case, we will learn, perhaps painfully, that parents of children cloned for certain abilities cannot just sit back and wait for the abilities to unfold, but will need to be just as involved as the ancestor's parents. If they are not, it will be easy to see where the blame should go.

Nevertheless, this argument emphasizes how bad parenting damages children and how society should not encourage bad parenting based on false expectations. This would be especially true if parents emotionally abandoned kids who did not meet their expectations.

On the other hand, this argument can go many places. Suppose the cloned child resembles the ancestor much more than expected and, because the parents already know what the child can excel at, encourage her in that direction. Would that be bad for the parents or child?

## Abnormalities

At present, a high rate of abnormalities plagues efforts to create primates by SCNT. Any such conception of a human baby by cloning would be an experiment on a child, and no such experiment is justified without a compensating benefit for the child. Such a benefit does not yet exist. As such, attempts to create a child by cloning the cells of a human ancestor and gestating it to birth are wrong.

Indeed, because a child is likely to be born with some genetic defect, conceiving a child from cloning might be a form of child abuse. If the motives of the parent were bad, then deliberately creating a child who was likely to be genetically defective would be like deliberately choosing to implant an embryo with cystic fibrosis.

Notice that this objection depends on the existing state of scientific knowledge. If scientists learn to originate baboons and chimpanzees by cloning without defects and learn how to originate all other mammals safely by cloning, then the chances of a defective cloned baby would drop drastically, and the force of this objection would correspondingly diminish.

Notice that when we discuss abnormalities, we need a baseline for comparison. Over 50 percent of embryos created sexually, half of which are chromosomally abnormal, do not implant successfully in the human uterus and are lost. About 2 percent of live-born babies have some genetic defect. Millions of babies are born after the mother smoked or drank during their gestation, yet we do not criminalize such smoking and drinking during pregnancy. (Perhaps we should, but why should we focus on the sensationalistic, remote cases of cloning and ignore obvious harm to babies around us?)

## Inequality

Some people, through no merit of their own, start out life much better than others. Some children get two parents, four grandparents, lots of gifts at holidays and birthdays, special pre-school and after-school tutoring, and the best private schools and universities. It seems unfair that some get so much, but others so little.

Over the last centuries, civilized societies have mitigated some of the more extreme effects of this *environmental inequality*: estate taxes have reduced how much can be inherited from parents, income taxes redistribute money from high earners to those on disability and public assistance, and expanding economies have created new opportunities for hard working and talented people to get ahead.

Even so, the gap between rich and poor is astonishing, having widened over the last decade. Given that gap, reproductive cloning could start a new kind of *biological inequality*, much deeper than our existing environmental inequality. Because reproductive cloning would normally involve a conscious choice to clone the genome of one person rather than another, it is likely that families would choose genomes with good qualities. If cloning could be done successfully, such families could create strong, clever, talented, energetic dynasties that outstripped normal humans. It would be a biological case of "the rich get richer, the poor get poorer." Princeton biologist Lee Silver calls the results the "GenRich" and the "Normals."[32]

This is something new in human evolution. Sexual reproduction randomly exchanges genetic material and, because of regression to the mean, makes sure that the great genetic norm of human nature never rises or falls too much. But in a single swoop, particular families single-mindedly devoted to raising their genetic stature could biologically out-distance normal humans over a few generations.

As such, reproductive cloning could endanger social justice. Moreover, because this danger is "written into biology," it would be much harder to undo. People without superior genes would find it much harder to compete against such superior people, even when competition was completely fair.

But is this the way we want the advanced countries of the world to go? Toward a deeply stratified society that divides into Superiors, whose genotypes were chosen by committed families bent on superiority, and Normals, whose genotypes were randomly assigned by the spin of the genetic roulette ball in sexual reproduction?

## Good of the Child

Almost all ordinary discussions of cloning beg two important questions: they assume bad motives on the part of parents or scientists involved in creating a child by cloning, and they assume the child would be harmed by knowing he was created this way.

We can see just how much is begged when we counter these assumptions. First, a child created through cloning would know that he was wanted by his parents. After all, creation of such a child would require in vitro fertilization, which at best is successful only 25 percent of the time. Thus, prospective parents probably would have to try several times to create the baby this way, and to pay for their efforts.

In contrast, all that many people know about the wishes of their parents is that their parents had sex and did not abort. They have no clear evidence that their birth was planned. This fact especially applies to children created before *Griswold v. Connecticut* in 1965, which made it legal for physicians to prescribe contraceptives.

To give this argument some play, assume that cloning children becomes safe. Because knowing she was wanted, is there anything about origination by cloning that would be in the best interests of the future child?

Well, for one thing, most likely no parents would knowingly re-create the genotype of an adult with a congenital disease. Insofar as possible, parents would choose children who would be healthy.

This in itself will be good for the child. Placing aside for the moment worries about eugenics, it is hard to ignore the good of a life where one is not constantly challenged by physical or mental disabilities.

Next, consider that certain traits might be genetically based. We already know that looks and physique are, because we see resemblances in a family. Suppose, too, that intelligence, wit, temperament, sociability, verbal ability, mathematical ability, and analytical ability are partly genetically based. To give the argument more rope, suppose that parents could choose children with some of these traits. Would doing so be good for the child?

It is hard to see why not. Although it may not be politically correct to say it, all other things being equal, it is better to live life as a beautiful, smart, healthy person than the reverse, and it is hard to see why such a life is not in the interests of the person created.

Of course, opponents will say that such a person has been created as a purchased commodity and is subject to the unrealistic expectations of the parent. We consider the objection about expectations later, previously but for now, notice that this general line of objections applies to any service that parents buy for present children with the same goals in mind, such as sending children to elite private schools. Yet no one considers the latter to be bad for the children.

Finally, we should notice that there is a dilemma that proponents of reproductive cloning encounter in which either way, they lose. If cloning is unsafe, then it hurts the child, and therefore it's wrong. If cloning is safe, then it improves the child and is eugenic and, therefore, wrong to do. Obviously, trapped in this false dilemma, proponents of cloning can never win.

At bottom, what may scare opponents of reproductive cloning the most is the possibility that it will work, be safe, and be in the best interests of the children created. Then some children will have more, biologically, than others, and some families may create biological dynasties. Be that as it may, these are not objections about the intrinsic evil of cloning, but indirect ones of public policy, focusing on harm to equality.

## Only Way to Have One's Own Baby

One of the main reasons to produce a child is to have a child with one's own genes. Whether it's to have one's family line continue or to have "a bit of me going into the future," no one questions the soundness of this parental motive.

Now in some rare cases, asexual reproduction will be the only method by which a parent can have a genetic connection to a resulting child. Men who are azoospermatic (producing no sperm) or women whose eggs are too old to conceive often still want a child who is genetically related. Reproductive cloning would allow each parent to have a child (assuming two children) with a strong (99.9 percent) genetic connection to the respective parent.

Although men with low sperm counts could reproduce sexually through intracyptoplasmic sperm injection (ICSI) into a donated egg, there is no option for a man who lacks sperm and a woman who lacks good eggs and who also want a genetic connection to a child. For either parent, the only route is the asexual one of using a cell from a nucleus of a differential cell, and using the genes inside it via cloning to create a human embryo.

The combination of two forces strengthens this argument in subtle ways. First, as they pursue careers, many women delay their first pregnancy, and when they marry so late that they cannot conceive, they are disappointed. At age 42, less than 10 percent of women carry healthy eggs; over 90 percent at this age will fail to bear a child with their own egg. Whatever child they adopt or create with donor eggs will have no genetic connection to them.

Second, it is easy to underestimate the urge to be genetically connected to a child. When government and private insurance refused to pay for in vitro fertilization in the late 1970s, everyone thought that few parents would pay cash for the experimental procedures, much less that struggling college professors with little money would forsake cars and a house in attempts to have a genetically related baby. But they did, and a $3 billion industry was born.

Hence, the millions of couples with women in their 40s who are trying to conceive a child, and who strongly desire a genetic connection to a child or two children, will be the prime movers in the quest to originate children by cloning. Hence, this argument will appeal to more people, and for different reasons, than might have been thought at first.

## Stronger Genetic Connection

A child created by cloning would have *all* the parent's genes, not just half, right? So he or she would have not the usual 50 percent genetic connection to a parent, but nearly 100 percent. But if half a genetic connection is good, why is double not also good?

See this as an onus of proof argument. Since people and courts assume in public policy that a biological connection makes for a bond between parent and child, why wouldn't a stronger bond be just as good? Whatever it is that makes genetic bonds good for children, is a stronger bond not also good? If not, why? If it's just the novelty of a stronger bond, that is not an argument against the bond, just a new item for empirical investigation.

Do our law and courts see the genetic connection this way? Indeed they do. In a dozen cases around the country, a baby who was adopted and who spent several years with an adopted family was returned to a parent with whom he shared a genetic connection. The point is not to judge the merits of the final resolution of custody of the child, but to emphasize how much weight the law puts on binding a parent to a child through shared genes.

In another context, countless talk shows feature unmarried women who have had sexual relations with more than one man, each of whom could be the father of the child. On these shows and often in life, the men say, "If it's mine, I'll support the child." And the law agrees, assigning paternity and requirements of child-support if a DNA test identifies a particular man as the father. All of these cases point to the power we assume of the genetic connection to the child.

But those are sexual connections, where only half a parent's genes are bequeathed to a child. Imagine a total, 100 percent genetic connection. Would that not bind males to sons in an incredibly strong way? Couldn't that be a good thing for some sons to have a father so tightly bound to him? Or for a girl to have a mother so tightly bound?

## Liberty

Those wishing to curtail reproductive cloning because it might increase social inequality need to speak honestly and not hide behind subterfuge. They rarely say exactly what they want to do, which is to decrease the liberty of the average person to have children and to create a family.

The liberty to create children and a family is not absolute and may be outweighed by a much greater social good. But in the rest of our lives, we prize liberty highly, especially when it comes to creating families and what goes on inside them.

In most areas of our personal lives, we are not willing to curtail our personal liberty to create more social-political-economic equality. For example, we could make private schools illegal and require all children to attend public schools. This would get the best parents involved in PTAs and community boards, which in turn would raise the level of all public schools, thereby helping equality. In the South, where private academies continue as the vestiges of racially segregated schools and where elite preparatory schools create a class of highly privileged students, equality is not furthered by giving the best students the most resources.

But few people favor mandatory public schools because it would take away freedom from parents about how and where their children are educated. It is for this reason that some people hate busing—because it forces some children to be bused across the city in the name of equality—and some people home-school their children

The point is not about busing and public education, but about how it is easy to pick on reproductive cloning, sacrificing it to equality, because so few people want to exercise this liberty. But the principle is the same: sacrifice liberty for equality. What justifies sacrifice in one area of reproductive life may be extended to another. For example, if only well-off people can afford IVF, shouldn't it be banned too?

## A Rawlsian Argument for Cloning and Choice

John Rawls argued famously that the principles of justice would be chosen in a hypothetical social contract where parties choose under a veil of ignorance about their position in society when the veil rises.

Under this veil, it is in the interest of all future children to possess as much natural talent as possible, with the best genes, and with the best chance at a long, healthy life. One could even argue, although this is controversial, that under this intra-generational, veil of ignorance theory of justice, people are not just *permitted* to improve the genes of future children, but are *obligated* to do so. Why? Because it is wrong to choose lives for future people that makes them much worse-off than they otherwise could have lived.

If it is true that embryonic cloning cannot be divorced from reproductive cloning, then other things also follow. If reproductive cloning is not bad, then neither is embryonic cloning. If reproductive cloning is not intrinsically bad, but bad only because of abnormal results, then we should study how to prevent abnormalities by funding research in embryonic cloning.

In other words, the preceding argument says that because reproductive cloning is evil, we shouldn't fund anything that would help us do it. But if that is false and reproductive cloning is just a tool—just another way to make a baby and start a family—then we should investigate ways to create such a tool.

## Links Between Embryonic and Reproductive Cloning

Leon Kass wrote, "And yet, as a matter of policy and prudence, any opponent of the manufacture of cloned embryos must, I think, in the end oppose also the creation of cloned human embryos."[33]

Because he fears that allowing cloning of human embryos will inevitably lead to implantation of a human embryo originated by cloning, Kass wants "an absolute and effective ban on all attempts to implant into a uterus a cloned human embryo to produce a living child."

To the criticism that the techniques of SCNT are not that complex and that someone in the world will eventually originate a child by SCNT, Kass would put the onus of proof on those who would permit the "horror" of such origination: "Perhaps such a ban will prove ineffective; it will eventually be shown to have been a mistake. But it would at least place the burden of practical proof where it belongs: on the proponents of this horror."

Not funding research on cloned embryos, or on ways to prevent abnormalities in reproductive cloning in primates, seems perverse. If abnormalities are the major reason for prohibiting reproductive cloning, then surely research to prevent them is justified. But if the real objection is the assumption of the intrinsic evil of reproductive cloning, then we should dispense with the cover argument about abnormalities and get to the real issue.

## FURTHER READINGS

Ronald M. Green, *The Human Embryos Research Debates: Bioethics in the Vortex of Controversy*, New York: Oxford University Press, 2001.

S. Holland et al., *The Human Embryonic Stem Cell Debate*, Cambridge, MA: Bradford/MIT Press, 2001.

Gregory Pence, *Who's Afraid of Human Cloning?* Lanham, MD: Rowman & Littlefield, 1998.

Gregory Pence, *Cloning After Dolly: Who's Still Afraid of Human Cloning?* Lanham, MD: Rowman & Littlefield, 2004.

Human Cloning Foundation, www.humancloning.org.

Francis Fukuyama, *Our Posthuman Future*, New York: Farrar Straus & Giroux, 2002.

Leon Kass, *Human Cloning and Human Dignity: The Report of the President's Council on Bioethics*, New York: Public Affairs Press, 2002.

## DISCUSSION QUESTIONS

1. Should cloning embryos be linked to reproductive cloning, or should the two issues be kept separate?

2. Is reproductive cloning now safe? How might it be made safer by studies of cloned non-human animals?

3. Should food from cloned animals be sold? Labeled as such?

4. Is a human embryo a person? A thing of value? Just tissue?

5. How has the discovery of IPS cells altered the landscape of the debate about research on human embryos?

6. If cloning babies were safe, how might it create more inequality in society?

# CHAPTER 8

# The Ethics of Treating Impaired Babies

*E*very issue in bioethics has a pedigree, and the treatment of impaired babies has a long one. That pedigree lies behind the cases of Infant Doe in Indiana in 1982 and Baby Jane Doe in New York in 1983, as well as the Baby Doe rules and the Baby Doe squads—this chapter's subjects. *Baby Doe cases* arise when parents of impaired neonates forgo treatment to let such babies die.

Just as respirators and feeding tubes during the 1960s allowed adult comatose patients to stay alive, so tiny respirators and tiny feeding tubes were used to save babies with congenital disabilities who otherwise would have died. During the same decade, neonatal intensive care units (NICUs) developed, where such babies were treated.

But heroic interventions at the start of life did not always create wonderful results. Many such babies were "saved" to suffer lives of chronic disability, making neonatologists wonder whether they had done the right thing to save them. Such is the context of the cases described here.

## 1971: THE JOHNS HOPKINS CASES

Down syndrome is a genetic condition that always causes mental disability and a characteristic facial appearance; it is often accompanied by cardiac or intestinal problems. In the early 1970s, physicians told parents that although the eventual IQ of a Down person could not be predicted at birth, it usually ranged between 25 and 60, with some severely impaired individuals below 25 (whether this information was correct will be discussed later).

In 1971, physicians sometimes omitted aggressive treatment from impaired newborns. Three Down babies then in the NICU at Johns Hopkins Hospital in Baltimore, Maryland, had life-threatening intestinal defects. Physicians and parents allowed two of them to die.[1]

One of the babies had *duodenal atresia*, a blockage between the higher duodenum and the lower stomach that prevents passage of food and water. The mother of this baby—a nurse who had worked with children with Down syndrome—knew that if she did not consent to surgery to open the atresia, her infant would die.

She refused to do so, as did her husband, a lawyer. Pediatric surgeons at Hopkins honored their decision and did not go to court to force them to operate.

Another mother, who already had children, allowed her Down baby to die. According to theologian James Gustafson, she explained her decision to forgo treatment by saying, "It would be unfair to the other children of the household to raise them with a mongoloid."[2] (Because of the facial characteristics associated in Down syndrome, it was previously called "mongolism," a term now considered prejudicial.) Gustafson describes this mother's decision as "anguished," but notes that when she learned her baby had Down syndrome, she "immediately indicated she did not want the child."

No one killed the two Down babies; they were simply allowed to die—physicians thought this course more morally acceptable and less likely to incur legal prosecution. One of these babies took 15 days to die; ordinarily, the baby would have died in about four days by dehydration, but some staff members surreptitiously gave the infant water.

The parents of the third baby eventually accepted treatment, and this baby lived. This baby's parents had originally been given a pessimistic prognosis for Down syndrome by the referring obstetrician. However—and perhaps significantly—the staff at Hopkins gave the third set of parents a more balanced view.

## 1970s: PEDIATRIC INTENSIVISTS GO PUBLIC

In the early 1970s, because of the increasing incidence of these cases, two well-known pediatricians, R. Duff and A. Campbell at Yale-New Haven Medical Center, admitted they had forgone treatment for 43 impaired infants, who then died early.[3] This caused a sensation and led to soul-searching by neonatologists at other NICUs, who wondered if they should also let some severely impaired newborns die.

English physician John Lorber then argued that some babies suffer such extreme impairment that they are better off being allowed to die without treatment.[4] Lorber specialized in spina bifida. *Spina bifida* literally means "divided spine" and is a hernial protrusion through a defect in the vertebral column. It is the most common serious neural-tube defect, occurring 3–5 times in 10,000 live births.[5] It may occur in the form of a *meningocele*, a protrusion of part of the meninges, or it may take the form of a *myelomeningocele*, a protrusion not only of part of the meninges, but also of the spinal cord (the nerve bundle).

A baby with spina bifida will almost always be paralyzed below the level of the opening and suffer bowel and bladder problems. The opening makes the baby vulnerable to infections such as meningitis. Quality of life depends on the level of the meningomyelocele and the degree of associated problems such as hydrocephalus—a swelling of cranial tissue that commonly accompanies spina bifida.

Hydrocephalus often increases intracranial pressure and decreases blood flow to the brain, resulting in mental deficiency. The probability of mental impairment can be reduced by aggressive surgical treatment involving tubes called *shunts* that decrease the pressure.

Lorber developed criteria to predict which spina bifida babies, if left untreated, would die: the higher the meningomyelocele on the spine and the larger the affected area of the spine and its coverings, the greater the probability of death. These criteria had risks and a dilemma: if left untreated, not all infants with spina bifida die, and for infants who live, nontreatment makes them worse off.

Lorber's criteria seemed to make it possible to identify babies who would die: all those in his lowest category did die. During the 1970s, criteria like Lorber's were apparently used at Oklahoma Children's Hospital, where it was decided not to treat 24 babies with spina bifida who were in the lowest category and all of whom subsequently died.[6]

## ANCIENT HISTORY

In ancient Athens, both Plato (in *The Republic)* and Aristotle (in his *Politics*) advocated killing impaired newborns. In ancient Sparta, a cyclops baby (i.e., an infant born with a single eye or with two eyes fused) would be left to die in a country field.

Exposure was practiced by ancient Romans, who also abandoned deformed babies in fields. During the next four centuries, exposure remained common: such letting die was legal and not considered infanticide. In contrast, the Bedouin tribes of Arabia, the Chinese, and much of India practiced female infanticide for two millennia.[7]

Around the year 300, Roman emperor Constantine converted to Christianity and as such, outlawed both abandonment and infanticide. However, the church had neither funds nor people to care for abandoned babies. Foundling hospitals for abandoned babies did not start until the eighth century in Milan.

During the Middle Ages, wet nurses acted as agents for parents wishing to rid themselves of children (a practice that would continue well into the nineteenth century). In the eighteenth century, when the population of Europe exploded, exposure-as-infanticide became a form of extreme birth control.

During the reign of Napoleon, women abandoned so many babies that Napoleon established his own foundling hospitals, where parents could deposit a baby on a turntable set into the front entrance, spin it to send the baby inside, and depart unseen. In France in 1833, mothers abandoned over 100,000 babies—20 to 30 percent of all births.[8]

## 1981: THE MUELLER CASE: CONJOINED TWINS

In 1981, twins joined at the trunk and sharing three legs were born in Danville, Illinois, to Pamela and Robert Mueller.[9] Robert Mueller, a physician, was in the delivery room when their family physician, Petra Warren, delivered the babies, who were named Jeff and Scott. The Muellers and Warren decided together not to treat the twins aggressively, so they could die.

Other physicians in Danville were divided deeply over the ethics of the Muellers' decision. An anonymous caller alerted Protective Child Services, which obtained a court order for temporary custody of the children.

Prosecutors charged the Muellers with neglect. Later a judge dismissed that charge, but he did deny the Muellers custody. In September 1981, they regained custody after pediatric surgeons testified that they would be unlikely to successfully separate the twins and that they had a bleak prognosis.

Subsequent events in this case tell a different tale. The twins lived, still joined, for about a year, at which time they weighed 30 pounds.[10] Shortly thereafter, they were separated in a long operation. Scott, the weaker twin, died at age 3; but Jeff, the stronger twin, survived, and later entered a regular school.

Some might also question the necessity of separating the conjoined twins in the first place. The desire for normality and to have singletons often creates an unstoppable force to turn all children into normal-looking singletons (a topic discussed in Chapter 12).

## 1982: THE INFANT DOE CASE

The Infant Doe case in Bloomington, Indiana, took place about one year after the Mueller case, but over the course of only a few days—from Infant Doe's birth on April 9, 1982, to its death on April 15. Infant Doe had Down syndrome with tracheoesophageal fistula, and once again, physicians split over forgoing treatment.[11]

The prognosis for tracheoesophageal fistula is more serious than for duodenal atresia and depends on the severity of the fistula, or gap. Infant Doe had a fairly small gap, and an early operation to close it would have had a 90 percent chance of success. However, in discussing the case with the parents, the referring obstetrician, Walter Owens, downplayed this fact and emphasized that some Down people are "mere blobs" and that the "lifetime cost" of caring for a Down child would "almost surely be close to $1 million." Infant Doe's parents decided not to allow the operation.

Hospital administrators and pediatricians disagreed with the parents' decision and contacted Monroe County judge John Baker. Owen testified before Baker that even if surgery were successful, "the possibility of a minimally adequate quality of life was nonexistent" because of "the child's severe and irreversible mental retardation."

Infant Doe's father, a public school teacher who had worked closely with Down children, agreed with Dr. Owens and felt that such children never had a "minimally acceptable quality of life." It is noteworthy that Judge Baker held this hearing late at night in a room at the hospital where no one recorded it and did not appoint a guardian *ad litem* for Infant Doe. The judge then ruled for the parents.

The county district attorney appealed to the County Circuit Court, and after losing there, to the Indiana Supreme Court. Both appeals failed: each time the court ruled for the parents. He then appealed to U.S. Supreme Court Justice Paul Stevens for an emergency intervention, but Infant Doe died, making the case moot.

Seven years later in 1989, the U.S. Civil Rights Commission cited the Infant Doe case as a landmark case of prejudice against disabled infants. Owens wrote about his role in the Infant Doe case, maintaining that he was "proud to have stood up for what I and a large percentage of people feel is right"; he also said he was glad that Infant Doe had died in only a few days and with little suffering and was glad that the parents were able to have another baby—a healthy child who, if the couple had been forced to treat Infant Doe, would not have been born. The commission concluded that Owens's evaluation was "strikingly out of touch with the contemporary evidence on the capabilities of people with Down syndrome."[12]

## 1982–1986: THE BABY DOE RULES

National media extensively reported the Infant Doe case, which prompted President Ronald Reagan to direct the Justice Department and the Department of Health and Human Services (HHS) to mandate treatment in future cases. Reagan, who opposed abortion, had appointed C. Everett Koop as Surgeon General. Koop had previously written a book opposing nontreatment of impaired newborns.[13]

Because states and not the federal government define crimes such as homicide and gross negligence, Reagan's Justice Department needed to find an indirect route to make nontreatment illegal. This department created a way to do so.

The executive branch can set social policy by reinterpreting prior congressional legislation. In the 1960s, President Lyndon Johnson reinterpreted old laws to fight racial discrimination. Institutions violating the new interpretations risk losing all federal funds.

Through similar executive orders, lawyers for the Justice Department in 1982 interpreted nontreatment to violate Section 504 of the Rehabilitation Act of 1973, which forbade discrimination solely on the basis of handicap. This interpretation saw imperiled newborns as handicapped citizens who could suffer discrimination against their federal civil rights. Congress had originally meant this act to apply to adults and children with handicaps, not babies.

HHS then required large posters to be displayed on the outer glass walls of every NICU:

DISCRIMINATORY FAILURE TO FEED AND CARE FOR HANDICAPPED INFANTS IN THIS FACILITY IS PROHIBITED BY FEDERAL LAW.

It also posted a toll-free 800 telephone number on the poster so anyone around an NICU could report abuses—including concerned nurses, disgruntled parents, ambulance-chasing lawyers, and anonymous cranks. New *Baby Doe squads*, composed of lawyers, government administrators, and physicians, investigated complaints.

In 1983, the American Academy of Pediatrics successfully sued in a federal district court to block the Baby Doe Rules. While this suit ran, the Baby Jane Doe case began.

Before we turn to it, we should describe the Baby Doe hotline and the Baby Doe squads. As long as they existed, the Baby Doe squads were ready on an hour's notice to rush to airports, fly across the country, and suddenly arrive—as a squad arrived one day at Vanderbilt University—like outside accountants doing a surprise bank audit. They seized records, took charts from attending physicians, and investigated all night. The squads thought they saved the lives of innocent babies.

Besides Vanderbilt, the University of Rochester also suffered (in the words used privately by some pediatricians) a "blitzkrieg by the Baby Doe Gestapo." Eventually, because of the objections by pediatricians and the national press, the squads were called off.

What was the ultimate effect of the hotline and the squads? One study discovered that Baby Doe squads did in fact *force* more treatment for six infants, who had operations they otherwise might not have had, but in no case did the squads *prove* a violation of the Baby Doe regulations.[14]

## 1983–1984: THE BABY JANE DOE CASE

On October 11, 1983, physicians delivered Baby Jane Doe at St. Charles Hospital of Long Island, New York. Because she had several major defects, they transferred her to a NICU at University Hospital of the State University of New York (SUNY) campus at Stony Brook.

Her parents—known only as Linda and Dan—worked hard to improve their lives as lower-middle-class people. Linda, 23, and Dan, 30, had been married four months when Linda became pregnant.

Baby Jane weighed six pounds and was 20 inches long. According to testimony, at birth she had spina bifida, hydrocephalus, a damaged kidney, and *microcephaly* (small head, implying a minimal brain or lack of most of the brain). Her defects surely traumatized her parents. For one thing, her spine was open with the meningocele protruding prominently.

At Stony Brook, surgeon Arjen Keuskamp recommended immediate surgery to minimize retardation by draining the hydrocephalus. When Baby Jane was examined by George Newman, a pediatric neurologist, he told Dan that Baby Jane would either die soon without surgery or could undergo surgery and be paralyzed, mentally impaired, and vulnerable to continual infections in her bladder and bowels. According to Newman's later court testimony:

> The decision made by the parents is that it would be unkind to have surgery performed on this child. . . . On the basis of the combination of malformations that are present in this child, *she is not likely to ever achieve any meaningful interaction with her environment, nor ever achieve any interpersonal relationships*, the very qualities which we consider human.[15]

Keuskamp withdrew from the case and did not testify in court. About midnight on October 11, 14 hours after Baby Jane's birth, Newman probably told Dan something like his testimony in court.

After a good deal of soul-searching, Dan and Linda decided not to allow the operation to drain the hydrocephalus. They acted on their understanding of the distinction between extraordinary and ordinary treatment, disallowing surgery but allowing "comfort care": food, fluids, and antibiotics.

Based on what they had been told, they naively assumed that Baby Jane would soon die, but four days later she was still alive. A social worker wrote at this time that Dan was in "despair" because Baby Jane had not yet died; she also noted that Linda was determined to give Baby Jane "as much love as possible" while the infant was still alive. "We love her very much," Linda said, "and that's why we made the decision we did."[16]

*Newsday* reporter Kathleen Kerr broke the Baby Jane Doe story nationally on October 18, 1983. Kerr, who had numerous firsts on the story, was also the only reporter at the time to interview the parents. She described the interview:

> Each time he began a sentence, Mr. A. let out a deep sigh, as though seeking strength to answer. Mrs. A. continually touched her husband's arm and rubbed it soothingly. Mr. A. shed his tears openly. . . . Mr. A. said, "We feel the conservative method of treatment is going to do her as much good as if surgery were to be performed. It's not a case of our not caring. We very much want this baby." . . .
>
> "We're not being neglectful, and we're not relying on our religion [Catholicism] to give us the answer to what we're doing here."[17]

Baby Jane Doe continued to survive, and—as occurs naturally in some cases of spina bifida—her open spinal wound closed.

## 1983–1986: BABY JANE'S CASE IN THE COURTS

On October 18, 1983 (the same day that Kerr broke the story), Lawrence Washburn, a municipal-bonds lawyer who lived in Vermont and who promoted right-to-life organizations, filed suit in a state court to force treatment for Baby Jane. Over the following weeks, the case sped through the courts because everyone wanted to avoid a repetition of the Infant Doe case, where the baby died while appeals bogged down.

Judge Melvyn Tannenbaum held an emergency lower-court hearing on October 20. Because Washburn lacked legal standing to sue, Tannenbaum appointed another attorney, William Weber, as Baby Jane's guardian *ad litem* ("for this action or proceeding") and empowered him temporarily to make decisions regarding Baby Jane's medical care.

At first, Weber supported the parents, but then an interesting fact surfaced. Having talked to Newman, Weber abruptly changed his mind when he read two items in Baby Jane's medical chart. First, he read that Newman had written that after surgery, Jane would be able to walk with braces.[18] Second, her chart said that the initial measurement of her skull was 31 centimeters, within normal limits. This measurement indicates that Baby Jane may have had a normal brain.

Yet Newman had testified that the baby had microcephaly and would never be able to recognize her parents. Weber concluded that what Newman had written on the chart conflicted both with what he had told the parents and with his testimony in court. So dramatically, Weber decided that Newman's claim of microcephaly was "a lie" and on October 20, authorized surgery.

The case ended up in the appellate division of New York courts. The justices there decided that the law left decisions up to parents when a choice was available between two *medically reasonable options*. Interestingly, previous rulings of courts had required a "medically reasonable option" to be an option that was not only supported by evidence, but was also in the interest of the child. The new judgment contradicted these precedents.

These court hearings splashed across front pages of American newspapers. Perhaps this immense publicity created too much pressure. The courts seemed to forget about the traditional doctrine of *parens patria*, according to which the state protects helpless people against those who might neglect them.

After these court proceedings concluded, the parents said:

> I just want [all this] to end. Just to have a baby like this and deal with it is so much to go through right now. Just let us be with our daughter and leave us alone. . . . If there's hell, we've been through it.

By this point, however, the federal government had begun to act.

In October, the Justice Department informed Stony Brook Hospital that federal investigators wanted to see Baby Jane's medical records. This intrusion outraged the parents: "They're not doctors, they're not the parents, and they have no business in our lives right now."[19]

Stony Brook's lawyer then announced that the hospital would block the government from examining the records. HHS turned the case over to the Justice Department, which sued the hospital in federal court, charging possible discrimination against the handicapped. Attorney General Edwin Meese and Surgeon General Koop personally led the suit.

Federal judge Leonard Wexler then ruled that the Justice Department could not have the medical record and that the parents had not decided against surgery for "discriminatory" reasons. (It is not clear if Judge Wexler had examined Baby Jane's hospital chart.)

The ruling pleased the parents. "I'm drained physically, mentally, and emotionally," Dan said; "I believed that you couldn't look at what we were doing and say we were wrong."

In 1984, the case reached the federal Court of Appeals for the Second Circuit, which again denied the government access to Baby Jane's records. This decision, which would presumably apply in similar cases, had the practical effect of making the Baby Doe rules useless: because the government could not obtain medical records from NICUs or hospitals, it could not enforce the Baby Doe rules.

The Justice Department appealed to the U.S. Supreme Court, but two years later in 1986, in *Bowen v. American Hospital Association et al.*, the Supreme Court declared that no records needed to be released and, in effect, ended the Baby Doe Rules, their national hotline, and their possible investigators.

## FOLLOW-UP ON BABY JANE DOE

Amazingly, during the court battles over Baby Jane, Linda and Dan actually changed their minds and permitted surgery to drain her hydrocephalus—a decision that became known only months later.[20] After contracting pneumonia, physicians gave the baby strong antibiotics, without which, she might have died. At that time, one physician predicted that she would "probably always be bedridden."[21]

Baby Jane continued to live and went home on April 7, 1984, at age five-and-a-half months. Her real name was Keri-Lynn and we will use that in this text from now on because using her real name makes her seem more of a person and less just a case.

Five years later, Keri-Lynn lived at home with her parents. According to Kathleen Kerr, whose stories about the case won a Pulitzer Prize for local reporting and who visited with the family over those years, Keri-Lynn was:

> . . . doing better than anyone expected—talking, attending school for the handicapped, and learning to mix with her peers. She still can't walk and gets around in a wheelchair but her progress has defied the dire predictions.[22]

In 1994, another reporter interviewed Keri-Lynn and her family:

> Now a 10-year-old, . . . Jane Doe is not only a self-aware little girl, who experiences and returns the love of her parents; she also attends a school for developmentally disabled children—once again proving that medicine is an art, not a science, and clinical decision making is best left in the clinic, to those who will have to live with the decision being made.[23]

She had seizures for her first 12 years, but these became more controlled when she became a teenager.

In 1998, Paul Gianelli, who represented the parents in their legal battles, told reporters that Keri-Lynn was 15 years old and still living with her parents, who guard her privacy and theirs. "It was a very sad case and yet satisfying," said Gianelli, who ultimately won in court for the parents.[24]

In 2003, Dan and Linda granted another interview when Keri-Lynn was 20.[25] A reporter saw Keri-Lynn with her father watching her sister cheerleading below and heard her say:

> "Nothing gets better than this, Dad," Keri-Lynn said to the man who carried her all the way up the steps [from her wheelchair]. "You and me, watching the football game."

At 20, Keri-Lynn loved to talk. She lived with her three teenage sisters, mother, and father on Long Island. A bus picked her up each day at 8 AM for a school for people with special needs and returned her at 3 PM, when she would often roll her wheelchair up the sidewalk.

At 5 feet tall, the 86-pound woman wore a cast to keep her back and legs strong. Her mother or a school nurse changed a catheter to drain her urine four times a day; they hoped that one day occupational therapy could teach her to change it herself so that Keri-Lynn could live independently in a group home. Surgeons operated repeatedly for infections in the shunt in her head and, later, to correct problems in her hips, calves, and heels.

At 20, she appeared more normal emotionally and socially than academically. She had learned only the alphabet and to count, but had not mastered reading books. She appeared very integrated with, and dependent on, her immediate family and on her strong publicly funded special school.

As of October 2012, Keri-Lynn was still alive.[26] From her picture then, she appeared to have aged prematurely, looking 60 rather than 29.

## MEDIA ETHICS AND BIAS

The reporting of Baby Jane's case in the print and visual media raised some disturbing questions, especially when we consider that Jane not only survived but also was able to live at home and even attend school. Recall that Dr. Newman had testified that Jane would never achieve any meaningful interaction with her environment or any interpersonal relationships. Why did Newman's opinion prevail? That should stimulate some thought.

During 1983, the momentum of the media in support of the parents—and with it the momentum of medicine and medical ethics—became so strong that the media portrayed dissenters as bigots. People read reports of the Baby Jane Doe case with their minds made up. In November, when Lesley Stahl grilled Dr. Koop on *Face the Nation*, her tone painted him as a fundamentalist, parent-baiting Big Brother. Ed Bradley on *60 Minutes* also did a similar hatchet job on Koop and the case.

From today's perspective, Koop's answers during these interviews are impressive: he said that the medical chart had discrepancies and that he merely wanted to see it to learn what was best for the child.

One pediatric neurosurgeon who had treated over a thousand patients with spina bifida said that children whose heads measured 31 centimeters (as Baby Jane's did) are among "the very brightest" of such children, presumably implying that Baby Jane's IQ could be normal or better.[27] The public also did not learn that although hydrocephalus generally accompanies spina bifida, if shunted immediately, it may not result in as much mental damage.

All the major media simply accepted George Newman's negative prognosis, and almost all dismissed William Weber, the child's court-appointed guardian, as a fanatic. The media's stance may have unduly influenced not only the general public, but even many physicians and medical ethicists, who took Newman's depressing prognosis as fact.

In retrospect, another astonishing aspect of the story escaped the public's notice. When Stony Brook Hospital resisted Koop's attempt to see Baby Jane's medical chart, the hospital's motives might have been not to protect the privacy of the family, but also to protect itself from a court suit. Given that what Newman had written in the chart contradicted what the parents had heard him say, one can see that the hospital had a big problem.

Beyond a doubt, pediatricians disagreed about which treatment was best for Baby Jane and about the "medically reasonable options" in this case. Unfortunately, the public never read about the two real sides of this medical controversy. As a result, the public came to believe that the case involved only moral questions about parental decisions and low quality of life, when in fact it raised questions about making decisions based on incomplete, biased information and a hospital protecting itself from suit.

It is astonishing that a story for which the journalist won a Pulitzer Prize has such major errors and omissions. It is astonishing that neither the *New York Times* nor the *Wall Street Journal* checked the story's facts independently. During this time, the media so much favored the parents that perhaps it was politically impossible for any reporter to present another side.

Perhaps, too, it shows how hard the story was to understand and how difficult it is for the public to get the real medical facts. Physicians usually will not talk to reporters about a controversial case and will not criticize their colleagues to reporters. So the public finds out only in court what is really going on about the case.

## ETHICAL ISSUES

### Selfishness

Theologian James Gustafson said Baby Jane Doe's parents selfishly did not want Baby Jane to live.[28] For him, Judaism and Christianity require us to live our lives for others. Dr. Koop argued similarly: "Why not let the family find that deeper meaning of life by providing the love and the attention necessary to take care of an infant that has been given to them?"[29]

In contrast, the late bioethicist John Fletcher said that he could "stand by the parents" in such cases and "would not want to come down real hard on them" for letting a baby die by forgoing treatment.[30] Also, if living for others is a religious value, should atheists and agnostics be forced to live by it?

Reluctance to raise a profoundly disabled child is not necessarily selfish and may be simply realistic. For a couple, raising a severely disabled child usually means that one parent must give up a job. Because people with Down syndrome had an average lifespan of 50 years in 2013, and some lived into their 70s, some adult Down children will outlive their parents. Is it really selfish for parents to decide that they are not called to spend their lives caring for such a person, especially if at birth they can choose a normal child?

Disability advocates argue that disadvantaged children cannot be allowed to die merely because they don't fit into their parents' plans. Part of the responsibility of having sex, and thinking about possible childbirth, is to accept whatever comes along. We can't let parents adopt the attitude of, "I'll only be a parent if my child is healthy and normal." They also stress that family values mean that everyone pulls together to help the least well-off member, whether that person is Baby Doe or Granny Doe. They reject the conceptualization of this case as parental autonomy versus Big Brother. Instead, they say it takes a village to raise a Down child.

On the other hand, if we do not consider the family's good in some way, are we not implying that every family must accept the birth of an impaired child, no matter what? As an institution, the family today seems shaky; how much can it take?

### Personal versus Public Cases

Was Baby Jane's case a private, personal family decision or a case of neglect that public policy must not tolerate? One critic argued that, "private individuals and private groups of individuals don't have the right to make life or death decisions in private in an unaccountable manner."[31] And we don't tolerate child-abuse in the private homes of citizens.

On the other hand, many people at the time argued that Baby Jane's parents should have been left alone to make decisions. As *Newsday* writer Fred Bruning wrote:

> Travelers familiar with Beirut claim it is a city lost to hope because consensus is impossible. Perhaps it can be said that parents of severely damaged children inhabit a Beirut of the spirit, a place where innocence has no armor, where there is no distinction between suffering and survival. The rest of us are strangers, and we ought to let the parents consult the doctors, reach their decisions, tend to their babies, grapple with their lives. We ought to respect their heartache and their wishes. We ought to leave them in peace.[32]

In 1983, Tennessee intervened over a father's religious objections to chemotherapy for his 12-year-old daughter Pamela Hamilton, who had leukemia. Another such case occurred in Boston in 1988, when a young child became ill; the child's parents, who were Christian Scientists, called a practitioner instead of a physician; after apparently improving for a while, the child suddenly died five days later. Boston district attorney Newman Flanagan charged them with manslaughter.

In the presidential elections of 2008 and 2012, Sarah Palin's son Trig, with Down syndrome, and Bella, Rick Santorum's daughter with Trisomy 18, became campaign issues.

Clearly society must strike a balance between allowing parents some choice about medical treatment of their children and protecting vulnerable children from misguided parents.

## ABORTION VERSUS INFANTICIDE

Today, many pregnant women undergo amniocentesis or sonograms, and if the results indicate a fetus with a chromosomal abnormality, many terminate the pregnancy and try again for a healthy baby. Such abortions can take place legally late in the second trimester, when the fetus is large and perhaps at a stage of development where some premature babies are saved.

When amniocentesis indicates spina bifida, the fetus will almost always be aborted. But if spina bifida justifies abortion, why doesn't it also justify letting a newborn with spina bifida die? Similarly, if an abortion is permissible because the fetus has Down syndrome, why shouldn't Down syndrome justify allowing a baby to die?

Birth, after all, does not change the medical condition: in this sense, it can be argued that the significance of birth is merely symbolic. Note that this logic is neutral between opposed moral conclusions about nontreatment. If there is no good reason why a neonate with, say, spina bifida should be allowed to die, then presumably there is no good reason why a fetus with spina bifida should be aborted.

If parents want to forgo treatment in these cases, then should they be required to justify the decision? Should they simply be left alone? When a woman decides to abort even a healthy fetus, she is not required to give good reasons. Why are we so much more concerned when an impaired newborn is involved?

Conceptually, the problem is to find a consistent position that includes accepting abortion but opposes letting parents decide to forgo treatment in a Baby Doe case. If one accepts choice with regard to abortion because of a Down fetus, should one also not accept choice about parents letting a Down newborn die? Or perhaps one should oppose both?

## Killing versus Letting Die with Newborns

As discussed in Chapter 3, the late James Rachels asked whether it would not be more compassionate to simply kill impaired and imperiled newborns than to let them die slowly by forgoing treatment.[33] Rachels argued this way: in both forgoing treatment and infanticide, the motive (death of the baby) is the same, and so is the result (death of the baby). If both decisions have the same motive, and if both lead to death, how can the two differ morally?

This might seem to be a matter of simple logic: whatever makes one decision good (or bad) should also make the other decision good (or bad). If so, the kind of action itself, as to its active or passive nature, should make no difference.

Some bioethicists disagree. People make mistakes and killing is too final. In contrast, allowing a person time to die leaves the door open for a while, during which mistakes can be corrected or opinions can change. Another argument for forgoing treatment is that it shows more respect: a quick end cheapens life, but forgoing treatment makes parents and professionals suffer through the ordeal of dying.

## PERSONHOOD OF IMPAIRED NEONATES

Before he became surgeon general, Dr. Koop wrote that, "each newborn infant, perfect or deformed, is a human being with unique preciousness because he or she was created in the image of God."[34] On the other hand, Catholic theologian Richard McCormick argued that an infant can realize some "good" of its own only if it can potentially form human relationships.[35] So Koop assumed that any human newborn is a person, whereas McCormick's criterion would rule out anencephalic (brain-absent) babies as persons.

McCormick's *potential-for-relationships standard* is a reasonable attempt to delimit personhood, but it has problems. It can be difficult to predict potential for relationships, which seems to depend on the attitude of parents. Associations of parents of babies with spina bifida hold that a person's potential cannot be known until his or her life is lived.

The *gradient view of personhood* (discussed in both Chapters 3 and 5) asserts that the developmental stage of the fetus/baby really does matter morally. A crying baby differs a lot from a two-day old embryo. Several neuroscientists and bioethicists believe that personhood develops along a gradient, such that the further along this continuum, the more the fetus is a person. This view rejects the all-or-nothing fallacy that an embryo or fetus is not a person one moment, but a person the next.

On the gradient view, it's worse to kill fetuses than embryos, and it's worse to kill fetuses just before birth than in the first trimester (which explains why many physicians are reluctant to perform so-called partial birth abortions). Similarly, a Down baby differs from a Down fetus: the former has more moral status and rights. The death of a baby requires more justification than the death of a fetus.

The distinctions of the gradient view drive some opponents to claim that no difference in personhood or moral status exists between human embryos and human babies. Both sides agree about the gradient and the continuum of personhood, but the sides disagree about the proper inferences to draw from this fact.

In Baby Doe cases, some bioethicists champion the *cognitive criterion of personhood*. It identifies certain characteristics, including reason, agency, memory, and self-awareness, and assumes that without them, personhood does not exist.

With regard to impaired infants, bioethicist Peter Singer once used the cognitive criterion to argue that children should not be regarded as persons until "a few months" after birth; physician and philosopher Tristam Engelhardt once held that infants are not persons until they form a self-concept, around the age of 2 (he has since given up this position). Philosopher Michael Tooley holds that they are not persons until they can use language.[36] For Singer, Engelhardt, and Tooley, newborns fail to meet the cognitive criterion.

Some families use the cognitive criterion in letting adult relatives die. However, its application to impaired newborns may be more questionable. Allowing parents to forgo treatment for an imperiled neonate is one thing; claiming that a child is not a person until age 2 seems to be quite another.

## KINDS OF EUTHANASIA

Cases of treatment versus nontreatment are often wrongly lumped together with assisted suicide and physician-assisted dying—all as "euthanasia." This is confusing and possibly dangerous. As argued in Chapter 3, we should differentiate physician-assisted dying, which involves terminally ill competent adults, from assisted suicide, which involves nonterminal competent adults; we should also distinguish these from nontreatment of incompetent adults in PVS, and distinguish the above from allowing impaired newborns to die.

One reason why such distinctions matter has to do with criteria for forgoing treatment. Criteria for nontreatment of *never-competent* patients should presumably be much higher than the criteria for competent or formerly competent patients whose own wishes can be known or inferred. We need to prove beyond a reasonable doubt that an impaired, presently incompetent patient would be better off dead than being treated to live some kind of life later as an adult.

## DEGREES OF DEFECT

In practice, criteria for nontreatment of impaired babies tend to be based on long-term prognoses and degrees of defectiveness in newborns.[37] Babies whose problems are "less serious" should be treated, whereas it would be permissible to let die babies who are "most serious" or "gravely ill."

Cases between these two poles—cases such as spina bifida and Down syndrome—create controversy because prognosis is far from absolute and may be influenced by moral frameworks.

Consider John Lorber's predictive criteria for spina bifida. One vocal critic of Lorber's approach is his colleague at the same hospital, pediatric surgeon R. B. Zachary. Zachary argues that the only options for babies with spina bifida are either to kill them or to do everything possible for each one of them. Basically, he is saying that there is no category of babies with spina bifida who can be "allowed to die."

Lorber and some other pediatricians say that the mortality rate is high for babies they place in the "worst" category of spina bifida, but Zachary maintains that these physicians do not simply withhold treatment. According to Zachary, they "push the infant toward death" by giving:

> . . . eight times the sedative dose of chloral hydrate recommended in the most recent volume of Nelson's *Pediatrics* and four times the hypnotic dose, and it is being administered four times every day. No wonder these babies are sleepy and demand no feeding, and with this regimen most of them will die within a few weeks, many within the first week.[38]

Prognoses about the intelligence of impaired people seem to be influenced by social views. Down syndrome is a good example, especially because of the external characteristics associated with it. Let's briefly consider Down syndrome in more detail.

During the last 50 years, a Copernican revolution has occurred in thinking about Down people.[39] Many earlier studies of IQ on Down people who were institutionalized were flawed. A sampling bias failed to take into account the higher IQs of Down people who lived with supportive families.

At present, although most Down syndrome people will have IQs below 70, less than one-third (some studies say only 10 percent) will have IQs lower than 25 (profoundly mentally deficient and untrainable).[40] Most Down people who receive good early care, maximum stimulation, and support will have IQs between 50 and 70.

What does this imply about quality of life for a Down person? IQ is a measure of intelligence, of course, and academics and physicians often associate intelligence with happiness. However, it is an unwarranted conclusion to infer that people with IQs between about 50 and 70 must be unhappy, unless we simply define unhappiness in those terms.

Given reasonable stimulation, love, and supervision, most Down people will, to use a phrase made important in ethics by philosopher Tom Regan in another context, "have a life."[41] Almost every Down person will have a narrative history and lives that will go (to use another famous phrase from Regan) "better or worse for them." Under almost any criteria of quality of life, most people with Down syndrome would not be better off dead.

Note the mention of early care, stimulation, and support; the prognosis for Down syndrome varies with treatment: early stimulation can raise IQ, whereas merely custodial care will lower it. At birth, we cannot predict whether a Down baby will be at the low or the high end of the IQ range; consequently, the best interest of these babies is maximal treatment. Whether maximal treatment best benefits their families is another question.

## WRONGFUL BIRTH VERSUS WRONGFUL LIFE

Parents can sue physicians in civil courts for allegedly causing babies to be impaired. Today, few parents simply accept birth defects as God's will; standards of health continue to rise, and couples expect healthy babies. Parents often blame physicians for the birth of impaired babies.

Both wrongful life and wrongful birth suits fall into the general classification of tort law, and in both kinds of actions compensation for a harm or "tort" is sought.

As discussed in Chapter 6, it is important to distinguish between different meanings of "harm." Like the concept of good, the concept of harm covers a broad range of meanings. For our purposes here, we can distinguish three broad meanings of harm.

In the first way, both a baseline and a temporal (time) component are necessary, so that a change occurs that makes someone worse off. *Baseline harm* requires an adverse change in someone's condition. With baseline harm, someone who doesn't yet exist cannot be harmed, because he or she has no baseline from which change can occur.

The second way of defining harm compares a present deficiency with what normally would have been. In this *abnormal harm,* someone is injured by being brought into existence with some defect that could have been avoided by taking reasonable precautions. Here, the event or omission that causes the defect is the cause of harm.

Third, harm may be defined as a life of total pain and injury, such that no hope exists. Perhaps this is the lot of many pigs raised in industrial factory-farms, confined their whole lives and squashed together for maximal profits in tiny metal pens with their tails cut off. Let us call this third harm *total harm.* To some of its critics, reproductive cloning would be so bad for the child as to constitute total harm.

Preventing abnormal harm underlies the belief that parents should do everything possible to have healthy, unimpaired babies; that anything less than the maximal effort is blameworthy; and that it is wrong for a woman to take risks with a future person's intelligence or health. In this sense, deaf parents harm their children when they implant only embryos genetically disposed to be deaf.

Total harm in the law is called *wrongful life*. In such cases, lawyers claim that the lives of some babies are so miserable that their existence is a tort. In contrast, *wrongful birth* assumes abnormal harm, and claims not that the child's life is totally miserable, but that the child has been damaged by being born less than normal, and that a physician's action or omission caused the relevant defect. Courts have almost always rejected wrongful life suits because courts have rejected the implication that killing a baby can benefit it.

Several well-publicized wrongful birth suits have been brought by parents against physicians. In New Jersey, parents of a baby with Down syndrome sued pro-life obstetrician James Delahunty, whom they say discouraged them from pursuing amniocentesis when a sonogram showed a fetus with a thick neck (a possible sign in utero of this condition).[42] The jury awarded the couple nearly

$2 million and found Dr. Delahunty guilty of "failing to recognize, appreciate, and discuss the results of the tests, particularly ultrasound" with his patients. The verdict may have stemmed partially from Delahunty's combative behavior in the courtroom.

At least 27 states allow parents to sue for wrongful birth, although Michigan and Georgia recently disallowed them. In a case in 1999, as well as another case in 1990, the Georgia Supreme Court ruled that a couple with a Down child could not sue their physician for failure to perform amniocentesis or other prenatal tests.[43]

## 1984: LEGISLATION

In 1984, Congress amended its Child Abuse Prevention and Treatment Act of 1974 (not the Rehabilitation Act) to count nontreatment in Baby Doe cases as *child abuse*. The Child Abuse Amendments (CAA) circumvented the injunction against the Baby Doe rules. They made states, not the federal government, responsible for such cases—getting Uncle Sam out of the neonatal nursery.

The only exceptions to the CAA were (1) when an impaired child is "chronically and irreversibly comatose," (2) when a child is inevitably dying, and (3) when treatment would be "futile and inhumane." These exceptions are often interpreted narrowly, so as to give parents few choices. As one law professor sums it up, "Since passage of the CAA, ethical and legal controversy over parental authority to withhold treatment from handicapped or disabled newborns . . . has largely ceased."[44]

Problems resulting from such narrow interpretation were illustrated dramatically in the Rudy Linares case, which took place in Chicago in 1989. Dan Linares held an NICU staff at gunpoint while he disconnected the respirator of his 16-month-old son Rudy, who—after swallowing a balloon at a birthday party—had gone into PVS nine months earlier. Rudy soon died, and Dan Linares was charged with first-degree murder.[45] Because there was no doubt that Dan Linares was a caring parent, a grand jury refused to indict him for homicide; he later received a suspended sentence on a minor charge arising from his use of a gun.

## 1992: THE AMERICANS WITH
## DISABILITIES ACT (ADA)

In 1992, the Americans with Disabilities Act (ADA) went into effect; this act protects Americans with a wide range of disabilities from discrimination.

In 1994, a federal court specifically cited ADA in mandating treatment for a 16-month-old anencephalic infant, Baby K, who had been brought to a hospital emergency room in Virginia in respiratory distress.[46] Baby K had been on a respirator since birth. Her physicians wanted to disconnect it and let her die, but for religious reasons, her mother insisted on continued care. At its heart, Baby K's case was about whether physicians may overrule parents' decisions about continuing futile, expensive treatment without incurring charges of discrimination against the handicapped. For over a year, Baby K continued to receive treatment, but she died in 1995.

After two decades of legal wrangling about Baby Doe cases, the results are equivocal. On the one hand, some impaired babies who would once have died as a consequence of nontreatment now survive to lead meaningful lives. On the other hand, the right of parents to make choices in cases of disabled newborns has declined dramatically. As a result of the amendment to the child abuse act, most NICU physicians usually *overtreat* severely impaired newborns.[47]

The ADA does not make it criminal for physicians to withhold treatment from impaired newborns. Rather, it threatens to withhold federal funding from a state for its programs. Even under this threat, *no state has ever been found to be out of compliance.* Moreover, although thousands of such infants have had life-sustaining treatment withheld or withdrawn, contrary to the guidelines in these regulations, *no legal charges have ever been brought against physicians, hospitals, or states for doing so.*

Nevertheless, while the ADA imposed no criminal charges on physicians who failed to comply with it, most obstetricians perceived it as requiring a presumption in favor of treatment. And subjected to a barrage of lawsuits with every disabled baby, obstetricians these days take few unnecessary risks.

## THE STRENGTH OF DISABILITY ADVOCATES

Many pediatricians claim that in the 1950s, it was rare for a baby with Down syndrome to live long.[48] Even after institutionalization, nontreatment intending death was the norm, not the exception. Babies who survived were sent to be warehoused in custodial institutions, where they were never stimulated or educated. They almost always developed with low IQs.

Within pediatric neurology, opinion about treatment in Baby Doe cases changed dramatically over the past decades. In the 1960s and early 1970s, the consensus was that many such cases should not be treated; today, all but the most hopeless cases are treated.[49]

For example, Lorber's criteria concerning spina bifida initially swung the pendulum toward nontreatment in many NICUs; but during the 1980s, right-to-life organizations and disability advocates swung the pendulum back toward treatment. Also, breakthroughs were made in urology, neonatology, neurosurgery, and CAT scan diagnosis, and these not only increased the accuracy of prognoses, but also improved quality of life for such children.

These changes have led to a new understanding:

> Mild to moderate degrees of microcephaly are compatible with normal or even exceptional intellect. This is particularly true in cases of untreated meningomyelocele in which loss of cerebrospinal fluid through the unrepaired hole in the back may decrease the total mass of the head. . . . Essentially all children with severe meningomyelocele have hydrocephalus. . . . Children with hydrocephalus who are treated reasonably early and who do not develop meningitis have a better chance than 50 percent of being intellectually normal.[50]

The Spina Bifida Association has stated:

> Since we have found it virtually impossible to predict at birth which infants with meningomyelocele will become competitive, ambulatory, and intellectually able,

we have not relied on arbitrary guidelines to determine which children should or should not be treated. On the contrary, we believe that all such children should be treated, and we feel that our data show this philosophy to be correct.[51]

The outcome in the Baby Jane Doe case, chosen for discussion because of its fame but otherwise typical of spina bifida, makes this statement seem reasonable. Moreover, the unexpected outcome of the Mueller case and the newer prognoses for Down syndrome suggest that similar reasoning may be appropriate regarding other defects.

## CONCEPTUAL DILEMMA: SUPPORTING BOTH CHOICE AND RESPECT

The parents of spina bifida child Leilani Duff-Fraker, born in 2004, love their daughter, but if their obstetrician had ordered the right tests, they would have aborted her and tried again for a healthy child.[52] Is that inconsistent? Can you love a child whom you might have terminated as a fetus?

In some aspects, this question is analogous to the Ayala case, where parents deliberately conceived a child to be a source of bone marrow for her older sister with leukemia. The Ayala parents claimed that they would and could love Marissa, and not just see her as a resource for her sister. Philosopher Francis Kamm observes that "love is for a particular," not a potential child, but once the particular child is born, love occurs.[53]

Public policy reveals a similar dilemma writ large. Is it consistent to do prenatal testing for genetic diseases while at the same time telling adults with the same diseases that they are respected? Is it consistent to test babies at birth for genetic conditions such as PKU and at the same time tell adults with PKU that they are valued? Do funds for prevention of disabilities compete with funds for services for disabled adults?[54]

> Abortion done after genetic tests have revealed undesirable conditions (mental deficiency or other disability) in the fetus. This topic is discussed in an excerpt from Gregory Pence's *Elements of Bioethics*. To read "Are Genetic Abortions Eugenic?," go to Chapter 8 in the Online Learning Center (OLC) at www.mhhe.com/pence7e.

## FURTHER READING

Fred Frohock, *Special Care: Medical Decisions at the Beginning of Life*, Chicago: University of Chicago Press, 1986.

Loretta Kopelman, "Are the 21-Year Old Baby Doe Rules Misunderstood or Mistaken?" *Pediatrics*, 115: 3, March 2005, pp. 797–802.

John Freeman, "On Learning Humility: A Thirty-Year Journey," *Hastings Center Report*, May-June, 204, 13–16.

John Robertson, "Extreme Prematurity and Parental Rights After Baby Doe," *Hastings Center Report*, July/August 2004, 32–39.

Peggy and Robert Stimson, *The Long Dying of Baby Andrew*, Boston: Little, Brown, 1983.

U.S. Commission on Civil Rights, *Medical Discrimination Against Children with Disabilities*, September 1989.

## DISCUSSION QUESTIONS

1. Suppose you were expecting a healthy baby and discovered that you were going to have a Down syndrome baby or a baby with spina bifida. Would you be able to care for the child?

2. Suppose you discovered the preceding issue in the first trimester of pregnancy. Would it be selfish of you to abort the baby then and try again for a healthy baby?

3. Is testing of fetuses for genetic conditions, followed by abortions, a new kind of eugenics? Should it worry people with disabilities?

4. Because it harms fetuses/babies so much, should it be illegal to smoke, drink, or use drugs during pregnancy?

# CHAPTER 9

# Medical Research on Animals

*T*his chapter discusses the ethics of using animals in medical research.[1] It surveys philosophical opposition to such research and focuses on the research of Thomas Gennarelli, who injured primates to model head injuries in humans, and Edward Taub, who injured primates to study stroke in humans. Publicity about these cases changed the way American researchers use animals.

## THE ANIMAL LIBERATION FRONT AND GENNARELLI'S RESEARCH

On Memorial Day 1984, members of the Animal Liberation Front (ALF) quietly entered the University of Pennsylvania Medical School in Philadelphia. They broke into a vacant laboratory, where they stole 32 audiovisual tapes documenting experiments on primates.

The team of neurologist Thomas Gennarelli had made the tapes. They hoped to produce exact brain damage in adult baboons. According to the *New York Times,*

> One sequence showed a monkey strapped to a table pulling against its bonds. The animal's head was encased in a steel cylinder to a pneumatic machine called an accelerator. Suddenly, a piston drove the cylinder upward, thrusting the animal's head sharply through an arc of about 60 degrees.

From 1970 to 1985, or for more than 15 years, Gennarelli had tried, but failed, to create reproducible head injuries.

The ALF edited the 70 hours of tape to create a 25-minute piece showing the worst abuses. People for Ethical Treatment of Animals (PETA) gave the tape to Congress and ABC News. (The Wikipedia article on this film "Unnecessary Fuss," contains free links to it.[2]).

Researchers claimed they sedated baboons prior to injury and that baboons felt no pain, but just before the pneumatic hammer smashes their heads, baboons struggled to free themselves, obviously not sedated.

On the tape, the male researchers sound adolescent and macho. As the *Times* reporter continues:

> . . . In another sequence, as an animal lay in a coma, a researcher's recorded voice was heard saying, "You'd better have some axonal damage, monkey," and calling him "sucker."[3]

Researchers used profanity and performed unsterile surgery. They held up conscious baboons with broken arms and laughed at them. Gennarelli's defenders claim the insensitive comments and behavior of researchers on the tapes resembled gallows humor among medical residents.

The National Institutes of Health (NIH) appointed a committee of animal researchers to review the tapes, which had no problem with Gennarelli's hypothesis: "The research, as proposed," it said, "is likely to yield fruitful results for the good of society."[4]

Nevertheless, it found Gennarelli guilty of 9 out of 10 charges against him: lack of anesthesia, inadequate supervision, poor training, inferior veterinary care, unnecessary multiple injuries to the same animals, smoking, statements in poor taste around animals, improper clothing, and overall "material failure to comply with the Public Health Service Animal Welfare Policy." So the NIH suspended Gennarelli's research—the first time it had closed a lab because of abuse of animals.

To ALF, this meant victory. One member of the original ALF team defended the break-in:

> We may seem like radicals to you, but we are like the Abolitionists, who were regarded as radicals, too. And we hope that 100 years from now, people will look back on the way animals are treated now with the same horror as we do when we look back on the slave trade.[5]

Six weeks after its Memorial Day raid, ALF struck the University of Pennsylvania's veterinary school, taking three cats, two dogs, and eight pigeons. The dean of this school said the raid "would set back research efforts, including a study to determine the cause of sudden infant death syndrome."[6] Another dean said the stolen cats modeled breathing during sleep, a missing dog had a steel plate inserted to study osteoarthritis, another dog had been given ear-canal infections to study cures, and the bones of pigeons had been broken to benefit all birds.[7] He said that the work on dogs would benefit other dogs, adding that such research had to be done and that more dogs would now need to be used as subjects.

In 1984, ALF struck in California, taking hundreds of small mammals from the City of Hope National Medical Center in Duarte. They painted inside the lab: "ALF Is Watching and There's No Place to Hide!" Ingrid Newkirk of PETA called City of Hope a "concentration camp" where animals were "being used for painful experiments."[8]

The associate director of City of Hope said the theft of these animals had disrupted $500,000 worth of research on emphysema, cancer, and herpes. ALF had targeted a study testing tobacco carcinogens in dogs. The dogs were forced to breathe air full of tobacco smoke, but this model has never been proven to give lung cancer to dogs.

The associate director said 36 dogs, 12 cats, 12 rabbits, 28 mice, and 18 rats had been stolen and that, "We're concerned that very important research work may not now be completed."[9]

In 1985, the ALF hit the biology and psychology laboratories of the University of California, Riverside, taking 467 animals, including a stump-tailed macaque whose eyes had been sewn shut to study a device to help the blind navigate. PETA said these animals had been used in painful, unnecessary experiments, some involving starvation. NIH investigated the charges but found no evidence of abuse. The university claimed $683,000 in damages.

In 1987, arson gutted the $2.5 million veterinary research animal lab at the University of California, Davis; ALF claimed responsibility. In 1988, ALF destroyed a new building for animal research at the medical school in San Diego and burned down a veal-packing plant in Oakland. In televised interviews, masked ALF spokespeople took credit, vowing to continue the attacks "until the killing of the innocent animals stops."

Also in 1988 in Connecticut, Stephanie Trutt planted a bomb outside a company that made surgical staples and that used animals to train surgeons in handling them. She was arrested for attempted murder.[10] About this time, the Federal Bureau of Investigation started to monitor and infiltrate the ALF, listing it as a terrorist, violent group.

Several experiments reviewed by NIH in the 1980s fared poorly. The City of Hope Medical Center was fined $25,000, lost $1 million in grants, and lost its Animal Care Assurance, a legal document whereby an institution promises to abide by federal regulations. After ALF released pictures of poor lab conditions and when inspectors made an unannounced visit, Columbia University lost grants involving vertebrates.

To prevent further abuses, Congress mandated in 1986 *Institutional Animal Care and Use Committees* (IACUCs) for all institutions receiving federal funds for research on animals. Although IACUCs are composed mostly of researchers themselves, they force experimenters to justify their projects to fellow scientists. The existence of IACUCs is directly attributable to the exposure of Gennarelli's and Taub's experiments by the ALF and PETA.

## EVALUATING THE PHILADELPHIA STUDY

Gennarelli can be described as working at the bottom of a pyramid of basic research on head injury. To him, it seemed obvious that the first step should be to produce one head injury precisely and reliably, so others could study it. Similarly, knowing how to produce different kinds of burns in animals is the first step in studying the physiology of burns and the metabolism of healing.

Activists held that Gennarelli had bashed heads for a decade and gotten nowhere. They argued that even if he had succeeded in devising a reproducible model of head injuries, such a model would offer little help in treating these injuries.

Critics said these conclusions papered over a lack of findings. Nedim Buyukmichi, an activist and veterinarian, argued that Gennarelli's studies were too inconsistent to result in a reproducible model of head injuries and too limited in scope to adequately mimic injuries sustained by human victims of accidents: "After 15 years and $11 million to $13 million, essentially nothing has come out of this research that hasn't already been known from studies of human head trauma."[11]

Defenders also ask: even if the animals were mistreated and the researchers were insensitive, does that necessarily affect the scientific value of the research? For activists, Gennarelli's treatment of his animal subjects proved that his project was immoral, but perhaps the two claims should be separated.

## PETA AND EDWARD TAUB'S RESEARCH
## ON MONKEYS

In 1981, Alex Pacheco volunteered in the primate lab of psychologist Edward Taub in Silver Spring, Maryland. Pacheco told Taub that he wanted to become a research scientist, but he really wanted to videotape Taub's research for PETA.[12]

Taub studied "somato-sensory deafferentation" in monkeys by surgically cutting all the nerves in one limb and trying to stimulate regrowth. Based on psychologist Martin Seligman's famous idea of learned helplessness, Taub hypothesized that voluntary non-use caused some damage in stroke. Each year, stroke disables a half-million Americans, who often lose the use of a limb.

Pacheco entered the lab late one night and photographed Taub's experiments. As a result, authorities tried Taub in Maryland on charges of cruelty to animals after drawn-out legal maneuverings in which various research organizations backed Taub.

Convicted of failing to provide proper veterinary care, a charge based on the fact that he did not bandage the animals' wounds, Taub testified that it was better to leave the wounds unbandaged. Years of experience had convinced him that the monkeys would only tear the bandages off, making their wounds worse.

Some veterinarians disagreed. In response, the American Psychological Association's Ethics Committee, the NIH, and an ad hoc committee of the American Physiological Society exonerated Taub of failure to provide good care. After its own investigation, the psychology department at UAB hired him as a full professor, but to work only on humans, not animals.

Pacheco's tactics here raised questions. To obtain evidence for the trial, Pacheco invited activists such as Donald Barnes, John McArdle, and Michael W. Fox to search Taub's lab at night. When warrants were served on Taub, several television stations recorded the event, while PETA leaders distributed press releases. During the trial, PETA's handling of the media was brilliant, and it orchestrated each element for maximal impact.

In 1986, the 15 surviving monkeys had been transferred to the federally funded Tulane Regional Primate Center in Covington, Louisiana. In 1990, in an experiment that PETA opposed, Timothy Pons examined the brain of a dying monkey before euthanasia. Pons was "flabbergasted" to discover that "the entire patch of the cortex corresponding to the arm—about half an inch wide—had been rewired to receive input from the face." Pons concluded, "The results offer hope that the brain can be coaxed into rewiring itself after injury." Data from other monkeys in the study supported this finding.

Neural rewiring is the Holy Grail in rehabilitative medicine, offering hope to victims of stroke and spinal cord injury. In 1991, the Story of the Year for ethics in *Discover* magazine concluded that four of Taub's monkeys showed:

> . . . dramatic new evidence of the adult brain's capacity to "rewire" itself, something previously thought to be impossible. And ironically, it was PETA's success at keeping the monkeys away from research for a decade that made the discovery possible.[13]

In 2000, Taub achieved a breakthrough, which CNN and ABC News reported extensively.[14] Taub declared that all stroke patients using his *Constraint-Induced*

*Movement Therapy,* or CI therapy, had significantly improved in function. For an affected arm, 30 percent of patients gained close to normal use.[15]

So can the brain reorganize after a stroke? Some people think that CI therapy jump-starts self-repair of surviving, healthy cells in the brain or spinal cord. CI therapy tries to "wake up cells that have been stunned," says Taub.[16] "CI therapy appears to produce a re-wiring in the brain that leads to improved motor function of the affected limb."[17]

In 2004, the NIH funded the first multi-center national trial to study the benefits of CI.[18] In 2006, a placebo-controlled study proved that CI therapy's benefits last two years after the intervention.[19] Taub claimed a separate result showed benefits five years later. In another study, 21 survivors of stroke underwent the standard CI therapy, while 21 other survivors merely had a general fitness program. Two weeks after CI therapy, patients in the treatment group had a "large to very large" improvement using the affected arm, but those in the control group had no change.

At present, the Taub Therapy Clinic at UAB offers constraint-induced therapy for victims of stroke and brain injury for two to three weeks.

## THE LAW AND ANIMAL RESEARCH

In 1992, the Farm and Animal Research Facilities Protection Act made it a federal crime to break into a research facility or the premises of a company that breeds research animals. Violators face prison sentences up to one year for illegal entry and fines up to $5,000. A vice-president at UAB Medical Center, which had originated the bill, hoped this legislation would protect scientists against "activists who use terrorist techniques to interfere with potentially life-saving research."[20]

In 1993, animal rights activists won a significant victory for dogs and primates used in laboratory research. Judge Charles Richey ordered the Agriculture Department to enforce the Improved Standards for Laboratory Animals Act of 1985, the act creating IACUCs. The judge concluded that the Agriculture Department had violated the act by giving all power to interpret it to local IACUCs. He implied that IACUC members, including veterinarians and one non-scientist member, too often protected their own institutions.

Richey also criticized the government for taking nine years to implement some of its own rules, and he implied that some of the rules increased profitability more than protected animals.

Judge Richey later affirmed the gradient and rejected the claim by Ingrid Newkirk of PETA that "a rat is a pig is a dog is a boy" and dismissed claims that American researchers had to keep detailed records for their 21 million rats and mice. He said researchers could treat rats and mice differently from dogs and primates. That is significant because medical researchers claim that rats and mice constitute 87 percent of animals they use.[21]

Animal activists see IACUCs as window dressing and claim they do little good. They say that the Department of Agriculture, which must inspect labs, has a too-cozy relationship with animal-abusing agribusiness. They lament that veterinarians on IACUCs are caught in the middle, charged with protecting animals but salaried by researchers.

During the 1980s, faced with what they perceived as devastating losses in public confidence, scientists went on the offensive, establishing the Foundation for Biomedical Research, a lobby for 350 universities, drug companies, manufacturers of medical devices, and commercial animal-supply companies. To counter PETA's lobbyists, it has its own lobbyists, as well as a paid member in most states to work with students in high schools and colleges.

## NUMBERS AND KINDS OF ANIMALS IN RESEARCH

Animal rights activists made two tests controversial: the LD-50 tests and Draize tests. LD stands for "lethal dosage." LD-50 tests determine what amount of a substance will kill 50 of 100 animals. Done routinely across species for substances ranging from soap to chemotherapies, these tests have been criticized as crude measures (one witness said they tell mice how much of something to take for mass suicide). Because of criticisms, since the early 1970s, use of LD-50s declined 96 percent and has been replaced by LD-10s.[22]

The Draize test estimates whether products irritate human eyes. Samples are dripped into rabbits' eyes, which are particularly sensitive. Activists seek alternative tests using cell cultures and computer models.

Over the last decades, activists and researchers agreed on the *3R's*, made famous by researcher Barbara Orlans, of replacement, refinement, and reduction. "Replacement" means using tissue culture instead of animal skin or a mouse instead of a dog. "Refinement" means improving the quality of life of research animals, as well as the methodology. "Reduction" means reducing the number of animals used, e.g, LD-10s rather than LD-50s.

As of 2010, the European Union banned use of animals to test cosmetics, so the Draize test is no longer done there. Instead, blush or eyeliner made by L'Oréal is tested on artificial human skin called Episkin and EpiDerm (the same skin grown for burn victims from a sample of their own skin).[23]

The Foundation for Biomedical Research claims that, "many people think that abandoned or stolen pets are used in research. This is completely untrue and is banned in this country."[24] However, a 2009 report by the National Academies of Science implied that, even though demand has declined and that the system should be phased out, some "Class B" dealers have previously been selling "random source" dogs and cats to researchers.[25]

Activists have claimed that researchers use a vast number of animals in research, with estimates in the past from 14 to 71 million.[26] The Foundation for Biomedical Research claims that the number has fallen from a peak in the 1970s of 5,500,000 to the present level of around 2,500,000. They attribute this reduction to the 3R's.

Whatever answer is correct, basic research uses far more animals than people realize. For every practical success in human medicine, such as cyclosporin or knee replacements, dozens of failures occur in studies with human subjects and dozens of failures occur in animal studies. To arrive at each success, the sad truth is that researchers use millions of animals each year.

## DESCARTES ON ANIMAL PAIN

Since prehistoric times, humans have used animals for many purposes, but experimentation on animals did not arise as a specific issue until the beginning of modern science. In the seventeenth century, Rene Descartes set the premises for the modern debate.

Not only a mathematician and philosopher, Descartes also studied physiology and the circulation of blood by dissecting live animals without anesthesia (which was not discovered until 1846). To understand why he considered that permissible, it is necessary to understand his basic philosophical approach, *Cartesianism*, which deeply influenced western science and philosophy.

Descartes is known for his famous argument *Cogito ergo sum*: "I think, therefore I am." According to him, what distinguishes human beings from other animals is *res cogitans*, or "thinking stuff," a substantial mind or soul. For Descartes, this mental substance held together transient mental states such as perceptions, feelings, thoughts, and dreams and served as a ground for free will, reason, and moral values. Non-human animals, Descartes believed, lack *res cogitans*, mind or soul, and are therefore ultimately only *res extensa*, or "extended, physical stuff." Thus, in Cartesian philosophy, animals were merely fleshy machines; their eyes reflected no soul and no pain lay behind their external "pain behavior."

Descartes' idea that animals lack a soul was not unique as this was also Christian doctrine. Descartes accepted Christian teaching that humans have souls created by God, whereas animals do not. Descartes assumed further that *soul* is identical to *mind,* so if animals have no soul, neither do they have a mind; and if animals have no mind, they are not conscious; and if they are not conscious, they cannot feel pain.

For Descartes, in order to feel pain, a mind is needed, and—to repeat—only human beings have minds. In Descartes' view, no middle ground exists between a human being, who has a soul and a capacity to experience pain, and an animal that has no soul and no capacity to experience pain.

Cartesianism represents an attempt to deal with the tension between science and religion by demarcating proper areas for each: the province of science is the study of matter, mathematics, animals, and the human body; that of religion and the humanities is mind, art, and ethics. Obviously, however, it has not come to represent a consensus, or even a widely accepted solution—even for Christians, who are still struggling with the concept of how mind and soul are related and whether animals count in the grand scheme of things.

Among Descartes' followers during his own century were an infamous group of early physiologists and *vivisectionists* (researchers operating on live animals without anesthesia) at the Jansenist seminary of Port Royal. Here is how eighteenth-century writer Nicholas Fontaine describes them:

> They administered beatings to dogs with perfect indifference, and made fun of those who pitied the creatures as if they felt pain. They said the animals were

clocks; that the cries they emitted when struck were only the noise of a little spring that had been touched, but that the whole body was without feeling. They nailed poor animals up on boards by their four paws to vivisect them and see the circulation of the blood that was a great subject of conversation.[27]

To some extent, the Cartesian concept of animals has persisted into modern times. Some behavioral psychologists argued against assuming rats were conscious and drew a distinction between "pain behavior" and the experience of pain. Rats and chickens, they said, exhibited "pain behavior," but whether they had mental states and thus had an experience of pain like humans, was another matter.

## C. S. LEWIS ON ANIMAL PAIN

The twentieth-century Christian writer C. S. Lewis tried to find a middle ground between the Cartesian view and a view equating animal and human pain. Lewis rejected the view that animals feel nothing and argued that animals indeed do feel. But in what sense? Lewis distinguished between *sentience* (the ability to feel pain) and *consciousness* (awareness of feeling pain). All mammals are sentient, he argued, but only humans are self-conscious.[28]

According to Lewis, animals feel pain, but not as humans do. A rat receiving three electric shocks feels the pain of each shock—the rat is sentient—but it does not think, "I have had three shocks." The thought, "I have had three shocks," requires what Lewis calls "consciousness or soul."

Lewis agreed with the eighteenth-century philosopher David Hume, who argued that self-identity requires a permanent self or mental substance which unites all of a person's thoughts as "his" or "hers."[29] For Lewis, a baboon would have a "succession of perceptions," but not the human experience of pain as "my pain."

Lewis identified consciousness with self-consciousness or soul (for which he also used the term "deep self"). Some critics have disagreed with this idea, particularly since Lewis assumed that memory depends on self-consciousness. These critics observe that if self-consciousness were needed for memory, animals would never remember anything, and studies of learning in animals would be senseless. But everyone knows that animals remember—a dog who has been given a treat by a human remembers that human.

### Philosophy of Mind and Ethics

Today, philosophy of mind and animal ethics agonize over answers to the following questions: How much pain do animals feel? To what extent is their pain like our pain? On the ladder of evolution from an amoeba to baboons, at what point does an organism become sentient? When can an animal remember pain as "my" pain?

These are not simple questions. They raise some of the deepest problems in philosophy of mind and lie behind many controversies about animal research.

As we consider various answers to such questions, do we, as a species, have a conflict of interest? Do we have any bias toward accepting some answers and rejecting others? Remember that for centuries, societies considered people of color and women to be "obviously" and "naturally" inferior to white men.

Finally, even if animals are not aware of pain, or do not remember pain as humans do, that does not mean they suffer less in medical experiments. When humans consent to be subjects of medical experimentations, we explain to them the purposes and risks of the study, so they understand the experiment. This does not occur with animals, who have no idea why they are being used. Having no way to understand the research, they may suffer more.

In discussing abortion and end-of-life care, we explored the gradient theory of personhood. To extend that theory to animals, we should note that on a cross-species gradient of characteristics of persons, adult baboons will possess more characteristics than newborn humans or profoundly brain-injured humans. Therefore, adult baboons will be more persons than human embryos or end-stage vegetative humans. As discussed later, this explains why use of chimpanzees, gorillas, and baboons in research troubles so many.

## PETER SINGER ON SPECIESISM

Before 1975, groups promoting animal welfare focused on humane treatment of research animals. In that year, Australian philosopher Peter Singer published *Animal Liberation*, where he argued that animals should count for something.[30] To say animals do not count because they are inferior by nature, Singer held, is like saying slaves or women do not count because they are inferior by nature. Just as racism and sexism are evil, Singer said, so is *speciesism*.

According to him, the argument that supports equal rights for minorities and women also supports animal rights. If our moral concern for children, women, and minorities stems from their sensitivity to pain, family ties, and ability to reason, why wouldn't these factors also be a basis for concern for animals?

Note that we treat humans with *equal* human rights despite the obvious fact that they are *unequal* in their ability to suffer, in their intelligence, strength, and character. Inequality of ability does not dictate inequality of treatment. Such arguments put speciesists on the defensive: if the principle of equality applies to all people, despite their obvious differences in ability and intelligence, why should it not apply to animals?

Singer emphasized how pigs are more intelligent than horses, dogs, and cats, which we revere as pets. Pigs suffer the sad quirk of fate that humans like the taste of their smoked, cooked flesh—a fact less true of deer, buffalo, and bison. Singer explained how farmer-businessmen raise pigs, veal calves, and chickens in small, confining cages in industrial-type farms. Singer argued that current factory farming is evil. Billions of animals suffer and die each year so humans can enjoy their flesh. Arguably, vegetarian eating is healthier for humans today than a meat-centered diet and, in addition, saves animals much pain.

Singer also argued that a medical experiment using animal subjects must be *speciesist* unless humans would be willing to substitute irreversibly comatose human subjects. This is an interesting approach. Most people who accept the idea of using, say, a chimpanzee in medical research would cringe at the idea of using an anencephalic baby (an infant born lacking a normal brain). But if the chimpanzee is active, gregarious, sensitive, and responsive, whereas the anencephalic baby is hopelessly mute, comatose, and dying, why should the chimp be the victim? If the answer is simply that the baby is human and the chimp nonhuman, that answer is mistaken because it assumes what it must prove; in other words, it's speciesist.

Let us put the point differently. Suppose an institution exists with hundreds of profoundly mentally challenged human children and adults who have been abandoned by their families to the State. They are so profoundly challenged mentally as to have virtually no recognizably human interactions with each other or the staff. Even so, most people would be horrified to learn that a drug company was using them as subjects to test promising drugs for toxicity in humans.

Now move to a large center for primates, such as one near San Antonio, Texas, that holds hundreds of chimpanzees and baboons. These primates are *more* social, interactive, and intelligent than the humans just described. Yet these are precisely the beings drug companies use to test new drugs for toxicity. Why do we tolerate such testing on them and not on the mentally challenged humans?

In addition to his argument about speciesism, Singer also used utilitarian reasoning. According to utilitarian ethical theory, right acts produce the greatest good for the greatest number; for instance, research on presently sick patients is right if it helps a greater number of future sick patients.

Singer maintains that stipulating that the "greatest number" must refer only to humans begs the key question. Once animals count for something, however small, in utilitarian reasoning, then radical conclusions follow. Experiments that inflict horrible pain on many animals cannot be justified on the grounds that they save a few human lives because the number of animals suffering outweighs the small good to humans. Suppose a mouse's suffering counts 1/1000th of a human and that it takes painful experiments on 50,000 mice to ameliorate the suffering of one adult with psoriasis. In that equation, the research would not be justified.

Yale philosopher Shelly Kagan pointed out that Singer often argued "a utilitarian view without limiting itself to utilitarianism."[31] That accurately sums up *Animal Liberation*, where Singer graphically described the many ways that animals suffer in vast, industrialized hog factories to become tasty flesh for humans.

## TOM REGAN ON ANIMAL RIGHTS

Underlying the controversy over Gennarelli's experimentation on primates is a more basic issue: whether scientific research on animals is *ever* justified. Tom Regan, an American philosopher and animal rights activist, thinks not:

> I argue that the whole system of animal experimentation [and] the whole system of commercial and sport trapping and hunting are morally bankrupt institutions. The only way you change these things fundamentally is by eliminating them—in much the same way as with slavery and child labor.[32]

Regan argues that human beings have rights because they *have a life*. That is, humans have lives that can go better or worse for them, and this is true for each human being independently of whether or not others value him or her.

In other words, people have inherent, not instrumental, value. Where Singer loosely applied utilitarianism to animals, Regan loosely applied a Kantian ethic to animals, asserting the rights-based idea that each animal's life should be treated as an "end in itself."

Regan condemns research on animals because it treats them as a means to the end of helping humans. For Regan, animals have rights not to suffer at the hands of humans, rights to be respected in their own habitat, and rights to enjoy a natural lifespan. So eating them is also immoral. In other words, each animal's life has *inherent value*.

Once the premise is accepted that each animal's life has inherent value, it follows that medical research to benefit humans is unjustified. For if a life has inherent value, no competing value trumps it.

Regan maintains that like humans, many species of animals have lives that can go better or worse for them, and he draws this crucial inference: "They too have a distinctive kind of value in their own right, if we do; therefore, they too have a right not to be treated in ways that fail to respect this value."[33] Regan reasons that if humans count in the moral calculus because they possess a quality, and if animals possess the same quality, then it is inconsistent not to count animals equally.

Regan's critics say that his argument runs several unjustified inferences together. First, they ask, if any being (human or nonhuman) has a life that can go better or worse, does that fact give every life a distinctive value? Second, and more important, just because an animal "has a life," that doesn't mean it is equal in value to that of humans.

Note, however, that Regan includes a qualification: he says that animals (like humans) have lives that can go better or worse *for them*. By qualifying his claim this way, no comparison is possible between human and animal lives. If fish in an aquarium "have a life" that can go better or worse *for them*, from that standpoint, we do not have a right to destroy them.

Consider the Lifeboat Test: only a dog or a man can remain in a lifeboat. Which should survive? Regan implies that because "animals aren't there to be used as our resources," it is wrong to kill the dog to save the man, and scientist Charles McArdle concurs—"I would seriously have to question whether I would allow an animal to die just to protect me."[34] On the other hand, pediatric researcher Carolyn Compton disagrees: "I love animals, but there's no question in my mind that if I were able to sacrifice an animal life to save a human being, I would do it."[35]

The philosopher Carl Cohen says, "Rights arise, and can be intelligently defended, only among beings who do, or can, make moral claims against one another."[36] For Cohen, because animals cannot make claims, they lack rights.

But this seems to assume that claims can be made only with vocal cords. When a dog pesters his owner to be taken for a walk, isn't he claiming a right to a walk? What about minimally conscious patients who can't interact but are still aware?

Cohen rejects the analogy among racism, sexism, and speciesism: although racism and sexism are bad, speciesism is not. "Speciesism is not merely plausible; it is essential for right conduct, because those who will not make the morally relevant distinctions among species are almost certain, in consequence, to misapprehend their true obligations." That is, they will take the dog from the burning building, not the child; give money in their wills to ensure that their pets are taken care of, but ignore their nephews and nieces; and support the Humane Society, but not famine relief.

## WHY WE NEED ANIMALS IN RESEARCH:
## THE OFFICIAL VIEW

According to the Official View, which federal law expresses, drugs must first be tested on animals to screen for toxicity and to indicate possible benefit to humans. Sometimes this view approaches religious fervor: "Every major medical advance of the century has depended on animal research," says a neuroscientist from Rutgers University.[37]

Since 1907, researchers have used mice for many reasons, including their small size, easiness to care for and breed, and genomic similarities with humans. For cancer research, mouse models have yielded extensive knowledge of the pathogenesis of different cancers, potential treatment for cancer, and the genetic background of cancers.[38] For example, scientists use mice to test extract of grapes to prevent cancer and also give mice cancer in order to test anti-cancer drugs.

Researchers studying the hepatitis C virus always use chimpanzees, because "HCV infects only humans and chimpanzees, using specialized molecules found in these organisms to establish infection."[39] Although mouse models are being studied, researchers studying HCV at present need to continue using chimpanzees.

As an NIH report concluded, "No single set of results from a particular model—whether animal, cell, or computer—can predict exactly what will happen, so researchers often ask the same questions in different kinds of studies. When different models yield similar results, the results are much more believable."[40]

In Phase I of testing drugs on humans, scientists strive to see how much of the drug can be given without producing toxic effects. Phase I is done only after extensive testing of the drug in animals. Without such testing, the Official View claims, many more toxic reactions would occur in humans.

The Official View argues similarly for how scientists test new heart pumps, artificial pumps, salves for burns, antibiotics, and new kinds of surgery. If they did not test these first on animals, making their mistakes and gaining skill, more humans would be injured or harmed.

If no animals were available, such tests would need to be done on humans. It is inconceivable that humans would be given cancer to have subjects to test anti-cancer drugs, so progress against cancer would slow.

As evolution teaches, humans evolved through primates from even lesser animals. As such, we share nervous systems, receptors for pain, and fight-or-flight reactions with our predecessors. Moreover, it is precisely because of sharing so much with primates and mammals that the latter make such good subjects for medical research: they predict well how drugs and surgeries will work in humans.

Finally, the Official View emphasizes Taub's research. Condemned originally as cruel, Taub's studies led to his breakthrough and stroke victims now benefit.

In sum, on the Official View, if we want medical research to continue, using animals in research is indispensable and also reduces harm to humans from medical research.

## CRITIQUING THE OFFICIAL VIEW

For too long, the Official View has not been challenged in medicine or science, but it is time to do so. Three different critiques of it can be made.

1. *Inherently wrong.* The most basic criticism of the Official View is that the infliction of pain on animals is inherently wrong, that just as we should not experiment on some humans to help the majority, so we should not harm animals to benefit humans. This argument assumes *equivalence*, that animal and human suffering are equivalent and that one should not be accepted to advance the other.

   Many people reject equivalence, believing that animals, compared to humans, are of either no moral value or inconsequential moral value. Others may believe that, although animals count for something, human welfare counts for so much more that animal suffering in research can be allowed.

2. *Bad science.* Some scientists think that the Official View is based on bad science. This objection has two parts: first, testing drugs, devices, and techniques on animals does not in fact predict harm to humans; second, some drugs, devices and techniques that harm animals may help humans, but are screened out, thus potentially beneficial tools are lost due to testing on animals. So testing these things on animals is both too broad and too narrow: it allows too many bad things to go through and wrongly screens out too many good things.

   Philosopher of science Niall Shanks and anesthesiologist Ray Greek studied whether testing of drugs on animals predicts their toxicity or benefits to humans, and have concluded that most extrapolations rest on shaky grounds:

   > Drugs such as Practolol, Opren, Fialuridine, Clioquinol, Zelmid, Troglitazone, and others (such as Avandia), came to market, in part, because they tested safe in some animal species. They went on to prove dangerous in humans. It is still difficult to induce lung cancer in animals from cigarette smoke. Animals that were fed a high fat, high cholesterol diet failed to develop coronary artery disease, and so this diet was thought safe for humans. Asbestos, benzine, glass fibers, and other environmental poisons were all proved "safe" in animals and consequently kept on the market long after epidemiological data proved them carcinogenic or otherwise dangerous.
   >
   > From 1976 to 1985, 209 new drugs were approved for use in the United States after extensive animal testing. . . . Of these, 198 were followed . . . by the FDA and 102, or 52 percent were either withdrawn or relabeled as having secondary to severe unpredicted side effects such as lethal dysrhythmias, heart attacks, kidney failure, and stroke.[41]

Such recalls make one wonder how well responses of drugs in animals predict responses of the same drugs in humans. Testing drugs on embryonic cells might be preferable and both save suffering in animals and prevent harm to adult humans.

What about Taub's study? Well, notice that Taub made his advance with humans only *after* he was banned from experimenting on primates (a condition of his hiring at UAB). What if he had directly tried to help humans overcome stroke? Were the animal studies necessary? One could argue that, if he had been blocked from using animals, he could have gone directly to using humans and more quickly have discovered his breakthrough.

What about evolution? Doesn't our common genetic history mean that drugs tested on non-human mammals will be likely to predict their effects on humans? Yes and no. Although we share 98 percent of our genes with apes and baboons, we also have many variations in the human genome, such that some drugs that work well in Caucasians do not work well in African Americans. Similarly, the variations between non-human primates and human primates mean there are many gaps in predictive drug testing.

Also, if we are 98 percent the same genetically as apes, shouldn't we regard apes as 98 percent persons? Shouldn't they have rights not to be kept in cages or to be used against their wills in research? Shouldn't they have 98 percent of the rights of persons, so virtually no benefit to humans justifies research on them?

Another problem is that many labs use mice or rats or primates bred to be a uniform type. In that way, the results are more easily reproducible by other scientists. But using only one genetic strain of mouse also limits testing of a new drug to that strain, whereas using many kinds of mice and animals would better mimic the variation in humans.

3. *Cost/benefit.* Most people do not understand how many animals scientists use in research or how much these animals suffer. If the benefits of using animals to screen drugs and devices are questionable, and if good arguments can be made that we should directly test human embryos or human volunteers, then using vast numbers of animals in research is morally unjustifiable.

So the argument is not whether a specific cost/benefit ratio is justified, but whether the meager, overall results for humans justify the immense suffering to millions of research animals. It is a bad argument to claim, as researchers often do, that *any* benefit to humans justifies this project, for that is tantamount to assuming that the welfare of animals doesn't count in the calculation, i.e., a small benefit to one human with a rare disease doesn't justify torturing a million pigs.

## CHIMPANZEES AND RESEARCH

In the twenty-first century, use of chimps in research became the flashpoint of activism for animal rights. Two things propelled this: the dismal failure of chimps to model HIV in humans and the rise of neuroscience, with a huge increase in basic research on chimps and monkeys. Pharmaceutical companies funded some of this research, but critics questioned whether anything like schizophrenia or Alzheimer's could be induced in primates or realistically studied with them. Neuroscience researchers such as Lawrence Hansen disputed whether decades of research with chimps had produced any significant results at all.[42]

The two largest collections of chimpanzees are a holding ground used in research outside San Antonio, Texas, and a retirement sanctuary northwest of New Orleans in Louisiana. The Humane Society of the United States joined Jane Goodall to push Congress to join all other developed countries in the world in banning research on chimpanzees. These groups wanted NIH to move all chimps to Louisiana. They all championed the Great Ape Protection and Savings Act in Congress, sponsored by Roscoe Bartlett, a congressmen and former Navy physiologist who once subjected chimps to painful tests for manned space travel and now regrets doing so.[43] Responding in part to Goodall's efforts, in April 2013, Harvard University announced it would close its New England Primate Research Center (NEPRC) in Southborough by 2015. In June 2013, Francis Collins, head of the NIH, announced that 300 of the 360 chimpanzees that NIH owned would be retired to sanctuaries.

## FURTHER READING

Deborah Blum, *The Monkey Wars*, New York: Oxford University Press, 1994.

Peter Carruthers, *The Animals Issue: Moral Theory in Practice*, New York: Cambridge University Press, 1992.

Gary Francione, *Introduction to Animal Rights: Your Child or the Dog?* Philadelphia, PA: Temple University Press, 2000.

R. G. Frey, *Rights, Killing, and Suffering*, Oxford, England: Basil Blackwell, 1983.

Jean Swingle Greek and Ray Greek, *What Will We Do If We Don't Experiment on Animals?* Bloomington, IN: Trafford Publishing, 2004.

Gil Langley, *Animal Experimentation: The Consensus Changes*, New York: Routledge, 1989.

Tibor Machan, *Putting Humans First*, Lanham, MD: Rowman & Littlefield, 2004.

Jim Mason and Peter Singer, *Animal Factories*, New York: Crown Publishers, 1980.

F. Barbara Orlans, *In The Name of Science: Issues in Responsible Animal Experimentation*, New York: Oxford University Press, 1993.

James Rachels, *Created from Animals*, New York: Oxford University Press, 1990.

Denise Radner and Michael Radner, *Animal Consciousness*, Buffalo, NY: Prometheus Books, 1989.

Richard Ryder, *Victims of Science: The Use of Animals in Research*, London: Davis-Poynter, 1975.

Tom Regan, *The Case for Animal Rights*, Berkeley: University of California Press, 1983.

Peter Singer, *Animal Liberation*, New York: New York Review of Books, 1975.

Susan Sperling, *Animal Liberators*, Berkeley: University of California Press, 1988.

## DISCUSSION QUESTIONS

1. If someone is against all use of animals in medical research, should he or she refrain from using medicines or products tested for safety on animals? Slaves built the White House. Should American presidents therefore refuse to live in it? Are the arguments properly analogous?

2. "I agree that animals suffer in being raised for my food, but I don't care. I enjoy eating bacon, barbecue, and ham, and I will never change." Does this person commit any mistake of reasoning in admitting that he doesn't care enough about suffering of animals raised for his food to become a vegetarian?

3. "I'd rather be your pet than your fetus." Do people concerned with animal rights too often discount the suffering of fetuses in abortion? Shouldn't pro-life people be against both kinds of suffering?

4. What about the dog and the man in the lifeboat? If only one can stay, should we draw straws to see who goes overboard? (And don't keep the dog to eat him!)

5. Would it be acceptable for humans to volunteer to spare animals? Could we imagine a scenario where, if enough humans volunteered to test, say, new vitamins, no animals at all would need to be used in testing?

# CHAPTER 10

# Medical Research on Vulnerable Human Subjects

*T*his chapter describes ethical problems of medical research on vulnerable human populations. It begins with a historical review of medical experimentation by Nazi physicians and secret American medical research. The first part of the chapter discusses the Tuskegee study of untreated syphilis in Alabama and studies in Africa to prevent mother-to-child transmission of HIV. The chapter ends with financial conflicts in research, especially with research sponsored by pharmaceutical companies, and medical research in vulnerable populations in developing countries.

## INFAMOUS MEDICAL EXPERIMENTS

### William Beaumont

In 1822, physician William Beaumont, the father of gastric physiology, treated patient St. Martin for a bullet wound in the stomach; St. Martin survived, but the wound healed strangely, leaving a hole. Beaumont then employed St. Martin as a servant and proved the previously unknown fact that stomach juices digest food. St. Martin ran away and Beaumont had him caught to continue to exhibit him. Hospitals today in Texas and Michigan bear Beaumont's name.

### Nazi Medical Research

Besides participating in the Holocaust, physicians during the Nazi regime conducted heinous experiments. They reasoned that if victims in concentration camps were going to die anyway, why not use them to benefit medical science?

From 1943 to 1945, gay men, convicted criminals, Russian officers, Polish dissidents, Jews, and gypsies on Ward 46 at Buchenwald in Germany got experimental vaccines against typhus. Physicians injected blood infected with typhus into 40 involuntary subjects, who served as a treatment group. Overall, they infected a thousand prisoners, 158 of whom died.

In experiments at Buchenwald, physicians tried to cure gay men of being homosexual with hormone shots, had inmates shot to study gunshot wounds, starved inmates to study the physiology of nutrition, and amputated women's bones and limbs to study regeneration. To study malaria, physicians used anopheles mosquitoes to infect subjects. Physician Ernst Grawitz infected legs of women with staphylococci, gas, and tetanus bacilli. In testing sulfa drugs, he rubbed into wounds particles of glass and stone.

In experiments at Ravensbrück, physician Sigmund Rascher devised his "sky ride wagon" to simulate rapid changes in altitude. Victims were locked inside an enclosed box on wheels with monitoring equipment inside.[1] Rascher froze a hundred nude Jewish and Russian prisoners in icy waters to study techniques to revive downed pilots in similar waters. He also forced nude Jewish women to revive the subjects sexually. This exercise simply degraded the subjects for the amusement of the guards.

## Josef Mengele

Josef Mengele, known as the Angel of Death, participated in the deaths of 400,000 victims in concentration camps. Ambitious, young Mengele sought fame and studied medical anthropology and genetics between 1930 and 1936, when eugenics movements swept Germany and America.

Contrary to some accounts, German medical schools did not resist, but led, Nazi eugenics and the killing of undesirables. To advance, Mengele joined the Brownshirts, a fanatical Nazi movement that promoted Aryan racial purity.

Mengele needed groundbreaking research to become a full professor. In 1943 at the Auschwitz concentration camp, he experimented to overcome the effects of genetics by modifying environments. He wanted to produce blue eyes, blonde hair, and healthy bodies free of genetic disease.

As subjects, he needed identical twins, natural controls. So he examined incoming trains of boxcars filled with Jews, looking for twins and other usable subjects, signaling his choices with a flick of his wrist.

He injected blue dye into children's eyes to see if he could create blue eyes. To see if twins could be produced, he forced female twins to engage in coitus with male twins. He interchanged blood of identical twins to observe results; he interchanged blood between pairs of twins.

One pair of fraternal twins consisted of a hunchback and a normal child; Mengele surgically grafted the hunchback to the normal child's back, creating the effect of conjoined twins. He accentuated this effect by sewing their wrists back to back. A witness reported that when these conjoined children returned to the barracks: "There was a terrible smell of gangrene. The cuts were dirty and the children cried every night."[2]

Mengele obtained between 150 and 200 twins, most of whom died. Mengele also tested endurance by subjecting 75 prisoners to electric shock; 25 of them died immediately. He subjected Polish nuns to high dosages of radiation to produce sterility.

He once found a hunchback and the hunchback's son; he had both of them killed, their bodies boiled, their flesh stripped, and their skeletons dipped in gasoline for preservation for his anthropological studies of body types. Coming upon seven dwarfs from a circus family, he exhibited them to visiting physicians.

When 300 Jewish children escaped a gas chamber, Mengele—cool, impersonal, and detached—had them recaptured, lit a gasoline fire set in a large pit, and had the children thrown in.

When the Russian army approached Auschwitz in 1945, Mengele escaped to Paraguay. He lived there for 40 years, eluding Israelis who tried to capture him as a war criminal. In later conversations with his grown son Rolf, he expressed no regret for his actions: it was not his fault that Jews had to die at Auschwitz, he said, so why not use them to advance medical knowledge and his own chances for a professorship? Never captured or tried as a war criminal, Mengele died in Brazil in 1985.[3]

## THE NUREMBERG CODE

After World War II, at the Nuremberg trials in 1946, German physicians defended themselves against charges of war crimes by saying that they had merely been following orders, that their experiments had been properly related to solving medical problems of war, and that what they had done did not differ from similar research done on captives by American physicians.

The judges at Nuremberg lacked a code of ethics for experimentation on captive populations, so they created 10 principles for ethical experimentation, known as the *Nuremberg Code*. Its most important principle was that people should freely consent to participation in any experiment.

### Questionable American Research

In 1941, American researchers experimented on orphans at the Ohio Soldiers and Sailors Orphanage, on inmates at New Jersey State Colony for the Feeble-Minded, and on patients at a mental institution in Dixon, Illinois.[4] To develop a vaccine against shigella, they injected deadened forms of the bacteria into subjects. None died, but many got sick.

Some questionable research used military personnel as subjects. Cornelius Rhoads, Director of Memorial Sloan Kettering Cancer Hospital in New York City, led the military's secret chemical warfare service. He exposed thousands of American troops to mustard gas, accidentally learning that the gas killed white blood cells and cancerous cells. After the war, he experimented with mustard gas as an anti-cancer drug.[5] About 4,000 to 5,000 subjects inhaled mustard gas in gas chambers. Altogether, in research conducted by the armed forces on poisonous agents, 60,000 subjects did not know what they were undergoing.[6]

During World War II, Franklin Roosevelt established the Committee on Medical Research, which approached its work with a wartime mentality that carried over after the war: disease was the enemy, researchers battled it, and victory could be won—with enough resources and enough will. As bioethicist David Rothman wrote, during the war, ethical concerns about experiments carried little weight:

> A wartime environment also undercut the protection of human subjects, because of the power of the example of the draft. Every day thousands of men were compelled to risk death, however limited their understanding of the aims of the war or the immediate campaign might be. By extension, researchers doing laboratory

work were also engaged in a military activity, and they did not need to seek the permission of their subjects any more than the selective service or field commanders did of draftees. . . . In a society mobilized for war, these arguments carried great weight. Some people were ordered to face bullets and storm a hill; others were told to take an injection and test a vaccine. In philosophical terms, wartime inevitably promoted utilitarian over absolutistic positions.[7]

When subjects of secret chemical research later applied for treatment at veterans' hospitals, the Veterans Administration (VA) denied that they had been exposed to these agents. This scenario recurred after the war in Vietnam and after Operation Desert Storm.

During the 1940s, radiation enthralled some physicians. Joseph Hamilton of the University of California at Berkeley injected plutonium into 18 unsuspecting patients diagnosed with cancer. According to Kenneth Scott, a scientist who later investigated these abuses, two patients were mistakenly diagnosed with cancer but nevertheless given "many times the lethal dose of plutonium."[8]

Physicians also studied radioactive isotopes used in diagnosis and research. In the late 1940s at Vanderbilt University, physicians injected 819 pregnant women with radioactive iron in a nutritional study. A study in 1960 found that three of their children died of rare forms of cancer.[9] In 1945, Eda Charlton entered Strong Memorial Hospital in Rochester, New York, with a mild case of hepatitis and was secretly injected with plutonium-239 to study how her body eliminated radiation. Physicians then secretly followed her for years to observe the effects (she died of a heart attack in 1983).

From World War II to the mid-1970s, physician-researchers subjected over 16,000 American patients to radiation experiments.[10] The Department of Energy or its predecessors conducted at least 435 experiments in 21 states. From the 1940s to the 1960s, physicians exposed 1,500 military aviators and submarine crewmen to encapsulated radium on the end of wires inserted high into their nostrils for several minutes.[11]

In another experiment, physician-researchers paid 130 male prisoners $200 to undergo X-ray radiation of their testicles; afterward, these men got vasectomies. In another, physicians injected plutonium into an indigent 36-year-old Texan's injured leg, which surgeons then amputated. In 1995, the President's Committee on Human Radiation Experiments investigated these experiments and concluded that the government should apologize to involuntary subjects and should compensate people who had been injured.[12]

In 1966, Harvard medical professor Henry Beecher criticized 22 specific medical experiments published in medical journals that had not obtained consent of subjects; he pointed out that this was the norm and criticized this fact.[13] About the same time, physician Henry Pappworth similarly criticized 500 medical experiments.[14] That year, the U.S. Public Health Service began to require informed consent of subjects, an important fact in judging the Tuskegee Study.

In 1991 in Operation Desert Storm, officers forced soldiers to take experimental vaccines against biological agents. Federal law stated that, under operational conditions, soldiers could not refuse such vaccinations. Subsequently, many soldiers became sick. For years afterward, the Pentagon and Department of Defense denied that their sickness was service-related. Yet the military's own records showed many causes of such sickness, especially acting in combination, with sand storms, biological weapons, oil fires, contaminated water, rare micro-organisms, the vaccines discussed earlier, chemical vapors from bombed Iraqi storage areas, unspent rocket fuel, and high levels of stress.[15]

## THE TUSKEGEE STUDY (OR "STUDY")

### Nature and History of Syphilis

Past victims of untreated syphilis included Cleopatra, King Herod of Judea, Charlemagne, Henry VIII, Napoleon Bonaparte, Frederick the Great, Catherine the Great, Christopher Columbus, Paul Gauguin, Franz Schubert, Albrecht Dürer, Johann Wolfgang von Goethe, Friedrich Nietzsche, John Keats, and James Joyce.[16]

Between 1900 and 1948, and especially during the two world wars, American reformers mounted the *Syphilophobia Campaign*. Reformers emphasized that prostitutes spread syphilis and that it rapidly killed. As an alternative for men to visiting prostitutes, they advocated clean, active sports, or "Muscular Christianity."

Anti-syphilis crusaders split twice over methods to prevent spread of syphilis: once during World War I over giving out condoms and again during World War II over giving out penicillin. In each conflict, reformers who wanted to reduce the harm of syphilis battled those who wanted to reduce illicit behavior.[17]

This conflict repeated over the next century in battles about venereal diseases, prostitution, alcoholism, drug addiction, gambling, and sex education. The *Harm Reduction Movement (HRM)* focuses on reducing the associated harms of these behaviors, not on moral censure or eliminating the behaviors. Moralists who oppose HRM attack the illicit behavior and view HRM as enabling it, for example, by teaching men how to use condoms.

During the world wars, the armed services adopted HRM. Commanders who needed healthy troops ordered the release of condoms in the first war and penicillin in the second. After the wars, returning troops continued to use both, normalizing these practices.

Physicians today treat syphilis with penicillin. Such treatment has been possible only since 1948, when penicillin became available to everyone.

Schaudinn discovered in 1906 the spirochete that causes syphilis. It is a chronic, contagious bacterial disease, often venereal and sometimes congenital. It has three stages. In the first, *primary syphilis*, spirochetes mass and produce a primary lesion, a chancre (pronounced "SHANK-er"). During this stage, syphilis is highly infectious. After the chancre subsides, the disease spreads silently for a time, but then produces an outbreak of secondary symptoms such as fever, rash, and swollen lymph glands.

In the second state of *latent syphilis*, spirochetes disseminate from the primary lesion throughout the body, producing systemic and widespread lesions, usually in internal organs. Syphilis may then spread silently from 1 to 30 years. During this stage, symptoms vary so widely that syphilis was once known as the Great Pretender.

In the last stage of *tertiary syphilis*, chronic destructive lesions damage the cardiac and neurological systems. Syphilis then may produce paresis (slight or incomplete paralysis), gummas (gummy or rubbery tumors), altered gait, blindness, or lethal narrowing of the aorta.

Beginning in the sixteenth century, to treat syphilis physicians applied the heavy metal mercury as a paste on the back. During the nineteenth century, they similarly administered another heavy metal, bismuth. Neither mercury nor bismuth killed the spirochetes, though they ameliorated symptoms.

In 1909, after the spirochete causing syphilis had been identified, two researchers—a German, Paul Erlich; and a Japanese, S. Hata—tried 605 forms of arsenic and discovered a "magic bullet" against it in combination 606 of heavy metals (which included arsenic). Erlich humbly called this Salvarsan (implying salvation from syphilis); its generic name is arsphenamine.[18] After finding that it cured syphilis in rabbits, Erlich injected it intramuscularly into men with syphilis.

At first, Salvarsan seemed to work wonders, and during 1910, physicians greeted Erlich with standing ovations. Later, syphilis recurred in some patients treated with Salvarsan, and some of them died, either from syphilis or from Salvarsan. Erlich maintained that the drug had not been given correctly, but he developed a less toxic form, Neosalvarsan.

Physicians injected Neosalvarsan intramuscularly in 20 to 40 dosages over a year, charging patients a dollar per visit. To get full treatment, patients needed both time and money. Neosalvarsan was no one-time treatment for syphilis, like penicillin later was.

Between 1890 and 1910, Norwegian Caesar Boeck studied the natural course of untreated syphilis in 1,978 subjects. He believed that heavy metals removed only the symptoms of syphilis. Because they killed some syphilitics, he studied whether subjects might fare better untreated.

In 1929, Boeck's successor, J. E. Bruusgaard, selected 473 of Boeck's subjects for further evaluation.[19] Bruusgaard learned that of subjects who had had syphilis for more than 20 years, 73 percent were asymptomatic. Because this discovery dramatically contradicted the Syphilophobia Campaign, the leaders of this movement resisted the fact that syphilis did not universally kill, much less did not do so rapidly (foreshadowing similar battles later about AIDS). Even more disturbing to the Syphilophobia Campaign, Bruusgaard confirmed that some latent syphilitics might never develop symptoms at all.

So when the Tuskegee study began in 1932, Boeck's and Bruusgaard's studies had caused physicians to question the received views about the natural course and treatment of syphilis.

## The Racial Environment

In the 1930s, American medicine was racist. Most physicians held stereotypes about African-American patients, as in this example from a 1914 *Journal of the American Medical Association*:

> The negro springs from a southern race, and as such his sexual appetite is strong; all of his environments stimulate this appetite, and as a general rule his emotional type of religion certainly does not decrease it.[20]

Physicians saw African Americans as dirty, shiftless, promiscuous, and incapable of personal hygiene. In 1900, a Georgia physician wrote, "Virtue in the negro race is like 'angels' visits'—few and far between. In a practice of 16 years in the

South, I have never examined a virgin over 14 years of age."[21] In 1919, a medical professor in Chicago wrote that African-American men were like bulls in *furor sexualis,* unable to resist copulation around females.[22]

Given such racism, white physicians around 1929 saw syphilis as a natural consequence of low character in African Americans, described by one white physician as a "notoriously syphilis-soaked race."[23] Such physicians also assumed that African-American men would not seek treatment for venereal disease.

## DEVELOPMENT OF THE TUSKEGEE STUDY

### A Study in Nature Begins

Physiologist Claude Bernard in 1865 distinguished *studies in nature* from normal *experiments*: in the former, someone merely observes what would have happened without any interventions; in the latter, scientists manipulate a variable. The Tuskegee Study was a study in nature.

The great physician William Osler once said, "Know syphilis in all its manifestations and relations, and all other things clinical will be added unto you."[24] Yet as of 1932, syphilis's natural history had not been documented, and because of Boeck/Brussgaard's results, physicians doubted the inexorability of its course.

This explains why the U.S. Public Health Service (USPHS) believed it needed a study in nature. Around 1929, six counties in America had high rates of syphilis—above 20 percent— and a charity, the Julius Rosenwald Foundation of Philadelphia, treated all syphilitics in those counties with Neosalvarsan. In 1930, this foundation surveyed African-American men in Macon County, Alabama, where Tuskegee is the chief town. It citizens were 82 percent black, and its rate of syphilis was then the highest in the nation, 36 percent. The foundation treated or partially treated some of these 3,694 syphilitics with Neosalvarsan.

Then something unforeseen happened: in 1929 the Great Depression began. Soon, funds for charity plummeted, and the Rosenwald Foundation left, hoping that USPHS would continue its program. Funds for public health also plummeted, and by 1935, the USPHS budget had fallen from $1 million to less than $60,000.

In 1931, USPHS repeated the Rosenwald Foundation's survey of syphilis in Macon County, testing 4,400 African-American residents, and found that 22 percent of men had syphilis, as well as a dangerous 62 percent rate of congenital syphilis. Of great importance for the Tuskegee Study, this survey identified 399 African-American men who had had syphilis of several years' duration, but who had never been treated.

The surgeon general himself, Raymond Vonderlehr, wrote in 1936 in the *Journal of the American Medical Association* that the Tuskegee study was "an unusual opportunity to study the untreated syphilitic patient from the beginning of the disease to the death of the infected person."[25] His decision began the Tuskegee Study.

Three points deserve emphasis. First, the 399 subjects had *latent* syphilis, not infectious syphilis. During this stage, syphilis is largely noninfectious during sexual intercourse. Second, researchers did not divide the 399 subjects into the typical experimental and control groups: they were all simply observed. There was, however, another group of natural controls, 200 age-matched African-American men living in Macon County who had never had syphilis.

Third, the 399 men with syphilis and the 200 men without it were perfect for a study in nature because they were *so vulnerable*: they were poor, illiterate, and tied to the land as tenant farmers. As such, unlike other people with syphilis over the next four decades, *they were unlikely to ever leave Macon County*. Partly because of this vulnerability, Vonderlehr implied, they presented an "unusual opportunity."

Vonderlehr had no sense that it might be wrong to use such vulnerable subjects in a life-long experiment. Like many of his time, he may have assumed that people with syphilis got what they deserved and that these poor black men would never have had the means, will, or opportunity to get treatment, even though the Public Health Service could have one day provided it.

## The Middle Phase: Poor Design

No one physician oversaw this study. It lacked written protocols, and later investigators often mixed up the subjects in the no-treatment group of 399 syphilitics with the 200 "controls" without syphilis. Nurse Eunice Rivers, an African-American nurse permanently assigned to stay in Tuskegee and keep track of the study, kept poor records, lost them, and because many of the men had the same last names, often confused one patient for another with the same common, last name.

Researchers assumed that controls would remain uninfected, but in a county where one in three people had syphilis, many controls eventually contracted syphilis. Unfortunately, when they happened, some were switched to the no-treatment group of syphilitics.

The study had gaps. Federal doctors visited in 1939 and then not again until 1948; seven years passed between visits in 1963 and 1970. Only Nurse Rivers held the shaky study together.

During the course of the research, many of the 399 syphilitic subjects, who were supposed to remain untreated, obtained Neosalvarsan or penicillin outside Macon County. James Lucas, a CDC physician, said, "effective and undocumented treatment had been given to the vast majority of patients in the syphilitic group."[26] As a result, researchers could not know whether any observed subject really represented the consequences of untreated syphilis or when the subject had contracted it.

Ultimately, the study proved nothing. Before it began, physicians knew that syphilitics had greater morbidity and mortality than nonsyphilitics, and from Bruusgaard's discovery, that not all men in the latent phase died of syphilis. The Tuskegee Study added nothing to that knowledge.

## Spinal Taps and Deception

When physicians returned, they wanted to know, first, if they had a subject in the study group; and second, if so, how far his syphilis had progressed. To determine progression, they did spinal punctures on 271 of the 399 syphilitic subjects.

In doing spinal taps, they inserted a 10-inch needle between two vertebrae into the cerebrospinal fluid to withdraw a small amount of fluid. Because this is a delicate and uncomfortable process, physicians warned subjects to stay still, lest the needle swerve and puncture their spinal cord or spinal nerves, causing infection and possible paralysis.

Some physicians then and now regard spinal taps as insignificant, justified by the need to prove a diagnosis. On the other hand, professionals who describe a spinal tap this way may be thinking about administering one rather than receiving one.

A spinal tap is not a minor procedure, like taking blood. Some patients experience side effects, such as being unable to stand for a week without a severe headache. One person in a million will become paralyzed or permanently comatose.[27]

Tapping someone involuntarily, without obtaining informed consent, is legally a form of battery. Researchers who need healthy volunteers for spinal taps offer as much as $1,000 for them.

To induce subjects to travel to town and undergo these painful taps, physicians offered a series of incentives: free transportation, free hot lunches, free medicine for any disease other than syphilis, and free burials. In return for these benefits, physicians did spinal taps and later, autopsies, to inspect for damage from syphilis.

But these freebies and the persuasion of Nurse Rivers failed to get all men to come to town for the "round-ups," so researchers resorted to deception. *Infamously, they told the black men that they had "bad blood" and that the spinal taps were treatment for their bad blood.* Researchers sent the subjects the following letter, under the imposing letterhead "Macon County Health Department," with the subheading "Alabama State Board of Health and U.S. Public Health Service Cooperating with Tuskegee Institute":

> Dear Sir:
> Some time ago you were given a thorough examination and since that time we hope you have gotten a great deal of treatment for bad blood. You will now be given your last chance to get a second examination. This examination is a very special one and after it is finished you will be given a special treatment if it is believed you are in a condition to stand it.[28]

The "special treatment" mentioned was the spinal tap to culture for neurosyphilis. The subjects were instructed to meet Nurse Rivers for transportation to "Tuskegee Institute Hospital for this free treatment." The letter closed, in capitals:

> REMEMBER THIS IS YOUR LAST CHANCE FOR SPECIAL FREE TREATMENT.
> BE SURE TO MEET THE NURSE.

To repeat, the researchers never treated the subjects for syphilis. *Although penicillin was developed around 1941–1943 and was widely available by 1948, the subjects in the Tuskegee Study never received it, even during the 1960s or up to 1972.* In fact, during World War II, the researchers contacted the local draft board, which prevented eligible subjects from being drafted, and hence from being treated for syphilis with penicillin by the armed services.

## Revelation of the Study to the World

In 1966, USPHS venereal disease investigator Peter Buxtun learned about the study. By this time, supervision of the study (and Buxtun) had moved to the newly created Centers for Disease Control (CDC) in Atlanta. When Buxtun asked about the study, the CDC threatened to fire him.

By 1969, Buxtun's protests led to a meeting of a small group of physicians at CDC to consider stopping the Tuskegee Study or revealing it. Ultimately, they voted to continue the study and to keep it secret.

In 1970, the American Public Health Association published a monograph on syphilis. It stated that treatment for late benign syphilis should consist of "6.0 to 9.0 million units of benzathine penicillin G given 3.0 million units at sessions seven days apart."[29] The first author was William J. Brown, head of CDC's Tuskegee section from 1957 to 1971. Brown had been on the CDC committee in 1969 and had argued for continuing the study, where subjects with late benign syphilis received no penicillin.

Buxtun eventually contacted Jean Heller, who worked for the Associated Press. On July 26, 1972, her story appeared on front pages of newspapers nationwide.[30] She described a study run by the federal government in Tuskegee, Alabama, where poor, uneducated African-American men had been used as guinea pigs. After noting the terrible effects of tertiary syphilis, she stated that in 1969 a CDC study of 276 of the untreated subjects had proved that at least seven subjects died "as a direct result of syphilis."

Heller's story stunned congressmen. Senator William Proxmire called it a "moral and ethical nightmare." In reply, J. D. Millar, chief of Venereal Disease Control at CDC, said that the study "was never clandestine," correctly pointing to 15 published articles in medical journals over 30 years.

After Heller's story appeared, the Secretary of Health, Education, and Welfare terminated the study. The CDC estimated that 28 syphilitics had died of syphilis during the study; it then gave penicillin to the remaining subjects.

In 1973, on behalf of the Tuskegee subjects, lawyer Fred Gray filed a class-action suit against the federal government. In 1974, the U.S. government settled out of court. According to the settlement, living syphilitics received $37,500 each; heirs of deceased syphilitics, $15,000 (since children might have had congenital syphilis); heirs of living controls, $16,000; heirs of deceased controls, $5,000. Controls and their descendants received compensation because they and their families had been deprived of antibiotics during the decades of the study. The government also provided free lifetime medical care for Tuskegee subjects, their wives, and their children.

In 1972, as a direct revelation of the study, the federal government required all institutions that conduct human medical experimentation and receive federal funds to have Institutional Review Boards (IRBs). Today, IRBs must scrutinize written proposals and defend against abuses in medical research.

In 1988, 21 of the original 399 syphilitic subjects were still alive, each of whom had had syphilis for at least 62 years.[31] In addition, 41 wives and 19 children had evidence of syphilis and had received free medical care.

In 1997, President Clinton met four of the eight living survivors to apologize for the Tuskegee Study, "What the United States did was shameful, and I am sorry."[32] The youngest survivor then was 87, the oldest between 100 and 109.[33] By then, the government had paid $10 million to the study's original 600 members or to their families or heirs, who numbered more than 6,000. Because of lack of treatment for syphilis of men in the study, any of these other people might have contracted syphilis.[34]

Perhaps the worst effect of revelation of the study was distrust by African Americans of medical experiments, a legacy that researchers still struggle to overcome.

## ETHICAL ISSUES OF THE TUSKEGEE STUDY

### Informed Consent and Deception

In the Tuskegee Study, the subjects did not know they were part of a government study lasting throughout their lives, did not even know what syphilis was, and did not know that they weren't being treated with available drugs. In other words, they had no informed consent, which many critics considered to be ethically outrageous.

R. H. Kampmeier, an emeritus professor of medicine at Vanderbilt Medical School, worked as a syphilologist during the decades of the study.[35] He argued that a study undertaken in the 1930s could not be faulted for lack of informed consent, which began only after 1966. Would it make sense, he argued, to judge Pasteur unethical because he, too, did not get consent?

Kampmeier cited another landmark study by USPHS in 1943 that studied giving penicillin to 35,000 syphilitics; it did not get consent from subjects. Medical historian and physician Thomas Benedek dismisses informed consent in the Tuskegee Study as "anachronistic," emphasizing that USPHS did not require informed consent until 1966.[36]

While it is true that informed consent in medical experiments was not mandated by court decisions until 1966, the presumption had always been that physicians would "First, do no harm" to their patients. Not obtaining consent for procedures that might benefit subjects differs from procedures that might *harm* subjects.

Finally, and granted that telling patients the truth was not *legally* required before 1966, was it *ethical* for the Tuskegee researchers to lie to their subjects for all those decades? Isn't the truth what one person owes another, especially as doctor and patient?

### Racism

The Tuskegee Study took place in Alabama and all its subjects were African American. Under such circumstances, was it only a coincidence that no subjects were white? Would white subjects have been deceived and left untreated the same way?

In his classic work, *Bad Blood*, medical historian James Jones saw the Tuskegee Study as a result of pervasive racism in American medicine during the 1930s.

It is true that some physicians then believed that syphilis ran a different course in different races, and this implied the need for a parallel study of untreated white syphilitics. That the USPHS did no parallel study of white subjects shows that it saw black subjects as expendable, but not white subjects.

## Media Coverage

In defending the Tuskegee Study, Kampmeier objected to the "great hue and cry" in the media in 1972 and to journalists' claims that "treatment was purposefully withheld to evaluate the course of untreated disease." He said about *Time* and *American Medical News*: "In complete disregard of their abysmal ignorance, members of the fourth estate bang out anything on their typewriters that will make headlines."[37]

With regard to the first objection, Kampmeier exaggerated the "hue and cry" of the media. Indeed, the media botched the story. Coverage shrank within days, and the story moved to the back pages, where only short paragraphs followed it.

To begin with the second objection, Kampmeier attacked the media for reporting the damaging aspects of the study, such as the withholding of treatment. In defense of the media, researchers *did* intend to withhold treatment. That was precisely the intention of the study.

The Tuskegee Study deserved far more attention. True, it had complex issues that involved racism at a time when racial turmoil upset Americans, but today such a story would receive weeks of nationwide scrutiny, and probably get a congressional hearing on television.

The relation then between medicine and the media can also be questioned. Before Heller's story broke, the Tuskegee Study had been reported repeatedly in at least 17 articles in medical journals between 1936 and 1972. Researchers did not conceal the study within medicine. Despite this, no professional publication, physician, or editor alerted the nation to the story.

Between 1966 and 1971, one African-American professional at the CDC mailed boxes of documents about the study to several national newspapers and magazines.[38] Nothing happened. Why is that?

The answer is important to understanding many issues in medical ethics and to whistleblowing about corruption. Print and television reporters need an expert to help them understand such complex stories and, equally important, to take responsibility for claims about wrongdoing. Virtually no reporters then or now have the medical background to understand such complicated stories and, without that, cannot risk charging physicians with possible crimes.

A natural tendency also exists to want *someone else* to be the whistleblower and to bear the brunt of retaliation. As a result, merely mailing information or passing it along conversationally is not enough for reporters to publicize wrongdoing.

## Harm to Subjects

Kampmeier argued that if the Tuskegee Study had never occurred, its subjects would have received no treatment and would have been no worse off. Such a claim can never be proved. If the Tuskegee study had not occurred, many things might have happened. Another charity might have provided Neosalvarsan. A writer like John Steinbeck might have soon written a novel about syphilis in Macon County, arousing national concern and getting penicillin to people there infected with syphilis.

So what harm, if any, resulted to subjects with syphilis from nontreatment? This question might seem even absurd: if subjects were left untreated, of course they must have been harmed! However, the issue is not that simple.

In 1931, penicillin was unavailable, so physicians withheld Neosalvarsan from subjects. Because Neosalvarsan was expensive and cumbersome to administer, even if this study had not occurred, subjects might not have received it. Boeck and Bruusgaard had also undermined claims about the benefits of heavy metals, so harm is difficult to prove. In a review of medical evidence available in 1940, medical historian Benedek concluded that in 1937, untreated syphilitics actually lived longer and better than those partially treated with heavy metals.[39]

Not everyone agrees. UAB Professor of Internal Medicine Benjamin Friedman, whose career spanned the decades of this study, countered that:

> In the 1940s it was known that patients receiving as few as 20 injections of arsenicals rarely developed symptomatic aortic disease. Since we could not determine in advance which of the latent syphilitics would, after 20 or 30 years, develop symptomatic aortic disease, it was necessary to treat all of them. One cannot maintain that some small number of syphilitics deprived of treatment did not therefore suffer injury.[40]

By 1934, the major professional organization of physicians treating syphilis in America, the Cooperating Clinical Group, proved that use of heavy metals improved Bruusgaard's statistics and recommended that all syphilitics get Neosalvarsan, mercury, and bismuth.[41] Even if many patients could not afford such therapy, they should have been told about it.

Later during the study, penicillin became available. Although Alexander Fleming discovered penicillin in 1929, the world did not appreciate his discovery until 1941, and only around 1946, as a result of wartime production to treat soldiers, did penicillin become available to most Americans. By 1948, anyone could get it.[42]

Kampmeier argued that withholding penicillin in 1946 did not harm subjects with latent syphilis, which he said was a "chronic, granulomatous, self-limiting disease" and not fatal. He argued next that proof of penicillin's effectiveness did not come until 1948 and then only for primary syphilis. So the study's subjects by 1948 could no longer have been helped by penicillin; the damage to them had already been done.[43]

Benedek disagreed. He concluded that giving penicillin to latent syphilitics in 1948 "might have exerted a definitely beneficial effect on the prognosis of only 12.5 percent of the subjects."[44] Still, that would have helped 50 subjects.

## Effects on Subjects' Families

"Virtually all subjects were or had been married" and had an average of 5.2 children.[45] Recall that Macon County had a rate of congenital syphilis of 62 percent.

When we consider the subjects' families, wouldn't the men in the study want to know they had syphilis? Even in latency, wouldn't they want to know they could become infectious again? Did the researchers withhold the truth because they thought these men couldn't refrain from sex?

These researchers subjected women and children in Macon County to harm. Either the researchers discounted this harm, or thought it didn't matter.

## Kant and Motives of Researchers

When physicians at CDC and USPHS debated the Tuskegee study in 1969, many assumed that if no harm could be proved, nothing unethical had been done. This is also Kampmeier's unstated assumption.

Focusing on consequences, however, is only one way to judge morality. We can also adopt, not a consequentialism or utilitarianism, but a Kantian ethics focused on motives or a virtue ethics focused on the character of researchers.

Although we cannot prove that being left untreated harmed the study's subjects, it may have been only good luck that the study caused no more harm than it did. Why is that?

Historical evidence cuts both ways. We cannot use differing historical standards at differing times to excuse lack of informed consent, but not pay attention to what else researchers believed at the time. Let us put ourselves in the minds of researchers in the late 1940s. *The crucial fact is that when penicillin became available, most physicians believed it would help latent syphilitics.*

So they believed that subjects would be harmed by not getting penicillin. For all anyone knew in 1948, penicillin could have helped patients with aortic heart disease or at least, would have ameliorated it.

For Kantian ethics, researchers deliberately willed harm on these subjects. They used them as "mere means," as guinea pigs, and could not universalize such behavior as a maxim for all physicians to act on. Not only did they lack what Kant calls a "good will," they had an *ill will* toward vulnerable subjects.

It is no good appealing to sophisticated knowledge that came later about how the damage from syphilis had already occurred. Researchers then believed they were depriving syphilitics of something likely to help them, or depriving them of something that could help them not pass syphilis on to their female partners. But out of a desire by researchers to prove the final ravages of syphilis, or lack thereof, researchers deceived subjects and believed they were allowing them to be harmed.

## HIV PREVENTION IN AFRICA: ANOTHER TUSKEGEE STUDY?

Unfortunately, research by physicians in wartime and the Tuskegee Study are not the only examples in the history of modern medical ethics of questionable research on vulnerable subjects. We now discuss a famous study in Africa that involved not syphilis but AIDS, and readers can see how the issues of the Tuskegee Study frame some of the criticisms of the African study.

In 1994, researchers had proved that giving the drug AZT (zidovudine) during pregnancy cut by two-thirds transmission of HIV from mother to child in North America.[46] In 1995, CDC, NIH, and the World Health Organization (WHO) began to study whether doing a similar study in Africa could prevent HIV in the 800 infected babies born there every day and started a randomized control trial (RCT).

One might well ask, "As the ability of AZT to block vertical HIV transmission had already been proven, why conduct such a study at all in Africa?" One answer: the strain of HIV in Africa differs from that common in North America. A second answer: in Africa, researchers felt that they needed a speedier proof that AZT could block mother-to-child transmission of HIV.

In 1997, Marcia Angell, executive editor of the *New England Journal of Medicine*, claimed that this research mimicked the Tuskegee Study because researchers gave pregnant, HIV-infected black women placebos (harmless sugar pills), and thus babies were born with preventable HIV infections.[47] Because giving AZT to all HIV+ pregnant women was the American *standard of care*, not giving AZT in a placebo group was unethical: "If it is unethical to do placebo-controlled trials in America, it should also be unethical to do them in third-world countries."[48]

This study had subjects who were highly vulnerable because they were (1) black, (2) female, (3) poor, (4) illiterate, (5) victims of sexually transmitted diseases, and (6) without other available treatment. Like the Tuskegee Study, magisterial but distant governmental agencies conducted the research. Like the Tuskegee Study, vulnerability and powerlessness characterized the subjects. Columnist Ellen Goodman noted that the Tuskegee Study had not ended, but had been merely exported.[49]

Apologists passionately retorted that, had their research not been done, infected mothers would not have gotten AZT and their babies would have been infected anyway.

African officials replied that Angell and Goodman were ethical imperialists imposing American ethical standards on African countries.[50] Such officials were also black and had lost children to HIV, unlike the white USPHS physicians of the Tuskegee Study.[51]

They also replied that if they could prove—via a placebo-controlled trial—that a shorter regimen of AZT could reduce HIV transmission by half, they could save 150,000 children a year. If skeptics such as Angell caused delays of proof, more children would die.

Officials also claimed that a placebo-controlled trial of HIV-transmission could be done faster and with fewer subjects than a AZT-controlled study, and that once they had good results, African governments would give all pregnant, HIV+ women the new, smaller dosage of AZT.

Researchers also argued procedurally that review committees in both countries had approved the studies and that, unlike the Alabama men, the women themselves had consented. Subsequent interviews by the *New York Times* cast doubt on how much the women understood.

Angell argued that researchers didn't need placebo-controlled studies; comparing dosages of AZT to other anti-HIV drugs could prove the same thing. Given the poverty of such countries, she denied that a proven, reduced dosage would later be given to all pregnant women because—even at $80—AZT costs 11 times more per year than that normally spent on such African women.

Both sides invoked justice.[52] One philosophical side invoked Bentham, utilitarianism, and public health ethics. The other hailed Kant, his axiom that people can never be used as a "mere means," and his belief that ethical principles are not local but universal.

For researchers, the risk/benefit ratio had to be different for poor, illiterate women in impoverished countries who otherwise would not have gotten treatment. For critics, the same reasoning had led to the Tuskegee Study and to Nazi experiments: "They're going to get die anyway, so we might as well study them to learn something."[53] As Angell retorted, "People can't be used as a means to a noble end."[54]

In 1998, CDC proved that $80 worth of AZT in the last four weeks of pregnancy cut transmission in half, and they suspended the study.[55] At this early cessation, both sides claimed victory.

## The Krieger Lead Paint Study

In 2001, after Ellen Roche died in a study of a drug to prevent asthma, the federal Office of Protection from Research Risks (OPRR) halted all federally funded research at Johns Hopkins Medical School. When she volunteered for the study, Ellen was healthy; soon, she was dead.

After its research stopped, a physician from Hopkins on television denounced suspension of Hopkins' research monies, claiming Hopkins had only killed one person in many decades of medical research and that lives would be lost from such a suspension because of delayed cures.

The Krieger case was a study by a branch of Johns Hopkins Medical School that studied mental handicaps in children from lead paint—which six of seven judges on Maryland's highest court likened it to the Tuskegee Study.[56] The study, conducted in the mid-1990s by Hopkins's Kennedy Krieger Institute, recruited 108 poor, vulnerable, black families to live in East Baltimore in houses with lead paint.

Ingesting lead-based paint is a known cause of cognitive disability in small children. According to the Krieger Institute, the study sought cheaper ways to reduce lead contamination in houses so landlords in East Baltimore would not abandon them.

Did the parents understand the nature of the study? Did they understand the risk to their children by living in these houses? "It can be argued that the researchers intended that the children be the canaries in the mines but never clearly told the parents," one critic said.[57] Moreover,

> Maryland Court of Appeals Judge Dale R. Cathell, who wrote last week's scathing opinion, said the board [had] instructed Kennedy Krieger researchers to write consent forms for study participants that skirted federal regulations requiring disclosure about risks.
>
> The Court of Appeals ruling ordered trials to be held in lawsuits filed against Kennedy Krieger by two women, Viola Hughes and Catina Higgins, whose children were involved in the study. Hughes's daughter now suffers from learning disabilities and cognitive impairments, both of which are often associated with lead poisoning. . . . Higgins says researchers withheld tests results that showed high levels of lead contamination from her. . . .
>
> Kennedy Krieger is a major institution in the study of lead paint abatement. Marc Farfel, who conducted the study, said today that it identified more effective ways to remove lead hazards and prompted legislation forcing landlords to remove those hazards.[58]

Amazingly, an investigation by OPRR revealed that the IRB at Johns Hopkins, which supposedly had reviewed and discussed the ethics of the Krieger study and all other research at the medical school, had rarely met face-to-face.

The Krieger study resembled the Tuskegee Study in that vulnerable, poor black people were deliberately recruited to a study where physicians foresaw harm to subjects. Researchers rationalized the harm by saying that if the study had not occurred, the subjects would have lived in such housing anyway. Revelation of the Krieger study further damaged already bad relations between Baltimore's African Americans and Hopkins.

## 1946–1948: The Guatemalan Syphilis Study

In 2011, Wellesley historian Susan Reverby, while researching the Tuskegee Study, chanced upon documents at the National Archives revealing that the U.S. Public Health Service between 1946 and 1948 paid syphilis-infected prostitutes in Guatemala to visit prisoners and inmates of mental institutions to study how easily syphilis could be transmitted and if penicillin could prevent transmission.[59] When men failed to become infected, researchers scraped penises and faces and injected infected pus, causing about 1,300 of the 5,500 enrolled men to catch syphilis or gonorrhea. Following this revelation, Secretary of State Hillary Clinton apologized to the Guatemalan people for the actions of the United States in this shameful episode of research on people even more vulnerable than those in the Tuskegee Study.

## Financial Conflicts and Twenty-First-Century Research

The Bayh-Dole Act of 1980 erased an ethical bright line between academic and corporate medicine and allowed universities and their researchers to patent and reap royalties together. Since then, scandals about money keep recurring in medical research.

Thirty-five years later, pharmaceutical companies fund most research into drugs and devices at universities. They do not fund independent peer review of their new drugs and do not publicize bad results. By indirectly paying physicians to test new drugs and by financially encouraging physicians to recruit patients for experiments, drug companies cause physicians to choose their drug and not the best drug for their patients.

In 1998, a study by the Department of Health and Human Services concluded that IRBs could no longer handle the job of protecting subjects from abuses in medical experimentation.[60] It found that IRBs were underfunded and overworked and that the volume of work expected of volunteers could not be accurately and conscientiously performed. Another study in 2002 by the Institute of Medicine reached similar conclusions.[61] Since then, several medical research centers improved their structures for reviewing research, although financial conflicts continue.

In 1991, the federal government adopted the *Common Rule*, under which universities' IRBs must review all protocols the same way, regardless of funding. This rule subjects all protocols to the same standards as those required by NIH and the U.S. Federal Drug Administration (FDA).

Several scandals erupted in the 1990s, wherein a few physicians appeared to have taken millions of dollars from drug companies for dubious research.[62] Some doctors in Georgia allegedly made $4 million over seven years from aggressively soliciting people with schizophrenia for drug trials; they made another $6 million over the same period from testing other drugs.[63]

In 1996, Apotex Inc. tried to suppress adverse findings by Nancy Olivieri, a Canadian hematologist.[64] When using its experimental iron chelating drug (deferiprone) on patients with thalassemia, a heritable blood disorder, in a clinical trial paid for by Apotex, she discovered serious risks and attempted to publish them, but Apotex threatened to sue her for doing so.

Because of its financial ties to Apotex, her employer, the University of Toronto, failed to support her. In 1998, she published her findings and UT terminated her employment. The case exposed the limits of academic freedom in Canadian medicine and the ties between medical universities and drug companies. An investigation in 2001 by the Canadian Association of University Teachers vindicated Olivieri.[65]

Some physicians who worked for drug companies made an extra $100,000 a year flying around the country giving talks to physicians to promote a drug for a pharmaceutical company.

Today, all medical journals run expensive ads from drug companies, and almost all medical practices allow drug representatives to buy them and their staff expensive daily lunches or dinners. Drug companies give these gifts because they work. Learning to take free stuff from drug companies begins in medical school, when students learn to expect free food at lunch paid for by drug companies. Everyone ignores the corrupting influence of taking these gifts on their later decisions about prescribing drugs to patients.

## TOWARD INTERNATIONAL STANDARDS OF RESEARCH ETHICS

Over the last 50 years, more and more medical research has been exported from developed countries to people in developing countries, although less than 10 percent of that research is intended to benefit poor people in those developing countries.[66] In North America and Europe, despite some famous exceptions, consensus has developed about standards of ethical research, such as the "Common Rule" mentioned earlier.

During the last 50 years, many thousands of people in third-world countries were subjects of studies, many of them placebo-controlled. One occurred in 1996 by Pfizer in Kano, Nigeria, during an epidemic there of deadly meningitis in children. Pfizer researchers flew there and gave half of 200 infected children either the low dosage of the standard antibiotic ceftriazone or Pfizer's experimental drug Trovan. Pfizer had never tested this drug in oral form in children.[67]

Researchers commonly create conditions most favorable to proving efficacy of their own drugs, such as giving low dosages of standard drugs or "washing out" all traces of previous drugs in subjects, making them worse off.[68] In this study, five children died who took Trovan, six died who took the lower dose of ceftriaxone, and "many others [were] blind, deaf, paralyzed, or brain-damaged."

Work over the last decade in bioethics has focused on four questions about such medical research in developing countries: (1) How can we prevent vulnerable patients from being exploited by research? (2) How can such patients give informed consent? (3) Is it right to apply standards of research of developed countries to research in developing countries, or can there be a double standard? (4) Are there special problems of context in doing research on poor, illiterate people in developing countries?

The first problem, of exploitation, can be illustrated by the fact that the 10 biggest pharmaceutical companies in 2002 had more combined profits than the combined profits of the other 490 companies on the Fortune 500 list.[69] Given that Big Pharma profits more than any industry in the world, isn't any drug testing by it on vulnerable patients likely to exploit them? The 2005 film *The Constant Gardener* chronicles one such case in Africa. Is there any way to adequately compensate poor Africans for being the guinea pigs for new drugs that will mainly benefit children in North America?

The second problem, of informed consent, has been contested by people who say it upholds an individualistic model of autonomous, educated patients not applicable to members of illiterate tribes in South America and Africa. In the vertical-HIV-transmission trial, consent of tribal leaders was the best that could be achieved.

Perhaps that is so, but it also resembles excuses of the U.S. Public Health Service in not telling the men of the Tuskegee Study about "bringing them to autopsy" because the men were too ignorant to understand.

The third problem, a double standard, vexes many people. In America, IRBs and the FDA monitor research, but nothing like these institutions exist in most developing countries. Who then monitors, say, Merck's research in Guatemala?

A problem here is where placebos can be used in developing countries. In developed countries, a new drug or device is generally tested against the traditional drug or device, not a placebo. Even where researchers did not originally do placebo-controlled studies, new drugs are usually only tested against currently used drugs, not placebos. Yet the vertical-transmission-HIV study on vulnerable African mothers did use a placebo before it was stopped.

One solution is to have domestic IRBs of researchers monitor overseas research and apply the same standards. In that case, the vertical-HIV-transmission research could not have been done because, as said, giving AZT to all HIV+ babies was the standard of care at the time.

The final dilemma concerns contextual problems of doing research overseas in poor countries. In America, should a problem arise in a Phase I study of a drug, emergency rooms, EMT personnel, and local hospitals are available to treat allergic reactions, but not in the middle of the savannah or jungle. Does that mean such research can never be done in the wild?

## The Collaborative Model

One widely discussed solution to most of these problems is for the institution sponsoring the research and the area of the developing country to develop a long-term partnership. Rather than an international company swooping down for a one-time research trial, both sides should think of an arrangement lasting for decades. In this way, both sides can potentially benefit.

First, research on vulnerable populations should not be done if such people cannot benefit from the research at all. Second, if the research is successful, the people on whom it has been tested should receive adequate supplies of the drugs as partial recompense for their participation.

Third, it might be necessary to help a developing country build infrastructure to facilitate a long-term partnership in research. When UAB built an AIDS hospital in Zambia, it was necessary to fund small refrigerators running on small generators to keep medicine cool in remote areas.[70] Similarly, it might be necessary to train and fund medical technicians, midwives, or local physicians to draw blood over a decade in order to study the long-term effectiveness of interventions. More radically, traditional tests for diseases depend on high-tech, faraway, diagnostic labs not available in developing countries. Lack of such labs and their results may affect the health of many people in poor countries. To overcome this gap, point-of-care testing with wireless transmission back-and-forth via satellites may be necessary to help indigent populations.[71]

The reverse of this seems obvious: if no partnership exists, researchers will be perceived as exploitive and countries will refuse to grant rights to investigate, to take samples, or to apply for patents. If something like SARS breaks out, this could be dangerous for the world.

Such collaboration is called the *Fair Benefits Model* and emphasizes sharing the benefits of successful medical research.[72] One good start is the third edition in 2002 of the *International Ethical Guidelines for Biomedical Research Involving Human Subjects* by the Council for International Organizations of Medical Sciences(CIOMS).[73] These are good guidelines for researchers in North American countries funded by multinational pharmaceutical companies, using vulnerable subjects in low-resource countries for the subjects, and include guidelines for compensating such subjects who are injured in research.

Medical research on vulnerable people with schizophrenia is discussed in an excerpt from Gregory Pence's *Elements of Bioethics* book. To read *Can Research Be Just on People with Schizophrenia* Go to Chapter 10 in the Online Learning Center (OLC) at www.mhhe.com/pence7e.

## The Death of Jesse Gelsinger

In 1999, the death of teenager Jesse Gelsinger from gene therapy, like revelations of the Tuskegee Study or Gennarelli's head-injuries on baboons, changed regulation of American medical research.

In 1999 in Tucson, Arizona, 17-year-old Jesse Gelsinger worked as a clerk and rode a motorcycle on weekends. He heard about experimental gene therapy at the University of Pennsylvania for his inherited disorder, ornithine transcarbamylase deficiency (OTC).

In the genetic disease OTC, the liver doesn't properly cleanse blood of ammonia, produced in normal metabolism, resulting in toxic levels. Many OTC newborns die around birth; half don't live to age 5. A new regimen of drugs and diet enabled Jesse to live to be a teenager, but without a cure, he would eventually die.

Jesse entered the study as a healthy research volunteer. A friend said he "wanted to prove he was a man."[74] Penn researchers claim they told Jesse that the experiment wouldn't help him, but that it might help OTC babies. Jesse wanted "to help save lives," his father said.

But why weren't studies done on dying OTC patients? Answer: Because OTC babies are born dying, their parents will consent to anything, no matter how dangerous the experiment.

So Penn researcher James Wilson sought adults with OTC whose livers still functioned. He wanted to inject an adenovirus into them that contained copies of the gene lacking in OTC patients. Quite common, adenoviruses can transmit genes to patients with genetic diseases.

What actually happened when Dr. Wilson injected his adenovirus into Jesse was quite grim:

> Four days after scientists infused trillions of genetically engineered viruses into Jesse Gelsinger's liver . . . the 18-year old lay dying in a hospital bed at the University of Pennsylvania. His liver had failed, and the teenager's blood was thickening like jelly and clogging key vessels while his kidneys, brain, and other organs shut down.[75]

The wrongful death lawsuit claimed that Wilson knew the virus had injured other OTC adults and that Wilson failed to use simple, direct language to explain this to the Gelsingers. As Penn bioethicist Arthur Caplan said,

> Not only is it sad that Jesse Gelsinger died, there was never a chance that anybody would benefit from these treatments. They are safety studies. They are not therapeutic in goal. If I gave it to you, we would try to see if you died, too, and if you did, OK.
>
> If you cured anybody, you'd publish it in a religious journal. It would be a miracle. All you're doing is you're saying, I've got this vector. I want to see if it can deliver the gene where I want it to go without killing or hurting or having any side effects.[76]

Doctor Wilson had a financial conflict of interest from his biotech company, Genovo, which owned patents on the adenovirus, should it prove therapeutic. Biogen Inc. had paid Genovo $37 million for rights to genetic therapies.

Wilson denies that money influenced his decisions, but that he wanted to be the first to cure a genetic disease.[77]

Wilson reported to the FDA only 39 of 700 problems about the virus, although the law required reporting all of them. In 2000, researchers concluded that adenoviruses should be used only as a last resort, not on healthy volunteers. Until it could be proved safe, they curtailed gene therapy.

After an investigation of Wilson's research, the NIH in 2000 suspended medical research at Penn. After a congressional hearing into Jesse's death, the NIH vowed to better monitor medical research. As a result, it suspended medical research at the University of Colorado Medical Center, the University of North Carolina, Johns Hopkins Hospitals, and at the University of Alabama at Birmingham. The Gelsinger family settled out of court with Penn for undisclosed monies.

After improving their regulation of medical research and conflicts of interest, these medical centers regained their grants, although Wilson's protocols were stopped.

## FURTHER READING

Thomas Benedek, "The 'Tuskegee Study' of Untreated Syphilis: Analysis of Moral Aspects versus Methodological Aspects," *Journal of Chronic Diseases*, vol. 31, 1978.
James Jones, *Bad Blood*, New York: Free Press, 1981.

## DISCUSSION QUESTIONS

1. Even if subjects can't be proven to have been harmed by not getting penicillin in the 1940s, explain how Kant would say they research was still wrong.
2. Were the studies to prevent vertical transmission of HIV in Africa really like the Tuskegee Study? What was the same and what differed?
3. Why did the controls without syphilis also get compensation?
4. Knowledge of the Tuskegee Study has prevented many black patients from participating in medical research. Is it time now to get over that? If blacks don't participate in medical research, will studies be done to help them?
5. Wasn't Mengele a sadist? Can you do such things just because of ambition?
6. Was the Krieger lead paint study like the Tuskegee Study?
7. What does the model of collaborative research with developing countries imply about licensing genetic versions of patented drugs for poor areas with HIV, malaria, and tuberculosis?

# CHAPTER 11

# Surgeons' Desire for Fame: Ethics of the First Transplants

*T*his chapter describes the race to be the first to transplant a human heart, implant an artificial heart, and perform hand and face transplants. Most people desire to be famous, but what happens to this desire in medicine? Do surgeons harm patients in trying to be first? Is that totally wrong or necessary for medical progress?

## THE FIRST HEART TRANSPLANT

In 1966, two American surgeons, Richard Lower of Virginia and Norman Shumway of Stanford University, had been trying for years to overcome the immune system's rejection of another person's heart.

After spending a decade transplanting hearts in dogs, Shumway announced on November 20, 1967, that he was now ready to transplant a heart and actively sought a suitable candidate and donor.[1]

Two weeks later, Christiaan Barnard, an unknown South African surgeon, transplanted a human heart on December 3, 1967, in Cape Town, but before he knew how to control rejection.

Barnard grew up in South Africa and attended medical school there. Between 1955 and 1957, he did a fellowship under famous surgeon Owen Wangansteen in Minneapolis-St. Paul. When Barnard returned to South Africa in 1967, Wangansteen gave him a heart-lung machine, expecting him to transplant kidneys.[2] Until surgeons overcame the problem of immune rejection, no one expected hearts to be transplanted.

However, Barnard had secretly decided to try to transplant a human heart. With his physician-brother Marius, he quietly assembled a team at Groote Schuur Hospital in Cape Town.

In 1967, Louis Washkansky, aka "Washy," suffered from end-stage cardiac disease. He had diabetes, coronary artery disease and congestive heart failure; his flabby heart extended across the inside of his large chest, from wall to wall.

As a young man, Washy had been a weightlifter and amateur boxer. A big, intelligent man with a ferocious desire to live, he had an exuberant, macho personality and liked to flirt with nurses.

Knowing that death approached and that his last two years had been hellish, when approached about the transplant, he did not hesitate. Barnard told him, "We can put a normal heart into you, after taking out your heart that's no longer good, and there's a chance you can get back to normal life." Washy replied, "So they told me. So I'm ready to go ahead."

After obtaining Washy's permission, Barnard waited three weeks for a donor. Meanwhile, Washy developed fulminant pulmonary edema—a sign of imminent death—and Barnard feared his chance would pass.

In California, Shumway also waited for the right patients and had to be especially careful that any donor was dead because brain death had not yet been legally defined. In Richmond the next year, Richard Lower narrowly missed criminal conviction for taking the heart of an African-American man for transplant when Virginia lacked any brain-death statute.

On December 2, 1967, as she walked with her mother to a bakery a half mile below Groote Schuur, a speeding car smashed into 25-year-old Denise Ann Darvall. The accident crushed her head, and a few minutes later, an ambulance took her up to Groote Schuur's emergency room. While driving up the mountain to visit her husband, Washy's wife passed the accident.

Shortly after Denise's arrival, Barnard spoke to Edward Darvall, who had just learned of his daughter's death. "We have a man in the hospital here, and we can save his life if you give us permission to use your daughter's heart. . . ." Edward replied, "If you can't save my daughter, try and save this man.'"

Denise Darvall was declared dead after her heart had stopped beating; surgeons then opened her body, preparing it for Barnard's excision. In an adjacent room, surgeons gave Washkansky drugs to produce paralysis and to prevent spontaneous breathing. They then placed him on the heart-lung machine that had come from Minnesota.

The operation took place during the early hours of December 3, 1967. At this point, everything almost failed. Washkansky's femoral artery, where a tube was attached, had been narrowed by buildup of cholesterol and the machine couldn't force blood into his heart. The pressure on the tube climbed to 290 mm/Hg, just below the point where the lines would blow, spilling liters of blood over the room. Barnard and other surgeons frantically reattached the line directly to Washkansky's aorta. Gradually, the pressure dropped.

Barnard walked to the next room and excised Denise Darvall's heart, leaving part of the wall attached to it like the lid of a jack-o-lantern. He put her heart into a basin of chilled fluid and walked 31 steps back to Washkansky's operating room, where he gave the heart to a nurse to hold. Barnard then cut out Washkansky's flabby heart. Peering down into Washkansky's empty chest cavity, he said, "This really is the point of no return."[3]

He next sewed Denise Darvall's heart with its attached wall into Washkansky's chest, where it looked small. After some false starts, the new heart started to beat. After working all night, the surgeons finished the operation at 7 AM on December 3. An hour later, Washy regained consciousness and tried to talk. Thirty-six hours later, he ate a soft-boiled egg.

He then had five rough days, when his urine output, enzymes, and heart rate seemed problematic. Worried about immunological rejection of the heart, Barnard flooded Washy with gamma ray radiation and administered the immunosuppressive drugs prednisone (steroids) and azathioprine, but Louis didn't tolerate them well. By day 5, he said, the constant tests were "killing me. I can't sleep. I can't do anything. They're at me all the time with pins and needles. It's driving me crazy."[4]

On the sixth day, Louis received more steroids to prevent rejection, and this began five good days when he laughed, visited with his family, and wanted to go home. At this time, Barnard told a press conference that if his patient's progress held, he would "have him home in three weeks."[5]

These five days were the eye of the hurricane because rejection soon started; Washy then felt terrible. He suffered from constant pain in the shoulders; dark circles formed under his eyes; his heart and breathing rates climbed; a shadow of unknown origin appeared on his lung X-ray. Soon this vibrant, forceful man became sullen and irritable.

In addition to the threat of rejection, dangers of infection loomed. At the time, most post-transplant symptoms could indicate either rejection or infection; treatment of one problem could exacerbate the other. Risking Washing's death, Barnard waited for a definitive diagnosis.

By the 14th day, Washkansky felt he was dying. He couldn't eat. He lost bowel control. He had such severe pain in his chest that he preferred to lay in his own feces than try to move. Barnard said that he was "constrained" to insert a nasogastric tube to feed his patient, but Washkansky didn't want it. To him, he didn't feel he would ever be normal again; he had lost his dignity and his will to live.

On the 15th day, mottled patches appeared on Washkansky's legs, indicating circulatory failure. He breathed with difficulty, and X-rays showed ominous patches on his lungs. As he gasped for breath, Barnard decided to place him on a respirator. Washkansky resisted. He had been on the respirator when he first woke up after the operation, and he knew that reconnecting it meant giving up speech. He also felt that he was near death.

Barnard disagreed; on December 18, he told Washkansky that there was "a chance" to be home by Christmas. Washkansky replied, "No, not now." His bed was in a sterile tent, and despite his extreme weakness, he grabbed its sides to prevent Barnard from entering to reopen his tracheotomy hole.

As Barnard entered, Washkansky persisted, saying, "No, Doc."

Barnard replied, "Yes, Louis," and put him on the respirator.[6] Washkansky never spoke again.

On December 19, new X-rays now showed that bilateral pneumonia—klebsiella and pseudomonas—had infiltrated Washkansky's lungs. Earlier treatment with penicillin had killed one organism but allowed others to grow. Barnard had guessed wrong: the immunosuppressants had allowed all these organisms to flourish.

On December 20, 17 days after the operation, Washy received 40 percent oxygen; then, as his breathing worsened, 100 percent. By day 18, infection overran his lungs and he suffocated.

After two hours of Washkansky's dying gasps, the transplanted heart went into wild fibrillation from lack of oxygen and stopped beating, but Barnard would not give up; he rushed a team together to put him on a heart-lung machine. Marius then screamed that it was "madness" to continue because Washkansky was "clinically lost." Reluctantly, Barnard agreed. On December 21, after having lived 18 days with a transplanted heart, Louis Washkansky died.

Meanwhile, a white, dying dentist, Phillip Blaiberg, waited for a heart transplant. Nevertheless, when invited to fly to America and to be on television, Barnard abandoned Blaiberg and the chance to build a cardiac unit of international quality. He skipped Washy's funeral to meet American President Lyndon Johnson and his face graced the cover of *Time* magazine.

Later back home, he transplanted a black heart into Blaiberg, who walked out of the hospital on his own and thus was considered a real success.

### Fame Cometh

Perhaps no physician will ever again get the kind of coverage by television, magazines, and newspapers that then came in 1968 to Barnard. Long before people talked of superstars, Christiaan Barnard became one. After 20 years of marriage, he soon divorced his first wife, Loki, who told reporters, "He was more famous than the Beatles and he loved it."[7]

Tall, physically fit, witty, worldly, ambitious, and lusty, he looked younger than his age. In his two autobiographies, he brags about bedding beautiful women, including actress Gina Lollobrigida. He admits that fame ruined his marriages to Loki, to a 19-year-old model in 1970, and at age 60 to a 19-year-old waitress who bore him two children before leaving.

In 1967, he had the beginnings of crippling arthritis and soon could no longer operate. In 1984, he took $4 million for saying that a facial cream named "Glygel" reverses aging in skin (it doesn't), for which he was expelled from the American College of Surgeons and a cardiology society. In 2001 he died of an asthma attack, alone at age 78 at a swimming pool in Cyprus, lured there in hopes of signing a contract for an olive oil bearing his name.

Barnard's fame influenced surgeons far more than his surgery. As journalist Donald McRae writes, "Which red-blooded cut-master among [surgeons] would not wish to bed Gina Lollobrigida, lunch with Sophia Loren, and then have Gregory Peck suggested as the perfect actor to play him on the big screen."[8]

In Plato's *Republic*, Socrates relates the story of the Ring of Gyges, a ring that made its wearer invisible. When Gyges found it, he killed the king, married the king's beautiful wife, and became king himself. The moral of Socrates's story is that when luck gives someone the opportunity to do anything he wants, that person's true character emerges. In Gyges's case and in Barnard's case, the character that emerged was not honorable.

### The Post-Transplant Era: "Surgery Went Nuts"

Following Barnard's success with Blaiberg, surgeons around the world went wild trying to transplant hearts. Magazines called 1968 the "Year of the Transplant." During that year, 105 hearts were transplanted. Of the 105 heart-transplant patients, 19 died on the operating table, 24 lived for 3 months, two lived for

6 to 11 months, and only one lived for a year. Of 55 liver transplants in 1968 and early 1969, in 15 months after Barnard's landmark operation, 50 of the patients failed to live even six months. These early transplants failed because the immune system rejected the organs.

Most reporters also missed the fact that in 1968, 25 percent of transplant recipients became not just depressed or irritable but *temporarily psychotic*. Massive dosages of immunosuppressive drugs produced initial euphoria, followed by catatonia, severe depression, hysterical crying, and even permanent psychosis. Few deaths could be more undesirable than as a psychotic patient in a post-operative bed.

One of the great figures of modern medicine, Francis Moore, chief surgeon at Brigham and Women's Hospital for three decades, says that the year 1968 saw "epidemics" of chauvinism and of surgeons' egos.[9] He says, "It was the only example I know in the history of transplant medicine where everyone went nuts."[10] Nobel Prize winner (1954) Andre Courmand of Columbia University called Barnard's operation a stunt: "Merely demonstrating that it is technically feasible" to transplant a human heart, he said, was unethical.[11] Physician Norman Staub said Barnard's operation was "grandstanding," a blatant grab for fame.[12]

Many cardiac surgeons criticized heart transplantation with reason. In animals or humans, heart transplants rarely lasted more than a month, let alone years, and the death rate in early heart transplants appalled knowledgeable observers. While 1968 may have been the "year of the transplant," the following two years were the years of transplanted patients dying in madness and agony.

Because of poor results, the Montreal Heart Institute in 1969 suspended heart transplants, followed by suspensions at Harvard and Pittsburgh. Despite pressure to do so, Surgeon John Kirklin at UAB (University of Alabama at Birmingham) refused to start them in the first place. Threatened with congressional action, by 1970 most surgeons stopped transplanting.

## BARNEY CLARK'S ARTIFICIAL HEART

Barney Clark practiced dentistry in Utah for decades. A Latter-Day Saint, he smoked cigarettes for 30 years.

After several years of feeling unwell, in 1978 at age 57, he was diagnosed with emphysema, an incurable, obstructive lung disease, and cardiomyopathy, a disease where the heart muscles weaken and quit pumping blood. Too late, he quit smoking.

Over the next four years, powerful drugs dilated his blood vessels and kept him alive, but by November 1982, he was dying. Initially scoffing an artificial heart, approaching death gave him a new perspective and he decided to go for it.

For two decades at the University of Utah in Salt Lake City, physician Willem Kolff had been working on an artificial heart. In many ways, Kolff's career symbolizes the pros and cons of the desire to achieve a medical breakthrough.

In 1943, Kolff invented the first hemodialysis machine in the Netherlands. He converted a fuel pump from an automobile to force blood through a semipermeable membrane to clean it before it returned to the body. His first patient, a woman who had belonged to the Nazi party during World War II, lived a few days. Unlike modern dialysis machines, his machine could not sustain patients indefinitely because each time it was used, physicians had to make new connections between arteries and veins for its cannulas. Only in 1960, when Belding Scribner of Washington invented a permanent indwelling shunt, could dialysis sustain patients for years (see Chapter 11).

Despite the simplicity of his machine, the world lauded Kolff as a genius and man of vision. Dubbed the "Father of Artificial Organs," Kolff received fame, honorary doctorates, and the Lasker Award for medical research. At Utah, he got his own research lab and didn't need to see patients to make a living. No wonder others emulated him.

In 1985, 40 years after inventing the dialysis machine, Kolff paired with Robert Jarvik, an ambitious young medical student whom Kolff got into Utah's medical school. After graduation, Jarvik immediately went to work exclusively in Kolff's lab, never did an internship or residency, and never directly cared for patients. Jarvik modestly named the first artificial heart after himself.

Another doctor who wanted to make medical history, William DeVries, looked the part: 36 years old, he was a tall, blonde-haired Nordic man with a lean, tanned face. Because of his rugged good looks and macho manner, reporters lionized him as a surgical John Wayne.

## The Implant

In a heart, the powerful, lower two chambers of the ventricles pump blood. The Jarvik-7 consisted of molded polyurethane with two chambers of plastic and aluminum holding an inner diaphragm. A wall of thin membrane separated these chambers, through which the diaphragm's contraction forced blood. An air compressor moved the diaphragm, brought by 6-foot tubes inserted through the upper abdomen. The compressor weighed 375 pounds and rolled around on wheels on a large metal cart.

The Jarvik-7 contained the same commercial valves used by heart surgeons, and as in a natural heart, so there were four of them (analogous to mitral, tricuspid, etc.).

DeVries operated on Barney Clark on December 1, 1982, almost 15 years to the day after Washkansky's transplant. On his way to the operating room, Clark joked, "There would be a lot of long faces around here if I backed out now."[13]

Upon opening the chest, DeVries found a flabby, enlarged heart. Twice the size of a normal heart, it merely quivered and didn't contract. One physician there described it as looking like "a soft, overripe zucchini squash." DeVries first cut away the lower part of the heart, the two ventricles; then he stitched two Dacron cuffs to the intact upper part, the atria. After using Velcro fasteners to connect Jarvik-7's plastic ventricles, the pressure of the pumped blood ripped out the stitches from Clark's paper-thin, atrial walls. DeVries then had to restitch the cuffs to a new section of heart wall and resnap the fasteners.

The cuffs then held, but when DeVries turned on the Jarvik-7, its plastic left ventricle didn't pump blood. Frustrated, DeVries tried for an hour to get it to work. Three times he opened the ventricle by hand, each time risking introduction of air into the blood and a stroke. At one point, DeVries reportedly exclaimed, "Please, please, please work this time!"[14]

DeVries finally replaced the faulty Jarvik-7 with parts from another one and got the rebuilt machine working, two hours late. The implant took all night and concluded about 7 AM on December 2. A heart-lung machine maintained Clark during this 10-hour operation, subjecting him to huge losses of memory from being under anesthesia so long and to stroke-causing clots.

About 10 AM on December 2, the anesthesia wore off and DeVries watched anxiously to see how Clark had fared. If he had had a stroke, Clark wouldn't be able to move his hands, so when Clark moved his hands, everyone felt relieved.

At a press conference, university physicians falsely described the operation as a "dazzling technical achievement," something "as exciting and thrilling as has ever been accomplished in medicine." Hospital administrators also called it "one of the most dramatic stories in medical history."

Back in the recovery room, Clark's condition, like that of most patients after serious cardiac surgery, shocked his wife, Una Loy. She saw a man pierced by five tubes: a breathing tube ran a hole in his throat, a feeding tube went into his stomach, a catheter emptied his bladder, and the two hoses connected the Jarvik-7 thumping through his upper abdomen to the 375-pound air compressor at his bedside. If she had pressed her ear to her husband's chest, she could have heard the valves' clicking as they opened and closed.

Like Louis Washkansky after his operation, Clark felt horrible. Though he had not suffered a massive stroke, he had experienced intensive care psychosis and felt confused, was delirious and amnesiac, and at times, was unconscious.

On December 4, DeVries operated to repair ruptured air sacs in Clark's lungs. On December 6, Clark felt better and asked DeVries how he was doing. DeVries replied, "Just fine." Seconds later, Clark had seizures—involuntary shuddering from head to toe—perhaps caused by the dramatic increase in blood flow from the Jarvik-7.

DeVries injected muscle tranquilizers and anticonvulsants. Clark lost consciousness for the next several hours and his seizures continued, though gradually the quivering became confined to his left leg and left arm. At this point, he had several small strokes. Throughout the next months, he continued to be confused.

During the following days, Clark asked DeVries directly, "Why don't you just let me die?"[15] His lack of energy, difficulty in breathing, and stupor depressed Clark; he told a psychiatrist several times, "My mind is shot."

On December 14, one of the $800 welded commercial valves broke inside the Jarvik-7. Clark's blood pressure dropped dramatically, threatening his life, and DeVries had to operate yet again to replace the valve. Each of these operations and anesthesias subjected Clark to more memory loss and more strokes.

Nineteen days after the operation, Clark improved, and DeVries hinted he might one day go home, but soon massive complications began. Devries gave Clark a blood thinner to prevent clots, but it caused severe bleeding. On January 18, DeVries surgically sealed a severe nosebleed. Clark's underlying emphysema created pneumothorax, escape of air from lungs into the chest cavity, which required DeVries to operate yet again to relieve pressure on Clark's weak lungs.

From January to March, Clark continually complained of conditions caused by his emphysema. He was suffocating and could never get a good breath. On February 14, he left the surgical ICU for a private room, but because he needed a respirator, he returned to the ICU the next day.

On February 24, he moved again to a private room and had a good week. On March 1, DeVries filmed several interviews with Clark. On March 2, Humana Hospital released a short, highly edited clip to the public. According to cardiologist Thomas Preston, this clip "came from an extensive interview in which, encouraged by Dr. DeVries, Clark issued a semblance of a positive statement."[16] Although the clip showed his best moment, even then, tethered to a huge machine, in pain, and not fully alert, Clark looked miserable.

The next day he developed severe nausea, aspirated vomit, contracted pneumonia, and ran a high fever. On March 21, his kidneys failed. On March 23, 1983, having lived 112 days with an artificial heart, Barney Clark died. Inside his body, after someone "called" the death, the Jarvik-7 continued to pump. Asked if she wanted to be present when DeVries turned off the Jarvik-7, Una Loy Clark said, "He's already dead," and left the room.[17]

Following Clark's death, public opinion varied. Some people called the operation "one of the boldest human experiments ever attempted"; others concluded that it had failed to prove its worth and that even if it had returned Clark to normal, it cost too much, both in money and suffering.

Predictably, Kolff defended the project: "A number of doctors were opposed to the artificial kidney and wrote articles against it. I decided not to respond at all. . . . I still have the same policy now for people [who] tell us that the artificial heart has no future."

DeVries surprisingly commented: "After the first two days, 95 percent of the issues we were dealing with concerned ethics, moral value judgments, communications with the press—problems I had never thought about."[18]

A few weeks after Clark died, the hospital disclosed that a valve had broken and killed Ted D. Baer, a 220-pound ram who had lived 297 days with a Jarvik-7. This was the most important model for the Jarvik-7 in a human, and the hospital had suppressed this lack of success. Heart surgeons understood this failure: even if Clark had lived a few more months, breaking valves would have killed him.

This is an important point for bioengineering students. Unlike hemodialysis, in which the machine can fail and the patient lives on by getting another machine, the challenge of creating a totally implantable artificial heart, such that patients could pass the "walk-on-their-own-out-of-the-hospital" test, is that the mechanical heart needs to be flawless, subject to no breakdowns, interruptions, or failures. Otherwise, when problems arise with patients with artificial hearts outside the hospital, they will immediately die.

## Post-Clark Implants

At Humana, on November 25, 1984, nearly two years after Barney Clark's operation, DeVries implanted a second Jarvik-7 into William Schroeder.

"Bionic Bill," age 51, younger and healthier than Clark, had no emphysema. Not surprisingly, he lived much longer than Clark, 21 months. But his quality of life suffered. Only 19 days after his operation, he suffered a stroke from a clot. Schroeder then had a cascade of strokes, repeated bouts of endocarditis, and eventually underwent a tracheotomy. On August 6, 1986, he suffocated to death.

On February 17, 1985, Murray Haydon received the third Jarvik-7. On the 17th day after the implant, he needed a tracheotomy. He experienced various infections and lived poorly for 10 months. His autopsy revealed that a hole from a catheter in part of his natural heart wall had not healed, allowing blood to pour into his lungs.

The fourth recipient, Jack Burcham, had a dreadful death. Going into surgery on April 16, 1985, Burcham thought he had nothing to lose by going for the implant, but he was wrong. During the operation, DeVries made the amazing discovery that *the Jarvik-7 wouldn't fit inside Burcham's chest.* When Burcham left the operating room, "his chest, draped with sterile dressing . . . [was] only partly closed around the device."[19]

Can a surgeon really take out a man's heart and not measure in advance whether a mechanical heart will fit inside? This is in the same territory as amputating a patient's leg rather than his diseased hand.

Burcham lived only 10 days. Afterward, DeVries admitted that surgery shortened Burcham's life.[20]

Three years later in 1988, after a long dispute, William DeVries left Humana Heart Institute. Divorcing his wife of 24 years, he moved to Humana Hospital in Louisville, Kentucky, a for-profit center where he hoped for a freer hand and was paid three times his former salary.

Over the next four years, he left three different surgery practices around Louisville before starting a risky solo practice in 1992. But because they saw only miserable outcomes, grandstanding, and obliviousness to clinical realities, physicians didn't refer patients to him. He still claimed that Jarvik-7s could work, but few believed him. Lacking referrals, he had no patients into which to implant Jarvik-7s.

William DeVries struggled as a cardiac surgeon between 1992 and 1999 and then retired. In 2001, at age 57, he joined the U.S. Army Reserve and completed the Officer Basic Course. He now teaches surgical residents at the Uniformed Services University of the Health Sciences in Washington, D.C.

After Barney Clark's death, Robert Jarvik modeled Hathaway shirts in ads and gave interviews to *Playboy*, with whom he discussed his sex life. In 1988, he divorced his wife of decades and, after having known her for only five days, married a columnist who calls herself Marilyn Vos Savant ("Marilyn the wise" in French). Billing themselves as "the world's smartest couple," Jarvik and Vos Savant say their children from previous marriages are their children "only in the biological sense." Marilyn once added, "I don't consider either of us to have children."[21] She writes a weekly column for *Parade* magazine.

In 2006, Jarvik reappeared in television ads for Lipitor, rowing across the screen (he does not row and a body double was used). In the intervening years, he founded Jarvik Heart, a small company developing not an artificial heart but a cardiac pump.[22]

Willem Kolff died at age 97 in 2009, lauded for his work in creating successful hemodialysis, but without success in creating a successful artificial heart, eye, or ear.[23]

## LIMB TRANSPLANTS

In 1998, surgeon Jean-Michel Dubernard performed the first hand transplant in France. The hand came from a 41-year-old man who had died in a motorcycle accident and went to 48-year-old New Zealander Clint Hallam. A year later, Louisville's Jewish Hospital did the first hand transplant in America on 38-year-old Matthew Scott, who lost his hand to a firecracker.

In 2001, Clint Hallam demanded that Dubernard amputate his transplanted hand. He felt pain and had no normal feeling in it. Because the antirejection drugs gave him diarrhea and influenza, Hallam had not taken them. He also ducked his required physical therapy.

In contrast and within a few months, Mathew Scott began to feel cold and heat in his palm as nerve growth reached his wrist. With his new hand, he could write his name, tie his shoelaces, and wear a new wedding ring. In January 2006, Scott had had his hand for six years. In an amazing video (posted on YouTube), Scott can later be seen throwing out a pitch at a baseball game.

In another case, which should have been front-page news in ethics, surgeons in South Africa considered but declined to try to be first in transplanting fingers in children.[24] Citing the significant dangers of taking immunosuppressive drugs over many decades, which include cancer, hypertension, opportunistic infections, and diabetes, the surgeons decided that the children might be able to adapt easier and live better without the transplanted digits.

In 2008, Karl Merk, a German dairy farmer who lost both his arms in a corn threshing machine, received the world's first double-arm transplant.[25]

In 2009, Jeff Kepner, whose hands and feet were amputated after a streptococcal infection, became the first American to receive a double-hand transplant at the University of Pittsburgh by a team led by W. P. Andrew Lee. Before the transplants, he had used prosthetics and worked part-time at a Borders bookstore. A year after having the hand-transplants, he had no control over his fingers and was frustrated by his slow progress in using his hands.

In 2010 and after she gave birth to a child, Texan Katy Hayes developed a Group A streptococcal infection that resulted in amputations of her arms above her elbows. Hayes received the first double-arm transplant in the United States, led by Dr. Simon Talbot of Brigham and Women's Hospital.[26]

By 2006, surgeons around the world had completed 30 hand-forearm transplants, including three in Lyon, France.[27] (In a video on YouTube, a successful patient after a double hand transplant can be seen threading a needle.) Double amputees reported the best psychological results. All patients survived, and after two years, none had rejected their new limbs. All had to endure immunosuppressant therapy, including steroids. Despite taking these medications, 12 had acute rejection episodes.[28]

## FACE TRANSPLANTS

In the early 2000s, history repeated itself as experienced surgeons around the world prepared to do the world's first face transplant, only to be startled when an unknown surgical team in France beat them. American surgeon Maria Seimionow of the Cleveland Clinic had been preparing for 20 years to do a face transplant and in April 2005 had been given permission by her IRB to go ahead.[29]

But in France in 2005, Jean-Michael Dubernard, the surgeon who had transplanted hands onto Clint Hallam seven years before, yearned for another victory before his upcoming mandatory retirement. In 2005, Isabelle Dinoire, an unemployed, divorced mother of two teenage daughters living in government housing, attempted suicide by taking sleeping pills, which caused her to pass out.[30] While unconscious, her newly acquired black Labrador retriever bit off her nose, chin, mouth, and supporting facial muscles (the dog later was inadvertently destroyed).

After several months in the hospital, Ms. Dinoire returned home. When outside, she wore a surgical mask. Without the mask, as she tried to talk, people could see her jawbone move.

At the university hospital in Amiens and at Dubernard's urging, Dr. Bernard Devauchelle, the head of maxillofacial surgery, decided to transplant onto Dinoire a triangular flap of a brain-dead cadaver's chin, nose, and mouth.[31]

Dr. Devauchelle had already identified a potential candidate in a hospital in Lille, Maryline St. Aubert, who had committed suicide by hanging and who was brain-dead. Importantly, the hanging may have damaged St. Aubert's facial veins and muscles. (Devauchelle claimed he did not know that St. Aubert had died by hanging.) He cut a triangle of facial tissue from St. Aubert, put it on ice, and then sewed it onto Dinoire.

Following the surgery, Devauchelle turned over Dinoire's care to Dubernard. Dr. Thomas Starzl, who performed the world's first liver transplant, said of Dubernard, "There's a big brain behind him and steely will to confront massive criticism."[32]

Dubernard, a former deputy mayor of Lyon, also served as an elected deputy in the French National Assembly. A self-described workaholic and chain smoker, Dubernard commuted from Lyon two days a week to Parliament and on other days doctored back in Lyon. Like Christiaan Barnard, he confessed to loving international publicity and to wanting a huge "first."

As we know from nearly 50 years of transplants, the key to success is preventing rejection of the transplanted tissue, not the surgery. Through a steady treatment of immunosuppressants, as well as use of hematopoietic stem cells from Dinoire's face and bone marrow, Dubernard tried to prevent her immune system from rejecting the new tissue. After a week, she could speak and drink.

In 2006, Dinoire resumed smoking, which jeopardized the healing and stability of her transplant by constricting blood vessels and increasing chances of infection. The same year, surgeons disclosed that the donor's face lacked a key nerve that controlled the lower portion of Dinoire's face. That same year in a visit to UAB, Dubernard revealed to this author that in the first weeks after the operation, he feared each phone call might tell him that the transplant had fallen off his patient's face.[33]

In 2007, Dubernard revealed pictures and video of Dinoire, who reportedly consented to this release. She looked much better than expected and was said to be satisfied with the results. Dubernard pronounced the surgery perfect and said her new face looks like, and moves like, her old face.[34]

In 2006, Chinese surgeons in Xian attempted a copycat 14-hour operation, transplanting two-thirds of the face of a man mauled by a bear.[35] When the operation occurred, the patient had been living as a recluse for two years.

French surgeons performed another face transplant in 2007 on Pascal Coler, who suffered from neurofibromatosis, which disfigured his face with large tumors. He suffered a life that is reminiscent of Quasimodo and felt himself a freak.

At the Cleveland Clinic in America, Dr. Maria Seimionow emphasized, "First, do no harm." She said, "The thing I'm worried about is, if it fails, what I'm going to be left with." Seimionow's protocol required good health, good personality, and good family support, none of which Isabelle Dinoire had.

In 2008, Seimionow performed the first American face transplant, at the time the largest and most extensive transplant ever performed, on Connie Culp, who had been shot in the face in 2004 by her husband. Over the next four years, Culp underwent 23 surgeries to reconstruct her face, without good results. Finally, the 46-year-old mother of two consented to a transplant of 80 percent of a face from Anna Kasper, a brain-dead nurse. Seven other surgeons at the Cleveland Clinic assisted Dr. Seimionow,

In 2009, Culp went on television with a swollen face but remarkably good speech and mental adjustment. In 2011, she rated her appearance 8 out of 10 and lived on disability, taking 29 pills a day to control rejection.[36]

In 2009, surgeons at Brigham and Women's Hospital in Boston performed a second face transplant. Though they did not disclose the patient's name, his "nose, upper lip, palate, muscles, nerves and some skin" had to be replaced.[37] In 2010 at the same hospital, 28-year-old Texan Dallas Weins became the first American to get a first "full face transplant" in a 19-hour operation and, over the next three years, 30 follow-up surgeries. After surviving an episode of rejection, in 2013 Dallas married burn-survivor Jamie Nash in a wedding that made national news.[38]

## ETHICAL ISSUES

### The Desire to Be First and Famous

In 1967, surgeon Norman Shumway at Stanford University Hospital in California had trained the longest and most rigorously in hopes of conducting a safe, successful, first heart transplant. After Barnard jumped the gun, a few months later, Shumway transplanted the first heart in America. But Shumway felt bitterly disappointed that Barnard had gotten the fame.[39]

A dozen heart surgeons around the world could have done what Barnard did. Isn't it arbitrary to glorify the surgeon who did the first heart transplant, but to ignore the great heart surgeons who laid the foundation but because of ethics waited before attempting a transplant?

Soon after Barnard's operation, Brooklyn surgeon Adrian Kantrowitz transplanted a heart into a newborn. Kantrowitz needed an anencephalic infant as a source of a heart and found one only the day after Barnard's operation. If he had found it sooner, Kantrowitz would be known today.

Reporters describe breakthrough surgeons as "brave," "brilliant," and "dedicated," but rarely do they report on those who were second or third or those who built the foundation for the breakthrough. Nor do reporters explain how many patients suffered before surgeons obtained good results or how hard the surgeon pushed these patients.

One factor in being first is the media, which feeds public hunger for medical breakthroughs. On the journalistic side, this hunger leads to inaccuracy and sensationalism. On the medical side, this hunger leads to haste and imprudence. In Brazil, a surgeon so raced to do the first heart transplant there that his patient learned of the event only when he woke up with another heart inside him.

Barnard wanted fame and seemed to relish it. He loved talking to reporters and held daily briefings. When leaving the hospital, he paused for photographers and shook the hands of waiting South Africans. For access to himself and Washkansky, he took money from American journalists, justifying doing so to supposedly raise money to benefit future patients.

Although Barnard wouldn't allow Washkansky's wife to touch him after the operation, citing dangers of infection, such dangers mysteriously vanished when Barnard allowed a film crew to tape the first conversation between Washkansky and his son inside the hospital room.

Reporters understandably focused on the symbolism of the operation: a heart that once lived inside one human now pumped inside another. But this symbolism and Barnard's resulting fame blinded them to clinical realities. Most reporters lacked medical background and the public wanted medical miracles, not messy clinical details.

Although DeVries criticized the "media circus," the media had changed since Barnard's operation and were now more skeptical. At one point, when told there would be no further briefings, reporters exploded. The hospital later relented, but reporters became angry as weeks passed and the hospital kept spinning the facts. *New York Times* physician-reporter Lawrence K. Altman especially held DeVries' feet to the fire.

What was going on? DeVries and the University of Utah had encouraged hundreds of television and print reporters to follow the operation, but when it didn't turn out well, they tried to stonewall them. The desire to manage the news conflicted with their desire for fame.

Medically, is it ethical to try to achieve a "first" when the essential, underlying problem remains unsolved? The artificial heart presented medical problems similar to that of heart transplants before cyclosporine in that poor trade-offs for the patient existed in both cases. Preventively treating one kind of problem worsened another.

With the first face transplant, French physicians seemed to have rushed Dinoire into surgery merely to be first. Admittedly, they feared the female American surgeon getting there first.

Problems of the desire to be first surfaced by examining selection of patients. Was Barney Clark, a life-long smoker, a good candidate to be the recipient of the first artificial heart? Obviously not. Was Clint Hallam, who wanted a quick, miraculous new hand without doing any physical therapy, a good candidate to receive the first hand transplant? Obviously not. Philip Blaiberg was a much better candidate for a heart transplant than Louis Washkansky, but he did not come early enough.

What about selection of Isabelle Dinoire for the face transplant? Was this case like Barney Clark's? In other words, "She's got nothing to lose, so why not try it?" A surgeon in Paris, who had been carefully preparing and playing by the rules, accused Dubernard of bypassing established ethical and legal guidelines for doing transplants.[40] Was St. Aubert selected, despite damage to her face from her hanging, in a rush to have a donor face so Devauchelle and Dubernard could be first?

As a mentally unstable smoker, was Dinoire a good candidate for the first face transplant? Obviously not. Would she adhere to rigorous post-transplant regimens? If her face sloughed off in the worst case, did she possess the mental health to continue?

## Concerns about Criteria of Death

In 1968 and after Barnard's operation, cardiac surgeon Werner Forssmann, publicly criticized Barnard for taking a beating heart out of one patient and transplanting it into another.[41] For Forssmann, before it became a candidate for transplantation, a heart should stop. Because of similar concerns, Japan banned heart transplants for many decades.

Although Barnard did not discuss this with Edward Darvall, he must have been concerned about whether Denise Darvall's death would be accepted. Critics scrutinized him for any sign of Dr. Frankensteinian overeagerness.

Barnard turned off Darvall's respirator and waited for her heart to stop. The longer he waited, the more her heart would be damaged. Washkansky needed a heart in the best possible condition, and Marius wanted to remove Denise's heart before it stopped beating.

But Denise Darvall had a healthy heart. Why did her heart stop at all? Well, first there was a problem. Because brain death had not yet been defined, death came only by *whole-body standards* when the heart and lungs stopped. As surgeon Thomas Starzl explained much later, "The steps to donation began with disconnection of the ventilator. . . . During the 5 to 10 minutes before the heart stopped and death was pronounced, the organs to be transplanted were variably damaged by oxygen starvation and the gradually failing and ultimately absent circulation.[42]

So recipients like Louis Washkansky received damaged hearts that could have been supplied in better condition. On the other hand, most transplant surgeons at the time realized that in this matter they had little choice. Transplant surgery depended entirely on altruistic, voluntary donations, and any suspicion of doubtful procedures would sabotage donations.

However, Marius kept secret a detail for nearly 40 years: that rather than wait for her heart to stop beating, at Marius's urging, Barnard had injected potassium into Denise's heart to paralyze it and thus, to render her technically dead (by the whole-body standard).[43]

Responding the next year to this emergency, Harvard appointed a committee to decide when beating hearts could be ethically removed from brain-damaged patients. This committee gave birth to the famous Harvard Criteria of Brain Death (discussed in Chapter 4 on comas), which requires the entire brain to be non-functioning before organs can be removed.

After Barnard's operation, in trying to be first in their area, surgeons hoarded possible donors and did not share them with other surgeons, even if they better tissue-matched a patient at another hospital. Everyone in the 1970s needed a system that matched donor organs and patients, but the United Network for Organ Sharing (UNOS) would not begin operating for another decade.

Even as late as 1985, a Gallup poll showed that 44 percent of Americans hadn't signed organ cards because they feared being declared dead prematurely. In the United States today, by law in all states, physicians who declare a potential organ donor brain-dead may not belong to the surgical transplant team.

## Quality of Life

An important ethical issue concerned the resulting quality of life for the recipients. In many cases of famous, first-time surgery, quality of life for patients has been poor.

In particular, life after a heart transplant does not live up to the wonderful life reported in the popular media. Taking cyclosporin for life often causes cancer, and many recipients are in and out of hospitals for repeated operations and complications.

With organ transplants, surgeons fought infections with antibiotics and by holding off immunosuppressive drugs, but this thereby increased chances of rejection of the foreign heart. If they gave immunosuppressive drugs, infections flourished. With artificial hearts, blood clots (thrombi) formed on joints and surfaces of mechanical surfaces. When such clots break free (embolism), they travel in the blood to the small vessels in the brain, lodge there, and cause brain damage (strokes). Blood-thinning medications such as Heparin reduced or prevented clots, but when given to post-operative patients such as Barney Clark, the patients bled out of their sutures.

In 1988, three heart experts reviewed DeVries's surgeries and concluded that his implants created clots and the longer patients stayed on it, the more clots they had.[44] So they wrote the epitaph of the artificial heart, a verdict that 20 years of subsequent work has not reversed.

With the first face transplant, criticisms focused on the fact that Dinoire had to take immunosuppressant drugs for life. Already in late 2005, surgeons had to give her increased dosages to prevent rejection of her new face. As we know, such drugs increased Dinoire's risk later of cancer, diabetes, and other medical problems. Estimates predict that 10 percent of such grafts will fail the first year and 30 to 50 percent within three to five years, so candidates must be prepared for failure. Because transplanted skin triggers more fierce rejection than any other organ, facial transplantation carries great risk of rejection and more risk of cancer from taking immunosuppressants drugs at higher levels.

Barnard, DeVries, and Dubernard emphasized that for the first case, the question was not how long the patient could live, but whether they could live at all.

But later criticisms set in. Did Washy have 17 days worth living? Did Clark have 112? Or was it merely, as the *New York Times* said, "112 days of dying"?[45] The *Times* dubbed research on the artificial heart, "The Dracula of Medical Technology," a phrase that stuck.[46]

In the early 1980s, Sandoz Pharmaceutical discovered cyclosporin, a drug that selectively blocks immune rejection of foreign tissue and that revolution- ized organ transplants. Thereafter, the number of organs transplanted soared dramatically.

In 2012, two-thirds of heart transplant patients survived for five years.[47] Dirk van Zyl, Barnard's sixth heart transplant patient, died in 1996, the longest-living heart transplant recipient at 23 years.

In 2001, a surgeon at Abiomed implanted AbioCor, a titanium artificial heart, into Robert Tools, who lived 151 days. Three other patients lived for 92, 78, and 32 days; another died on the operating table. Tom Christerson lived 17 months. By 2005, Abiomed had tested 14 patients, two of whom died immediately, the rest of whom lived for an average of 5 months. The widow of James Quinn sued because her husband went through two months of hellish dying and constantly worried about who would pay for his round-the-clock nursing care.[48] Abiomed asked to implant another $250,000 device, but the FDA refused.[49]

In 2001, Norman Shumway doubted whether artificial hearts would ever be successful. "An artificial heart is a tremendously difficult problem because the human body is living tissue. . . . [The body] always is going to be opposed to plastic materials."[50]

In 1998, the FDA allowed cardiac surgeons to insert left ventricle assist devices (LVADs) into patients as bridges to heart transplants. Being on the pump, which costs about $60,000, gave patients 408 days of life compared to 150 on drugs.

Early patients on LVADs fared poorly. About half returned to the hospital within six months, and a year after surgery, only 30 percent were alive. Worse, many complained of pain and poor quality of life; some turned off their power, committing suicide, or requested physicians or ethics committees to let them die.[51] Patients today still suffer strokes from clots, fungal and viral infections, and the usual problems caused by immunosuppressant drugs.

By 2005, "the workhorse of mechanical support for patients with heart failure today is the left ventricle assist device, which piggybacks onto the native heart, pumping blood directly out of the left ventricle into the aorta."[52] In 2008, about 2,000 American patients a year got LVADs.[53] In 2010, surgeons gave former vice- president Dick Cheney an LVAD, although reporters downplayed any risks or complications (and he later got a heart transplant)

In one large, multi-institutional study in 2009 of 281 patients after 18 months on LVADs, 157 had undergone transplants, 58 continued on LVADs, 7 had the LVAD removed because their heart recovered, and 56 had died.[54]

One wonders about LVADs as a final destination. Is this a good way to live? In any given year, 5 million Americans live with heart failure, with a half a million new cases diagnosed each year. One study in 2001 estimated that the five-year cost of an LVAD was $223,000.[55] To give all patients with heart failure LVADs would cost over a trillion dollars.

## Defending Surgery

Surgeons are criticized for their desire for glory in pushing the boundaries of medicine to achieve a first. But what is so wrong with that? If no one aggressively tries to make advances, no progress occurs.

Yes, Barnard pushed Washkansky, and yes, Washy didn't know what he was in for, but had Barnard guessed the other way, Washy might have lived much longer. And because Barnard proved it could be done, today thousands of people are living with heart transplants.

The same is true with hand and arm transplants, which are making more and more progress. Face transplants are also coming along; they rescue horribly deformed people from lives as outcasts.

True, the artificial heart failed, but LVADs and other heart-assist devices continue to improve and keep hundreds of people alive. One day, surgeons will achieve breakthroughs here, too. It's just a matter of time. Until then, "No guts, no glory" should rule in surgical research, even if it sometimes gets messy for patients.

## Cosmetic versus Therapeutic Surgery

When someone awakes to a different face, it is natural to ask, "Who am I?" Although personality is not physical appearance, many people could find themselves with an altered personality when their face changes. With better surgical techniques, will some patients seek face transplants for merely cosmetic reasons? What exactly is "cosmetic"? Neurofibromatosis?

What about transplanting an arm, hand, or finger? When does wanting to improve appearance slide into wanting to improve function and both into the therapeutic realm? With these transplants, skeptics debated the ethics of transplanting non-vital limbs. Unlike hearts and livers, humans do not need a hand to survive. More important, recipients must take anti-rejection drugs for life, increasing their lifetime risks of cancer.

Right now, the consensus is that face transplants should be done only in cases of lack of physical function, such as not being able to eat or speak. The risk associated with surgery and drugs is too high for face transplants to be done merely to improve appearance.

Hand and arm transplants are another matter. American wars in Iraq and Afghanistan resulted in thousands of soldiers suffering amputations from roadside bombs, which in turn amped up research into artificial limbs. Progress with such limbs has been so striking that in many cases, artificial limbs outperform transplanted limbs and carry no long-term risks from immunosuppressant drugs of cancer, bone loss, and heart damage.

## Expensive Rescue versus Cheap Prevention

Yearly, surgeons transplant about 2000 hearts in America, the country that performs the most heart transplants. What about costs? Was the program cost-effective? How much is one more year of life worth? Is every life worth the same amount? What's the opportunity cost of spending so much money this way?

Artificial hearts could cost society dearly. NIH invested over $8 million in research leading up to the Utah project and over $200 million nationally in similar projects between 1964 and 1982.

According to Transplant Living, a website of UNOS, the cost of one heart transplant for the first 180 days is about a million dollars.[56] A double-lung transplant costs about $800,000, a kidney about $263,000, and a liver about $577,000. Most insurance plans and state Medicaid plans cover transplants. The End-Stage Renal Disease Act mandates Social Security Disability to pay for kidney transplants (see next chapter).

If artificial hearts were successful, could society afford to pay for them? The now-defunct Office of Technology Assessment estimated in 1990 that 60,000 Americans might use artificial hearts, at a cost to Medicare of $5.5 billion a year.[57]

All of which is a lot of money and effort to rescue a damaged heart. Glamorous, high-tech operations are dramatic, but might not the money spent do more good for more people if spent to prevent smoking, promote exercise, and create healthier hearts?

*Progressive* magazine complained that a "medical establishment grown fat on chemicals and technological wizardry is not willing to empower people so they can prevent illness."[58] *Progressive* argued that artificial hearts would benefit only the small number of cardiac patients who could afford them and hence were "qualitatively different from the basic advances in immunology which have saved millions of lives, even among populations not directly treated."

Saving bad organs illustrates again the rule of rescue. Our society cares more about saving an identifiable life than about preventing future deaths from heart failure.

One way to prevent such deaths is to tax cigarettes out of existence. Around 2002, New York and Washington put high state sales taxes on tobacco. A pack of cigarettes in New York City in 2013 costs $12 to $15. Such taxes discourage smoking in people when they are young—just when cigarette companies want them to become addicted. Another way is to make cities, hospitals, and campuses smoke-free, making it socially unacceptable for smokers to thrive.

## Real Informed Consent?

How much does a candidate for a new kind of transplant understand about its experimental nature? How much can such candidates understand, given that they are seriously ill and desperate? In their situation, how is *informed* consent obtained?

As for consent, one hopes any possible patient understands the risk of cancer from taking drugs for life to suppress rejection.

With face transplants, there is also risk of the entire face sloughing off and ending up with a gigantic hole where nose, mouth, and chin should be. When asked about the face transplant, Ms. Dinoire supposedly consented. A French national ethics committee dismissed her consent: "the very notion of informed consent [in this case] is an illusion."[59]

The media paint a sunny picture of organ transplants, typically citing only one-year survival rates. Within surgery, transplants have grown from being described as *experimental* not poor ten-year rates to being routinely described as *therapeutic*.

Nevertheless, laypeople believe that healthy, transplanted organs will function for a lifetime. The reality is different. If the recipient lives long enough, almost all recipients will reject their organs. One-third to one-half of recipients reject their heart transplants after five years. Kidney transplants began in 1951 and today are closest to being truly therapeutic rather than experimental. But even so, over 50 percent of patients reject transplanted kidneys after 10 years.

To prevent rejection, surgeons prescribe cyclosporine, which over years often causes malignant lymphoma and which often destroys kidneys, the liver, or the brain. Cyclosporine also makes women grow facial hair. After several years, its efficacy fades.

Medical sociologists Rene Fox and Judith Swazey argued that reclassification of organ transplants in the 1990s as "therapeutic" stemmed not from medical progress, but to make transplants eligible for reimbursement and to obtain publicity to increase donors. So organ donation was framed as a "gift of life" and "making a miracle happen," ignoring "the darker emotional and existential implications of what it involved.[60]

After miserable results from heart surgery, one wonders about the relationships between surgeon and patient. One surgeon confesses: "It is sometimes hard to meet the eyes of patients who have improved enough to have been moved to the regular post-op floor and finally become alert enough to communicate their despair and disappointment. . . . Often, after entering the experience with great hope, patients for whom transplantation has been a series of setbacks clearly articulate their feelings of betrayal: 'No one ever told me it could be like this.'"[61]

## CONCLUSION

Norman Shumway, regarded inside surgery as the true "father of heart transplant surgery," died at age 83 in 2006, but his passing attracted little notice. Doctors called him "one of the twentieth century's true pioneers in cardiac surgery." Philip Pizzo, M.D., dean of Stanford School of Medicine, said of Shumway that "he developed one of the world's most distinguished departments of cardiothoracic surgery at Stanford, trained leaders who now guide this field throughout the world and created a record of accomplishment that few will ever rival. His impact will be long-lived and his name long-remembered."[62]

Maria Seimionow will not be remembered for doing the first face transplant, but should be remembered for doing the first *ethical* face transplant. And when it comes to heart transplants, the name we really should remember is "Shumway."

## FURTHER READING

Philip Blaiberg, *Looking at My Heart*, New York: Stein and Day, 1968.
Christiaan Barnard and Curtiss Bill Pepper, *One Life*, New York: Macmillan, 1969.
Donald McRae, *Every Second Counts: The Race to Transplant the First Human Heart*, New York: Putnam, 2006.

Renée Fox and Judith Swazey, *The Courage to Fail: A Social View of Organ Transplants and Dialysis*, 2d ed. rev., Chicago: University of Chicago Press, 1978.

Thomas Starzl, *The Puzzle People: Memoirs of a Transplant Surgeon*, Pittsburgh, PA: University of Pittsburgh Press.

National Institute for Health and Clinical Excellence (UK), "Interventional Procedure Overview of Left Ventricular Assist Devices as a Bridge to Transplant or to Recovery," December 2005.

## DISCUSSION QUESTIONS

1. Was surgeon Barnard correct to force Washy to go back on a ventilator one last time? In terms of Margaret Battin's ideas, did Washy get a "least worst death?"

2. How did the first heart transplant lead to the first definition of brain death at Harvard? Why was this definition so conservative?

3. What were the medical trade-offs in the first heart transplant and first artificial heart between treating two different things? Do such trade-offs suggest that each operation was premature?

4. Is it wrong for people to want to be famous? For surgeons? Isn't that how great things are accomplished, by people pushing themselves? What's wrong with fame that is deserved?

5. Is the fact that so many famous surgeons got divorced after becoming famous relevant to judging their accomplishments?

6. Why is it so hard to put money into preventing heart disease rather than expensively trying to cure it after it develops?

7. If one is dying and hope is offered, is it possible to get real informed consent? Won't a dying man grasp at any offered hand?

8. The Baby Doe chapter and this one suggest that many reporters may not have the medical background to inform readers of the true issues of a breakthrough. Has this situation gotten better or worse with the demise of some famous newspapers?

# CHAPTER 12

# Just Distribution of Organs: The God Committee and Personal Responsibility

*T*his chapter focuses on two questions: just allocation and personal responsibility for health.

Every day, someone gets expensive medical resources and someone does not. In 1962, the famous God Committee in Seattle decided which patients received dialysis and which not. In distributing such scarce resources in medicine, does it make sense to ask: "Who *deserves* it?" Should smokers with emphysema get lung transplants? Should alcoholics get liver transplants?

Several distributive standards conflict in answering that question. We can adopt an impartial Kantian approach and distribute by an impersonal lottery, or we can be utilitarian and focus on maximizing the years lived per machine or organ. At another level, we can focus on personal characteristics of the recipient either to exclude one class or to identify the most deserving: we can exclude smokers from a list of eligible patients for a lung transplant or we can identify the patient most likely to die without a lung transplant, regardless of how that patient became needy. Finally, we can let the media identify a patient for the organ or machine, a way called the "Rule of Rescue."

## THE GOD COMMITTEE AND ARTIFICIAL KIDNEYS

The kidneys remove toxins accumulated by normal cellular metabolism in the blood. When both kidneys fail, toxins accumulate to lethal levels. Hemodialysis (literally "tearing blood apart") substitutes for the kidneys: it removes blood from the body and sends it through cannulas, where a surrounding solution absorbs toxins by osmosis through a semipermeable membrane; then the cleansed blood is returned to the body. Patients in renal failure must undergo hemodialysis (more simply, "dialysis") for several hours, two or three times a week.

The process doesn't cure kidney (renal) failure and leaves patients tired and cranky, with lives revolving around appointments. To get off dialysis, most patients want to get a kidney transplant.

Dutch physician Willem Kolff invented the hemodialysis machine in the Netherlands in 1943 and later worked on artificial hearts with Robert Jarvik. Kolff converted an automobile's fuel pump to force blood to and from the body for cleansing. Each session of dialysis required surgeons to connect cannulas to arteries and veins. Because an artery or vein could be used only once, surgeons soon exhausted all sites.

In 1960, physician Belding Scribner in Seattle invented the permanent indwelling shunt, a piece of tubing permanently attached to one vein and one artery, which allowed blood to flow continuously. The shunt could be shut off between dialyses, like a spigot.

At first, Scribner did not realize that the combination of a workable dialysis machine and a permanent shunt meant that he and Kolff had created an artificial kidney, a machine that could sustain life.

This breakthrough led to something wonderful: thousands of dying renal patients would now live. It also led to a new ethical issue: given the scarcity of machines, what criteria of distributive justice would be used to select who would live and who would die?

When Belding Scribner developed his shunt, inpatient dialysis cost $20,000 a year. Because it was experimental, insurance companies refused to pay for it. Such companies do not cover experimental treatment in order to hold down costs; when proven therapeutic, the treatments are covered.

Scribner's Swedish Hospital dialyzed its first patients without charging them, but in 1962 told Scribner he could admit no more patients for dialysis inside the hospital. By then, Scribner had a year's experience with dialysis and decided that patients could undergo it outside the hospital in clinics staffed by nurses. In 1963, Swedish Hospital started an outpatient dialysis center.

That center could serve 17 patients, but many more were eligible. From the beginning, the ethical problem arose: *who shall live when not all can?*[1]

Instead of leaving this problem of distributive justice to physicians, Swedish Hospital, Scribner, or King's County Medical Society, they all took the unusual step of creating an Admissions and Policy Committee to decide who would get a dialysis machine. Scribner wrote in 1972, "As I recall that period, all of us who were involved felt that we had found a fairly reasonable and simple solution to an impossibly difficult problem by letting a committee of responsible members of the community choose which patients [would receive treatment]."[2]

They created this committee to take the burden of moral decision away from physicians, assuming that physicians would naturally want their patients to be accepted.[3] The committee of seven members represented the community: a minister, a lawyer, a housewife, a labor leader, a state government official, a banker, and a surgeon. Two physicians familiar with dialysis served as advisers and screened applicants for medical unsuitability. The committee worked anonymously and never met candidates.

The committee first limited candidates to residents of the state of Washington who were under 45; candidates had to be able to afford dialysis or have insurance that covered it. Almost immediately, too many patients applied and additional criteria became necessary. Famously, the committee then considered personal characteristics about possible recipients: employment, children, education, motivation, achievements, and promise of helping others—criteria somewhat like those used by committees to admit students to medical school.

The committee eventually asked for analyses of a candidate's abilities to tolerate anxiety and to manage medical care independently; it considered whether a candidate had previously used symptoms to get attention from relatives and physicians. It evaluated the personality and personal merit of the candidate and the family's support for a patient on chronic dialysis. Elderly curmudgeons without siblings or children fared badly.

## SHANA ALEXANDER PUBLICIZES THE GOD COMMITTEE; STARTS BIOETHICS

This committee agonized over distributive justice before bioethics began. In 1962, no philosophers had written about ethical issues of allocating organs; indeed, no one had written about bioethics at all.[4] At least, they had not in the modern sense in which cases are analyzed to find a just public policy. The major previous writings were in Catholic medical ethics.

In May 1962, Dr. Scribner took a patient to Atlantic City for a newspaper convention to lobby publicly for more dialysis machines. In the process, he described to reporters his Admissions and Policy Committee, and it was his account of that committee, rather than his appeal for more machines, that made the front page of the *New York Times* the next day.[5]

*Life* magazine assigned its first woman reporter, Shana Alexander, to write this story and she spent three months in Seattle doing so.[6] Her article appeared in November 1962 and carried the term "God Committee"—a term that stuck.[7] She described the committee as playing a godlike role in deciding who would live and who would die. She described in detail the committee's criteria, which came to be called *social worth criteria*, or criteria about a person's worth to society.

In the spring of 1963, the *Seattle Times* ran on its front page a picture of nine of the center's dialysis patients, with the heading, "Will These People Have to Die?"[8] As a result of this "rescue in the media," the Boeing Corporation and the U.S. Public Health Service offered temporary financial support for the patients identified by the newspaper.

In 1965, television reporter Edwin Newman narrated an NBC documentary on the God Committee, *Who Shall Live?* That year, Congress had added to Social Security two national medical programs—Medicare for the elderly and Medicaid for the indigent, but neither covered dialysis. In *Who Shall Live?* a congressman asks why, if America could have a program to explore space, it couldn't have a dialysis program to save Americans. National interest grew about the story and, indirectly, about bioethics.

The media mattered greatly in this case. Shana Alexander said that when Scribner went to Atlantic City, he had been "angling" to get the story into the magazine with the largest circulation. Medical sociologist Judith Swazey agrees that Scribner set out to get publicity.[9]

Thirty years later, Scribner said that he had been "totally naive" about the national publicity; that a 1968 article in *UCLA Law Review* gave him "a lot of flak";[10] that he had had nothing to do with the committee, which had been created and supervised by the King's County Medical Association, and that when he had a dying patient who wasn't selected, he tried to circumvent the committee.

The story in the *Seattle Times* about his work could not have been written without the initiation and cooperation of Scribner and other physicians at Seattle hospitals. These physicians manipulated the *Seattle Times*, *Life*, and NBC News to obtain funds for their patients. Their success began a pattern of using the media when patients needed organ transplants, a pattern that came to be called the *rule of rescue*.

## THE END-STAGE RENAL DISEASE ACT (ESRD)

The God Committee continued to select and reject candidates for dialysis for nearly a decade. By 1971, many stories had dramatized the plight of patients in renal failure, and that year Shep Glazer, the president of the American Association of Kidney Patients, testified before Congress. As the story goes (it may be exaggerated), Glazer dialyzed himself before the House Ways and Means Committee, disconnected a tube from the machine, let his blood flow onto the floor, and said, "If you don't fund more machines, you'll have this blood on your hands."

In 1972, Congress legislated for Americans a one-organ right to medical care. The End-Stage Renal Disease Act (ESRD) mandated the federal government to pay for a dialysis machine for any American who needed one. Faced with the problem of distributive justice, of deciding which patients should be funded and how to select them, some critics believe that Congress took the easy way out and funded all patients. Others say that Congress showed compassion, allowing everyone to live in times of prosperity and passing the buck to later generations about how to pay for it all.

Congress passed ESRD in a session lasting only 30 minutes. The impetus came from a coalition of kidney patients, lobbyists for some physicians, concerns over high rates of kidney failure in people of color, and concerns that too much money was being spent on space and the war in Vietnam but too little on dying people who might be saved.

By making dialysis available to all patients, ESRD ended the problem of allocating machines and ended the need for the God Committee.

In retrospect, ESRD was hastily conceived, and it set an unfortunate precedent. Other groups, such as hemophiliacs, pressed for similar coverage.

Senator Vance Hartke of Indiana predicted that ESRD would cost $100 million the first year, but its cost would then drop sharply because of later efficiencies in production. Willem Kolff said his machines could be mass-produced for $200 each. These predictions are textbook lessons in how classical supply and demand fail in medical finance.

Under *cost-plus reimbursement* under ESRD, in effect during the 1970s and 1980s, hospitals could buy as many dialysis machines as they wanted and charge the cost *plus* a percentage of profit to ESRD. So ESRD incentivized them not to buy $200 machines, but to buy $20,000 machines. The larger the cost, the greater the profits they made.

In 1983 to rein in out-of-control costs, government tried reimbursement by *diagnostically related groups (DRGs)* instead of cost-plus funding. Hospitals got around DRGs and costs continued to soar. As yet another way to control costs, *managed care* started in the 1990s.

By 2010, instead of costing $100 million, the 594,000 Americans on dialysis in ESRD cost ESRD $47 billion a year, making ESRD one of the most expensive medical programs in North America.

Under ESRD, Congress also reimbursed kidney transplants. After the approval for use of cyclosporin in 1983, renal transplants jumped from 3,730 in 1975 to 9,000 in 1986 and to 15,000 in 2003.[11] This development raised new questions: Should every dialysis kidney patient get a kidney transplant? If so, where should the kidneys come from?

One thing is certain: what drove the expansion of people on dialysis and people getting kidney transplants was the fact that federal funds paid for all treatments for the kidney, a situation that existed for no other organ or disease. In contrast, during the next half-century, over 40 million Americans lacked basic medical coverage. At the same time, any American suffering kidney failure had all medical expenses covered and, frequently, could go on disability.

## THE BIRTH OF BIOETHICS

For complex reasons, Belding Scribner did something that went against a medical practice that was centuries old: he made public a moral dilemma that hitherto had been discussed only privately among physicians. Bringing this issue to the public's attention created controversy within medicine. As in Karen Quinlan's case, physicians felt that such ethical issues should be handled quietly within the profession.

By making this move, Scribner began a new process—the education of the American public about ethical problems in medicine. Scholars now began to publicly discuss problems such as brain death, assisted reproduction, and just allocation. With these articles and new courses, the new interdisciplinary field of bioethics began.

## SUPPLY AND DEMAND OF DONATED ORGANS

Over the last half-century, organs available for donation have never matched demand: the number from cadavers hovers around 4,000 a year. Second, the need for transplantable organs has steadily increased, especially as more Americans on dialysis desire kidney transplants and as Americans live longer.

A new source of organs has been so-called *live donations* from friends and relatives ("live" here contrasts to "cadavers" or "brain dead patients"). In a milestone in 2003, more transplantable kidneys came in America from live donors than from cadavers.

*Mandated choice* requires adults, in obtaining a driver's license, to indicate whether they want to be organ donors. Most American states require this choice. *Required request* mandates that someone at a hospital ask a relative upon admission of a patient. About 47 percent of Americans are potential organ donors.

Confusion over the definition of brain death decreases organ donation. For this reason, America has not moved beyond the conservative Harvard criteria of brain death to broader criteria.

Of course, without a signed donor card, a family may still donate organs of a brain-dead relative. Even if the brain-dead patient has a signed card, if the family refuses, surgeons usually do not take organs because they fear lawsuits and bad publicity.

Some African Americans refuse to sign donor cards because they consider themselves more likely to be declared dead prematurely. In 1968, surgeon Richard Lower transplanted the heart of African-American Bruce Tucker using the new Harvard criteria of brain death. When Tucker's heart was removed, he was not legally dead by the old, whole-body criteria, but it took a tense trial for a judge and jury in Richmond, Virginia, to decide that the new criteria excused a transplant surgeon from charges of murder.[12]

At least 14 European countries follow France and Spain and adopt *presumed consent*: anyone who has not declined to be a donor in writing to a national agency is presumed to be a donor. This is also called an *opt-out* policy. Most American states follow an *opt-in* policy, where only those citizens who consent to donate are potential donors.

## ETHICAL ISSUES

### Social Worth

The God Committee took *social worth* into account (although it did not use this phrase) in distributing machines. Medical sociologists Renée Fox and Judith Swazey, who spent 40 years studying artificial kidneys and transplantation, reviewed the minutes of the committee's meetings and criticized its criteria:

> Within these very general criteria, the specific, often unarticulated indicators that were used reflected the middle-class American value system shared by the selection panel. A person "worthy" of having his life saved by a scarce, expensive treatment like chronic dialysis was one judged to have qualities such as decency and responsibility. Any history of social deviance, such as a prison record, any suggestion that a person's married life was not intact and scandal-free, were strong contraindications to selection. The preferred candidate was a person who had demonstrated achievement through hard work and success at this job, who went to church, joined groups, and was actively involved in community affairs.[13]

Any standard of social worth implies that some people are worth more than others. Is it therefore unjust? Immanuel Kant argued that every human should be treated as an "end in himself" with absolute moral worth. To judge that one human deserves to live more than another is to treat some wrongly as a "mere means."

How then would Kant treat everyone the same? The key question is what rule or maxim could be universalized. For Kant, that would be impartial, random selection by lot, say, by drawing straws.

Two critics of the God Committee, a psychiatrist and a lawyer, raked social worth over the coals:

> [*Life*] magazine paints a disturbing picture of the bourgeoisie sparing the bourgeoisie, of the Seattle committee measuring persons in accordance with its own middle-class suburban value system: Scouts, Sunday school, Red Cross. This rules out creative conformists, who rub the bourgeoisie the wrong way but who historically have contributed so much to the making of America. The Pacific Northwest is no place for a Henry David Thoreau with bad kidneys.[14]

Boston University law professor George Annas criticized the committee for preferring housewives over prostitutes, working men over "playboys," and scientists over poets.[15] Annas argued that some criteria of social worth can be just at some stage of the selection process, but these criteria must be made public. If the rule is going to be "always prefer housewives to prostitutes," this should be explicit. Secret rules allow discrimination based on race, sex, class, wealth, or other arbitrary qualities.

In fairness to the God Committee, everyone today prefers that patients dialyze as outpatients because six patients can be supported outside the hospital for the cost of one inside.

## PERSONAL RESPONSIBILITY FOR ILLNESS AND EXPENSIVE RESOURCES

Kant's ethics may also be contradictory because Kant also stresses personal responsibility for health. Should someone who behaves irresponsibly get a scarce medical resource?

Take the famous case considered by the God Committee of the half-Sioux Ernie Crowfeather. A small-time criminal and a charmer, he received dialysis for 30 months, but refused to follow the regimen, hated his quality of life, drank, imposed his childlike needs on the staff, and finally turned down further therapy and died.[16] Scribner confessed that to get dialysis for Ernie, he went around the committee.[17]

As a matter of public policy, why should the medical system reward a lifetime of unhealthy behavior by giving patients expensive medical resources? Overweight patients with high blood pressure often later get diabetes and suffer strokes or heart disease, all expensive to treat. Should the system spend so much on people whose own unhealthy behavior caused their problems?

Consider giving liver transplants to alcoholics. By far the most expensive organ to transplant, a liver transplant requires a highly skilled team and takes a long time. The most common cause of liver destruction, or end-stage liver disease (ESLD), is alcoholism. When alcohol is a factor, the condition is actually called *alcohol-related end-stage liver disease (ARESLD)*.

In the 1990s, physicians debated whether patients with ARESLD should be equally eligible for liver transplants. This is partly a medical issue, since it can be analyzed in terms of which patients will benefit most from such a transplant, but it also concerns personal responsibility. Is a nondrinker more deserving of a donor liver? Can someone with ARESLD be blamed for the loss of his liver? Would a drinker keep on drinking, thereby destroying the new liver, or would drinkers be transformed by receiving the gift of life?

With ARESLD, this question is complicated by disagreement over whether alcoholism is a disease or a chosen behavior. The disease model of alcoholism has prevailed for some time, but has recently been attacked by philosopher Herbert Fingarette, who in turn draws on themes in Kant's ethics.[18]

In 1992, two teams of clinical medical ethicists conflicted over this point. In Chicago, physicians Alvin Moss and Mark Seigler argued that as ARESLD principally causes liver failure, because not enough livers are available for transplant, and as recidivism is likely among alcoholics, patients who develop liver failure "through no fault of their own" should have a higher priority for donor livers than patients with ARESLD, whose condition "results from failure to obtain treatment for alcoholism."[19]

Two medical ethicists at the University of Michigan, Carl Cohen and Martin Benjamin, disagreed. They maintained that alcoholics are not morally blameworthy and, after liver transplants, survive as long as non-alcoholics, and so should not be penalized.[20]

> Free will and medical ethics in the context of alcoholism are discussed in an excerpt from Gregory Pence's *Elements of Bioethics*. To read *"Kant On Whether Alcoholism Is a Disease,"* go to Chapter 12 in the Online Learning Center (OLC) at www.mhhe.com/pence7e.

At the very least, the medical system sends out contradictory messages: first, eat healthy, exercise, and take responsibility for your health; second, we will rescue you in illness and do everything possible to keep you alive, regardless of cost or time expended by medical staff.

## KANT AND RESCHER ON JUST ALLOCATION

Kantian ethics pulls in two directions on the question of penalizing alcoholics for liver transplants. On the one hand, Kant believes that people choose to drink and should be held responsible. For him, the claim that, "The alcoholic's actions are caused by a disease" treats the person as a "mere means," as if he were the passive vehicle of causal forces over which he has no control. Herbert Fingarette's research shows that most so-called alcoholics drink voluntarily. Given proper incentives and contexts, they can moderate their behavior. Fingarette also emphasizes that Alcoholics Anonymous assumes that drinkers can choose not to drink.

As said, all other things being equal, Kantian ethics also pulls for a lottery in distributing a scarce liver, to treat each person equally and as having equal moral worth. Can these two strains of Kantian ethics be reconciled?

Perhaps. In 1969, philosopher Nicholas Rescher argued that the God Committee had been correct to use criteria that included social worth.[21] Rescher favored considering life expectancy, number of dependents, potential for future contributions to society, and past achievements. Less controversially, he supported screening candidates for medical problems that were likely to make them do poorly on dialysis and waste machines. He suggested that such a system might be based on points, with ties broken by a lottery.

Kant might be sympathetic to Rescher's two-tiered approach. Those who had injured themselves through voluntary behavior do not deserve the same chance as those who lost kidneys through a genetic disease. Once such people are screened out, however, everyone should be considered equally by lottery.

## WEALTH, CELEBRITIES, JUSTICE, AND WAITING LISTS FOR ORGANS

In the 1970s, no system existed for distributing donated organs, and surgeons with organs in one medical center did not always share them with surgeons elsewhere. This was wasteful. Some hoarded organs soon were lost.

The National Transplantation Act (1984) and the federal Task Force on Organ Transplantation (1986) were combined in 1987 to create the United Network for Organ Sharing (UNOS). UNOS alleviated some regional competition and established national standards about which patient would get the next available organ. UNOS continually grapples with the crucial philosophical question: *what is the most just way to allocate organs*?

UNOS deals only with candidates who are already in the system. Thus, how and when applicants get onto waiting lists for donor organs remains a pressing issue. Specifically, if you don't have medical insurance or a hospital willing to take you as a charity case, you won't get on the UNOS list.

The practice of *multiple listing* raises questions about wealth and injustice.[22] Some patients get appointments with surgeons at more than one transplant center and have themselves worked up at each; but only people who can take time off from work, afford to travel, and have generous medical plans can arrange for multiple listings.

In 2009, Apple co-founder Steve Jobs illustrated the advantages of multiple listing when he traveled from California to Memphis to get a liver transplant. Having the money to get himself worked up in Tennessee, he became the sickest patient on the hospital's list and got the transplant.

For a patient who needs a kidney, being on several lists may not be necessary to get one, but for a patient who needs a heart or a liver, a multiple listing may be a matter of life and death. One criterion for receiving a heart or liver is locality: a candidate must be within the area of the transplant center or have the money to get there fast. A patient who registers at half a dozen such centers could significantly increase his chances of being selected.

Imagine that you are going to die in Memphis of liver failure, but you know that a hundred other patients want a liver for the same reason. Then you learn that Californian Steve Jobs received a liver because he gamed the system to get on the right list. It's one thing to feel unlucky because you're in a life-threatening condition, but another to feel that you are going to die because someone else managed to get into line in front of you.

When former baseball star Mickey Mantle came to Baylor University Medical Center in Dallas on May 28, 1995, decades of alcoholism, as well as Hepatitis C, had destroyed his liver. Physicians diagnosed him with end-stage liver disease.[23] A CT scan found a large tumor on the center of his liver, compressing his common bile duct.[24]

Mantle went on the UNOS waiting list for a liver transplant classified as a Stage 2, the second most urgent.[25] Two days later, he received a liver.[26]

Many felt that Mantle's celebrity had vaulted him to the top. The transplant team was also criticized for giving a transplant to a person with (1) liver cancer and (2) lifelong alcoholism. Many felt that Mantle had destroyed his liver on his own and that someone more deserving should have received the transplant. Three months after his transplant, Mantle died from cancer.[27] His case rocked the public's trust in UNOS and its methods of selecting candidates.

Similarly in 1993, the governor of Pennsylvania from 1987 to 1995, Robert Casey, was diagnosed with Appalachian familiar amyloidosis, a rare genetic disease. Seemingly within 10 hours of entering the waiting list, Casey got a combined liver-heart transplant, even though many other candidates were ahead of him.

It was later claimed he had been on the list for a year but did not want his disease known for political reasons. Pittsburgh's famous transplant program also defended Casey's selection, saying he was the only person needing both a liver and a heart. After the outcry, UNOS revised its criteria to say that a successful candidate must be at the top of one of the lists for single organs (which Casey had not been) in addition to his place on any list for two transplants.

In 1990, New York banned multiple listing. In 1992, some patients who were multiple-listed argued in a hearing before UNOS that forbidding the practice denied their "liberty right" to contract for medical care.[28]

There are two powerful arguments against multiple listing. First, a primary attribute of a just medical system is equality of access, and the use of wealth to jump the line violates this norm. Second, multiple listing compromises the entire UNOS system because some people are getting listed above others arbitrarily. UNOS should be impartial not only in dealing with candidates who are already listed, but also in the actual process of deciding who gets listed.

A similar problem surfaced in the early 1990s, when it was revealed that candidates for neonatal heart transplants were being identified prenatally and then being placed on waiting lists immediately, while they were still fetuses.[29] Because time accumulated on a waiting list gives a candidate extra points, such a practice would offer a significant advantage. In this case, prenatal listing was made possible by the ability to diagnose hypoplastic left heart syndrome (HLHS) in utero; but such early diagnosis is not uniformly distributed in the United States, and early listing of babies diagnosed in utero seemed unfair to babies who were not diagnosed until birth. Moreover, fetuses with HLHS remain relatively safe while they are in the womb, whereas at birth HLHS babies are almost always at great risk and are in NICUs. For these reasons, UNOS changed its policy in June 1992 and put fetuses on a separate list from babies. UNOS also decided to allocate a heart to a fetus only when no baby could use it.

## RETRANSPLANTS

Retransplantation of the same patient raises other issues about justice. Since patients often reject transplanted organs, a second or third transplant can be done. But is it fair to rescue a particular patient with a second heart or kidney when thousands of others never get a first one? Shouldn't patients get a second organ only when everyone has had a chance at one?

As we shall see later, retransplants raise a profound conflict about justice. The rule of rescue involved here (discussed soon) is really a particular instance of the general conflict between impartial ethical theories and partial ones.

UNOS treats patients waiting for retransplants as first-time patients. This does not lead to the best outcomes. Nearly 82 percent of first-time transplants survive one year, but only 57 percent of re-transplants do. Retransplanted patients fare worse than first-transplant patients because they usually are sicker.

Let us call *organ-utilitarians* those who see justice as creating the greatest years of life per donated organ. Under such constraints, UNOS should give first-time patients priority over retransplant patients.

But maximal years per organ is not the only thing to value. Shouldn't medicine save those who are about to die? Shouldn't others, who are less sick, wait?

Transplant teams bond with patients and find it difficult not to save them. Consider a hypothetical 41-year-old Judy Rogers, a former bank teller now on dialysis and disability who suffers severe depression. This is understandable: the medical team has worked very hard over many years to save Judy's life, and when she rejects an organ, the team does not want to be forced by UNOS to watch her die. Medical staffs would see this as *patient abandonment*. More simply, nurses, medical students, and the surgeon know Judy personally, whereas new patients are abstractions to them.

But it is reasonable to ask why identified patients should take priority over new patients: a new patient may benefit more and be more meritorious. Moreover, if the medical teams are allowed to select who gets a new organ, patients who are better at forming relationships with transplant teams will be favored.[30] And it may be true that patients who are beautiful, charismatic, privileged, white, and socially connected fare better with staff than those lacking these characteristics.

Although transplant teams identify with retransplanted patients, others may identify with the patients who are waiting. Consider a hypothetical Max Loftin, a 53-year-old accountant with severe depression and a dialysis patient waiting for a kidney transplant. A new kidney might cure his depression. But if present patients in hospitals get all next month's available kidneys as second or third retransplants, Mr. Loftin will die, a nameless victim never known to the hospital's staff.

An actual patient named Ronnie DeSillers in Miami, who received *three* liver transplants, caused bitter feelings among patients waiting for a liver. Because his father knew how to work the system, Danny Canal of Wheaton, Maryland, in 1998 received *three quadruple* organ transplants (the first due to multiple-listing). Did 11 other people deserve never to get an organ so Danny could get 12?

## THE RULE OF RESCUE

The rule of rescue, named by bioethicist Albert Jonsen, refers to giving scarce medical resources to an identified patient, rather than to equally deserving and equally endangered anonymous people.[31] We can cite countless examples of this rule.

Frequently, the media identify the person. If reporters cover the plight of a small girl trapped in a deep well, thousands will send dollars for her rescue; meanwhile, reporters may not cover the plight of another young boy in peril, he is not rescued, and he dies. Is this just?

In 1982, hospital administrator Charles Fiske interrupted a televised news conference to successfully plead for a liver donation for his daughter, Jamie. For more than 25 years since, desperate parents have used such methods to save their children in organ failure. Belding Scribner illustrated this in rescuing Ernie Crowfeather.

In 2013, the mother of 10-year-old, cystic fibrosis patient, Sarah Murnaghan, worked national media to draw attention to UNOS's practice of listing children under 14 on a separate list from adults for lung transplants.[32] UNOS had excluded such children because adult lungs must be cut down to fit children, but a judge overruled UNOS. Subsequently, an exception was made and Sarah received not one but two lungs.

From the perspective of distributive justice, why is the rule of rescue problematic? Why is it an unjust way to distribute organs?

First, television often identifies the rescued person, but who gets to live shouldn't be decided by who gets on television. But the media favor people who look good, which means cute, articulate people and families who know how to work reporters. It is not a trivial fact that Sarah M was a cute white girl. But who gets to live shouldn't be decided by who is most photogenic.

The rule of rescue makes journalists and their editors the gatekeepers of life and death. The rule of rescue replaces the God Committee with the assignment editor ("Oh, we just did a child transplant story. Let's wait a month before we do another.")

And for every identifiable person who is saved, there are a dozen anonymous patients who are lost. If one life is worth the same as another, why is identification by a newspaper important?

When a physician admits a hypothetical Karen Smith to a hospital, Karen becomes identified as a candidate for rescue. The medical team then bonds to the smart, gregarious Karen and bestows on her a million dollars of publicly funded resources. Again, if there are many worthy candidates for a scarce medical resource, who gets to live shouldn't be decided by the likes of hospital staff or the whims of physicians in admitting patients.

Hospitals frequently set up rules and committees to prevent just this sort of thing. Left-ventricle assist devices (LVADs) can be bridges to heart transplants, but if hearts don't materialize, how long can a hospital keep patients on LVADs, especially if the patients have no coverage? The physician who initially admits his patient for an LVAD may feel like he's saved a life and is a hero, but he may be a villain to the hospital's administration, which must pay for the resulting care.

As said, the conflict here lies between impartial ethical theories and partialist ones. On one side, we have Kantian ethics and utilitarianism, which treat everyone the same and which oppose the rule of rescue. On the other side, we have the Ethics of Care that values "partial" or particular relationships. Our moral intuitions stem from both kinds of theories, which explains why they pull us in different directions. (The Ethics of Care, Kantian ethics, and utilitarianism are discussed more in chapter 1 on ethical theories.)

It is precisely the pull of partialist theories that attracts us to rescuing the patient before us in the hospital bed. It is precisely that pull that impartial theories urge us to resist in seeking a more impartial way of deciding who gets into the hospital bed in the first place. Partial theories implicitly discount the value of unidentified people not in the circle of concern of the medical team.

## SICKEST FIRST, UNOS, AND THE RULE OF RESCUE

As we have seen, utilitarianism clashes with the ethics of care over retransplants and the same clash looms larger in how UNOS allocates organs. One partialist theory is to allocate organs according to "sickest first" or "give the organ first to the patient most likely to otherwise die."

A utilitarian wanting to maximize human life in the lifeboat for the long row to Africa selects the strongest rowers, tosses the weak, sick, and elderly overboard, and eats the dog. Similarly, utilitarians wanting maximal years per organ allocate organs only to first-timers and allow no retransplants. For impartial ethical theories such as utilitarianism or Kantian ethics, one human life counts as much as another, regardless of whether that life is my father, my neighbor, my patient, my fellow citizen, or a complete stranger.

Piggybacking this logic on some facts leads to a surprising conclusion: giving organs to the sickest patients does not maximize the most years per life per organ. Why? Because some patients are too near death. When they die, the organs are wasted.

"But what if they don't die?" others reply. "Then they have been rescued and saved." And some patients will, in fact, be saved this way.

But the best way to get the most organs per life is to give the organ to moderately sick people just experiencing organ failure. In that way, with a limited supply, more people live longer.

Congress, many surgeons, and the families of many patients rejected the impartial system. As their loved one grows closer to death, they grasp for life. Even if it wastes an organ, they feel that after waiting for years on the list for an organ, they deserve their one chance to live.

So strong is this feeling that in the fall of 2000, Congress *mandated* that the UNOS allocate organs on the basis of *sickest first*. As the Fact Sheet on the UNOS website states: "For heart, liver and intestinal organs, patients whose medical status is most urgent receive priority over those whose medical status is not as urgent."[33]

Howard Eisen, head of Temple University Hospital's heart transplant program, disapproves, "What you're doing is giving hearts to people who will do less well with them. People are waiting longer, so they get sicker, and end up getting two operations when they would otherwise need one."[34]

Personal responsibility for health also could enter here. "Give first to the sickest patients" is a standard of distributive justice, but is fair to others down the line who took better care of their bodies and therefore are not now as sick?

## LIVING DONORS

For many decades, an ethical bright line existed in transplant surgery of, "First, do no harm," which in part meant "Do not harm one person to benefit another." In 1954, Dr. Joseph Murray successfully transplanted a kidney from Ronald Herrick, a 23-year-old man, into his identical twin Richard, who was dying of kidney disease. Since the transplantation involved identical twins, immunological rejection posed no problem, and Richard accepted the transplanted kidney. Since no compatibility barriers existed, and since a brother's life was saved, the benefits of this surgery appeared to outweigh possible harms to the donor, and consequently ethical concerns were overridden. This precedent demonstrated the viability of live organ transplantation and paved the way for alternatives to cadaveric transplantation.[35]

By 2003, the number of live donors had surpassed the number of cadaver donors (brain-dead patients whose relatives consented to harvesting their organs). In that year, transplant surgery leapt from making one exception—an exception from a traditional rule in order to save a life—to letting people volunteer to have surgeons risk harm to them to benefit another. By 2013, organs from cadavers had again surpassed live donors, due to increased efforts to get drivers applying for licenses to indicate their organ-donor status.

In 1989, the first transplant occurred from a healthy parent (a mother) to a daughter—from Teri Smith to Alyssa Smith. While he was removing the lobe of Teri's liver, surgeon Christoph Broelsch of the University of Chicago nicked Teri's spleen and had to excise it. Broelsch called the loss of Teri's spleen a "major complication," saying it gave him "the sickest feeling to have trouble with the first patient."[36]

Also in 1989, Marissa Ayala was conceived to provide stem cells for her sister Anissa, who had leukemia.[37] Pre-implantation genetic diagnosis (PGD), the practice of analyzing artificially fertilized embryos, allowed Anissa's parents to choose an embryo that could serve as a compatible bone marrow donor for Anissa. Should Marissa have been conceived as a resource for Anissa, what is now called a *savior sibling*? Jodi Picoult's novel *My Sister's Keeper* brought to life the tensions in this scenario. Marissa's bone marrow was taken and given to Anissa, which saved Anissa's life, but does one happy result justify creating a thousand more children to serve as resources for dying siblings?

In 1993, transplant centers accepted and recruited adult relatives of children for organ transplants, and Nilda Rodríguez gave one-quarter of her liver to her sick granddaughter. In the same year, James and Barbara Sewell each donated part of a lung to their 22-year-old daughter, whose own lungs had been damaged by cystic fibrosis, a genetic disease that is typically fatal by age 30 (the patient usually dies from infection and collapse of the lungs). By 1997, as the practice became more accepted, California surgeon Vaughn Starnes had taken lobes from 76 donors for 37 recipients. One commentator in the same year noted that the practice was "ethically problematic," implying that a norm had not yet been established.

From 1990 to 2002, surgeons in St. Louis performed 207 lung transplants on 190 children.[38] All 190 children were under age 18, 121 were ages 10–18, and the most common reason for transplantation was cystic fibrosis. This means that surgeons took lung lobes from 207 healthy adults for these children. Italian surgeons reported similar results for 1996 to 2002, giving 55 people of mean age 25 years a lung transplant.[39]

Something similar happened with liver transplantation among relatives. From a few isolated cases in 1993–1994, such requests eventually became the norm: "There now exists an ethical imperative to develop this [live-donor donation of livers]," said Jean Edmond, M.D., director of liver transplantation at New York Presbyterian Hospital in 1999.[40] Between 1996 and 1999, surgeons performed over 70 transplants among adult relatives, with 45 in the first half of 1999, showing exponential growth.

In 1999, officials confirmed the first death from adult-to-adult liver donation and they estimated that two to three other adults had died from donating parts of organs to their children.[41] By 2003, at least five people had died.[42] Exact figures are unknown.

The surgical journal *Transplantation* reported in late 2002 that 56 people who had previously been living organ donors later required a kidney transplant.[43] Of the 56 people, only 43 received transplants, and of these, 36 worked. Of these 56 candidates, two died while waiting for an organ and one died after the operation.

Consider the sad case of Walter Wood, 45, who donated to his brother under the impression that kidney transplants were relatively safe and done only to save a life. Wood experienced an unexpected outcome during surgery: his abdominal muscles ruptured. He has since been in constant pain and has been unable to perform the simplest of tasks. As a result of his severe disability, Walter lost his job, had to sell his house, and approached bankruptcy. "I'm in constant pain from the surgeries I've had. I can't even move around in bed," Wood says.

Protecting patients such as Walter Wood is a problem in the system because the transplant team understandably focuses on the sick recipient of the organ, not the donor. Not only that, transplants occur only on people who have medical coverage, so the transplant team and its hospital get paid for medical services to the recipient. In contrast, they receive nothing for caring for donors and give such care at a financial loss. In sum, transplant teams have asymmetrical relationships to donors and to recipients.

After he donated part of his liver to his brother in 2002, reporter Mike Hurewitz of Albany, New York, died a gruesome death at Mount Sinai Hospital in New York City (because he was a reporter, his death generated lots of publicity). Also, 69-year-old Barbara Tarrant from North Carolina disastrously donated a kidney to her mentally retarded son and wound up paralyzed on her left side and without coherent speech.[44]

Widely regarded as heroic in the popular media, living donor transplantation carries real dangers. Until recently, no one then knew how many donors have ended up like Mike Hurewitz, Barbara Tarrant, or Walter Wood. Why? Because living-donor transplant centers then had no obligation to report deaths or injuries to the UNOS, nor did UNOS have any legal obligation to monitor such deaths and injuries.

Previously, no hospital, transplant center, or medical department tracked deaths and injuries from live donors such as Walter Wood. Once donors leave the hospital, they were on their own—for medical care, for insurance, for follow-up.

Given the lack of such studies, an obvious question arose then of how donors could give *informed* consent about the risks of donation. Finally, after nearly a decade of uncertainty, a 2009 study at the University of Minnesota that tracked mainly white, middle-class donors found only slightly more problems with donors than non-donors, although non-white donors seemed to fare worse.[45] In 2010, UNOS started to track problems of live organ-donors and to provide more realistic data to potential donors.

> Adult organ donation is discussed in an excerpt from Gregory Pence's *Elements of Bioethics* read "Kant's Critique of Adult Organ Donation," go to Chapter 12 in the Online Learning Center (OLC) at www.mhhe.com/pence7e.

## COSTS AND THE MEDICAL COMMONS

According to Transplant Living, a service of UNOS, the total cost of a liver transplant is $577,100.[46] This includes the cost of pre- and post-transplant care and testing, surgery, procurement of organ from donor, immunosuppressants, and more. The total cost in 2011 of a kidney transplant was $262,900. The total cost of a heart transplant was $997,700, and the cost of a heart-lung transplant was $1,148,400.

During the 1970s, the biologist Garrett Hardin discussed the *tragedy of the commons,* a situation in which no one reduces his or her consumption of some public resource until the resource becomes so ravaged that it disappears. The concept originated centuries ago in England, when pastures held in common were overgrazed: in each town, each shepherd increased his own flock until there were so many animals that the commons could no longer support them. The lesson is that the unregulated pursuit of self-interest leads to destruction of public resources.

Former Colorado governor Richard Lamm agrees. He has emphasized that Americans cannot continue such extravagant policies and do well. In particular, as a matter of intergenerational justice, America cannot fund extravagant care for the elderly on the backs of the working young: "When a society faces fiscal reality and seeks to optimize its dollars, it not only starts on the road to financial sanity, but it also brings dramatic change to existing medical practices. Dialysis and transplantation will undoubtedly undergo major change."[47]

Lamm continues, "Dr. Thomas Starzl recently gave a liver transplant to a 76-year-old woman. It cost $240,000. Dr. Starzl should understand that with the average U.S. family making $24,000 a year, he has sentenced 10 U.S. families to work all year so that he could transplant a 76-year-old woman." (Chapter 18 discusses ethical issues in medical finance.)

## NON-HEART-BEATING ORGAN TRANSPLANTATION

The issue of exactly how a patient, whose body is a potential source of organs, gets declared dead has simmered in the background of organ transplantation for nearly half a century. Between 1954 and 1967, organs for transplantation either came from living, related donors (e.g., a kidney from one twin to another) or from patients who had died (cadavers). Physicians then declared patients dead by cardiopulmonary criteria—that is, the hearts of patients stopped beating and the patients stopped breathing. These criteria were not ideal because when tissue no longer receives blood, damage occurs very fast, and such damage often occurs while the heart is stopping.

With the Harvard definition of brain death in 1967, declaration of death in cadavers switched to neocortical criteria, allowing retrieval of organs from cadavers who had their breathing and circulation maintained artificially by ventilators. Because obtaining organs from patients declared dead this way did not injure organs, and because all states passed neocortical brain-death laws, procurement of organs for transplantation switched almost entirely to use of the neocortical standard. After that, surgeons obtained organs in better shape for the receiving patient.

In recent years, improvements in automobile safety have reduced the pool of such bodies, while burgeoning numbers of transplant programs have learned to transplant sicker people. Supply has dropped, while demand has soared.

In 1993, the University of Pittsburgh Medical Center developed a protocol to start obtaining organs from patients who were declared dead by the old cardiopulmonary criteria. Their novel idea was to manage death in the small class of patients where the underlying illness causing death has not damaged the organ and where the patient or the family has signed a "do not resuscitate" (DNR) order.

In this protocol, a patient on a respirator is moved to the operating room where his respirator is removed, breathing stops, the surgical team waits a few minutes for breathing to resume, the patient is declared dead, and then his organs are removed.

The official name of this protocol. is the non-heart-beating cadaver donor (NHBD). This phrase is not felicitous, for it seems to be an oxymoron (can a cadaver be a "donor"?).

The NHBD protocol declares death after two minutes during which no pulse is detected and after ventricular fibrillation, asystole, or electromechanical dissociation occurs. It allows drugs to be administered, such as vasodilators and anticoagulants, which are given solely to maximize health of organs to be transplanted. It declares that death occurs when there is irreversible loss of *cardiac function*, as opposed to the neocortical standard, which declares that death occurs when there is irreversible loss of *all brain activity*, including brain stem activity.

A 1997 study requested of the Institute of Medicine (IOM) by the Secretary of Health and Human Services distinguished between *controlled* and *uncontrolled* NHBDs. Before the Harvard, neocortical definition of death was adopted, patients died in "uncontrolled" ways as their hearts stopped beating and injured their other organs. In the Pittsburgh protocol, the IOM said, "the (deaths of) donors are controlled because the timing and thus the process of donation are controlled through the timing of (withdrawal of) life support." These patients generally suffer from severe head injuries or progressive neurological illness.

One aspect of the new protocol that some people have trouble accepting is that the judgment of irreversibility differs from the judgment about lack of neocortical activity. The only way to know if such changes truly are irreversible is to start cardiopulmonary resuscitation (CPR), but in the Pittsburgh protocol, of course, the family and/or competent patient must explicitly decline CPR.

This point must be stressed. Consent of the patient distinguishes physician-assisted dying from murder. If the family has not consented to the Pittsburgh protocol, staff might be charged with accelerating death to harvest organs.

Another point to stress here is that CPR on a dying or elderly patient is a brutal way to die and often involves breaking chest bones. It is a peculiar form of torture practiced today. Fewer than 15 percent of hospital patients who receive CPR ever leave the hospital.[48] If a family understands these facts, it might elect to forgo CPR and allow the Pittsburgh protocol.

Hence the essential idea of the NHBCD protocol: because the family, the patient, and the physicians believe the patient is going to die soon, why not manage the death to create life for others? For the family, something good may come out of the death—the gift of life to another person.

A 1993 conference explored the ethical issues of the Pittsburgh protocol but did not achieve a consensus. Although all agreed that the dead-donor rule should continue—that is, that organs should be taken only from dead patients—they could not agree on whether families should be allowed to consent to organ procurement under the new protocol. "The Pittsburgh protocol gives an interpretation of irreversible that comes down to a low probability of auto-resuscitation and excludes the possibility of interventions that could restart the heart."[49]

But what about the ethical issue where families consented but did not understand the issues? Critics object on Kantian grounds that the patient is not being treated as "an end in himself." Alan Weisbard argued that the Pittsburgh protocol "indirectly brings about the death of some people to benefit others." Medical sociologist Renée Fox thinks it "morally offensive" to ask families, nurses, and residents to be involved in this effort, and criticizes the "macabre" public policy of championing maximal organ transplantation.[50]

In 1997, the controversy made national news in the worst way when a bioethics professor in Cleveland went to a district attorney, charging that transplant surgeons at the famous Cleveland Clinic were about to violate the law. The headline of the *Cleveland Plain Dealer* was "'Murder, She Said" and a few days later,

*60 Minutes* interviewed Mary Ellen Waithe and broke the story nationally. Other bioethicists criticized Waithe's elevation of a dispute in public policy to charges of illegal activities with overtones of criminal mischief.

The *60 Minutes* story on the Cleveland Clinic revealed that the University of Wisconsin Medical Center had been using an NHBD controlled-death protocol to harvest organs for more than 20 years. During this show, a point of contention was whether the administration of heparin and regitine accelerated the death of donors. Heparin, a blood thinner, prevents clot formation, and regitine dilates blood vessels, keeping organs perfused with blood.

Surgeons at centers using NHBD hotly deny the claim that administration of heparin and regitine hastens death. The Institute of Medicine study vindicated such surgeons, noting the NHBD protocols across the country divided evenly between allowing the use at some stage in the donation process of one or both of these agents and expressly prohibiting or not mentioning them.

In most cases, the IOM report allows careful administration of these drugs. Nevertheless, because under certain circumstances in certain patients, there is a concern that these agents might be harmful, this report recommends case-by-case decisions on the use of anticoagulants and vasodilators and consideration of additional safeguards such as involvement of the patients' attending physician in prescribing decisions. The Institute of Medicine also recommended waiting five minutes, rather than two, after life-support was removed, before declaring death.[51]

The Scientific Registry of Transplant Recipients, a branch of the U.S. Department of Health and Human Services, compiles data on transplants and wants us to distinguish between "living donors" and "deceased donors."[52] The latter refer to "an individual whose tissues or organs are donated after his or her death. Such donations come from two sources: patients who have suffered brain death and patients whose hearts have irreversibly stopped beating. The latter group is referred to as non-heart-beating or donation-after-cardiac-death (DCD) donors. Throughout this report, we have used the term deceased donor instead of cadaveric donor." Because not all "deceased donors" are brain-dead by the Harvard criteria, "deceased donor" covers more sources.

## THE GOD COMMITTEE, AGAIN

It's easy to criticize the way other people think about justice and allocate scarce medical resources. Critics of the God Committee probably couldn't themselves do a better job. After all, problem drinkers like Ernie Crowfeather, immature people, and people with poor personal hygiene fare poorly on dialysis and dialysis nurses often hate them.

Moreover, life on dialysis is not great. It has a high symptom burden, meaning that quality of life is low. As one nephrologist reports about daily life on dialysis,

> Insomnia is extraordinarily common and many [patients] experience severe muscle cramping and pains of different sorts. Itching is an equally common phenomenon, along with nausea, vomiting, and poor spirits. Our data indicates that among the roughly 300,000 patients undergoing dialysis in any given year, about 65,000 (or 23%) will die.[53]

Maybe the God Committee correctly considered which people had the strength to endure these procedures. Today, when everyone gets dialysis, many patients indirectly commit suicide by failing to comply with regimens or by missing appointments. The life expectancy for dialysis patients falls between one-eighth and one-third of the rest of the population, in part because too many patients who are old and sick get dialyzed.[54]

In 2006, a new form of home dialysis became available called *Rogosin dialysis* or *nocturnal dialysis*.[55] It requires a $13,000 dialysis machine and a $5,000 water purifier, but it can be done at home, six nights a week for eight hours each night. Complying with nocturnal dialysis means not needing to go to dialysis clinics three times a week for outpatient dialysis under nursing supervision.

As with outpatient dialysis, nocturnal dialysis requires cleanliness and personal hygiene. Pet hair may clog the machine, so pets are out. At present, patients with poor hygiene, or those who cannot part with pets, cannot use Rogosin dialysis. Because personal responsibility for health is an important criterion for getting this kind of dialysis, the same ethical issues arose 50 years later here as in 1962 with the original machines in Seattle.

## FURTHER READING

Renée Fox and Judith Swazey, *The Courage to Fail: A Social View of Organ Transplants and Dialysis*, 2nd ed. rev., Chicago: University of Chicago Press, 1974, 1978.

Institute of Medicine, *Non-Heart-Beating Organ Transplantation—Medical and Ethical Issues in Procurement*, Washington, D.C.: National Academy Press, 1997.

Renée Fox and Judith Swazey, Spare Parts: Organ Replacement in American Society, New York: Oxford University Press, 1992.

Thomas Starzl, *The Puzzle People: Memoirs of a Transplant Surgeon*, Pittsburgh, PA: University of Pittsburgh Press, 1992.

## DISCUSSION QUESTIONS

1. In getting a transplanted organ that saves your life, which of the following should a just system of allocation consider?

   Whether the patent smoked; whether the patient drank alcohol extensively; whether the patient has medical insurance; whether the patient is rich and get herself listed in several medical centers; whether the patient has already received one organ transplant.

2. Isn't it human nature to rescue the sickest first? To stave off death from someone you know? Do we want surgeons to be bureaucratic robots or to have a heart? What's wrong with the rule of rescue and caring for patients who are known?

3. Even if people have a small amount of free will, shouldn't the system act as if they had lots of it? By rewarding good behavior and punishing bad behavior, doesn't the system itself become a major causal factor in how people behave? On the other hand, if it rescues unhealthy behavior, doesn't the system undermine healthy behavior and reward unhealthy habits?

4. Who is going to pay for organ transplants if more and more people keep getting them? When 40 million Americans lack basic coverage, isn't this luxurious medicine for the well-off?

5. If you are a physician or a nurse and a patient doesn't want to cooperate—if he keeps smoking, eating five sausage sandwiches for breakfast each day, and drinking a bottle of wine with dinner each night—and his health gets worse and worse, are you justified in getting mad at him? Or does getting mad at him just cause him to avoid coming back to see you? Is moralism a tool for changing behavior or is it a primitive venting of feelings by the health provider?

6. Do families of the NHBD protocol understand what's going on? Do they believe that not every possible effort will be made to keep their son alive and that his death is being managed so that his organs can be transplanted in the best shape? Even if they don't understand all this, is that bad? If the patient is going to die anyway, isn't this a way of getting something good out of the process?

# CHAPTER 13

---

# Using One Baby for Another:

## Babies Fae, Gabriel, and Theresa and Conjoined Twins

*T*his chapter discusses the case of Baby Fae, who briefly lived with a baboon's heart; the case of Baby Gabriel, an anencephalic baby whose heart went to another infant; the case of the anencephalic Baby Theresa, whose parents wanted to donate her heart to another baby; and sacrifice surgeries, cases about separating conjoined twins where one is sacrificed to help the other. This chapter discusses whether dying babies should be used in experimental medicine, even to help another baby.

### 1984: BABY FAE

On October 14, 1984, doctors delivered Baby Fae in California. Three weeks premature, she weighed five pounds. Noticing her pallor, the pediatrician transferred her to Loma Linda Hospital, a Seventh-Day Adventist facility near Riverside. Physicians there diagnosed her with hypoplastic left heart syndrome (HLHS).

Affecting one in 10,000 babies, HLHS leaves the normally powerful left side of the heart and aorta underdeveloped and too weak to pump blood. HLHS almost always kills infants within two weeks.

Fae's mother, a 23-year-old, unmarried, unemployed Roman Catholic with no medical insurance, lived with the baby's father, a 35-year-old laborer. The two had a son and had lived together for five years, but at Fae's birth, they separated.

At Loma Linda, doctors told the mother that Fae would soon die; they kept Fae overnight in the hospital and then released her. The mother had Fae baptized and took her to a motel to wait for death. Leonard Bailey, the 41-year-old chief of pediatric surgery at Loma Linda, then suggested that Baby Fae could receive a xenograft from a baboon.

Transplantation of an organ from one species to another is called a *xenograft*. In 1964, James Hardy implanted a chimpanzee heart into a 68-year-old man, who lived 90 minutes.[1] During the 1960s, Thomas Starzl and Keith Reemtsma performed six transplants each with simian kidneys, but eventually abandoned the projects because such kidneys worked at best only two months.[2] In 1975, a British cardiologist connected veins and arteries of a dying 1-year-old boy to a live baboon, neither of whom lived through the operation. In 1977, Christiaan Barnard piggybacked a baboon heart next to the heart of a 25-year-old Italian woman, who lived 300 minutes; he later used the same technique to implant a chimpanzee heart in a 59-year-old man who lived four days.

Bailey had been aggressively pursuing heart xenotransplants for seven years, performing about 160 of them, "mostly on sheep and goats, none of whom survived more than six months."[3] During the previous year, Loma Linda's Institutional Review Board (IRB) had granted Bailey permission to perform five xenografts.

On October 19, Bailey readmitted Baby Fae and placed her on a respirator, then discussed the operation with Fae's mother, father, and grandmother. Both parents then signed a consent form, which had been reviewed in great detail by the IRB.

Bailey's immunologist, Sandra Nehlsen-Cannarella, began antigen-typing tests to find the best match for Fae among potential baboon donors. These tests took six days. Using Fae's reaction to her own blood and tissue as a control, Nehlsen-Cannarella tested various beings for compatibility: Baby Fae's mother (who had a weak immune reaction), some lab workers (strong reaction), herself (strong reaction), three baboons (strong reaction), and three additional baboons (weak reaction). A baboon named Goobers, a 9-month-old female from the Foundation for Biomedical Research in Texas, had a "very, very weak" reaction, so she became the source of the xenograft.[4]

Human blood strongly resembles other primates' blood, thus we might expect to find some close matches of blood types between humans and primates. The fact that a baboon heart could be used at all indicates a common ancestor of humans and primates. Moreover, one-third of humans have a preformed anti-body against tissue from other humans. About 70 percent of humans also have a preformed antibody against baboon tissue; Baby Fae was among the 30 percent who did not. Bailey gave this fact considerable weight, arguing that previous ignorance about human–baboon matching explained Hardy's earlier failures with xenografts.

But because chimpanzees are closer to humans in evolution, Bailey was once asked why he had picked a baboon rather than a chimpanzee. He replied, "Er, I find that difficult to answer. You see, I don't believe in evolution."[5]

On October 26, the tissue-typing tests arrived, and Bailey said Baby Fae's heart was dying and her lungs were swelling with fluid. Whether Fae was dying at this point is important: according to the hospital's spokesperson, a baboon heart was used because there was no time to find a compatible human heart, so the transplant had to take place immediately.

Bailey placed Fae on a heart-lung machine that lowered her blood temperature to 68 degrees. Meanwhile, he sedated Goobers and excised her walnut-sized heart. He then removed Fae's defective heart and replaced it with Goobers's healthy one.

Over the next four hours, he connected the transplanted heart and transplanted arteries. Then the heart-lung machine raised Fae's temperature to 98 degrees, and Goobers's heart began to beat spontaneously inside Fae.

On October 29, nurses weaned Fae from her respirator. On November 5, Bailey predicted that the animal heart would grow with Fae, and that she might celebrate her 20th birthday.

Two other surgeons who had grabbed fame chimed in. Christiaan Barnard predicted that soon medicine would have baboon farms for simian xenografts. William DeVries, said, "I really have sympathy for what [Bailey and his colleagues] are going through."[6]

Two weeks after surgery, Fae showed the first signs of rejection of the donor heart. Soon she deteriorated and went back on a respirator.

On November 15, Fae developed a heart blockage and renal failure; Bailey started closed-heart massage and dialysis. She then died, having lived 21 days with her baboon heart.

Bailey attempted no more xenografts, but other surgeons did. In 1992, Thomas Starzl at the University of Pittsburgh transplanted a baboon liver into a 35-year-old man with hepatitis B. He lived 70 days. The same year, a woman waiting for a human liver at Cedars Sinai Medical Center in Los Angeles received a pig liver as a bridge to a transplant, but she died 32 hours later. In 1993, a man with hepatitis B received a baboon liver at the University of Pittsburgh; he was 62-years-old and died during the operation.

Surgeons hope that transferring human genes into pigs will allow porcine xenografts, but none have worked to date. Even when drugs suppress immuno-rejection, a more lethal *hyperacute rejection* soon occurs in all xenografts. Since 1905, surgeons transplanted organs of baboons to humans in 33 operations, but none have succeeded.

## 1987: BABY GABRIEL AND PAUL HOLC

Like the Terri Schiavo case two decades later, the media extensively covered Baby Fae's story, making Bailey and Loma Linda household names. When the xenograft failed, Bailey used his new fame to create a center for infants with HLHS and hoped to get donated hearts from anencephalic babies.

In 1987, surgeons and medical ethicists who were sympathetic to Bailey's goal met at a conference in Ontario, Canada, and created guidelines, known as the *Ontario Protocol*, for using anencephalic babies as organ donors.

Anencephaly is a congenital neurological disorder characterized by absence of the cerebrum and cerebellum, as well as the top of the skull, resulting in exposure of the brain stem.[7] However, anencephaly "does not mean the complete absence of the head or brain."[8] Because there is a brain stem, an electroencephalogram can be taken, and autonomic functions such as breathing and heartbeat may be present. Anencephalics at birth do not usually meet the Harvard criteria of brain death.

Anencephaly is perhaps the most serious of all birth defects, because the baby essentially lacks the higher brain necessary for personhood. Anencephalics are born dying. There is no hope of growth into childhood or adulthood. The open skull is vulnerable to infection, and most anencephalics die within one week, though in rare cases some have lived for a year.[9]

Anencephalics are the major potential source of organs for other babies born needing organs, creating a major bioethical issue about whether to use anencephalic babies as such sources. When the recipient is an infant, a donor organ must be very small, so an infant donor is needed. However, few infants are involved in accidents that leave them brain-dead but with healthy organs. Babies who die as a result of abuse or from sudden infant death syndrome usually have damaged organs that are unsuitable for transplantation.

The most important guideline of the Ontario Protocol stated that an anencephalic baby could become a donor only after being pronounced dead by the classical criteria of brain death. Another guideline was that the potential donor could not be expected to live more than one week; this standard was meant to ensure that the donor was born dying. At birth, an anencephalic baby was to be put on a respirator to preserve its organs, then taken off every six hours to see if it could breathe on its own. If a baby failed to breathe for three minutes, it could be declared brain-dead by three physicians independent of the transplant team.

It should be noted that the respirator is necessary in this protocol because the normal course of anencephaly is for the heart gradually to stop beating. This diminishes blood flow, so the organs become anoxic and start to deteriorate; by the time the brain stem is dead, the heart and kidneys are no longer useful for transplantation.

Because maintaining the brain stem may prevent a potential donor from becoming brain dead, the Ontario Protocol was ill-conceived.

UCLA pediatric neurologist Allan Shewmon, an authority on anencephaly, criticized the Ontario Protocol. He held that anencephalic babies should not be used as donors at all, because there was no consensus in neurology about determining brain death in them.[10]

In October 1987, a Canadian couple, Karen and Fred Schouten, learned after eight months of pregnancy that their fetus was anencephalic. They decided to bring it to term and to donate its organs. When her heart began to fail after birth, the baby, a girl named Gabriel, was ventilated. The United Network for Organ Sharing (UNOS) was alerted, but no potential recipients were found in Canada or the northeastern United States.

Meanwhile, at Loma Linda Hospital, Bailey was working with another couple, Gordon and Paul Holc, also Canadian, whose eight-month fetus had HLHS and needed a heart transplant and who had come to Loma Linda because of publicity about Bailey's new program. The Schoutens and Gabriel flew to Loma Linda. There, the Holcs' baby, Paul, was prematurely delivered by cesarean section to get the donor heart. Three hours later, Gabriel Schouten's heart was excised and transplanted into Paul Holc's chest.

This was the first time a transplant from an anencephalic baby to another infant resulted in a baby who could grow up and lead a normal life. In gratitude to the Schoutens and to Bailey, the Holcs named their baby Paul Gabriel Bailey Holc. Karen Schouten later said that she felt good about her decision and how it had benefited Paul Holc: "Paul is very special to me because he has a part of our baby inside him. One day maybe I'll see him. I hope he comes to me when he's 30 years old and says, 'Hi. Guess what? I made it.'"[11]

In 1994, NBC aired a TV movie about the case, which ended by showing the real Paul playing in first grade and hugging the real Karen Schouten. Paul Holc, aka "The Incredible Holc," turned 13 in 1998 and was healthy and doing well.

In 2011, Karen Schouten thought that the 23-year-old was living in Vancouver, Canada, and Bailey had heard he was a mechanic there.[12]

Bailey never applied the Ontario Protocol in the Schouten-Holc case. Its first application came at Loma Linda in 1988 with Michael and Brenda Winners and their anencephalic baby. That case had a sad result: no recipients were found.

This was the first of 12 unsuccessful attempts by Bailey to transplant organs from anencephalic babies to other babies.[13] Of these 12 potential donors, 10 lived beyond the one-week limit, one could not be matched to a recipient, and in the remaining case, the physicians decided against a transplant. In 1988, Bailey suspended his transplant program. There was a de facto moratorium on transplants from anencephalics until the 1992 case of Baby Theresa raised the issue again.

## 1992: BABY THERESA

In 1991 in Fort Lauderdale, Florida, unmarried Laura Campo and Justin Pearson conceived a child. Like Fae's mother, Laura had no medical insurance and did not see a physician until her 24th week of pregnancy. During her eighth month of pregnancy, she learned that her fetus was anencephalic.

Because the diagnosis of anencephaly was made so late in Laura Campo's pregnancy, and because Campo's health was not in danger from the fetus, no legal abortion could be performed. Campo said that if she had known the diagnosis earlier, she would have aborted.

After hearing a talk show about organ donation from anencephalic babies, Campo brought the fetus to birth. Because an anencephalic is likely to have a swollen head (hydrocephalus), vaginal delivery may kill it, so Laura underwent a cesarean delivery to keep the organs healthy for transplantation.

Anencephaly occurs today in 1 in 5,000 pregnancies. Over 95 percent of these fetuses identified prenatally are aborted. Of those carried to term, 60 percent are stillborn.

In the United States, 2,000 babies a year need organ transplants; this number includes 600 babies with HLHS, about 500 with liver failure, and another 500 with kidney failure.

Since 1968, it has been technically possible to use anencephalics as organ sources. A few days after Christiaan Barnard's transplant, Adrian Kantrowitz transplanted a heart from an anencephalic baby to another infant, who died six hours later.[14] Kantrowitz had almost performed a transplant 18 months earlier, but had to wait for the anencephalic donor's heart to stop beating, and then restart it, which proved impossible.

In 1992, Laura Campo had her baby girl and named her Theresa Ann Campo Pearson. Pictures of Theresa showed a beautiful baby wearing a pink knitted cap that covered the top half of her head. Removing the cap revealed the brain stem inside a partial skull.

Under Florida law, before Theresa's organs could be donated, she had to be brain-dead. Like most states, Florida used the Harvard standard. Unless Baby Theresa was brain dead, no one would remove her organs.

The parents asked Judge Estella Moriarty to rule Theresa brain dead. But Judge Moriarty correctly ruled against the couple: "[I am] unable to authorize someone to take your baby's life, however short—however unsatisfactory—to save another child. Death is a fact, not an opinion."[15]

The couple appealed to Florida's District Court of Appeals, which affirmed Judge Moriarty's decision. The baby then began to experience organ failure. At this point, the neonatologists said, "We had to tell the parents [that] all they were doing was prolonging the baby's death."[16] They removed the respirator and Theresa died the next day. By then, surgeons couldn't use her organs.

The next day, the parents appeared on television to plead for a change in Florida's laws regarding brain death. Upset and depressed, Campo probably shouldn't have been allowed on the show. A calm, eloquent surgeon joined them and discussed the need for donor organs.

Even though Baby Theresa died, the Florida Supreme Court decided *not* to change the law and that anencephalic newborns should *not* be considered dead for organ donation.[17]

## 1993: THE LAKEBERG CASE: SEPARATING CONJOINED TWINS

Cases often occur where twins conjoined at birth are separated in long surgeries. The media often cover these cases extensively and lionize the surgeon who separates the twins. Although not generally known, the surgeon understands that she will usually sacrifice the weaker twin to create a singleton.

For example, in separating conjoined twins Angela and Amy Lakeberg in 1993, Amy Lakeberg died. Bioethicist and historian Alice Dregger writes, "Yet no matter how justified the ends, it is troubling to see surgeons actively cause the death of a child like Amy—who was obviously conscious and as entitled to the conjoined heart as her sister."[18]

In 2002, UCLA surgeons separated 1-year-old Guatemalan craniopagus (conjoined at the head) twins in a 22-hour operation. The story received saturation coverage nationwide. In 2006, Dr. Ben Carson announced he would separate 10-year-old craniopagus twins from Delhi, India.

Dregger argues that separation surgery is a modern freak show, the kind of thing that people once paid to see in exhibits.[19] In the eighteenth century, physicians paid such people to exhibit themselves. But as Dregger argues, at least back then such people got paid and were allowed to exhibit their bodies with dignity. Today, the only message they get is: "You're abnormal. We can surgically normalize you, even at risk of killing you. Be grateful."[20]

Separating conjoined twins, especially adults, may often be a reach for fame by the hospital and by the surgical team, saying, "Hey. We can do this and nobody else can! We're the top dogs!" More charitably, it may be just another version of the rule of rescue: we can separate these two conjoined babies, give them separate lives, and feel good about doing so.

In lionizing these cases and their surgeons, the media often describe twins undergoing separation as "brave little fighters," the surgeons as "heroes," and the hospital as performing operations that are "medically necessary." But is this really so?

Johns Hopkins's Ben Carson became famous in 1987 for successfully separating 7-month-old German craniopagus twins (joined at the head and sharing part of the same brain). Since then, he has written several best-selling books about his surgeries on conjoined twins and his life.[21] In 1994, he and his team tried to separate 7-month-old South African craniopagus twins, who both died during the operation. In 1997, he traveled with a 50-member team to successfully separate two Zambian craniopagus twins who faced in opposite directions and did not share any organs.[22]

In 2004, Carson attempted to separate the German craniopagus twins Lee and Tabea Block. His surgery was only partially successful, as Tabea died during the surgery.[23]

## ETHICAL ISSUES

### Use of Animals as Resources for Humans

In the case of Baby Fae, animal activists criticized Leonard Bailey: "This is medical sensationalism at the expense of Baby Fae, her family, and the baboon," said People for the Ethical Treatment of Animals (PETA).[24] Activists protested outside Loma Linda Hospital, claiming that Fae's life was not worth more than Goobers's. Philosopher Tom Regan claimed the operation had "two victims," Fae and Goobers.

Regan argued that beings who "have a life" have a *right* to life. He held that Goobers had a biographical life in that it mattered to her whether she would live or have her heart cut out: "Like us, Goobers was somebody, a distinct individual." Regan argued that all primates have equal moral value, so Goobers did not exist as Fae's resource:

> Those people who seized [Goobers's] heart, even if they were motivated by their concern for Baby Fae, grievously violated Goobers's right to be treated with respect. That she could do nothing to protest, and that many of us failed to recognize the transplant for the injustice that it was, does not diminish the wrong, a wrong settled before Baby Fae's sad death.[25]

Regan argued that even if human beings had obtained benefits in the past from using animals, it was wrong to continue using other primates this way as our resources.

Other animal rights philosophers emphasized that Baby Fae and Goobers, considering their youth and individual potential, differed more than Baby Fae and an anencephalic baby.[26] Anencephalic babies lack potential cognitive ability, whereas Goobers has more cognition, agency, and consciousness than such a dying human baby.

Some philosophers contemplated the large breeding facility from which Goobers had been bought and offered the image of a similar facility supplying anencephalic babies as sources of organs. If this image shocks, they asked, why do we tolerate such a facility for non-human primates, especially when such primates resemble us more than mentally challenged humans?

So why not use an anencephalic newborn as a donor? As we saw, this logic prevailed in the later cases of Baby Gabriel and Baby Theresa.

Bailey retorted that, "People in southern California have it so good that they can afford to worry about this type of issue."[27] Moreover, he claimed, "When it gets down to a human living or dying, there shouldn't be a question" of using an animal to save that human.

The director of Loma Linda's Center for Christian Bioethics agreed:

> On an ethical scale, we will always place human beings ahead of subhumans, especially in a situation where people can be genuinely saved by animals. That is the story of mankind from the very beginning. Animals, for example, have always been used for food and clothing.[28]

Of animal-rights activists, Fae's mother said, "They don't know what they're talking about."[29]

## ALTERNATIVE TREATMENTS?

In the Baby Fae case, was alternative treatment possible? One alternative to a xenograft for Fae was a human donor heart. Loma Linda claimed that the xenograft was necessary because Baby Fae was dying and no human heart was available. Bailey argued that it would be impossible to find a heart because the donor would have to be less than 7 weeks old, and criteria for neonatal brain death were problematical (Bailey: "You can have a flat EEG on a newborn, and yet the baby will survive").[30]

Most neonatal transplants come from anencephalic babies, and Bailey maintained that most parents of such infants would refuse to accept the fact that their baby was brain dead and would not agree to donate the baby's organs in time. He described the baboon heart as Baby Fae's "only chance to live."

An associate surgeon at Loma Linda defended Bailey:

> It would have to be the sort of case where an infant fell out of a crib and was declared brain dead but the heart was okay. Then all these tests would have to be done to insure a proper matching. With Baby Fae, we had five days to do those tests, getting the best possible [animal] donor. With a human heart, we might not have been able to keep the recipient alive.[31]

In his memoirs, surgeon Thomas Starzl describes Paul Teraski as a "symbol of integrity" in the transplant community.[32] Teraski, director of the Southern California Regional Organ Procurement Agency, said that an infant heart had been available *on the day* of Baby Fae's xenograft. Teraski added, "I think that they [the Loma Linda team] did not make any effort to get a human infant heart because they were set on doing a baboon."[33]

Bailey agreed that he didn't look for a human heart:

> We were not searching for a human heart. We were out to enter the whole new area of transplanting tissue-matched baboon hearts into newborns who are supported with antisuppressive drugs. I suppose that we could have used a human heart that was outsized and that was not tissue-matched, and that would have pacified some people, but it would have been very poor science. On the other hand, I suppose my belief that there are no newborn hearts available for transplantation was more opinion than data or science, but it is scientific to

acknowledge that the whole area of determining brain death of newborns is very problematical.[34]

Another alternative existed. Pediatric surgeon William Norwood had developed surgery for HLHS that attempted to repair the left ventricle. He had performed his operation many times at Children's Hospital in Philadelphia, with a success rate of 40 percent. Bailey claimed that children did not do well enough after the Norwood procedure to justify this operation for Baby Fae. But given Bailey's interest in xenografts, was he an impartial judge?

What about conjoined twins? What's the alternative?

Some adult conjoined twins claim surgeons and parents are prejudiced against life as conjoined adults, thinking that their quality of life is so low that likelihood of death for one during surgery to free the other is preferable.[35] Alice Dregger calls these *sacrifice surgeries* and argues that they pose challenging ethical questions. Surely they raise the most controversial assumption of all: that a chance of normalcy for one twin is worth the death of the other.

Conjoined children can live and grow into late adulthood while conjoined. Eng and Chang famously lived into their 70s; each married and fathered several normal children. Despite being conjoined at the waist, they had good lives.

But don't conjoined twins do better when separated to live separate, independent lives? This is like the problem with involuntary commitment of homeless people with mental illness: from our point of view, they'd be better off in institutions, but they themselves may not agree (see Chapter 15). Also, "conjoined twins almost invariably state that, from their point of view, they don't need to be separated to be individuals, because they do not *feel* trapped or confined by their conjoinment."[36]

Perhaps the most spectacular issue here is how little is known about long-term survival for conjoined twins who were separated and about their subsequent quality of life. As Dregger notes, the one extant study merely asked whether separated twins were later alive or dead, with no other questions asked. How can surgeons get informed consent without real data? The assumption always is: anything is better than living like as a conjoined twin.

Perhaps the best outcomes occur where physicians discover conjoined twins in utero and can separate them before birth or shortly thereafter. In one study of 20 twins (10 pairs) from 1978 to 2000, 14 survived and 4 graduated from college. All twins had several additional surgeries to correct orthopedic, neurological, and urologic problems.[37]

But is surgery better? What is the resulting quality of life for survivors? In retrospect, what do the separated twins think of the operation? Would they do it for their own children, if they were conjoined? How many mourn the loss of a twin killed in the operation?

## BABIES AS SUBJECTS OF RESEARCH

Critics objected to Bailey's surgery not because of risk or experimentation but because Bailey *used a baby*, who could not consent. In the decades since the earlier attempts at xenografts, the only new developments had been the discovery of cyclosporin and better matching of tissue, but both could have been used in a consulting adult.

In addition to questions about whether using Fae made sense medically, a more general question is whether parents should volunteer children for experiments. Protestant theologian Paul Ramsey argued that it is always wrong for parents to volunteer their children for *nontherapeutic* research.[38]

Catholic theologian Richard McCormick demurred, holding that parents can volunteer children for "low-risk" nontherapeutic research.[39] Based on the Roman Catholic tradition of natural law, he argued that just as adults should volunteer for low-risk, nontherapeutic research, infants should be volunteered for the same kind of research.

Neither Ramsey nor McCormick used the utilitarian justification of the greatest good for the greatest number. To many people, though, utilitarianism offers the most natural justification. If no one volunteered for such research, progress would halt, so for the general good, both adults and babies should participate. Because HLHS is a congenital defect of babies, how can treatment for it advance unless some HLHS babies participate?

## INFORMED CONSENT

Many people wondered whether Dr. Bailey had carefully described the Norwood procedure to Baby Fae's mother. Was she also informed that a human donor was available?

Fae's mother had no medical insurance. Bailey offered her the xenograft for free. Fae's mother had no money for the Norwood procedure or for a human heart transplant. Costs for such a transplant can be $250,000, with immunosuppressive drugs costing $20,000 a year for life.

Law professor Alexander Capron summed up this criticism:

> Doubts linger, not only about the adequacy of the information supplied to Baby Fae's parents but about whether their personal difficulties made it possible for them to choose freely, and whether the realization that their child was dying may have left them with the erroneous conclusion that consenting to the transplant was the only "right" thing to do.[40]

In most respects, the mother's poverty and lack of insurance rendered her consent meaningless. Faced with the death of her baby and no other realistic options, what else could she choose?

And was the mother informed about the probable outcome of the xenograft? Did Baby Fae's mother understand that Bailey's xenograft was a shot in the dark, unlikely to work, and a procedure that might merely extend her baby's dying?

Historically, lack of informed consent was always a problem with xenografts. Boston University law professor George Annas emphasized that in previous attempts to implant animal hearts in humans, patients were poor, vulnerable, and rarely consented.

In 1963, Keith Reemtsma at Columbia University implanted chimpanzee kidneys in a 43-year-old African-American man who was dying of glomerulonephritis. In 1964, James Hardy at the University of Mississippi implanted a chimpanzee heart into a poor deaf-mute man who was dying, was carried to the hospital unconscious, never consented to the operation, and survived for only two hours. These operations were experimental, not therapeutic, and were characterized by exploitation and lack of consent. Annas saw Baby Fae's case as a continuation of such practices. Calling Bailey the champion of the "anything goes" school of experimentation, he concluded:

> This inadequately reviewed, inappropriately consented to, premature experiment on an impoverished, terminally ill newborn was unjustified. It differs from the xenograft experiments of the early 1960s only in the fact that there was prior review of the proposal by an IRB. But this distinction did not protect Baby Fae. She remained unprotected from ruthless experimentation in which her only role was that of victim.[41]

What about conjoined twins? In 2003, Ben Carson joined the team of surgeons separating the adult Iranian women, Ladan and Laleh Bijani, who both died during the operation. Before the operation and in consenting, did they really understand the high probability that they might both die?

Alice Dregger criticizes what Carson said he told the twins in obtaining consent, that a 50 percent chance existed that one of them would die or be disabled from the surgery:

> But as a leading expert in the field, Carson surely knew of the most comprehensive study of craniopagus separations, which had concluded that "mortality and morbidity after surgical separation of craniopagus twins is horrendous: of the 60 infants operated on, 30 died, 17 were impaired, 6 were alive but ultimate status unknown, and only 7 were apparently normal."[42]

As Dregger points out about the Iranian women, at their advanced age, experts agreed that their skulls had thickened and hardened, their brains had matured and were less resilient, thus making their chances of success even worse than the dismal statistics given earlier.[43] Dregger wonders whether these women were given true information about the dismal prospects of the surgery.

The issue here resembles getting informed consent from live organ donors during the decades when no one did medical follow-up on such donors. Without evidence of long-term harm (or lack thereof), how can there be *informed* consent? Similarly, without long-term follow-up of the results of separating conjoined twins at birth, how do we know that life as a conjoined twin isn't better? Especially when society might be prejudiced against such a life?

## THE MEDIA

In 1984, the media sensationalized the Baby Fae case. True, Loma Linda tried to protect the family's privacy and confidentiality, but both the hospital and Bailey withheld more than identifying details. Their account of events leading up to the surgery was confusing, hospital spokespersons gave occasional misstatements of fact, and Loma Linda refused to release a copy of the consent form that Fae's parents had signed. Journalists complained about secrecy and the public's right to know.

This situation formed an interesting contrast to the case two years earlier of Barney Clark's artificial heart. Just as many reporters came to Loma Linda as to Utah, but they got much less information. William DeVries had held daily press briefings; Bailey held fewer. Reporters accused Loma Linda of ineptitude and said that aspects of the case begged for clarification.

While journalists accused Bailey and Loma Linda of reticence, they also accused them of publicity seeking, self-promotion, grandstanding, and adventurism.[44] In contrast, Keith Reemtsma at Columbia University gave no news conferences until his patient had been discharged from the hospital and until he had prepared and submitted a scientific paper. Reemtsma argued:

> Science and news are, in a sense, asymmetrical and sometimes antagonistic. News emphasizes uniqueness, the immediacy, the human interest, in a case such as [Baby Fae's]. Science emphasizes verification, controls, comparisons, and patterns.[45]

Law professor Alex Capron argued similarly:

> There was a time when the public learned of biomedical developments after they had been reviewed by, and generally reported to, the researchers' scientific and medical peers [a procedure that protected everyone's dignity and meant that the public would learn only of genuine advances] rather than merely being titillated by bizarre cases of as yet unproven import.[46]

Separation of conjoined twins also raises issues about use of babies in risky surgery and about surgeons seeking fame. On any given day in any major children's hospital, surgeons operate on two desperately ill infants and no one notices. Spectacular surgery occurs, teams spend weeks nurturing each child back to health, but the public is indifferent.

Now make one change and have the two infants enter the hospital as conjoined twins, connected at the head, sternum, or pelvis, and everyone takes notice. Why is that?

Can we imagine a surgeon saying to two 20-year-old conjoined twins, "If you are reasonably happy with your life together, go home and enjoy life. Don't worry about what others think or about people staring. That is their problem, not yours. You are wonderful as you are."

## THERAPY OR RESEARCH?

Was Fae's xenograft therapy or research? Was alternative treatment available? Did the xenograft have a chance to help Fae, or was she just one sacrifice among thousands on the altar of medical research?

A *therapeutic* procedure offers a patient a reasonable chance of benefit; a procedure which offers uncertain or unknown chance is *research* and *experimental*. This medical distinction can be expressed in Kantian ethics as the difference between treating people as "ends in themselves" and using them as "mere means." Essayist Charles Krauthammer wrote:

> Civilization hangs on the Kantian principle that human beings are to be treated as ends and not means. So much depends on that principle because there is no crime

that cannot be, that has not been, committed in the name of the future against those who inhabit the present. Medical experimentation, which invokes the claims of the future, necessarily turns people into means.[47]

Was Bailey's best scenario possible? Was there a probability that Fae could have lived to 20 with a baboon heart? At one point, Bailey phrased his claim differently, saying that Fae had a chance to "celebrate more than one birthday with her new heart."[48] Was this modest scenario possible?

Bailey claimed his operation had *therapeutic intent*:

> I have always believed it would work, or I would not have attempted it. . . . There was always therapeutic intent. My dilemma has been educating the university and the medical profession.[49]

He made these comments nine days after the operation, when Baby Fae was still alive and seemed to be doing well. He also said that xenografts might soon be preferable to human transplants.

Immunologist Nehlsen-Cannarella argued that, if a perfect match had been found with the best-matched lymphocytes, the operation could have been therapeutic. With such a perfect match, Fae could have accepted the heart.

Other surgeons castigated Bailey, rejecting the idea of *therapeutic intent* and saying that Bailey needed *therapeutic probability*. Almost any experimental surgery has a remote chance of being therapeutic, but that's not enough.

These surgeons also rejected Bailey's and Nehlsen-Cannarella's claim about tissue typing. In 1970, Paul Teraski had discovered that while tissue typing can improve transplants within families, it couldn't outside of families. Surgeons resisted Teraski's findings, but accepted the limitations his results suggested. Thomas Starzl wrote in 1992:

> Twenty years later the only controversy is whether matching under all circumstances means enough to be given any consideration in the distribution of cadaver kidneys. By exposing the truth, Teraski had made it clear that the field of clinical transplantation could advance significantly only by the development of better drugs and other treatment strategies, not by vainly hoping that the solution would be through tissue matching.[50]

Most transplant surgeons agreed. The American expert on pediatric transplants, John Najarian at the University of Minnesota, said of the Baby Fae case: "There has never been a successful cross-species transplant. To try it now is merely to prolong the dying process."[51] He also said that Fae's death on November 15 was "reasonably close to what could be expected," because three weeks was about how long it usually takes for rejection to do its damage.

In a review of this case, the editor of *Journal of Heart Transplantation* concluded:

> From the experimental data and past clinical attempts, there is nothing to indicate that a human infant will tolerate a primate heart for months or years using today's means to induce and control tolerance. The Loma Linda surgical team has not informed the medical community, as yet, of any new evidence that might suggest the contrary.[52]

The case against Baby Fae's transplant as "therapy" may be summed up as follows:

First, it had been known since 1970 that better antigen matches between donor and recipient would not improve transplants.

Second, even the best matches required long-term maintenance on cyclosporine, which selectively prevents the immune system from rejecting transplanted organs. Bailey claimed that infants could be given larger dosages of cyclosporine than adults, but cyclosporine eventually produces toxic side effects.[53] The autopsy on Baby Fae indicated that her kidneys were probably poisoned by the massive dosages of cyclosporine she received.

Third, Bailey argued that since an infant's immune system is not fully developed, babies might initially tolerate xenografts. But this is not certain; and even if it were true, an initial success would be followed by failure as the baby's immune system developed and rejected the xenograft.

Fourth, only one heart xenograft had been tried previously, and this had a disastrous result.

Fifth, Loma Linda was a small medical institution. In their zeal to perform a xenograft and be famous, the staff was blind to their own limitations.

Sixth, Bailey himself was an amateur: he had never performed a human heart transplant, and he had never published about xenografts.

Taking all this into account, Baby Fae had no chance of surviving one year, let alone reaching her 20th birthday. Thus, the surgery was not therapeutic but experimental. *Nature* concluded that "the serious difficulty over [Bailey's] operation . . . is that it may have catered to the researchers' needs first and to the patient's only second."[54] In his essay in *Time*, critic Charles Krauthammer said that Baby Fae had lived and died in the realm of experimentation:

> Only the bravery was missing: no one would admit the violation. Bravery was instead fatuously ascribed to Baby Fae, a creature as incapable of bravery as she was of circulating her own blood. Whether this case was an advance in medical science awaits the examination of the record by the scientific community. That it was an adventure in medical ethics is already clear.[55]

In a review of the case, the American Medical Association and top medical journals criticized Bailey, concluding that xenografts should be undertaken only as part of a systematic research program with controls in randomized clinical trials.[56]

## ETHICS AND TERMINOLOGY: INFANTS AS "DONORS"

The cases of babies Fae, Theresa, and Gabriel, as well as most separations of neonatal conjoined twins, raise ethical questions about using one infant as a resource for another. One argument against using infants as organ donors is their vulnerability. In general, the more vulnerable people are, the less defensible it is to do something to them without their consent, and babies are some of the most vulnerable humans.

In this regard, a question of terminology arises. When an infant's organ is used as a transplant, who is giving what as a "gift"? Terms like donation and "the gift of life" seem to be inappropriate in this situation; since no baby ever consents to donate his or her organs, a baby cannot really be described as providing a gift.

More accurate terms are "organ transfer," "organ recovery," "organ reassignment," and so on. Such terms seem cold, and this connotation suggests why people resist using infants' organs as sources for other infants and why organ procurement agents prefer phrases such as "gift of life."

## ANENCEPHALICS AND BRAIN DEATH

One vital question in the debate over anencephalics as donors has to do with brain death. Shewmon argued that there are no good criteria for brain death in infants, and whether or not this is true, brain death in anencephalic infants is unclear.

*Anencephaly* is a medical term describing a range of gross congenital brain deficits, all of which entail no chance of normal brain function but some of which do not entail immediate brain death.[57] The fact that most babies do not die the first week—and thus could not be donors under the Ontario guidelines—illustrates this problem, because some kinds of anencephaly are similar to a persistent vegetative state (PVS); therefore, with maximal supportive care, some anencephalic infants could survive indefinitely. One critic said, "I have an uneasy feeling that what lurks behind the anencephalic issue is the vegetative state issue."[58]

Some commentators have suggested creating a new category of legal brain death, or an exemption from the usual legal criteria of brain death, to allow for transfers of organs from anencephalic babies. Such a new category or exemption is needed for organ donation because anencephalic infants are neither dead nor about to die quickly enough, and allowing them to die naturally could destroy their organs.

So the question boils down to this: Should we change our criteria of brain death for infants to get more organs from other dying infants? Disability advocates agreed: "Treating anencephalics as dead equates them with 'nonpersons,' presenting a 'slippery slope' problem with regard to all other persons who lack cognition for whatever reason."[59]

Two physicians considered a proposal to adopt a system used in Germany, where anencephalics are considered "brain-absent" and therefore brain dead. They rejected this proposal for America:

> Not only are the brains of such infants not completely absent, but there is also a remarkable heterogeneity of morphologic and functional features in the infants considered anencephalic. . . . The causes of the neural-tube defects, including anencephaly, are complex and multiple—a fact that confounds the issue and supports the concept that the condition is quite variable. It is worrisome, but not surprising, that the diagnosis of anencephaly is occasionally made in error. Indeed, too many errors have been made for the diagnosis to be considered reliable as a legal definition of death. We conclude that anencephalic infants are not brain-absent and that the condition is sufficiently variable that the establishment of a special category is not justified.[60]

Another problem is that diagnosis of anencephaly, even as a range, is often problematic. Diagnosing brain size or brain function at birth is controversial (see Baby Jane Doe case). Will overzealous physicians and parents, wanting to bring some good out of a tragedy, declare babies anencephalic when they have some lesser defect—say, microcephaly? These media sometimes report cases of developmentally delayed children allegedly diagnosed as anencephalic but who now function well.

A slippery slope might occur here: if borderline anencephalics can become a source of organs, there might be a tendency to use infants with closely related disorders such as atelencephaly (incomplete development of the brain) and lissencephaly (unusually small brain parts). It has been argued that "the slippery slope is real," because some physicians have proposed transplants from infants with defects less severe than anencephaly."[61]

Judge Moriarty wrote in her medical review for her decision, "There has been a tendency by some parties and *amici* to confuse lethal anencephaly with these less serious conditions, even to the point of describing children as 'anencephalic' who have abnormal but otherwise intact skulls and who are several years of age."[62]

Some critics have asked whether less was being done for anencephalic babies when these babies were seen as potential organ donors. Alex Capron described the situation as follows: "By far the most fundamental problem . . . was trying to sustain an anencephalic's liver, heart, and kidneys without temporarily giving life to its brain stem, the one organ that needed to die for transplant to begin."[63]

According to the Ontario Protocol, a potential anencephalic donor is to be maintained on a respirator, but periodically removed from the respirator to see if independent breathing will occur. Is this removal in the best interest of the infant? Is the anencephalic infant really being seen as a patient? Or as an organ source? (The Pittsburgh Protocol raises the same questions.)

A counterargument here is that with anencephaly, birth is not morally relevant. That is, most fetuses diagnosed as anencephalic are aborted (indeed, anencephaly is one of the best reasons for aborting a fetus during the second term), and the birth of an anencephalic does not make a moral difference. If abortion is appropriate in anencephaly, why should it be considered immoral to do less to prolong the life of an anencephalic who is a potential organ donor? It might be argued, along these lines, that since anencephalics almost always die a few days after birth, why not allow physicians to kill them painlessly and transplant their organs at the optimal time?

Another question concerns keeping an anencephalic fetus alive to be a later source of organs, a neonatal version of the non-heart-beating donor protocol. There seems to be a real distinction between keeping a fetus alive for this purpose and simply using the organs of a baby who has accidentally become brain dead or who has unexpectedly been born anencephalic. Some critics say we shouldn't cross this line.

So how many anencephalic organ sources are we talking about? Most anencephalics are identified in utero, and most are aborted. Between 1999 and 2004, about 2,116 anencephalic babies were born, or about 423 a year.[64] If 423 anencephalics are born alive and survive immediately after birth, about half will be possible donors of hearts, kidneys, and livers; the others will be unacceptable for various reasons, including organ malformation, low birth weight, and lack of consent by family. The number of possible donors would be further reduced after blood and tissue matching. Taking all this into account, one study in 1988 estimates that *only about 30 recipients a year* would benefit from using anencephalics as sources of organs.[65]

Given that serious problems exist using anencephalics as organ sources, is even 50 babies a year a large enough number to benefit? Would it justify changing our criteria of brain death? Would it justify a departure from the so-called *dead donor rule*—that patients must be dead, must be cadavers, before organs are harvested? Most ethicists and doctors decided negatively: the numbers were too small for so big a change.

## SAVING OTHER CHILDREN

Something has been missing in the discussion so far. As mentioned, thousands of children die each year waiting for an organ. All anencephalic babies are born dying, and even near-anencephalic babies will never have lives with any cognitive awareness. Both the parents of Baby Teresa and her doctors tried to create some good out of these tragic births. Paul Holc stands as an example of a child saved who otherwise would have been lost to overzealous concern for ethics. What is wrong with that?

And, yes, dangers exist of misdiagnosis and "inclusion creep," where more and more near-anencephalic babies are used as sources. But even 50 anencephalic babies a year could save another 50 babies.

Meanwhile, the opportunity cost of doing nothing is staggering. Each day, babies who could be saved will die. Can ethical concern sometimes be a bad thing, if it blocks us from saving lives?

Another argument in favor of using infants' organs for transplants would be analogous to McCormick's argument: parents should choose for a child as the child ought to choose in adulthood. Such organs should be used for transplant if that resulted in the greatest good for the greatest number and if otherwise the organ would be wasted.

Even if, on average, 400 anencephalic babies are born each year, and even if only half of them have usable organs, why not save 200 other dying babies with transplanted hearts, livers, kidneys, and corneas?

## COSTS AND OPPORTUNITY COSTS

In the Baby Fae case, many critics questioned whether expensive resources should be spent on a single case when the same money could have done more good for many others. Although Loma Linda never revealed the cost of Fae's surgery and the associated treatment, it probably cost at least $500,000. Would it make sense to perform a thousand such operations a year, at cost of maybe $1 billion, while thousands of babies are born deformed because their mothers could not afford prenatal tests like amniocentesis and sonograms?

In the case of Baby Gabriel and Paul Holc, the surgery alone cost $140,000; in addition, there were costs of flying everyone to Loma Linda and, for the Schoutens and the Ontario hospital, the cost of keeping Gabriel Schouten alive for a week. Consider that thousands of pregnant women in the United States get no prenatal care and that as a result, many babies are born with preventable defects. Isn't the system biased in favor of dramatic surgical cases and against these anonymous women and their children?

With conjoined twins, what about costs of separating conjoined twins in 14-hour operations with dozens of surgeons? Millions of dollars can easily be spent on one case. Why is so much free care given on these dramatic cases, while other babies are ignored?

## CONCLUSIONS

There is an old saying, "Beware the surgeon with one case." That summarizes the ethics of the cases in this chapter. As Alice Dregger states, "Unlike drugs and many nonsurgical medical procedures, surgeries, at least in the United States, are largely exempt from systematic review."[66]

When experimental surgery is done, it should be in a well-conceived research design. One surgeon grandstanding for fame should not be allowed. Should Loma Linda be proud of Leonard Bailey and what happened there? Should Hopkins boast of separating conjoined twins? What's the opportunity cost of all these surgeries?

## FURTHER READING

George Annas, "Baby Fae: The 'Anything Goes' School of Human Experimentation," *Hastings Center Report*, vol. 15, no. 1, February 1985, p. 15–17.
Alice Dregger, *One of Us: Conjoined Twins and the Future of the Normal*, Cambridge, MA: Harvard University Press, 2004.
"Baby Fae: Ethical Issues Surround Cross-Species Organ Transplantation," Scope Note 5, Kennedy Institute of Ethics, Washington, D.C., Georgetown University.
Denise Breo, "Interview with 'Baby Fae's' Surgeon," *American Medical News*, November 16, 1984.
Charles Krauthammer, "The Using of Baby Fae," *Time*, December 3, 1984.
Thomasine Kushner and Raymond Belotti, "Baby Fae: A Beastly Business," *Journal of Medical Ethics*, vol. 11, 1985.

## DISCUSSION QUESTIONS

1. Was Baby Fae used as a guinea pig to advance a medical experiment? Did she have a chance to live to age 21?

2. Was it right to treat Goobers as a thing when a human donor heart was available?

3. Should anencephalic babies born dying be allowed to be used as heart donors for babies who might live?

4. How can separating conjoined twins be seen as good for the parents and the surgeons but not good for the twins themselves?

# CHAPTER 14

# Ethical Issues of Intersex and Transgender Persons

*T*his chapter begins with the case of "John/Joan" or David Reimer, who was born a boy and raised as a girl. Citing this case and others, advocates for intersex people during the last 30 years argued that surgeons and psychologists mistakenly assigned gender to children so often that such children would be better off unchanged. But the traditional view argues that a child, for happy adjustment in school and in a family, *must* leave the hospital as a boy or a girl.

This chapter generally explores cases of, and ethical issues surrounding, physicians who assign a gender to babies at birth and of intersex teenagers and of transsexual people, who often seek gender reassignment from endocrinologists and surgeons.

## DAVID REIMER

When Ron and Janet Reimer had twin boys in 1966 in Winnipeg, Canada, the Mennonite-raised couple felt joy. Eight months later, Bruce and Brian developed problems urinating from phimosis (a minor problem where the foreskin cannot be fully retracted from the head of the penis) and their pediatrician recommended circumcision. Bruce went first and his physician botched the operation, leaving him without a penis.

Devastated by this malpractice, Ron and Janet forewent surgery on the other twin, Brian, and took Bruce home, saddened that he would never be able to reproduce or have sex. Ten months later in 1967, they saw psychologist John Money of Johns Hopkins Hospital in Baltimore, MD, on television discussing the success of gender-assignment surgery.

Money, a brilliant, iconoclastic psychologist, pioneered the field of sexology. At the time, behaviorism ruled in psychology, and Money strongly believed that the early experiences of the child constructed its later gender identity.

On television, Money described how Hopkins had just performed two male-to-female sex-change surgeries and had opened a clinic for further operations. Based on his [alleged] studies of 151 pairs of hermaphrodites who had been raised male or female, Money concluded that, "The psychological sex in these circumstances does not always agree with the genetic sex, nor with whether the sex glands are male or female."[1] Money claimed that whether an adult lived as a female or male depended on how each was raised, not on their biological sex.

Money, who co-founded the field of sexology, taught at Johns Hopkins Medical School for 55 years and co-founded its famous clinic for sex reassignment surgery. He created important concepts, such as the distinction between gender identity and biological sex. *Gender identity* refers to how one sees oneself and how one behaves as male, female, or in-between. *Gender role* refers to how one acts in public, or how the public expects one to act, as a male, female, or in-between. Both differ from the idea of a *biological sex*, which is determined by one's chromosomes.

Money believed that intersex children were experiments in nature for understanding whether biology or upbringing determined an adult's gender role and sexual attraction. For centuries, this *nature–nurture debate* has been ongoing in the field of human development.

Sigmund Freud famously quipped that for women, "Biology is destiny," but Money believed Freud was wrong and that what really mattered was conditioning, early rehearsal, and socialization. Contacted by the Reimers, Money welcomed the chance to see their son and promised his help. In this embrace, Money had another motive. New evidence had appeared that exposure of the fetus to hormones during gestation organized sexual differentiation. If this were true, then people born male could not escape their sexual orientation. What Money needed was a human who was born male, made into a female, and then happily lived as an adult female.

Ideally, there would be a control, for otherwise too many factors might influence the outcomes. So for Money, the Reimers' call was a godsend, as Bruce Reimer had an identical twin brother, Brian, who was being raised as a boy.

Money convinced the Reimers to raise Bruce as a girl, calling him "Brenda," and they agreed to surgical removal of his testes. They also agreed to later create through surgery a vagina for Brenda.

But first, according to Money, it was important to create a gender identity for Brenda. Money believed that a *gender identity gate* was open only between 2 and 3 years of age, after which it closed, locking the child into a male or female gender.

At home in Canada, Brenda resisted being a girl and wanted to do the same things as Brian, such as climb trees, play with soldiers, and urinate standing up. She disliked wearing dresses, sitting with girls, playing with dolls, and going to Girl Scout meetings. The parents hid Brenda's true identity from neighbors, teachers, and relatives, who thought of Brenda as only a disruptive tomboy and who didn't suspect that Bruce was being forced into a new gender identity as Brenda.

Money stipulated that he had to see the twins twice a year in therapy sessions at Hopkins, which the parents were barred from attending. He believed it important for Brenda to self-identify as a female, and he tried to push her into femininity.

In 1972, quite ahead of any true results, Money caused a sensation at a meeting of the American Association for the Advancement of Science (AAAS) by making stupendous claims about his research. Unfortunately, his claims were fraudulent.

Whether Money knew or admitted that he committed fraud is unclear. He appears to have been a true believer and was totally committed to his view about the primacy of nurture and role rehearsal in childhood in forming later gender identity. Those who knew him suggest that some of his intensity about this issue stemmed from his own troubled early childhood in a repressive Christian sect in Australia.

Money lied about Brenda being happy as a girl and falsely claimed that her successful gender reassignment validated his theory. He also claimed that anyone could be raised male or female and be happy as a gender reassigned adult. Unfortunately, subsequent investigation showed that he committed many self-serving errors in his studies, including his study of 151 pairs of hermaphrodites.

Feminists and psychologists loved his results, for they destroyed sex-role stereotypes and raised the importance of psychology in the eyes of the world. Unfortunately, like other frauds later, this deceit had major consequences on how others acted: "Money's case was decisive in the universal acceptance not only of the theory that human beings are psychosexually malleable at birth, but also of sex reassignment surgery as treatment of infants with ambiguous or injured genitalia."[2] Money's work also helped establish Johns Hopkins as a worldwide center of gender reassignment.

Back home, Brenda increasingly resisted being treated as a female and refused to consent to upcoming vaginal surgery. When the twins saw Money, the psychologist made them strip and—in what now would be regarded as child abuse—made Brian mimic sexual copulation with Brenda as s/he was made to lie on her back with her legs spread. Nude Brian was forced to mount nude Brenda from behind. Understandably, years later, both twins felt traumatized by these sessions. Of course, Money justified these sessions by his claim that later sexual orientation stemmed from childhood sex play and behavior rehearsal.

The twins then resisted visiting Money, who always saw them in private in a building apart from the regular hospitals of Johns Hopkins. Impressed by Money's credentials, his appointment at Hopkins, and the august reputation of that institution, the parents naively trusted Money in private with their children. The twins mistakenly thought that their parents knew and had consented to what Money was doing with them.

To see if a change in school or neighbors would help, the parents moved to another city, but that move proved disastrous. As Brenda approached her 11th birthday, she fought off surgery. Things worsened for the couple: Ron drank and Janet attempted suicide. Amazingly, in published accounts, Money portrayed the parents as happy with their decisions about Brenda. He wrote about the case often, calling it the "John/Joan" case.

Like many children sexed surgically one way or the other at birth, Brenda was not told during these sessions what had been done to her. Today, some adults assigned a sex at birth by surgeons still do not know they were born with ambiguous genitalia.

Like intersex children, Brenda increasingly suffered feelings such as, "I'm a boy in girl's clothes," and resisted starting hormone shots to feminize her appearance. For six months, Money had convinced pediatricians in Winnipeg to give Brenda estrogen shots.

On a visit to Baltimore and alone with Brenda, Money introduced the child to an adult male patient who had undergone a sex change. Brenda/Bruce ran from the room, pursued by Money and staff, down a flight of stairs and out of the hospital, and was finally helped by a sympathetic employee to get back to her parents in their hotel room. There, the child vowed that, if ever forced to see Money alone again, she would kill herself.

After a team of reporters from the British Broadcasting Corporation unearthed problems with Money's optimistic reports about Brenda, doctors in Winnipeg and Hopkins grew increasingly suspicious about the case. After a crisis, Brenda's father told her the truth about her origins. Rather than being shocked, the child said, "I was *relieved*. Suddenly it all made sense why I felt the way I did. I wasn't some sort of weirdo. I wasn't crazy."[3]

Brenda almost instantly decided to live as a boy. Almost 15 years old, he started dressing as a boy and took the name "David." He switched from getting injections of estrogen to getting injections of testosterone.

As a boy, David soon started hanging out with girls and starting dating. He found a girl he liked and told her the truth about his life. She already had figured it out. She was unmarried with kids from two different men, and wanted to marry David. In 1990, they married.

David learned that false reports about his happiness were letting Money and surgeons change other children. David eventually went public and attempted to refute Money's claims. In 2002, his twin brother, who claimed he had been neglected during his childhood as "the normal one," died of a drug overdose.

David made money from a book about him, *As Nature Made Him: The Boy Who Was Raised as a Girl*, and from an attendant movie, but he squandered the money in bad investments. Then his wife left him, and all these losses—his twin, his wife, and his money—drove him to commit suicide in 2004 at age 38.

## INTERSEX PEOPLE

David Reimer's case was *not* typical of intersex people because it was entirely caused by humans: first by human error, then by human decisions. Ninety-nine percent of people undergoing sexual reassignment surgery were not made so by surgical mistakes.

In contrast, most intersex babies are born because of deviations in anatomical development of the fetus and because of exposure during fetal gestation to hormones and chemicals. Throughout history, some babies have always been born with ambiguous genitalia, partially formed sex organs, micro-organs, or organs of both sexes (historically called "hermaphrodites" from the combination of the Greek gods Hermes and Aphrodite.) To describe such people, sexologists later used the more neutral phrase *intersex* children or children with developmental sex disorders.

As in many areas of bioethics, the terms used to refer to people are controversial and in flux. Here, some advocates prefer "people with developmental sex disorders." Advocates push this broader definition to include more people. People with developmental sex disorders may be more common than often assumed and have an incidence as high as 1 per 5,000. Because of shame and secrecy, such people may be underreported.[4]

Physicians prefer the phrase "intersex people." "Intersex" includes anomalies of sex chromosomes, the gonads, the reproductive ducts, and genitals, including congenitally ambiguous genitals, contrasting internal and external sex anatomy, incomplete development of sex anatomy, and disorders of gonadal development.[5]

*Transgender* differs from *intersex* in a way that might be called internal versus external. The former usually are people who feel they live in the body of the wrong gender and as teenagers seek hormones and surgery to change to the right gender. They feel dysmorphia about their bodies. Intersex people are usually identified externally because they have non-normal sex organs.[6] Both kinds of people want the right to choose their gender and both may seek hormones and surgery to do so.

Intersex and transsexual people especially create problems in sports where athletes must compete either as female or male. In the 1970s, Yale ophthalmologist Richard Raskind underwent surgery to become Rene Richards and controversially competed on the professional women's tennis circuit against Martina Navratilova and other women. At age 76, Dr. Richards now believes it's not fair for transsexuals to compete because "it's not a level playing field" and that "maybe not even I should have been allowed to play on the women's tour."[7]

In 2009, 18-year-old South African runner Caster Semenya had been running as a girl, but gender tests showed the teenager had neither ovaries nor uterus and had internal testes producing testosterone.[8] She was allowed to keep her previous prize and some prize money, but her professional future running was unclear.

Around 1931, surgeon Magnus Hirschfield in Berlin attempted the first known surgical sex reassignments. Rudolf Richter became Dora ("Dorchen"), and another patient, Lili Elbe, had five operations, unfortunately resulting in her death. In 1952 American George Jorgensen went public after his male-to-female sex-reassignment surgery in Copenhagen to "Christine Jorgensen" and caused a sensation (*Daily News*: "Ex GI Becomes Blonde Beauty").[9] Unlike the German cases decades before, Christine received hormone therapy, which created much more successful results. By this time, endocrinology had begun to flourish as a medical field.

## CONGENITAL ADRENAL HYPERPLASIA

The most common cause of intersex is congenital adrenal hyperplasia (CAH), an autosomal, recessive, gene-based disease affecting the adrenal glands. CAH babies lack the adrenal enzyme, 21-hydroxylase (21-OH), and therefore don't produce enough cortisol and aldosterone, while overproducing androgens. Due to an excess of androgens during fetal development, females with CAH tend to have ambiguous genitalia.

Without enough aldosterone, which regulates salt retention, CAH children experience vomiting due to "salt wasting." This results in severe dehydration and, if untreated, death. Newborn screening in many states picks up this condition and it can be corrected at birth by adding or subtracting hormones or by giving salt.

Without proper treatment, CAH girls may be incontinent or have life-long urinary problems. Treatment includes medications such as hydrocortisone or fludrocortisones to boost levels of hormones. In some cases, female fetuses have been treated in utero, to which we now turn.

## FETAL DEX

In 2010, controversy erupted between bioethicists over a program using of prenatal dexamethasone (aka fetal dex) for CAH fetuses.

For the prior 25 years and in a program pioneered by physician Maria New at Mt. Sinai Hospital in New York City, fetal dex had been given to pregnant women with CAH fetuses. Dexamethasone prevents androgens from reaching the fetus, and hence, prevents development of ambiguous genitalia. Research also suggests that women with CAH treated with dexamethasone "show more typical gender behavior" as adults than untreated fetuses. Without intervention, CAH females tend to be tomboyish and more sexually oriented toward other females.

Once a woman learns of her CAH pregnancy, she must receive daily doses of dexamethasone. Treatment with fetal dex starts only if tests show a female baby affected with CAH. This often occurs with a mother who has already had one CAH baby. Treatment cannot wait until after birth because virilization will have already occurred (in other words, the female fetus has been exposed to masculinizing factors).

In 2010, bioethicists Alice Dreger, Ken Kipnis, Hilde Lindeman, and others sent a "Letter of Concern" to the FDA and NIH, suggesting that Maria New's studies were immoral and questionable.[10] In the fall of 2010, other bioethicists, led by Larry McCullough and Ben Hippen, retaliated, accusing Dreger and others of (1) improperly using their positions as bioethicists in challenging this protocol and (2) not having evidence-based beliefs.[11] Subsequent exchanges back and forth have been among the most heated in the history of bioethics.[12]

Dreger and others raised many issues about this protocol. First, why was it necessary to normalize CAH females? What's wrong with being a masculinized female? Is this some anti-butch lesbian protocol? Must medicine be used to normalize every deviance? As one involved physician puts it, "To say you want a girl to be less masculine is not a reasonable goal of clinical care."

Second, was this protocol safe? Because fetal dex was being used "off label," it was in some sense experimental. Though it's legal for physicians to prescribe off-label treatment, it's wrong for them to do research on patients without IRB approval. But it was not clear that this research was actually done. Was Dr. New doing unethical experiments on our most vulnerable subjects?

Third, was there possible long-term harm from fetal dex? For women who received fetal dex in utero, we really won't know until their lives are over.

Finally, intersex advocates such as Cheryl Chase and Sheri Groveman argued that CAH and intersex teenagers should decide later how they want to be, not have decisions made for them at birth as trumped-up emergencies by scared, misinformed, prejudiced people.[13]

In reply, traditionalists say that, if they are right, it will be too late for teens to decide their gender because by then (as Money put it) the "gender gate will be closed."

Finally, Dr. New's treatment appears to actually work and to prevent all CAH-linked birth defects in women. In 2010, federal regulators sided with Dr. New and upheld her research on fetal dex for CAH fetuses, absolving her of any charges of unethical behavior.[14]

## ETHICAL ISSUES

### What Is Normal and Who Defines It?

Eng and Chang Bunker (1811–1874), conjoined twins born in Siam, now called Thailand, traveled with P.T. Barnum's circus as "The Siamese Twins." Because they were treated with dignity and paid well for exhibiting themselves, they earned enough to buy a farm, marry two women, and have many normal children.

In 1990, conjoined twins Abigail and Brittany Hensel were born in Minnesota and now live happily together as adults. The Hensel twins had parents who taught them that the world was abnormal for rejecting them and that they were perfect as they were born. Attitudes of parents and medical staff obviously affect the self-esteem of any children born with anatomical anomalies.

In ordinary life, anatomy matters greatly. Our anatomy limits what we can do and how we experience the world. Socially, we expect behavior based on other people's anatomy. We normalize ourselves each day by cutting hair, dressing, etc. Our chaotic social world is also more predictable because of gender normalization.

John Money distinguished between biological sex and gender identity. In the transgender community today, the Gingerbread Person (a picture used to explain ideas about gender and sex) represents more choices: a picture of a heart denoting sexual orientation, a picture of a brain denoting gender identity; an arrow to the crotch, denoting biological sex; a penumbra around the person, denoting gender presentation.[15] Some intersex people orient heterosexually with the gender identity of a female, but with androgynous sex organs, and present as a man. Other biological males orient as gay males, have female sex organs, and present themselves as men. Still other biological males present as females and orient (are attracted to) to females.

Therefore, people of ambiguous anatomy frustrate us: we don't know what to expect from them or where they fit in. They create a problem for us, for society, so we seek to normalize them or regard them as freaks.

Currently, to get insurance to cover hormones for teenagers or sex-assignment surgery, patients must be diagnosed with "gender identity disorder," and it is recommended that applicants for surgery have "a year of experience living entirely as a member of the new sex."[16]

## SECRECY IN THE CHILD'S BEST INTEREST

Most families cannot accept a child with ambiguous genitalia or mixed reproductive organs. In elementary school, bathrooms do not exist for males, females, and others. For normal development, a child must have a gender identity. Therefore, it is best for the child to have a clear gender assigned, one way or the other, than to have a mixed one or none at all.

Consider normal social expectations: everyone who knows a pregnant woman wants to know the gender of her baby at birth. Many people learn the gender of the fetus before birth, setting up a definite expectation. Families express disgust at going home with, not a boy or girl, but an "it."

Intersex children are often bullied or battered when they try to use the "wrong" bathroom in public places.[17] Androgyny, having the appearance and affect of neither gender, is not a good option. If the person's sexual orientation is heterosexual, others will mistakenly interpret the lack of a clear gender as evidence of homosexual orientation.

Furthermore, most children do not need to know about their problems at birth with ambiguous genitalia. If such problems can be corrected, or given a better appearance, then the adult can live and function normally. In fact, some people may not even know they were "sexed" at birth and still live happy lives.

Finally, surgeons and parents at birth do the best they can. They believed that lack of gender at birth was a social emergency and that decision had to be made. It is wrong to second-guess them years later.

## ENDING THE SHAME AND SECRECY

In his 20s, David Reimer met Cheryl Chase, who soon became the leading advocate for intersex people and who argued that everyone should know his or her true origins and make their own decisions about their gender and sexuality.

At birth, Cheryl had ambiguous genitalia and was first sexed as a boy, but after 18 months and an unusual appearance, doctors decided to make her a girl. Cheryl's life refuted Money's claim that professionals can assign gender with happy results. Like some other intersex teenagers and adults, Cheryl never felt completely male or female and lived between genders.

Cheryl argues that, "What most harms the intersex child is the attitude that the child suffers from something shameful that must be concealed and never publicly acknowledged."[18] She argues that such children would be better off being told the truth and being allowed to choose, in early adolescence, which gender they want to be. Ideally, the parents would embrace the child as he/she is and not be ashamed.

In the late 1990s, Cheryl Chase and other intersex people challenged the view of Hopkins/Money that early surgery and hormones were good for intersex children. They picketed a meeting in 1996 of the American Academy of Pediatrics. With David Reimer's public testimony falsifying Money's claims that biology doesn't matter to gender, other intersex people emerged and claimed they were wrongly assigned a gender at birth and irreversibly harmed by it. Some who were absent had committed suicide.

During the same period, a more sophisticated view was emerging in endocrinology, genetics, and medicine about normal sexual development and intersex. Behaviorism was fading and biology was ascending.

This situation of intersex children parallels that of conjoined twins. As bioethicist and historian Alice Dreger argues, most parents consider such births an emergency at birth and ask surgeons to normalize conjoined twins into singletons, even at the cost of killing both children.[19]

Alice Dreger and Cheryl Chase argued that (1) physicians and families should wait until the child/adolescent can decide for itself what gender it wants to be; (2) physicians should help families understand that a child with intersex can be happy with an ambiguous gender; (3) if physicians and families guess wrong about gender, intersex children can be irreversibly harmed; and (4) such crises at birth about gender were socially constructed and mediated by ignorance and fear.

The American Academy of Pediatrics disagreed. In its 2000 guidelines on how to deal with intersex children, it wrote, "The birth of a child with ambiguous genitalia constitutes a social emergency."[20] By sexing a child immediately at birth, it hoped to prevent later harms, such as uterine infections, cancer, and infertility. It also hoped to provide the child with working genitalia for later sexual satisfaction and a stable gender identity. It wanted to foster parental bonding with a gender-defined child and help the child to avoid being different.

## TRANSGENDER/INTERSEX AND CIVIL RIGHTS

In the last 20 years, a remarkable change has occurred in North American culture. Not only have gay men and lesbians been increasingly accepted as normal, but transgendered people have also been accepted. Popular television shows such as *Glee* and *DeGrassi: The Next Generation* portray "trans" people. *People* magazine has done feature stories on Chaz Bono's female-to-male (F.T.M.) transition[21] and of supportive parents who allow the same transition to start by giving puberty blockers to a group of 30 transgendered children as young as 10 years old in the Los Angeles area.[22] A child of Warren Beatty and Annett Benning, born Kathlyn, transitioned to Stephen, making a video of himself in the popular series, "WeHappyTrans."

Various singers present as sexually ambiguous: Lady Gaga, Freddy Mercury, David Bowie, Elton John, George Michael, Melisa Etheridge, the Indigo Girls, K. D. Lang, and many others. Children's books such as *Parrotfish, Luna,* and *I am J* help intersex kids understand who they are at an early age.[23]

In *The New Yorker*, Margaret Talbot portrays the female-to-gay-male transition of Skylar, a precocious child living around Yale University whose parents supported his transition at a young age. She writes:

> Transgenderism has replaced homosexuality as the newest civil-rights frontier and trans activists have become vocal and organized. Alice Dreger, a bioethicist and historian of science at Northwestern University, says, "The availability of intervention and the outspokenness of the transgender community are causing a lot more people to see themselves as transgender, and at younger ages."[24]

But, as the parent Danielle of a trans (F.T.M) child named Anna worries in Talbot's essay, is this just a social fad, like tattoos and breast implants for teen-age girls?[25] Should parents be eager to support such irreversible changes before children know who they really are, and when they are subject to all kinds of peer pressure?

## NATURE OR NURTURE, OR BOTH?

When it comes to feeling attracted to members of the opposite sex, or one's gender identity, things may be more complex than either having certain chromosomes or being raised as a boy or girl.

As a graduate student in the 1970s, Milton Diamond of the University of Hawaii discovered that exposure to hormones of a region of the Y chromosome (the SRY gene) organizes pluripotent anatomical tissue into male or female sex organs.[26] Now we know that testosterone organizes formation of the Wolffian ducts, which then become the internal, male reproductive system. Mullerian Inhibiting Hormone (MIH) simultaneously tells the precursor to Mullerian ducts, out of which the internal, female reproductive system is formed, to disintegrate, allowing the fetus to develop the male sex organs.

Diamond came to believe that biology and hormones made gender identity, not childhood socialization, and hence, became skeptical about Money's claims about Brenda/David.

The work of Diamond and others explains how intersex children come to exist. A biologically female fetus over-exposed to androgens from a mother's unknown tumor, from her using steroids, or from CAH-type conditions. This will give the child and adult a masculine, or androgynous, unfeminine appearance. So "biology may be destiny," but it's a biology that's part genes and part what happens to the fetus in utero.

Diamond then became a life-long critic of John Money's views on the social construction of gender. He was also horrified by Money's attempt to use David's case for similar attempts to construct gender with other intersex babies.[27] Money attempted to suppress Diamond's criticisms and, at one convention, assaulted Diamond.

### An Alternative, Conservative View

Not everyone agrees that transsexual people should be warmly accepted or that sexually ambivalent children should be encouraged to explore alternate sexual orientations and presentations. Social and religious conservatives generally abhor such acceptance and encouragement, regarding intersex people as deviant, morally wrong, and even perverted.

One flashpoint, as with being gay or lesbian, concerns whether individuals can choose their gender identity and second, whether society doesn't push some confused adolescents into sexual orientations that are not really theirs.

## Ken Kipnis' Proposals

In 1998, Professor Kenneth Kipnis, a prominent bioethicist in Hawaii, made three recommendations with Milton Diamond about sex reassignment surgery:[28]

1. Impose a moratorium on surgical assignment of gender:
    a. without the consent of the patient and
    b. until evidence-based medicine proves that such surgery helps more than it harms.
2. Do not restart such surgery until comprehensive look-back studies show how and when benefits of such surgery can be obtained.
3. Undo the deceptions by past physicians to living patients about such surgeries imposed on them as infants. Tell them the truth.

Before agreeing to surgery on their children, Kipnis thinks that parents should be given "bullet-proof" informed consent and understand that reassignment surgery may compromise sexual sensation, end ability to have children, conflict with the later adult's feeling of true gender identity, lack proof of benefit, and be opposed by some experts.

Kipnis argued that because so few intersex children were told the truth, many don't know what happened as adults. Because of such secrecy, no long-term outcome studies have obviously been done. Like the juggernaut to normalize conjoined twins without evidence, what has been done to intersex babies has been done in "an epistemic black hole." In other words, when we ask, "How many adults seeking sex reassignment surgery were sexed at birth and never told by their parents?" we do not know the answer.

Whose responsibility is it then to tell intersex adults what happened to them? Physicians? Parents? In cases of androgen insensitivity syndrome (previously called "testicular feminization syndrome"), a couple sometimes comes to an infertility clinic to figure out why the wife can't get pregnant. Detailed, anatomical inspection then reveals that the wife is a chromosomal male. The genetic counselor then experiences the problem of how to tell the husband he's married to a biological male and how to tell the wife that she's biologically male.

Do they both have the right to know the truth? Most geneticists think they do. Of course, such revelations must be made gently and with care.

## MEDICAL EXCEPTIONS

Where not intervening to treat intersex children will be medically harmful to these children, it is morally imperative to intervene. But the definition of "medically harmful" must be very tight and not stretched to appearance to conform to social norms.

CAH is the obvious case for intervention. Another similar case is complete androgen insensitivity syndrome (CAIS), which also creates intersex children.

Some medical conditions have not achieved consensus. Although not medically threatening, not everyone seems comfortable reducing the size of a very large clitoris (clitoromegaly) to give the girl a more normal appearance later as an adult. Some people argue that this should be left alone.

Medically speaking, the long-term risk of cancer, heart disease, and other diseases are unknown from sex-change surgery and a lifetime of taking the necessary hormones. Serious questions remain unanswered about how early hormones can safely be started and whether they should be stopped after a certain age.[29]

## THE DUTCH APPROACH: DELAYING PUBERTY

In contemporary Holland, long considered a progressive country about sex, intersex children attend a special clinic where they are given hormones to delay the appearance of their sexual organs.[30] Without such delays, intersex children attempt suicide at high rates and, loathing their gender, mutilate their bodies. They frequently report feeling trapped in the wrong body, or having feelings of no clear gender.

Puberty creates a crisis for intersex children because their bodies start changing, seemingly irreversibly, into a gender they reject. It can create tremendous anxiety for a gender-identified girl to suddenly have her voice drop lower and to sprout facial hair.

Dutch professionals seek delays to enable such kids to explore their sexuality and choices about gender in a supportive atmosphere, in contrast to the one most were raised in. In such a context, some may choose surgical assignment but some may choose to live as they are, like adult conjoined twins.

## CONCLUSIONS

No parent expects an intersex child, but no parent expects a child with any disability, noticeable difference, or aberration. From this fact, it doesn't follow that physicians must try to normalize each child, guessing which way is right.

Between 2000 and 2006, the American Academy of Pediatrics revised its views on intersex babies. Its 2006 Consensus Statement no longer considers the birth of an intersex baby to be a surgical emergency.[31] Few pediatric surgeons or pediatric endocrinologists today take a decision lightly to sex a child at birth, and even fewer would sex a child against its biological gender.

Still, most parents have trouble accepting an intersex child and are uncomfortable with an ambiguous gender or ambiguous sexuality. Sex assignment before leaving the hospital may seem like a magic wand, making the problem go away— at least for a while. It is also possible that most people so sexed are happy and that only unhappy ones speak out as advocates.

## FURTHER READING

Consortium on the Management of Disorders of Sex Development, *Clinical Guidelines of the Management of Disorders of Sex Development in Childhood*, 2006, Intersex Society of North America.

Alice Dreger, *One of Us: Conjoined Twins and the Future of the Normal*, Cambridge, MA: Harvard University Press, 2005.

David Benatar, ed., *Cutting to the Core: Exploring the Ethics of Contested Surgeries,* Lanham, MD: Rowman & Littlefield, 2006.

Linda Geddes, "Puberty Blockers Recommended for Transsexual Teens," *New Scientist,* December 10, 2008.

Louis Gooren, "Care of Transsexual Persons," *New England Journal of Medicine,* March 3, 2011, 364:13, pp. 1251–1258; letter, "Care of Transsexual Persons," Walter Booking, June 30, 2011, 364:26.

Merle Spriggs and Julian Savulescu, "The Ethics of Surgically Assigning Sex for Intersex Children," in Benatar (ed.), *Cutting to the Core.*

Margaret Talbot, "About a Boy," *The New Yorker,* March 18, 2013, pp. 56–65.

Leslie Feinberg, *TransGender Warriors: Making History from Joan of Arc to Dennis Rodman,* Boston: Beacon Press, 1996.

L. Sax, "How Common is Intersex? A Response to Ann Fausto-Sterling, *Journal of Sex Research* 39 (3): 174–8.

Ken Kipnis and Milton Diamond, "Pediatric Ethics and the Surgical Assignment of Sex," *Journal of Clinical Ethics,* 9 (3), 1998.

Jane Allison Sitton, "Introduction to the Symposium: (De)Constructing Sex: Transgenderism, Intersexuality, Gender Identity and the Law," *William and Mary Law Journal of Women and the Law,* 7 (1), 2000.

Heather Draper and Neil Evans, "Transsexualism and Gender Reassignment Surgery," in Benatar (ed.) *Cutting to the Core.*

Jeffrey Eugenides, *Middlesex*, New York: Picador, 2003.

## DISCUSSION QUESTIONS

1. Could most families handle raising an intersex child of ambiguous gender? Most schools?

2. Would an intersex child with ambiguous gender be subjected to ridicule and abuse by other children?

3. One family reportedly was wrongly told their fetus was male and planned the nursery in blue. When told at birth that the child was female, the parents demanded the child be sexed as a male. When surgeons there and at another hospital refused, they went to another hospital in another state, where the operation was done. Was this wrong?

4. Is sex reassignment surgery a good thing for adults not told of their unique origins? If told, might some adults decide not to seek such surgery?

5. Are physicians and parents correct in intervening with fetal dex to prevent a female fetus from later developing masculine tendencies?

6. Should physicians and parents wait and let CAH children decide which gender they later want to be?

7. Is society prejudiced in making every teenager either a female or male, with nothing in between?

8. How does the controversy about fetal dex reflect the nature–nurture controversy about human traits?

# CHAPTER 15

# Involuntary Psychiatric Commitment

## The Case of Joyce Brown

*T*his chapter describes a homeless woman living on the Upper East Side of Manhattan who psychiatrists committed against her will for treatment for schizophrenia. Defended by the ACLU, her case raised issues about paternalism, political psychiatry, rights of mental patients, and compassion.

This chapter's key discussion question concerns whether people with mental illness who are unlikely to harm others should be committed for their own good.

### THE CASE OF JOYCE BROWN

In the 1980s, mentally unstable, homeless people overwhelmed Manhattan; mental health professionals and the public wanted something done. In 1987, New York City started Project Help to assist such needy, homeless people, but they resisted. Could Project Help seize them anyway, for psychiatric evaluation and involuntary commitment? Or should they just be left (as some defenders of Project Help criticized) "to die with their rights on"?

The first person picked up was Joyce Brown, a 40-year-old African-American woman. For 18 months, she slept outside a Swensen's ice cream parlor on Second Avenue and 65th Street, near Gracie Mansion, where Mayor Ed Koch lived. During the day, she panhandled for money to buy food, cigarettes, and toilet paper. Mayor Koch spoke to her on the street sometimes and helped Project Help choose her as a test case.

Controversially, Project Help broadened its standards for involuntary commitment beyond the standard, legal requirements of mental illness and dangerousness. It added two new criteria: "self-neglect" and a "need to be treated for mental illness."

Joyce's physical appearance suggested mental instability. Her teeth needed care; she tucked her hair under a bulky, white, knit cap. She looked disoriented, muttering to herself as she panhandled. She sometimes sang, "How much is that doggie in the window?" When residents of the block threw her money, she tossed it back. One neighbor described her as "full of rage." She cursed approaching men, but liked babies. She sometimes defecated and urinated in gutters. On bitterly cold nights, police tried to take her to shelters, but she resisted.

Project Help forcibly brought her to the emergency room of Bellevue Hospital, where against her will, psychiatrists injected 5 mg of Haldol, an antipsychotic drug, and 2 mg of Ativan, a fast-acting, short-term tranquilizer. They then took her to a new 28-bed, locked psychiatric unit on the 19th floor.

## The Legal Conflict

After psychiatrists evaluated Joyce Brown at Bellevue, they informed Mayor Koch that she was neither sufficiently insane nor sufficiently dangerous to legally commit without her consent. Although schizophrenic, Brown did not pose danger to herself or others. New York state law allowed involuntary injections only in emergency rooms; in the psychiatric unit at Bellevue, Joyce Brown refused further drugs.

Once police bring people to a psychiatric facility, their release rarely happens until a judge holds a hearing. Before her hearing with Judge Robert Lippman, Joyce called the American Civil Liberties Union (ACLU). If she would waive confidentiality and agree to publicity about her case to help other homeless people, which she did, the ACLU agreed to represent her.

Her three sisters from New Jersey testified at the hearing. Married, working, and middle class, they had been searching for Joyce for 18 months. All four girls grew up in Elizabeth, New Jersey, well-churched daughters of a Methodist minister.

They described Joyce as a "bright, attractive, and happy-go-lucky child." She had graduated from both high school and business school and had held several jobs at Bell Laboratories. During these years, she had been a "big, healthy girl" who wore nice clothes and jewelry and "always drove around in a new Cadillac."

They said that Joyce had started taking heroin in her 20s and later cocaine. She worked for 10 years as a secretary for the New Jersey Human Rights Commission (HRC). In 1982, her mental health and her job performance plummeted. In 1985, at age 38, because of absenteeism and use of drugs, the HRC fired her. She then left her family and went to a shelter in Newark, but after she assaulted someone there, the shelter expelled her.

Her sisters then tricked her into a voluntary commitment in the psychiatric ward of East Orange General Hospital in New Jersey. When Joyce was diagnosed as psychotic, psychiatrists forced antipsychotic drugs on her. She resisted and attendants put her in an isolation room. Altogether, she spent two weeks locked up there, after which she fled to East 62nd Street in Manhattan, living under various aliases. She avoided shelters for the homeless, considering them dangerous for unattached women. She shunned her sisters, fearing they would commit her again.

At her hearing, Brown spoke well, called herself a "professional street person" and answered probing questions:

Q: Why had she torn up paper money given to her? A: "I only need $7 a day to live on. I tore up additional money given to me to prevent being robbed of it at night."[1]

Q: Why did she defecate on herself? "I never did," she replied, although she had used the streets because no local restaurant would let her use its restroom. "I offered to buy something and they still refused."

Four psychiatrists testified for the city that Brown suffered from schizophrenia, should be treated in an institution, and, if left on the street, would deteriorate. They denied that this was "political psychiatry" and stated that Brown's "self-neglect" was "so severe" that she should be helped against her will. They noted that people with schizophrenia are often bright and have periods of rationality.

Three psychiatrists testified for ACLU that she was not psychotic, not dangerous, not unreasonable in her answers, and not incapable of caring for herself on the streets. In his summation, an ACLU attorney said the city had not proved that Brown showed danger to herself or others: "The only evidence the city had is that she goes to the bathroom in the streets. I see that in New York City every day, because there's a lack of public restroom facilities."

In her rebuttal, the city's attorney replied: "Decency and the law and common sense do not require us to wait until something happens to her. It is our duty to act before it is too late."[2]

Judge Lippman ordered Brown freed. He had found her "rational, logical, and coherent" throughout her testimony;[3] he said that she "displayed a sense of humor, pride, a fierce independence of spirit, [and] quick mental reflexes"; and he noted that she met none of the conditions set forth in *O'Connor v. Donaldson* (to be discussed later).

Even if all psychiatrists had considered her psychotic, he stressed that the city had not proven her dangerous to others or herself:

> I am aware that her mode of existence does not conform to conventional standards, that it is an offense to aesthetic sense. [Nevertheless] she copes, she is fit, she survives . . . [s]he refuses to be housed in a shelter. That may reveal more about conditions in shelters than about Joyce Brown's mental state. It might, in fact, prove she's quite sane. [Also] there must be some civilized alternatives other than involuntary hospitalization or the street.[4]

After the hearing, Brown's sisters called the judge's decision "racist" and "sexist." They argued that if his own wife or mother were sleeping on the streets, "he would not stand for it." They insisted that Joyce needed treatment.

The sisters then revealed that after Joyce had been hospitalized, they had gotten her declared mentally disabled and she had accordingly received $500 a month in Social Security disability payments, which they had been holding for her. Brown had refused the money, rejecting the "lie" that she was mentally disabled.

After her victory, Brown and her ACLU lawyers held a press conference, where she said, "I didn't want to play the game before, but now I am. . . . I am going to get an apartment, go back to work, and get my life together." She criticized the city for spending $600 a day on her care: "I could be living at Trump Tower."[5]

Why did Brown appear so different at her hearing than on the streets? Her psychiatrists claimed she had improved rapidly in the hospital. She dismissed their claim, asserting she had never been crazy. She resented being taken into Bellevue like "cattle" and affirmed that living on the street was a rational choice. Her sisters dismissed this assertion: "You might be able to survive one winter, or even two, but you can't survive that way forever."

Mayor Koch blasted Judge Lippman's decision: "If anything happens to that woman, God forbid, the blood of that woman is on that judge's hands." Reminded by a reporter that Lippman had found Brown lucid, Koch replied, "This woman is at risk. When she lay on the ground in the rain, in the snow, uncovered—was that lucid?"[6] When asked if Brown's commitment was "political psychiatry," Koch asked, "*Who* would claim that?" When told that it had been Brown herself, he replied, "*That alone* proves she's crazy."[7]

The city and Koch appealed to a five-member New York State Appellate Court, before which the ACLU argued that Brown would not return to the streets but would live in a supportive residence for the homeless. The city argued that where she would live was irrelevant: "She was not hospitalized because she was living on the streets [but because] three psychiatrists said she needed medical and psychiatric help."

The appellate court reviewed the testimony of a social worker who said she had observed "fecal matter" on the sheets in which Brown wrapped herself. The appellate court reviewed the testimony of another psychiatrist who said that Brown had told him she often defecated and urinated on herself. It found that "the evidence presented in this case clearly and convincingly demonstrated her past history of assaultive and aggressive behavior."[8]

The appellate court overruled Judge Lippman, saying he had placed too much emphasis on Brown's testimony instead of that of the psychiatrists. Surprisingly, the majority noted that this case required the high standard of proof of "clear and convincing evidence" rather than the weaker one of "preponderance of evidence," and that the city had met that higher standard.

After the appellate decision, Koch said, "Up until this moment, the only treatment has been a loving, safe environment. Now we will seek to treat her medically." But New York state law required the city to get a court order to medicate her against her will. In 1988, a state judge ruled against forced medication. Bellevue Hospital then released her, saying there was no point in still holding her.

After being held for 84 days and then released, Brown said:

> I was incarcerated against my will. . . . [I was] a political prisoner. The only thing wrong with me was that I was homeless, not insane. You just can't go around picking everyone up and automatically label them schizophrenic. I'm angry at Mayor Koch, the city and Bellevue. They held me down and injected me . . . They took my blood against my will. . . .
>
> I need a place to live; I don't need an institution. . . .
>
> People are treated differently just because of your economic status, [because of] what you look like and where you live. . . .
>
> I was mistreated, mentally abused, and I will never, ever, forget this.[9]

Released to live in a hotel for women run by a nonprofit agency, Brown worked temporarily as a secretary in the ACLU office. In early 1988, she became a celebrity. She received half a dozen offers for books and movies, and dined at Windows on the World, a restaurant atop the World Trade Center. She appeared on *The Donahue Show* and *60 Minutes*. She loved the attention.

She lectured to law students at Harvard on "The Homeless Crisis: A Street View." She observed, "It looks like I have been appointed the homeless spokesperson."

Then things worsened. Her roommate at the hotel said Joyce had "a lot of anger inside." While walking to work, she muttered racial slurs and obscenities to herself. By March 1988, Joyce began begging in Times Square, shouting obscenities at passersby. Asked about herself, she insisted, "I'm not insane."[10]

In September, police charged her with possession of heroin and two hypodermic needles in a Harlem housing project.[11]

During 1989, Joyce lived in a supervised residence for formerly homeless women in Manhattan. Unconfirmed reports indicated that she entered and left psychiatric hospitals between 1989 and 1994. After a decade of interventions, her physicians discovered that addiction to drugs was her main problem, not schizophrenia. At last report, she had thrown off drugs and lived on her own, and attended a daily support group for former drug users. Thus, she may never have been truly schizophrenic, and hence, never met the commitment standards of *O'Connor v. Donaldson*.

In 2000, a newspaper reported that Brown attended a talk sponsored by the Institute for Community Living and described her as "formerly homeless," as continuing to receive drug counseling, and having recently suffered a stroke.[12] According to the Social Security Death Index, Joyce Brown lived her last years in Kings County, Brooklyn, and died on November 29, 2005, at age 58.

## IDEOLOGY AND INSANITY

Early humans believed that the voices characteristically heard by people with schizophrenia came from the gods. Psychologist Julian Jaynes claims that the first humans to have identifiable thoughts experienced them as terrifying internal voices and argues that the human brain evolved as bicameral to control them.[13]

Hippocrates held that mental disorders had natural causes. Plato thought an imbalance between parts of the mind caused insanity. Roman physician Galen continued this naturalistic concept.

The Middle Ages abandoned this naturalistic approach, substituting demonic possession and exorcism. The insane sometimes were forced to live on a *ship of fools*, which sailed from port to port to take on food and water, but which never was allowed to disembark its human cargo.

From the fifteenth to the eighteenth centuries, the public saw the insane as possessed by demons, or as witches, and often killed them.

The sixteenth century saw the founding of Bethlehem Royal Hospital in London, based on naturalistic principles. It had more patients than it could handle, and hence, a slurring of its name lies behind "bedlam."

The French physician Philippe Pinel (1745–1826), head of the Bicàtre Hospital for the Insane in Paris, unchained his patients, used compassion, and looked for natural causes, all with therapeutic results.

In the nineteenth century, Quaker institutions practiced "moral treatment," allowing patients to roam the grounds, work in gardens, and live in a homelike atmosphere.

In the twentieth century, psychiatry embraced pharmacological treatments. Psychiatry then faced two related, ethical issues: commitment for political or social deviance and patient rights against involuntary treatment.

## PATIENTS' RIGHTS

If one accepts that the insane need therapeutic help rather than criminal justice, then they need no trial to commit them for treatment. In a benevolent system, committing psychiatrists act in the best interests of patients.

In the 1960s and 1970s, movies such as the Oscar-winning *One Flew over the Cuckoo's Nest* (1975) attacked such benevolent commitment as unjust. Lawyers who defended patients' autonomy argued that psychiatric diagnoses were biased, that large public mental institutions abused patients, and that psychiatry needed checks and balances. These lawyers eventually battered down the locked doors of psychiatric wards.

In this battle, psychiatry saw itself as benevolent and argued that liberal lawyers had deprived the insane of necessary treatment. It emphasized that biochemical imbalances caused schizophrenia, which could be rectified pharmacologically. However, some people with schizophrenia had to be forced to take their medications or they would fare poorly.

Thomas Szasz, a famous gadfly in psychiatry, saw no problem with patients who voluntarily sought help, because psychiatrists properly should help them. He criticized forcing psychiatrists on people like Joyce Brown—people who did not see themselves as mentally ill and who resisted intervention. Szasz held that such involuntary commitment rarely benefited the patients and politically existed to rid society of strange people.

Szasz essentially argued that a physical disease, such as AIDS or cancer, has a physical cause. Some mental illnesses have a physical cause in the brain, and these mental illnesses are real. But pseudo mental illnesses have no physical cause and merely result from problems in living. A mental illness with no physical cause, Szasz famously held, is a *myth*, not a disease. (Szasz did not claim, as some critics say, that most mental illness is a myth.)

Szasz concluded that psychiatry could not be objective, or value-free, in social cases. He held that it is "much more intimately related to problems of ethics than is medicine in general."[14] Consider that interpersonal relations—relationships between wife and husband, between the individual and the community, among colleagues, among neighbors—inevitably involve stress, conflict of interests, and strain. Much of this disharmony has to do with incompatible values, and to pretend that psychiatrists can offer value-free approaches to resolving them is ludicrous: "Much of psychotherapy revolves around nothing other than the elucidation and weighing of goals and values—many of which may be mutually contradictory—and the means whereby they might best be harmonized, realized, or relinquished."

Szasz wonders who truly defines norms of "correct" and "psychotic" behavior. He opposed classification of personality disorders as mental illness. According to him, psychiatry presumes that love, continued life, stable marriage, kindness, and meekness indicate mental health, whereas hatred, homicide, suicide, repeated divorce, chronic hostility, and vengefulness indicate mental illness. These presumptions are evaluative, not factual.

A famous study by D. Rosenhan, "On Being Sane in Insane Places," figured famously in movements for rights of patients. In this study, several sociologists, psychiatrists, and others voluntarily entered mental hospitals, saying they heard voices—a major symptom of schizophrenia.[15] Once committed, they acted normally and no longer mentioned their voices. Because of the label "schizophrenic" in their medical charts, the staff continued to see them as schizophrenic. Ironically, although the staff did not see through the sham, several of the genuine mental patients did.

## LEGAL VICTORIES FOR PSYCHIATRIC PATIENTS

In 1972, in *Wyatt v. Stickney*, Alabama federal judge Frank Johnson ruled that a committed mental patient must either receive treatment or be released. Johnson's decision specified the institutional conditions necessary to ensure minimal treatment: at least two psychiatrists, 12 registered nurses, and 10 aides for every 250 patients. Even in 2000, many states for years had not met this minimal standard.

Johnson required state mental institutions to provide individualized treatment plans, to allow patients to refuse invasive electroconvulsive therapy and lobotomies, and to establish the least restrictive conditions necessary for treatment.

Johnson's ruling prefigured the *O'Connor v. Donaldson* decision by the U.S. Supreme Court in 1975.[16] In 1943, at age 34, Kenneth Donaldson got into a fight with coworkers over politics and someone knocked him out. His parents considered him crazy and petitioned a Florida judge to commit him. Committed, he underwent 11 weeks of electroshock treatment and was then released.

In 1956, while he was visiting his parents in Florida, his father asked for a sanity hearing for Kenneth, saying that his son had a persecution complex. The judge then committed Donaldson to the Florida State Mental Hospital, where he was held against his will for 15 years. During those years, he constantly petitioned the courts for a new hearing. All the while, he rarely saw a physician and never received treatment. Inside the institution, staff presumed him insane and—like Rosenhan's impostors—he could not prove otherwise. In 1971, when his case was about to be heard, officials released him.

A lawyer then helped Donaldson sue for damages against the superintendent of the institution, J. B. O'Connor. The case reached the Supreme Court, which decided for Donaldson, ruling that he should not have been held against his will, even if he was mentally ill, unless he had been dangerous to himself or others and had no means of existing outside the institution.

*O'Connor v. Donaldson* established two necessary conditions for involuntary commitment:

1. Suffering from mental illness (being "insane").
2. Being dangerous to others or being dangerous to oneself.

Note that both conditions—insanity and danger to oneself or others—must be met for involuntary commitment. Judges later interpreted dangerousness as imminent risk to life or imminent risk of bodily harm; "imminent" means within days or hours. Two psychiatrists arbitrate. Evidence of dangerousness to oneself can consist of attempted suicide, threats of suicide, and gross neglect of basic needs.

With these legal changes, the courts moved from a medical model of civil commitment, which had been used in the early 1960s, to a patient's rights model in the 1970s.

In the 1990s, many states added a third requirement for involuntary commitment:

3. Provision of the least restrictive environment by the institution.

Conditions 1 (mental illness) and 2 (dangerousness) applied in all states, since the Supreme Court had established them; two-thirds of the states also applied condition 3 (least restrictive environment).[17]

In some states, the *O'Connor* criteria have been interpreted to mean that a person must commit an *overt act* before a hearing occurs for involuntary commitment. This interpretation is controversial and has been opposed by relatives, who can often perceive a pattern of threats and hostility and do not want to wait until someone is injured or killed before a hearing takes place. At present, courts and legislatures are struggling with the implications of this "overt act" requirement.

## DEINSTITUTIONALIZATION

These legal decisions entailed the release of many mental patients from large state institutions because such institutions often could not provide individualized treatment (as required by *Wyatt*) and they were not the least restrictive environment for patients.

Other factors also contributed to *deinstitutionalization*. New psychotropic medications allowed more outpatient treatment. In 1963, the Kennedy administration advocated small, community-integrated facilities rather than large, impersonal state institutions. In the words of President Kennedy, "Reliance on the cold mercy of custodial isolation will be supplanted by the open warmth of community concern."[18] Other factors pushing deinstitutionalization in the 1970s included tight budgets, psychiatrists who sought lighter workloads, and a general distrust of authority.

All these factors emptied American mental institutions. By 1980, state institutions released 50 to 75 percent of their mental patients. In 1955, nearly 560,000 patients lived in state mental institutions; in 1988, only 130,000 did so. All levels of government saved money, this pleased the ACLU, and mental patients flooded into communities.

But the "warmth of community concern" envisioned by John Kennedy did not appear. Communities rejected halfway houses. Mental patients scraped by on warm-air grates more often than in group homes. Bag ladies suddenly appeared on city streets. Charities set up soup kitchens for hungry street people. In the

1980s, Reaganites hailed soup kitchens as proof that the homeless didn't need government housing, rather than seeing it as a Band-Aid.

Fifty years after Kennedy began it, deinstitutionalization has failed to help people with mental illness because governments never allocated funds for community homes; because communities rejected half-way homes; because mental health services were fragmented among county, state, and federal agencies; because housing was scarce; and because the legal pendulum had swung toward patients' rights.[19]

During the month psychiatrists released Joyce Brown from Bellevue, under its expanded criteria, Project Help helped 466 homeless mentally ill people. It estimated that 800 to 1,000 such people still lived on Manhattan's streets.

When New York City officials planned Project Help, they assumed that people such as Joyce Brown would stay for a few weeks in psychiatric hospitals and would then be moved into community facilities, where they would live under supervised conditions. When Project Help picked up these people, however, they were far sicker than had been expected. Many more places were needed in psychiatric hospitals than had been expected.

## VIOLENCE AND THE MENTALLY ILL HOMELESS IN THE CITIES

In 1977, Juan Gonzalez, a homeless man suffering from symptoms like Joyce Brown's, went berserk on the Staten Island Ferry and, with a sword, killed two people. As a result, the public clamored for incarceration of potentially dangerous mentally ill people.

The concept of potential danger soon came to be used to justify holding someone temporarily for a cool-down observational period. Gonzalez had been picked up for just such a period just before the killings and diagnosed as a paranoid schizophrenic, but he had not been considered imminently dangerous to others, so he was discharged.

In 1991, Keven McKiever, a homeless man who had gone to Bellevue Hospital seeking care and had been turned away, stabbed to death Alexis Walsh, a former Radio City Rockette. In 1993, Christopher Battiste, a homeless mentally ill drug abuser, murdered an elderly woman in the Bronx

Larry Hogue, a homeless, mentally ill African-American Vietnam veteran, sometimes lived peacefully on a street corner in the Upper West Side of Manhattan, but when he took illegal drugs, he became hostile, violent, and what *60 Minutes* called the "wild man of 96th Street." A judge ruled that he could be involuntarily committed for detoxification, but that would need to be released "as soon as he decides to seek outpatient care."[20]

In 1999, two schizophrenic men not taking their prescribed medications pushed innocent people in front of oncoming subway trains in New York City, killing a young woman named Kendra Webdale and leaving the other victim without legs. Both men had a history of violence. In previous years, similar events had occurred:

Reuben Harris, who suffered from paranoid schizophrenia, had 12 hospitalizations and a history of violent behavior, pushed Song Sin to her death in the same manner in 1995. Jaheem Grayton, who also had a history of violence and severe mental illness, pushed Naeeham Lee to her death after struggling to steal her earrings in 1996. Mary Ventura pushed Catherine Costello into the path of a subway train in 1985, three weeks after being discharged from a psychiatric hospital.[21]

These cases resulted in passage in New York in 1999 of *Kendra's Law*, where a psychiatrist or relative can force hospitalization for a mentally ill person who has been hospitalized within the last three years, who has a history of violence, and who will not take his medication. Forty-five states have passed laws implementing such Assisted Outpatient Treatment programs, where outpatients can be forced to take medications and remain under supervision (Maryland, Massachusetts, New Jersey, New Mexico, Connecticut, and Tennessee have not).[22]

The courts and the general public have come to expect psychiatrists to be able to predict dangerousness among the mentally ill, but can they? To assess the potential for violent behavior, emergency-room psychiatrists simply ask patients about their own tendencies toward violence and their own past acts of violence.[23] This is not a sophisticated tool, although in practice this question seems to work better than any other test.

The famous legal decision *Tarasoff* should be noted here.[24] In this case, Prosenjit Poddarin confided in 1969 to his psychotherapist at the University of California that he planned to kill Tatiana Tarasoff, which he did. Tarasoff's parents sued the therapist and claimed the university should have broken confidentiality and warned the girl and her parents of Poddarin's threat. The actual decision has been misinterpreted to say that therapists must breach confidentiality to warn potential victims when life is at stake. In fact the 1976 decision merely said that, in such situations, therapists have a duty to take "reasonable steps" to protect potential victims, such as notifying police or seeking involuntary commitment of the person making the threat.

## ETHICAL ISSUES

### Paternalism, Autonomy, and Diminished Competence

*Paternalism* in medicine is treatment of adult patients as incompetent children who do not know their own best interests. Under which conditions might paternalism be justified? One condition is *temporary incompetence*, followed by a return of competence. In these situations, if patients later agreed with paternalism, for example, where people prevented from committing suicide later agreed that they were glad to be alive, it could be justified.

Questions about patients' competence underlie any discussion of paternalism. The American legal system tends to treat mental patients as if they were either totally competent or totally dysfunctional and thus subject to involuntary treatment. Many observers argue that this is a false dichotomy. Competence is not an either-or capacity, but a matter of degrees on a gradient.

Another question concerns proof of competence and incompetence. This issue is not necessarily clear-cut: psychiatrist Virginia Abernethy argues, for instance, that "disorientation, mental illness, irrationality, [and] commitment to a mental institution do not conclusively prove incompetence."[25]

Abernethy describes the case of "Ms. A," a highly intelligent, independent woman who lived alone in a large house with six cats, in an unheated garbage-strewn room.[26] After a fire in her house, Ms. A was hospitalized but found competent and released. As winter came, a concerned social worker investigated; her feet were black, ulcerated, and bleeding. When he tried to take her to a hospital, she chased him away with a shotgun. The police later came and forcibly hospitalized her. Her feet were diagnosed as gangrenous, and surgeons wanted to amputate; when she refused, psychiatrists began to evaluate her.

It turned out that Ms. A's feet had blackened once before, a few years earlier, and she had recovered. She now hoped for another recovery, but the psychiatrists interpreted this as "psychotic denial" and tried to get her to say that she wanted to live, so that they could amputate. She refused, avoiding their questions. Ms. A was faced with a dilemma: either she had to let the surgeons amputate, or she had to let the psychiatrists conclude that she was in denial and therefore psychotic. It might seem unfair to present a patient with such a choice, and trying to avoid the choice would seem to be reasonable. Amazingly, according to Abernethy, "Her rejection of the two-choice model became the grounds, finally, for concluding that Ms. A was not competent to refuse amputation."

Abernethy analyzed the psychodynamics of this process. First, a false aura of medical emergency "pervaded the psychiatric consultations and judicial process." Second, "Ms. A herself was quick to anger and regarded most interactions with medical personnel as adversarial." Third, Ms. A's anger created anger in those evaluating her competence: "Professionals who think of themselves as altruistic, or at least benevolently motivated, may be particularly sensitive to hostility because they feel deserving of gratitude." Abernethy says that psychiatrists are outcome-oriented and cannot tolerate a patient's self-destructiveness, even in the name of autonomy and even when self-destruction results from an underlying disease that they cannot stop. Abernethy emphasizes that "hope is not a criterion of psychotic denial."

In some ways, Joyce Brown resembled Ms. A. Like Ms. A, she rejected her diagnosis, hoped that she was sane, and thought she could take care of herself. She saw psychiatrists as enemies. Though psychiatrists acknowledged both women to be generally competent, the doctors claimed both women had a *focal incompetence,* a specific ineptitude to make decisions about their own treatment. Abernethy notes, "The criterion of a focal delusion is dangerously liable to error because a patient can easily be seen as delusional in an emotionally charged interchange, when in other circumstances he addresses the same issue appropriately." Abernethy sums up: "Competence is presumed and does not have to be proved. Incompetence has to be proved."

## HOMELESSNESS AND COMMITMENT

What really mattered in the Joyce Brown case—insanity or homelessness? The ACLU, noting that Brown did not want to leave the street and had never been proven dangerous, argued that her presence embarrassed the rich people in her neighborhood. New York City had thousands of people like her, so why was there no outcry about others? Why did no one write letters to the *New York Times* about the Joyce Browns in the Bronx? Once Brown was gone, how many of her former neighbors on the Upper East Side inquired about her?

Norman Siegel, executive director of ACLU, extended this argument to Koch and the city as well: "In sweeping up the homeless, the Mayor is attempting to place these people out of sight and out of mind and hide the crisis from the public consciousness." Siegel claimed that Project Help targeted areas seen by tourists and inhabited by the rich.

Mayor Koch emphasized that homeless people were picked up for treatment, not to remove them from public places. Homeless people gravitated to rich areas because they were safer there and such places offered them better opportunities for begging.

Koch claimed that Brown's insanity was the true issue and her homelessness merely a side issue. Her ACLU lawyers disagreed: "The Joyce Brown story has captured the issue of the homeless that a lot of people have been trying to deal with for years."[27] Koch's goal, the ACLU implied, was to get homeless people off the streets, not to treat the mentally ill; Koch didn't seem worried about people with schizophrenia who camped out in bad neighborhoods.

The ACLU suggested reinstating public baths (which had been widely available in the city during the Depression) and using condemned housing as temporary shelters. Incarcerating the homeless "for their own good" was cheap; building homes for street people costs much more.

No one could deny that affordable housing was rare in New York City. The problem of creating permanent housing for the city's homeless had frustrated many good minds. The city maintained thousands of families in squalid welfare hotels at exorbitant rates. Critics feared that providing rented housing would encourage more people to depend on such government handouts. They also pointed out that the city was one of the most expensive places in the United States in which to subsidize public housing.

## PSYCHIATRY AND COMMITMENT

During this case, ACLU lawyer Robert Levy and psychiatrist Robert Gould, both of whom testified for Brown, emphasized the political dangers of involuntary roundups, handcuffing, forcible injections of medication, and confinement in locked wards. Levy and Gould said that Brown had been examined at least five times previously and had been found "not to require involuntary hospitalization." They claimed that nearly half of the 215 people brought to emergency rooms by Project Help did "not require involuntary hospitalization." They argued that to allow "preventive detention based solely on nebulous predictions of 'future self-destructive behavior'" would invite abuse. They warned of "totalitarian regimes" using psychiatry for control of dissidents.[28]

When confronted with arguments like this, Mayor Koch replied, "This is not political psychiatry! This is not Russia! We're trying to *help* this woman!"

On the other hand, how broadly should standards of commitment sweep? In cases like Brown's, how many people might be forced into mental hospitals by relatives? (Isn't this what Barbara Streisand portrayed in *Nuts*?) How many psychiatrists might use medication, time-out rooms, restraints, and continued commitment not as treatment but as punishment for patients who thwart their will?

Part of the debate about Brown's case concerned the ability of psychiatry to help people with schizophrenia. Judge Lippman noted that the four city and three ACLU psychiatrists had disagreed dramatically, and concluded, "It is evident that psychiatry is not a science amenable to the exactness of mathematics or the predictability of physical laws."

Most psychiatrists objected. They pointed to people with schizophrenia who were dysfunctional, but who gained years of ability after being forced to take medication. They said that such patients stabilize and become free from delusions and that many patients, if they take their medication regularly, can return to life outside institutions. The psychiatrist Paul Chodoff defended limited involuntary commitment as follows:

> Is freedom defined only by absence of external constraints? Internal physiological or psychological processes can contribute to a throttling of the spirit that is as painful as any applied from the outside. The "wild" manic individual without his lithium, the panicky hallucinator without his injection of fluphenazine hydrochloride and the understanding support of a concerned staff, the sodden alcoholic—are they free? Sometimes, as Woody Guthrie said, "Freedom means no place to go."[29]

In fact, many people suffering from paranoid schizophrenia can be improved by treatment. The big issue here is whether some should be forced to be so improved.

## SUFFERING AND COMMITMENT: BENEFIT AND HARM

Columnist Ellen Goodman argued that the ethical questions in this case boiled down not to whether people like Joyce Brown would harm themselves, but whether they suffered. Brown should be taken off the streets, she argued, before she dies there "with her rights on."[30]

But was the matter so straightforward? To say that commitment is justified to end suffering assumes first that a person is really suffering, and second that involuntary psychiatric commitment will stop that suffering.

Consider the first assumption, that the person suffers. When someone like Joyce Brown protests that she does not need or want help, it can be asked, as Thomas Szasz asked, who determines—other than the patient herself—that she is "suffering" enough to be locked inside a psychiatric ward? Who bears the onus of proof, the patient or the psychiatrist?

With regard to the second assumption, that involuntary commitment can help, it is important to consider the nature of involuntary commitment. What Brown feared most was another commitment to an inpatient unit like the one at East Orange Hospital. Would she really be helped by involuntary psychiatry, involuntary medication, and involuntary therapy in a locked unit within a large public institution? In another time-out room?

Brown's court-appointed psychiatrist found that she suffered from "serious mental illness" and would benefit from medication—but that she would suffer more from forced treatment than from the mental illness itself. In such a situation, she might harm herself while trying to resist the administration of antipsychotic medications and tranquilizers.

Moreover, the long-term side effects of antipsychotics of this period were as bad as the original disorder: administered over years, they created tardive dyskinesia in 10–25 percent of patients. This condition impairs voluntary movement, is untreatable, and when the medication is stopped, persists in two-thirds of the affected patients.

It can also be argued that the potential benefits of involuntary treatment cannot be defined objectively. Most psychiatrists think that people such as Brown benefit from living on medication and by losing their inner voices. But aren't benefit and harm, above the level of basic needs, defined by each person's own self-concept and life plans? As three lawyers write:

> When faced with an obviously aberrant person, we know, or we think we know, that he would be "happier" if he were as we are. We believe that no one would want to be a misfit in society. From the very best of motives, then, we wish to fix him. It is difficult to deal with this feeling since it rests on the unverifiable assumption that the aberrant person, if he saw himself as we see him, would choose to be different than he is. But since he cannot be as we, and we cannot be as he, there is simply no way to judge the predicate for the assertion.[31]

Isn't it a shaky application of paternalism to say that Joyce Brown had to be treated so that she could obtain someone else's idea of a benefit? Psychiatrists imply that mentally ill patients suffer internal pain, but if that is so, why don't all patients want to get rid of it? Isn't it illogical—isn't it begging the question—for psychiatrists to explain that patients don't want to get rid of this pain because they're crazy?

What makes us go round and round on this issue is that schizophrenia *is a disorder of thought*. So some people with such disorders of thinking will in fact fail to understand their obvious best interests.

## HOUSING FOR THE MENTALLY ILL AS AN ETHICAL ISSUE

Recently, the term "homeless" has been attacked by a new wave of critics as inappropriate for the wandering mentally ill; instead, "substance abusers who lack housing" has been substituted. Critics challenged the ACLU's view that people like Joyce Brown are primarily victims of a greedy or indifferent society which failed to provide affordable housing; they say there is evidence that as many as 85 percent of panhandlers are alcoholics, substance abusers, or mentally ill—and that all of these people need treatment.[32] These new critics advocate mandatory treatment and police intervention to prevent panhandling. They urge people not to give money to beggars, saying that those who do give money are "enablers of addiction."

Supervised group homes remain an elusive ideal, except in a few enlightened states such as Vermont and New Hampshire. Whether we are discussing severely physically disabled people like Larry McAfee, welfare reform, or the mentally ill homeless, the best living facility for many people is a supervised group home. Living in such a home is much better than being warehoused in a large institution or being left to fend for oneself. Supervised group homes in safe neighborhoods are the perfect compromise between institutionalization and independence.

Deinstitutionalization has continued. In 1993, in New York, 2,400 new group home beds had been planned in preparation for the release of 1,000 more people with mental illness from large institutions in 1994, but the number of new beds was later cut to 800. When New York's highest court ruled in 1993 that the city must provide housing for homeless mentally ill patients discharged from city hospitals, the city estimated that it would cost $300 million to do so and disputed the ruling. Nine years later, a study by the *New York Times* exposed widespread failings in the city's adult homes for mentally ill people, "allowing some of its most vulnerable citizens to be exploited in a system plagued by inept, wasteful and fraudulent services."[33]

Many cities emulated New York City's mayor Rudolph Giuliani, who forced homeless people off the streets in the 1990s and into city-funded shelters away from tourists and the affluent. Cities such as Sacramento, Seattle, and Atlanta forced homeless people to move out and did not build new shelters. After the recession of 2007–2009, many of America's largest financial institutions almost failed, saved by a $700 billion bailout. The effects of this collapse are still being felt in the collapse of public services for the poor, and housing for people with schizophrenia has been especially hard hit.

When cities tried to build group homes, fights ensued. Residents on Earle Street in Greenville, South Carolina, one of its oldest neighborhoods, sued in 1994 when charities tried to open a sixth group home there. In Alabama, Birmingham's Southside, Forest Park, and Avondale neighborhoods had too many group homes, while surrounding, affluent suburbs had none. All around the country, certain neighborhoods in each city became categorized as the preferred area for group homes, where too many were built. Such identification made other neighborhoods passionately resist having even one such home there, lest more follow.

In the twenty-first century, lack of housing remains a problem for mentally ill homeless people, who are often also plagued by drugs, dysfunctional families, and poverty.

Medical research on vulnerable people with schizophrenia is discussed in an excerpt from Gregory Pence's *Elements of Bioethics*. To read "Can Research on People with Schizophrenia Be Just?" go to Chapter 15 in the Online Learning Center (OLC) at www.mhhe.com/pence7e.

## MASS SHOOTINGS AND THE MENTALLY ILL

The shootings at Columbine and Aurora, Colorado, at Sandy Hook Elementary School in Connecticut, and of Representative Gabby Giffords and staff in Arizona by mentally ill people with semi-automatic weapons have made Americans afraid of people with schizophrenia. At the same time, one study in 2000 found that nearly half of "rampage murders" were committed by mentally ill people.[34] Another study found that the number of state hospital beds for the mentally ill has declined, because of cuts to funding, to a rate per capita comparable to the year 1850 in the United States.

## FURTHER READING

Alice Baum and Donald Burnes, *A Nation in Denial: The Truth about Homelessness*, Boulder, CO: Westview, 1993.

Paul Chodoff, "The Case for Involuntary Hospitalization of the Mentally Ill," *American Journal of Psychiatry*, vol. 133, no. 5, May 1976.

Saul Feldman, "Out of the Hospitals, onto the Streets: The Overselling of Benevolence," *Hastings Center Report*, vol. 13, no. 3, June 1983.

Charles Krauthammer, "How to Save the Homeless Mentally Ill," *New Republic*, February 8, 1988.

J. Livermore, C. Malmquist, and P. Meehl, "On the Justification for Civil Commitment," *University of Pennsylvania Law Review*, vol. 117, November 1968.

The video "Brown v. Koch" from *60 Minutes* may be available for purchase for a reasonable fee.

## DISCUSSION QUESTIONS

1. "The easiest way to become homeless in America is to lose your job, lose your medical insurance, and be unable to afford housing. It can happen to anyone." Is this true, or do people usually screw up, say, by using drugs, when they lose their jobs and places of living?

2. "When faced with an aberrant person, we think he would be happier if he were as we are. . . . But since he cannot be as we, and we cannot be as he, there is simply no way to judge the predicate for the assertion."[35] This "problem of other minds" in psychopathology has its limits. Shouldn't some crazy people be helped for their own good?

3. Are most problems of psychotherapy problems of values, as Szsaz says, about which psychiatrists have no special training or insight, and for having different values should people be involuntarily committed?

4. During his administration as mayor of New York City, Rudy Giuliani used heavy-handed police tactics to rid Times Square and other tourist areas of Manhattan of homeless people. Was he justified in doing so by the greater good? Today, you see maybe 1 percent of the number of homeless people that one saw in Joyce Brown's time on the streets.

5. Has destitutionalization worked for the best interests of people with mental illness, especially as community centers never came about?

# CHAPTER 16

# Ethical Issues in Testing for Genetic Disease

$T$ his chapter discusses two large themes: (1) is it wise to test in advance for genetic disease, and (2) can at-risk people do anything to avoid genetic diseases? The chapter focuses on two strong women, Angelina Jolie and Nancy Wexler, and their decisions to take or not take such presymptomatic tests. It discusses such testing for Huntington's disease, breast and ovarian cancer, Type 2 diabetes, and Alzheimer's disease.

## CASE 1: ANGELINA JOLIE AND GENETIC TESTING FOR CANCER

In 2013, movie star Angelina Jolie wrote of a personal medical decision in an op-ed essay in the *New York Times*.[1] For a decade, her mother, Marcheline Bertrand, had fought both breast and ovarian cancer and died of it at age 56. Bertrand's own mother had died of ovarian cancer at age 45.

Jolie paid $3,000 for presymptomatic tests for analysis of BRCA1 and BRCA2 genes, which have lethal variants that carry an 87 percent risk of breast cancer and a 40 percent risk of ovarian cancer. Her tests came back positive for the bad variant or, as she put it, the "faulty" gene.

Given how her mother died, and given her results, Jolie decided at age 37 to have a preventive double mastectomy. Three months after the private operation, she went public and caused a sensation. Actor Brad Pitt, her partner, supported her decision.

She wrote that, after the mastectomy, her risk of developing breast cancer had dropped from 87 percent to under 5 percent.

In 1990, Mary Claire-King discovered a mutation in a single gene, BRCA1 (BReast CAncer1) causing one form of breast cancer and ovarian cancer. In 1995, Alan Ashworth discovered another variant in another gene, BRCA2. In 2002, researchers discovered a third gene, CHEK2. Mutations in any of these genes can cause breast cancer.

As said, women (and some men) in families expressing mutations in these genes run an 80 percent risk or higher of developing breast cancer, compared to a

9 percent risk for other women. Both BRCA1 and BRCA2 are autosomal dominant genes, meaning that if the women live long enough, they carry a high chance of getting breast cancer.

Is most breast cancer caused by one gene? No. Indeed, 95 percent of breast cancer is *not* caused by a single gene.

But Angelina Jolie was at risk for the 5 percent that is caused by a mutation in BRCA1/BRCA2, which is more prevalent among Ashkenazi Jews and families with a history of breast/ovarian cancer.

The same mutation also put Jolie at a 50 percent risk of ovarian cancer, a very lethal disease, so Jolie planned to have her ovaries removed before she turned 40, after which she will likely experience early menopause.[2]

## BACKGROUND: BASIC GENETICS

The gene is the basic unit of heredity. Packed inside each of the 46 chromosomes in humans is a complicated strand of interwoven DNA, the famous double helix. The number of genes varies on each chromosome.

The Human Genome Project, one of the greatest projects in the history of science, began in 1993, cost $3 billion, finished in 2003, and mapped all the human genes.

Knowing which parts of DNA are genes, and where they are, begins genetic knowledge. In the next steps, scientists must identify what genes do, how they interact with other genes, and through which mediating proteins. Genetic diseases stem from harmful variants in standard genes, such as Angelina Jolie's variant of BRCA1.

Varying environmental inputs determine how genes express themselves. Exposure of the fetus to drugs, nutrition in childhood, and use of tobacco affects how genes control bodily characteristics. This is called the *norm of reaction*.[3]

*Genetic diseases* are inherited disorders. Some genetic diseases are caused by a dominant mutation, e.g., Huntington's disease, where just one copy of a gene causes a disease. However, most of us carry recessive forms of genes, but we do not develop genetic disease. That is, we are *homozygous recessive*; heterozygotes have a dissimilar pair of genes for an inherited disease and do not normally experience a disease, but can pass the gene for it to their offspring. Heterozygotes of autosomal dominant traits develop the disease because only one copy of the dominant variant of the gene causes the disease. If two parents who are heterozygous for a disease both confer the gene for the disorder to an offspring, that person has a 75 percent chance of developing the autosomal dominant disease—as either a homozygous dominant or heterozygous individual.

## CASE 2: NANCY WEXLER AND HUNTINGTON'S DISEASE

After a 10-year deterioration and catatonia, clinical psychologist Nancy Wexler's mother died of Huntington's disease, a fatal neurodegenerative disease. Because the Huntington's gene is dominant, Nancy and her sister Alice each had a 50 percent risk of inheriting the disease. Because the average age of onset is 36, victims often have children before learning they are affected.

In this progressive disease, neurons in the caudate nuclei region rapidly shed. Although age of onset varies, the gene is completely *penetrant* by age 65.

Huntington's progresses through several stages (about five years each). First comes loss of muscular coordination and changes in personality, making victims angry, hostile, depressed, and sexually promiscuous. Next comes slurred speech, distorted facial expressions, constant muscular jerkiness, and staggering and falling. The third stage brings incontinence, dementia, and dependence on others, usually in an institution. In the last stage, victims are vegetative.

At present, 25,000 Americans have Huntington's, and about 100,000 Americans have an afflicted parent. Most victims are white. People at risk of Huntington's constantly wonder if each stumble augurs onset of the disease.

Unlike others at risk for genetic disease, who remain fatalistic about their risk, Wexler helped both to discover the gene for Huntington's and to develop a predictive test for it. Around 1800, a European sailor with Huntington's jumped ship around Lake Maracaibo in Venezuela. He had 14 children, and because families there were large, by 1981 he had 3,000 descendants. Of these, 100 had Huntington's and another 1,100 were at risk. In 1981, Wexler led an expedition there to obtain blood samples from these descendants and to test them to find a genetic marker for Huntington's. In 1983, Wexler and co-researcher James Gusella found such a marker.

In 1987, although the actual gene had not yet been discovered, Gusella developed a *linkage test* for Huntington's, meaning he could test for a batch of genes that tended to be inherited (or "linked") together. The linkage test allowed people such as Wexler to know their risk, for example, 5 percent versus 80 percent.

In 1986, Nancy Wexler taught as a professor of clinical neuropsychology at Columbia University and often predicted that when the test became available, she would take it. Later, she changed her mind, deciding *not* to take the test.

The implications of her decision stunned people. She had been a leading advocate for testing and had decided at the last minute not to test. She had spent a decade developing the very test she now refused to take. She was a clinical psychologist who should have known her own heart.

Indeed, not only did Wexler not take the test, but she also became an advocate of not testing: "What are you going to do if you're positive? Spend the rest of your life waiting to be a patient?" To people who wanted to be tested so that they could decide to go to law school, she said: "Go to law school! Develop your mind! Get on with your life!"

Over the next decade, other researchers discovered single genes for muscular dystrophy, cystic fibrosis, neurofibromatosis ("elephant man" disease), colon cancer, ataxia, and sickle-cell anemia. In 1993, six laboratories discovered the exact location of the Huntington's gene.[4] Now at-risk people such as Wexler could directly test themselves for it.

By then, Nancy Wexler had become even more convinced that people should not take the test. In 2008, at age 63, she led the successful fight to get the FDA to approve tetrabenazine, the first drug that can ameliorate Huntington's symptoms.[5] In 2013, at age 68, she still actively speaks on Huntington's and presumably did not inherit the gene.

# THE EUGENICS MOVEMENT

The *eugenics movement* (or *"Eugenics"*) flourished from 1905 to 1935 and hoped to improve hereditary characteristics through voluntary, selective breeding. In the late 1880s, Charles Darwin's cousin, Francis Galton, coined the term "eugenics."

By "survival of the fittest," Darwin meant "best adapted," so "fit" referred to the adaptation between an organism and its environment—in other words, how well adapted the organism is to reproduce and pass on its genes to its offspring.

Unfortunately, social Darwinists mistakenly saw evolution in terms of competition among social groups. Elitist, white social Darwinists believed that their social advantages stemmed from their alleged biological superiority over Africans and Asians.

Social Darwinism was more ideology than fact-based. It overlooked the vast numbers of organisms involved in attempts to survive, the enormous length of time over which these attempts evolve, and the ongoing role of adaptive mutations.

Eugenics flourished around the globe, but its "headquarters was at Cold Springs Harbor on Long Island, New York. . . ."[6] A prominent New York urologist, William Robinson, proclaimed about people born mentally challenged: "It is the acme of stupidity to talk in such cases of individual liberty, of the rights of the individual. . . . They have no right in the first instance to be born, but having been born, they have no right to propagate their kind."[7]

Eugenics enjoyed popularity because of pervasive bigotry. The newspaper magnate William Hearst and Theodore Roosevelt thundered against "yellow niggers" who had invaded America from Asia. When Henry Ford ran for president in the 1920s, he promised to rid the country of the "Jew bankers," whom he accused of causing America to enter World War I and, later, causing the Depression.[8]

While the Nazis sterilized 225,000 "mental defectives," America also sterilized such people. Indiana required sterilization in 1907 of the "retarded and criminally insane," and 30 other states soon followed, led by California, Virginia, and Indiana.[9] By 1941, 36,000 Americans had sometimes been sterilized for a catch-all condition called "feeblemindedness," or being born into large families on welfare.

In 2012, we learned that North Carolina sterilized 7,600 Carolinians between 1929 and 1974.[10] In 2013, North Carolina legislators approved $10 million to compensate the living victims, but as this book went to press, its governor had still not signed the bill into law.

Eugenics underlay U.S. Supreme Court's (1927) *Buck v. Bell* decision. Supposedly mentally challenged like her mother, Carrie Buck had been committed at age 18 to a state mental institution in Virginia. Pregnant when committed, Carrie gave birth inside to a daughter.

Harry Laughlin, an influential geneticist who worked at Cold Springs Harbor, read a social worker's report that Carrie had a "feeble look" and concluded that her low intelligence was hereditary. Laughlin then declared that Buck "lived a life of immorality and prostitution" and that all the Bucks belonged to the "shiftless, ignorant, worthless class of anti-social whites of the South."

The U.S. Supreme Court upheld the Virginia law permitting Carrie Buck's sterilization. Justice Oliver Wendell Holmes wrote the majority opinion:

> It is better for all the world, if instead of waiting to execute degenerate offspring for crime, or to let them starve for their imbecility, society can prevent those who are manifestly unfit from continuing their kind. The principle that sustains compulsory vaccination is broad enough to cover cutting the Fallopian tubes. (He concluded that) Three generations of imbeciles are enough.

Eugenics motivated the Immigration Restriction Act of 1924, which restricted entry to America of "inferior" peoples from Asia, Africa, Greece, India, Ireland, Poland, and Italy, and promoted entry by English, Dutch, Scotch, Scandinavians, and Germans. President Calvin Coolidge enthusiastically signed this act into law. As vice president he said, "America must be kept American. Biological laws show . . . that Nordics deteriorate when mixed with other races."[11]

Although the Statue of Liberty today symbolizes freedom, after 1924, thousands of the world's "huddled masses" had only a glimpse of it before being sent back home. Although today we use it positively, "melting pot" in 1924 was a phrase that scared Americans about unwanted immigrants.

Eugenics had so many false ideas that it takes a long time to enumerate them.[12] After 1935, it declined in the United States. Geneticist Hermann J. Muller said that it was "hopelessly perverted," a cult for "advocates for race and class prejudice, defenders of vested interests of church and State, Fascists, Hitlerites, and reactionaries generally."[13] Another leading geneticist, J. B. S. Haldane, said about its sterilization programs that "many of the deeds done in America in the name of eugenics are about as much justified by science as were the proceedings of the Inquisition by the Gospels."[14] Advances in population genetics prompted Haldane to famously remark, "An ounce of algebra is worth a ton of verbal argument."[15]

## CASE 3: TESTING FOR DIABETES

In 2006, Maria Lopez, a 30-year-old woman, had Type 2 diabetes and struggled to control it.[16] Her extended family in East Harlem in New York City included many diabetic relatives. At 5 feet, 6 inches, she weighed 267 pounds. She had always fought to control her weight, found it hard to exercise, and liked French fries and soft drinks. Diagnosed with diabetes at age 15 after she was hospitalized for spells of fainting, she had once lost 100 pounds, but had later gained it back.

Diabetes mellitus is a disease of high blood sugar levels (hyperglycemia) caused by insufficient secretion or function of, or response to, insulin, a hormone produced by the pancreas, which regulates metabolism of sugar. *Type 1 diabetes,* once called juvenile onset diabetes or insulin-dependent diabetes mellitus, involves low or no secretion of insulin. *Type 2 diabetes,* once called adult-onset diabetes, obesity-related diabetes, or non-insulin dependent diabetes mellitus, involves bodily cells that are resistant to insulin.

Diabetes may soon reach epidemic proportions: The Centers for Disease Control estimate that 21 million Americans suffer from diabetes and another 41 million are pre-diabetic.[17] As they adopt Western diets high in fats and processed corn sugars, more people worldwide succumb each year.[18] Americans of Chinese, Korean, and Japanese ancestry develop Type 2 diabetes at a rate 60 percent higher than whites.[19]

In 2006, epidemiologists discovered that over 800,000 New Yorkers, more than one in eight, had Type 2 diabetes.[20] This incidence is a third higher than the rest of the nation. In East Harlem, as many as one in five people had diabetes.[21]

Maria Lopez said her diabetes made her miserable. "I have never wanted this disease to control my life." Since first diagnosed, she had denied her disease and that it could lead to her death. "I'm a traditionally-built woman from a culture of strong, big women," she said. "I eat what I like. To hell with needles and machines."

Diabetics should monitor their blood sugar several times a day. In the past, they did so by drawing blood with real needles, but now new, small kits allow miniscule, almost painless sticks to do the same, greatly reducing the hassle of checking blood sugar. Nevertheless, Maria found it annoying to use such kits.

Diabetics should give up beer, cokes, French fries, potato chips, pies, cakes, and "everything else that tastes good," Maria said. But many diabetics in East Harlem live in poverty and experience great stress. Public health educators urged Maria to exercise daily and to eat a low-fat diet high in fresh fruits and vegetables. "That's not so easy to do," she says. "And my two daughters (aged 10 and 8) like to go to McDonalds."

Uncontrolled diabetes leads to kidney failure, retinal damage and blindness, gangrene (especially in legs, leading to amputation), damage to nerves, and heart failure.

Research to cure diabetes gets far less funding than cancer or HIV/AIDS. Most medical care for diabetics merely manages crises rather than trying to prevent them.

In 2006, scientists at DeCode Genetics discovered a variant in a gene that increases one's susceptibility for Type 2 diabetes. If you have one copy of this variant, your risk of developing Type 2 diabetes is increased by 40 percent. If you have two copies your risk increases by 140 percent.[22]

In understanding this result, it is important to distinguish between *relative risk* and *absolute risk*. Consider these statements:

Women who smoke have a 50 percent increase in risk of Type 2 diabetes.

One glass of wine a 3day increases the risk of Type 2 diabetes by 20 percent.

These two statements tell us about the increased risk of two behaviors to women in one group compared to another group. In other words, the first statement provides the *relative risk* of a group of women who smoke or drink compared to a group of non-smoking or non-drinking women. But neither statistic tells us anything about the overall likelihood of women getting Type 2 diabetes, the *absolute risk*.

If the absolute risk of Type 2 diabetes is low, say, in Africa, then having a few more people with this diabetes gene doesn't mean that huge numbers of Africans will get diabetes. On the other hand, about 38 percent of the world's people have one copy of the variant of the gene for Type 2 diabetes, so a lot of the world is at risk for developing Type 2 diabetes. And where does that risk come from? Alterations in lifestyle and changes in diet alter the norm of reaction of underlying genes, such that over decades, Type 2 diabetes emerges.

## CASE 4: TESTING FOR ALZHEIMER'S DISEASE

Alzheimer's creates fear in most people because it strikes at their identity. Consider Roy Smith, a 22-year-old male whose father suffered early-onset Alzheimer's disease at age 58 and who, one year later, no longer knew Roy's name. Both of Roy's paternal grandparents had Alzheimer's disease, so Roy's father probably got two copies of the ApoE4 gene (discussed later).

Two biomarkers in cerebral spinal fluid may identify Alzheimer's: one tests blood for beta amyloid, the protein fragment that builds up the plaque that clogs arteries in the brains of Alzheimer's victims.[23] The second tests for tau, the "tangles" in the brain of Alzheimer's patients. Another test uses a dye to stain the same plaques so a PET scan can measure them.[24]

Another assessment test for the ApoE4 gene where "the risk conferred by ApoE4 was most marked in the 61 to 65 age group. Individuals with two copies of ApoE4 had a significantly lower age at onset than those with one or no copies."[25] Some individuals with two copies showed symptoms in their 30s and 40s.[26] Individuals with this gene have three times the risk of getting Alzheimer's than other people. However, having the gene does not guarantee getting the disease, which makes self-testing problematic, as someone could test positive and develop a presymptomatic sick identity (discussed later).[27]

These tests come at a time when understanding of Alzheimer's is being refined.[28] Some scientists classify it as falling into three broad phases: a preclinical phase when it begins destroying the brain (and which a presymptomatic test could identify); a middle phase characterized by lower cognitive skills in language, memory, attention, or visual-spatial recognition than is normal for a person's age; and the final symptomatic phase characterized by two major symptoms that, surprisingly, need not at first include memory problems but can include problems with recognition of names, faces, or objects, as well as changes of personality and declines in ability to reason. In 2011, about 6 million Americans were in the middle phase, another 6 million will soon be in the final phase, and an unknown number fall in the first phase. The Alzheimer's Association has a more nuanced classification and lists seven phases.[29]

Most of his adult life, Roy's father had a tremor in his right hand and at age 17, Roy already had a similar tremor. Roy's father drank heavily during his life, although he was never considered an alcoholic. For the last five years, at fraternity parties in college, Roy also drank heavily.

One common pattern was seen with Roy and his father: when the father forgot a name or where he put his keys, Roy would quickly supply the answer. This helped his father mask his problem and kept Roy and his mother in denial about the father's failing mind.

Should Roy test and find out if he inherited a gene for Alzheimer's? What if he discovers that, like his father, he got two copies?

# ETHICAL ISSUES

## Preventing Disease

For some genetic diseases, no matter what people do, they will get the disease. Both BRCA1 and BRCA2 mutations are autosomal dominant genes. These genetic diseases are like Huntington's in that, even if women live completely healthy lives, they will still get breast cancer. For such women, double mastectomy may be the only action they can take to reduce their chances of getting breast or ovarian cancer.

Things are more complex with diabetes. Consider whether Maria is *responsible* for getting diabetes. Do we want a moralistic physician saying, "You should have eaten better! Now you have nobody to blame but yourself." Even if her disease is partly environmental and due to poor diet, didn't something cause her to *crave* bad foods? If a genetic mutation makes her more susceptible to Type 2 diabetes, does that relieve some of the responsibility she has in developing the disease?

And given Roy's two copies of the ApoE4 gene, there isn't much he could have done to avoid Alzheimer's, right? Evidence suggests that drinking alcohol accelerates the decline of people with this gene. Moreover, taking cognitive enhancers such as donepezil (one trade name is Aricept) may prevent onset of severe symptoms of Alzheimer's by six months. Furthermore, the most significant way to maintain brain activity is by increasing blood flow, and the best, safest way to do that is through exercise. If we discovered that Roy had done nothing to prevent his Alzheimer's, could we say that he should have delayed some of it?

Recall that when a person has two copies of the gene rather than one, risk of developing Type 2 diabetes jumps from 40 to 140 percent above normal. A large amount of evidence in genetics suggests that this *one-hit, two-hit model* explains many things. If you have two "hits" or copies of BRCA1, your chances of getting breast cancer jump from low to high. The same is true with diabetes and Alzheimer's.

Most people with genetic components of conditions will have only one gene or one copy of a genetic variant. That means that what happens in their environment, or how they behave, will play a major role in whether or when they develop the condition. This one-hit, two-hit model has major implications for personal responsibility, motivation to be healthy, genetic fatalism, and presymptomatic testing.

# TESTING AS SELF-INTEREST

Testing for breast cancer genes may benefit an affected woman, such as Angelina Jolie. Even with surgery, radiation, and chemotherapy for breast cancer, about 20 percent of women will still die from the disease. For this reason, some women testing positive for mutations in BRCA1 or BRCA2 decided to remove both breasts in hopes of living to an old age.

This is a significant ethical issue that requires some explanation. In the 1960s, many women under 50 with breast cancer elected to have a bilateral mastectomy to remove both cancerous and precancerous tissue from their breasts.[30] In the 1970s and 1980s, studies showed that for women with breast cancer, getting a lumpectomy fared no worse than women getting bilateral mastectomies. Because significant percentages of women after their mastectomies experienced loss of femininity and self-esteem, sparing them this surgery was thought to be a benefit.

Even before clinical trials finished, large numbers of women testing positive for BRCA1 and BRCA2 mutations had preventive bilateral mastectomies. In 2002, a clinical trial proved that, five years after surgery, women with a BRCA1 or BRCA2 mutation undergoing prophylactic bilateral mastectomy had a statistically significant lower risk of breast cancer.[31]

However, if there is any lesson in the ethics of genetic testing, it is that everything is complicated. Later studies suggested that the figure of 80 percent risk was exaggerated. Women with breast cancer initially recruited for studies of the two breast cancer genes came from families with breast cancer in grandmothers, mothers, daughters, and sisters, resulting in a selection bias.[32]

If a woman has mutations in BRCA1, BRCA2 or CHEK2, the benefits of knowing early are that one can take measures to reduce one's risk of having breast and ovarian cancer. Taking birth control pills reduces risk of ovarian cancer by 60 percent and taking the drug tamoxifen reduces risk of breast cancer by 50 percent. And more radically, there is the option of mastectomy. These same benefits apply to men, who account for about 2 percent of cases of breast cancer.

Similarly, testing for the gene that increases likelihood of getting Type 2 diabetes could lead to benefits for Maria Lopez, especially if she could adopt a healthy lifestyle. For Maria and especially her daughters, it will be important to eat a low-fat, low-processed sugar diet and to exercise to keep their weight normal. In some cases, a positive test for the Type 2 gene could be a wake-up call to adopt a healthy lifestyle.

Testing for Alzheimer's could lead to some benefits, even for people with two copies of the gene. Knowing he will need someone to take care of him in old age, Roy might marry early. He might avoid all alcohol and take donepezil. He might exercise daily to maximize blood flow, the primary preventive of early dementia. He might enroll in a trial of bexarotene, which reduced amyloid plaque build-up in mice by 50 percent.[33]

## TESTING ONLY TO HEAR GOOD NEWS

When people take genetic tests, do they really understand what they're doing? One genetics counselor says, "When people say they want this test to find out if they have the gene so they can make decisions, they really want to find out that they don't have it."[34]

Yet half of people at risk for Huntington's will have the mutated gene, and some people will have mutations associated with diabetes, Alzheimer's, and cancer. And there's no way to prepare them for this terrible news.

In the first study of presymptomatic testing for Huntington's, most people at risk originally said they would take the test, but after counseling, some changed their minds.[35]

The same study reported that "[p]articipants found to be probable gene carriers reported being surprised or shocked by the test result."[36] They had not expected to have the lethal gene.

Another consideration is that self-knowledge is seldom perfect. As the SUPPORT study showed, people simply cannot predict how they will react to bad news, like testing positive for a terrible genetic condition.

Because Huntington's or Alzheimer's cannot be cured, a positive test will tell someone that she is going to die a terrible death. Not everyone can deal with such knowledge. As Nancy Wexler says, for some people, especially teenagers and young adults, such knowledge could be toxic, warping their lives.

Moreover, when little treatment is available, is it wise to give people such a diagnosis? Perhaps people should not be burdened with more truth than they can bear.[37]

On the positive side, testing for genes for breast cancer or diabetes allows intervention at an early stage. In one family, one of two sisters at hereditary risk worried about developing breast cancer and had planned to have her breasts removed as a preventive measure; she took the test for breast cancer genes, which turned out to be negative and she canceled her plan. Her sister did not think she was at risk and had refused mammograms but discovered she had the bad BRCA1 variant. A previous examination of her breasts had found nothing, but a reexamination found a minuscule node, and a biopsy determined that cancer had already begun, so a radical mastectomy was performed. Without the genetic test, this second sister might not have discovered her cancer until many years later.

## TESTING AS A DUTY TO ONE'S FAMILY

Knowing one's likely genetic fate isn't just a concern of individuals. People are not atomistic; they come embedded in families, with children and parents, brothers and sisters.

The major argument favoring testing for serious genetic disease concerns childbearing. Nancy Wexler did not have children for fear that one might inherit Huntington's, yet perhaps her decision was misguided. If she had taken the test and been negative, she could have had children unaffected by Huntington's. Angelina Jolie had children with Brad Pitt, and adopted others, but probably passed on her "faulty" gene to some of her biological daughters..

On the other hand, people who test positive should not have children or should test embryos and implant ones lacking the Huntington's gene. Why is that? Because parents should want the best lives for their children, and such lives start with freedom from genetic disease. No parent should willingly inflict a serious genetic disease on his or her child.

A second argument for testing concerns spouses and caretakers. Consider the following example. A man who was at risk for Huntington's had decided not to take the test and discussed his reasons before a large medical class. His reasons were greeted with respect; but as the class ended and the students started to file out, a woman cried out from the back of the room, "What about me and the kids? What about my view about testing him?" It was the man's wife.

She wanted to be able to plan for the future. If her husband was positive, she would be taking care of him. She might also have been thinking of money: if her husband was positive, he would eventually need custodial care, and they would have to start saving up for that or, if possible, arrange for more extensive life or health insurance. Moreover, when these neurological diseases strike, the family, as well as the victim, will suffer emotionally; they should prepare themselves for this. Finally, they might try to make the most of whatever time remains before onset.

Besides a strict duty to one's family, compromises are possible. For instance, middle-aged people who do not want to know may feel that they have escaped the disease and that they can now take the test as a gift to their children. Another compromise is to have blood samples taken and stored for later testing. Finally, as John Hardwig famously wrote, some people with lethal genetic diseases may feel they have a "duty to die" to spare their families the burden of caring for them.[38]

## TESTING ONE'S FAMILY BY TESTING ONESELF

One advocate for families afflicted with genetic disease believes that:

> First and foremost, genetic testing must be viewed as a family issue, not an individual one. The person who enrolls in a testing program should be strongly encouraged to involve other family members, within reason. Testing one member of a family will affect other members. Persons who refuse to involve their families may not have considered fully the consequences for other members or for themselves.[39]

It is important to keep in mind that in testing for dominant, single-gene diseases, such as Huntington's and the breast cancer genes, there is no such thing as testing only a fetus or testing only a parent: a positive fetus reveals a positive parent; a positive parent reveals that any children are at risk.

Helping families understand genetic testing is difficult. Catherine Hayes, President of a support group for families with Huntington's, notes, "Many medical professionals have difficulty viewing genetic issues in a family context. . . . Most researchers cannot possibly know what it is like to grow up in a family haunted by a genetic disease. . . . "

Testing may tear families apart. Consider the right to know. Even in a life-or-death situation, judges have ruled that relatives cannot be compelled to be tested for compatibility as bone marrow or organ donors. Such decisions indicate that judges will not force genetic tests on relatives.

If a person tested positive for Alzheimer's and concealed it from a prospective spouse, could that be grounds for annulment? Does a prospective spouse have a right to know about such a test? Or does marrying "for better or worse" cover such questions?

Can one parent have a child tested in order to find out if the other parent is affected? Suppose that a father tests positive for Huntington's and refuses to tell his teenage daughter, Laura. Suppose that a genetic counselor is aware of the father's result. When Laura gets married, what should the counselor do? Recommend general genetic tests to her? Suppose she refuses. If she knew that her father was positive, would she agree to testing? If so, should the counselor violate the father's confidentiality? To many people, the good of preventing another child with Huntington's outweighs the harm of violating privacy, especially where there is a strong sense that the affected parent had an obligation to reveal his result in the first place.

## PERSONAL RESPONSIBILITY FOR DISEASE

Let us return to the question of whether Roy, Joan, and Maria can do anything to *prevent* getting these diseases.

Type 2 diabetes is an especially good candidate for prevention because we know that many Asian people do not get diabetes until they adopt Western lifestyles. (Similarly, for Asian men immigrating to North America, incidence of prostate cancer jumps from 1 per 100,000 to 70 per 100,000.[40]) The prevailing view about preventing diabetes is this:

> What is especially disturbing about the rise of Type 2 [diabetes] is that it can be delayed and perhaps prevented with changes in diet and exercise. For although both types are believed to stem in part from genetic factors, Type 2 is also spurred by obesity and inactivity. This is particularly true in those prone to illness.[41]

So are 21 million Americans "failures" in personal responsibility because they have diabetes? Are another 10 million "successes" because they staved off the genetic predisposition?[42] Perhaps.

In 2007, researchers followed 91,000 women and discovered that those who drank one or more cans of soft drinks a day, compared to those drinking less than one can a month, were twice as likely to develop Type 2 diabetes. If nothing else, women who carry genes for diabetes can stop drinking soft drinks. Maybe Mayor Bloomberg was right to try to limit extra-large sizes of soft drinks at fast-food restaurants.

Let us take a larger perspective with cancer. Cancer occurs when tumor-suppressing genes or DNA repair mechanisms cease to work, resulting in wild, uncontrolled growth of cells. Diabetes occurs when the body fails to allow cells to take up glucose from the blood.

Both diseases occur when environmental inputs trigger potential in an inherited genetic template. At the very least, avoidance of the inputs can delay onset of disease and perhaps avoid it altogether. For example, people with genetic dispositions to alcoholism do not become alcoholics in countries where alcohol is banned. As a person ages, her immune system and organs deteriorate, and mutated cells in her body accumulate, making her more vulnerable to cancer and diabetes, so many people, despite healthy lifestyles, will eventually succumb to their genetic risk.[43]

Society can exert some control over how many carcinogens people ingest: it can ban tobacco in schools and hospitals, forbid smoking in public, and steeply tax tobacco. Similarly, it can ban junk foods and sodas from schools. Individuals at risk for cancer and diabetes can eat low-fat diets high in fiber, fresh fruits, and vegetables. In this way, both societies and individuals can reduce the incidence of cancer and diabetes.

But what if a daughter gets cancer or diabetes anyway? Should she be blamed? Probably not. To say that these diseases can be partially prevented by healthy living is not to say that some cases aren't, like Huntington's disease, genetically inevitable. Second, other factors in a person's life may have prevented healthy living such that a person truly could not have done otherwise. In these cases, blame would be wrong.

## TESTING AND SICK IDENTITIES

Nancy Wexler rejects an attitude she found dominant among the medical community about testing, which might be expressed as: "Come on! Take your knowledge like a man and don't be a sissy!"

This attitude benefits the medical community and family more than the individual affected. If there is no cure for Huntington's or Alzheimer's, what's so good about knowing?

Nancy Wexler thinks that people who test positive for a disease long before they experience any symptoms may develop a *sick identity* about it. If you're going to get Huntington's, she argues, you will in fact get it, so there's nothing you can do about it. Why burden yourself being self-identified as "sick" long before you are?

Moreover, some people are highly suggestible. People who are concerned about suicide often focus on the consequences of testing teenagers—a population that is already highly suicidal. Youngsters at risk for Huntington's, breast cancer, or diabetes already agonize about going to college and spending their parents' money, and those who learn for certain that they have these genes may be even more vulnerable.

Should girls under 18 years of age be tested for these genes if these genes run in their families? At first glance, the answer seems no, for a positive answer might take away the fun of childhood and adolescence. Moreover, great danger exists of developing a sick identity as a "woman with breast cancer" or a "woman who will get diabetes." On the other hand, eating junk food and smoking start early in many teenagers, so early testing might be beneficial.

One study published in 2011 of 3,639 clients of direct-to-consumer (DTC) genetic testing found no increased psychological problems after these people learned results of their genetic tests.[44] After such results, *Reason* magazine's science editor, Ron Bailey, challenged the author of this text, accusing him of mollycoddling consumers and thinking them too fragile to handle the truth.[45]

The movie *GATTACA* (which is recommended to watch with this chapter), illustrates the power of labeling by oneself and others. *GATTACA*'s real theme is about the effects of labeling on a family, individual, and society. A label such as "schizophrenia," "precancerous," or "precardiomyopathy" may affect a person so profoundly that it cripples his ambition and makes him a quasi-invalid decades before he has any symptoms. And how horrible such toxic labeling would be if it were based on mistakes, such as assuming a variable genetic disease was autosomal dominant.

## PREVENTING SUICIDE BY NOT KNOWING

Because 25 percent of people with Huntington's consider suicide and 10 percent carry it out,[46] scientists have debated whether tests for such diseases should be given. Nancy Wexler said, "We have to understand that the day you tell someone he has this gene, his life and view of himself change forever. We're worried about the potential for suicide."[47]

Is suicide an adequate reason for not testing? Even if some percent commit suicide, most will not. Nancy Wexler says, "Suicide is not unreasonable. It's not so awful that we can't discuss it or consider it." She observes, "For some of my friends who have Huntington's, knowing that they can commit suicide gives them a certain sense of control. They want to feel that if it gets too bad, they can have a way out. They can do something."[48]

Some scientists argue against paternalism: "I think we can trust people to make these decisions. I'm not so convinced we researchers should be dictating how the technology gets used."[49]

After watching his father quickly forget how to use e-mail or take a shower, Roy swears he would rather be dead than succumb to Alzheimer's, nor does he want to burden his mother or sister with caring for him. So Roy might test with the aim of discovering when to plan to kill himself or leave an advance directive asking that he be allowed to die when Alzheimer's starts.

---

For a paradox about dementia and advance directives, go to Chapter 3 in the Online Learning Center (OLC) at www.mhhe.com/pence7e where you will find "A Duty to Die?" and its section on Ronald Dworkin's discussion of a paradox about following the advance directives of Alzheimer's patients. From Gregory Pence's *Elements of Bioethics*.

---

## TESTING ONLY WITH GOOD COUNSELING

Experts agree that testing should be offered only *with good counseling*. The President's Commission on Bioethics (1983) emphasized that counseling should be guaranteed: "A full range of prescreening and follow-up services . . . should be available before a program [of genetic testing] is introduced."[50]

This is true; for most diseases and most people, the results will be probabilistic. Not "You don't have the gene," but, "You have a 10 percent chance of getting gene-related urologic cancer."

Besides the three mutations of BRCA1, BRCA2, and CHEK2 that cause breast cancer, hundreds of variant mutations are now known, each conferring a different risk. Moreover, the risk of each variant may differ with the peculiarities of each family. Conveying all this information accurately requires sophistication by a genetic counselor.

But the history of genetics shows that sophistication and understanding of subtle, complex issues are not strengths of the public and policymakers. Women are likely to think, "I have the breast cancer gene" and fear death in a few years.

This is, of course, paternalistic. However, it is true that some of those who test positive will wish they hadn't taken the test and some may develop emotional problems, and counseling can help such people.

Today, commercial companies aggressively market direct-to-consumer genetic testing. Although such companies say genetic counseling is available *after* they test, this seems like the wrong time to offer such testing. For the reasons stated earlier, after good counseling, many people decided *not* to be tested, but commercial companies surely won't pay counselors to give that kind of advice to prospective clients.

Most people are going to obtain such information without a genetics counselor for two reasons. First, finding a trained genetics counselor is not easy, and many people do not live near a major medical center that has skilled counselors. Second, only the very best medical coverage today reimburses patients for genetic counseling.

## GENETIC TESTING AND INSURANCE

Genetic testing raises financial issues. In 2000, when one woman had a preventive radical mastectomy like Angelina Jolie, she feared her insurance company would cancel her policy if they knew her reasons. Because this company didn't know anything, it thought she was being irrational and wouldn't pay for her surgery.

For decades, an important issue about genetic testing and medical insurance was confidentiality. Several national companies told insurance companies about applicants for policies who posed risks.[51] For people who take presymptomatic genetic tests and test positive, insurers could raise premiums for families. Worse, they could consider the result to be evidence of a pre-existing condition and exclude that disease from future coverage.

Congress in 2008 finally passed GINA, the Genetic Information Non-discrimination Act. This fed eral law bans insurers from using knowledge about a person's genes to determine eligibility for insurance or rates of premiums, or employers from using the same as a basis for hiring, firing, or assigning jobs.[52] Because of the likelihood of adverse selection, GINA does not apply to people applying for life insurance or for coverage for disability or long-term care.

Genetic testing for diabetes exposed problems in our medical system before the Affordable Care Act (ACA). Almost no money was spent by hospitals to prevent diabetes because doing so loses income. In contrast, and because insurance reimburses physicians well for doing surgical procedures, waiting until crises develop and then amputating gangrenous legs produces profits.[53] Similarly, before the ACA, insurance companies curtailed benefits to diabetics to discourage them from enrolling in their plans: in a 2003 survey, 87 percent of health insurance actuaries . . . said that "if they were to improve coverage [for diabetics] with richer drug benefits or easier access to specialists, they would incur financial problems by attracting the sickest, most expensive patients."[54]

## PREMATURE ANNOUNCEMENTS AND OVER SIMPLIFICATIONS

Almost every year, a newspaper headline announces startling discovery of a gene for a disease. For example, in 2007, researchers identified a gene that was a "risk factor" for heart disease.[55] Yet for previous announcements of 85 factors in

75 genes, when scientists examined the proof that they caused heart disease, they concluded that exactly "zero of the genes were more common in heart patients than in healthy people."[56]

In 1987, researchers retracted an earlier claim that manic-depression was linked to a gene on the X chromosome.[57] By this time, earlier claims about genetic causes of schizophrenia and alcoholism had been retracted.

Today, geneticists believe that psychiatric disorders such as schizophrenia will not be found to be single-gene disorders. According to one leading researcher, common forms of mental illness may be caused by three to five genes acting together, probably with environmental co-factors.[58]

Like eugenics, much of the news about genetics in today's mass media is simplistic, alarmist, and premature.

## CAVEAT EMPTOR: MAKING MONEY FROM GENETIC TESTING

In 2002, Myriad Genetics of Salt Lake City expanded its sales force from 85 to 600 agents to market BRCA1 testing directly to doctors and their patients. The tests, which cost between $750 and $2,750, would benefit only the 5 to 10 percent of people with breast cancer caused by these genes. Presumably, Angelina Jolie paid for a test for BRCA1 controlled by Myriad Genetics.

Unfortunately, BRCA1's discovery offered hope of a screening test only for women with hereditary breast and ovarian cancer—not for the 90 to 95 percent of women who develop non-hereditary breast cancer.

In some ways, marketing such tests was a win–win situation for Myriad Genetics. For the people who tested positive, they got their money's worth and advance news. People who tested negative got relief and did not complain about the money spent. The ethical issue arises when thousands of people seek relief who are really not at risk: they waste their money in getting a negative result. But it would be patronizing to say they can't spend their money as they choose, even irrationally.

In 2010, the Government Accountability Office chastised DTC genetic-testing for "deceptive marketing practices, erroneous medical management advice from DTC genetic testing companies, and a lack of standardization of results among companies."[59]

In 2013, the U.S. Supreme Court reversed a decision by the U.S. Patent Office and ruled that genes, as bits of life, could not be patented.[60] Thus Myriad's stranglehold on tests for breast cancer was broken and physicians became free to develop tests for BRCA1 and BRCA2 without paying Myriad $3,000. Indeed, this decision opened up a new world of genetic testing.

The hot item today in commercial genetics is a $99 test, which will get you assessed for 240 health conditions, 40 hereditary diseases, and the origins of your distant ancestors.[61]

For some people, such sequencing may give good information, especially if genetic co-factors of disease are accurately identified. For them, learning that they have two genes for Type 2 diabetes may cause them to keep their weight in check, to eat healthfully, and exercise. But as Angela Trepanier, president-elect of the National Society of Genetics Counselors, says, many people are genetic fatalists and will say, "To hell with it. I'm doomed anyway. Where's the cheesecake?"[62]

The other great danger of such an overall test is contained in the aphorism, "Be careful what you wish for." A person buying such a test may expect a certain kind of news, but he may get unexpected news that is traumatic—that one of the people he believed to be his parent is not really his biological ancestor. Or he may test to rule out cancer and heart disease but discover he carries two copies of powerful genes for Alzheimer's. Obviously, buyers should study these issues and carefully discuss their "emotional intelligence," i.e., whether they can handle unexpected bad news.

## PREVENTING GENETIC DISEASE: FINAL THOUGHTS

Genetic testing may lead each of us to think more carefully about causes of gene-associated diseases. Presymptomatic testing may give some people a small window of preventive control. People at risk for cancers can avoid smoking and secondhand smoke (exposure of children to secondhand smoke is strongly associated with adult development of diabetes).[63]

Previously, three standards of evidence were discussed that are used in the law: preponderance of evidence, clear and convincing evidence, and beyond a reasonable doubt. These standards can be used to make a point. We know beyond a reasonable doubt that no one with Huntington's disease can do anything to prevent this disease from destroying his brains and killing him. We also know that for people with single genes for breast cancer or Huntington's, or with two genes for Alzheimer's, diabetes, and other cancers, many will develop the disease.

This brings us to people with one gene for a disease like diabetes. One might think that the best chance we have to prevent diabetes is with children and adolescents, before they become overweight and have high levels of blood sugar. If they enter young adulthood overweight and accustomed to eating lots of processed sugars, the probability that they will develop diabetes is high.

But lifestyle interventions in the Diabetes Prevention Program (DPP), a 10-year clinical trial on 3,234 overweight or obese pre-diabetics, worked best in participants 60 years and over, proving it's never too late to change.[64]

So can people prevent genetic diseases? The flip side of this question is whether we can *blame* people for getting genetic diseases. This is a profound philosophical question, with many implications in family life, ethics, and public policy.

Consider the claim that alcoholism is a disease, and even more controversially, a *genetic* disease. Consider the fact that people of East Asian descent carry gene variants that rapidly convert alcohol to toxic acetaldedhyde, which—some researchers claim—makes them averse to drinking.[65] Between 10–20 percent of Americans carry a "tipsy gene," making them drunk after one to two drinks.

What are the correct inferences from these facts? This goes to the heart of the debate. Why would getting drunk fast *protect* people against alcoholism, rather than *encourage* it? Is there something else involved here? Culture? Free will?

Education? Certainly such "tipsy genes" have famously been devastating to Native Americans from Oklahoma to Alaska.

> [For more on alcoholism and free will, see online Supplement #5, "Kant on Alcoholism and Free Will."] From Gregory Pence's *Elements of Bioethics*.

To hand out blame, we would need to know, at least with clear and convincing evidence, that they could have acted otherwise and eaten or exercised differently. It may be true that they could have, just as it may be true that the presumption of innocence allows some of the guilty to go free.

Also, people who do not have genes for Type 2 diabetes cannot really know what it's like to crave fats and sugars and to be tormented by these cravings. Yes, everyone is tempted, but some are tempted so much more intensely and continually than others! Until we have evidence that pre-diabetics could have acted otherwise, we should not blame them as individuals or in public policy. We would need evidence beyond a reasonable doubt to do so, evidence we are unlikely to ever have.

Nevertheless, as with the hero of *GATTACA*, we should educate the young to think they can transcend their genetic dispositions. We want to give people hope. At the same time, when they turn out to be less-than-ideal, we don't want to condemn them.

Responsibility exists on a gradient, corresponding to a gradient of free will. Two people with the same genes, placed at birth in different families (like Dickens's *The Prince and the Pauper*) may have differing degrees of free will and responsibility for their health or disease. This makes sense. Even so-called identical twins are identical for disease only 60 percent of the time, proving that having a specific DNA sequence doesn't doom one to a disease.[66]

If responsibility exists on a gradient, then poor people from dysfunctional families and with no medical insurance are less to blame than well-educated young adults from loving, well-off families. If responsibility exists on a gradient, then people with genes predisposing them to diabetes or cancer are less to blame than those blessed with good genes. If responsibility exists on a gradient, there is some room for free will, but free will is not the only vector on the graph.

In the end, we need to avoid both simplistic genetic fatalism ("I've got a gene for X, so I'm doomed!") and also simplistic moralism ("You could've done X and prevented this!"). Neither attitude seems compatible with the emerging, complicated facts. The history of eugenics shows that we always oversimplify issues. We will do so again.

## FURTHER READING

Catherine Hayes, "Genetic Testing for Huntington's—A Family Issue," *New England Journal of Medicine*, vol. 327, no. 20, 1993.

Daniel Kevles, *In the Name of Eugenics: Genetics and the Uses of Human Heredity*, New York: Knopf, 1985.

Lenny Moss, *What Genes Can't Do*, Cambridge, MA: MIT Press, 2004.

Matt Ridley, *Genome: The Autobiography of a Species in 23 Chapters*, New York: Harper Collins, 2000.

## DISCUSSION QUESTIONS

1. How could some presymptomatic testing be considered toxic for the individual testing, especially testing at an early age?

2. Are couples testing their embryo or fetus for Down syndrome, with the possibility of abortion, practicing eugenics?

3. To what degree, if any, are pre-diabetics like Maria Lopez and her daughters responsible for getting diabetes?

4. How do most claims about genetics oversimplify complex kinds of causation?

5. Why will most people taking genetic testing not get good value for their money?

6. Is it true that some people are too suggestible and that knowledge of increased risk for genetic conditions will torture them? What if, as likely, the knowledge is not, "You will get bone cancer." but "You have a 50 percent greater risk of getting bone cancer than most people?"

# CHAPTER 17

# Ethical Issues in Stopping the Global Spread of AIDS

*B*locking the spread of AIDS around the world presents a challenge for bioethics. Since the start of this scourge, over 60 million people have contracted HIV, the virus that causes AIDS, and nearly 30 million have died of HIV-related problems.[1]

This chapter's introductory sections discuss past epidemics, medical facts about AIDS, scandals about HIV infection of the blood supply, Kimberly Bergalis, homosexuality, contact tracing, mandatory screening, and needle-exchange programs.

This chapter's key ethical issue involves four approaches to stopping AIDS. Part of our problem stems from conflicts between these approaches.

## BACKGROUND: EPIDEMICS, PLAGUES, AND AIDS

Throughout human history, epidemics have terrified humans. In 1348 in Europe, the deadly bacterial disease known as the *Black Death* or simply, the *plague,* erupted. *Bubonic plague,* the most common and classic form of the disease, displayed inflamed swellings of the lymphatic glands in the groin and armpits and was transmitted by fleas. Rats and other small mammals carried fleas to humans, and bites of fleas transmitted plague to humans. The bacillus *Yersinia pestis* causes bubonic plague. Untreated bubonic plague killed 50 percent of its victims. Today, antibiotics treat its earliest stages.

A virulent complication of untreated bubonic plague, *pneumonic plague,* involved the lungs. Easily transmitted by coughing, the microbe killed almost universally. Because of it, many physicians of the fourteenth century found their calling elsewhere.

In the same century, astrologers claimed that plague resulted from the conjunction of Saturn, Mars, and Jupiter; others claimed it resulted from sulfurous fumes released by earthquakes. Clergy taught that God had sent it to punish humans for great sins.

Historian Barbara Tuchman tells us that during medieval epidemics, "Organized groups of 200 to 300 . . . marched from city to city, stripped to the waist, scourging themselves with leather whips tipped with iron spikes until they bled.

While they cried aloud to Christ and the Virgin for pity, . . . the watching towns-people sobbed in sympathy."[2] In so marching, they spread infected fleas.

The fearful ignorance of the times required *scapegoats* (in the Bible, goats are sacrificed to atone for bad things and as sacrifices to ward off worse things). So people accused Orthodox Jews, with their distinctive dress, of poisoning wells and spreading plague. When atonement processions reached cities, they often attacked the Jewish quarter, trapped Jews inside, and set the area on fire. When plague followed, Jews were blamed, but not the procession (which had brought the fleas).

Leprosy, cholera, and syphilis also terrified people. Leprosy, or Hansen's disease, creates lesions on the skin and kills slowly over years. Twentieth-century medicine learned that people get infected only through exposure over many months through the skin or mucosa. Before then, society banished lepers and forced them to live in isolated lepers' colonies; if a leper walked outside the colony, they were required to ring a cowbell to warn people away.

Great epidemics of cholera from infected water also created fear in its victims. During the epidemic of 1813, Americans blamed those who fell ill, especially wanton prostitutes, drunken Irish, lazy people of color, and the dirty poor—many of whom lived along creeks used for both drinking water and defecation. Ministers praised God for cholera for "cleansing the filth from society."

In 1854, London physician John Snow realized that cholera only broke out in the district served by the Broad Street pump. He correctly inferred that infected water spread cholera and that clean water could prevent it. Nevertheless, many Americans clung to the belief that sin and being Irish caused cholera, so many Americans died needlessly in the third great cholera epidemic in America of 1862.

Everyone also blamed victims of syphilis for their disease. As discussed in Chapter 10, moralists blamed vice for the disease, whereas scientists blamed spirochetes.

Not until acceptance of the germ theory of disease after 1900 did public health prevent epidemics of cholera. It took a half a century for officials to translate a medical insight into public policy to save lives.


## A BRIEF HISTORY OF AIDS

In 1959, a blood sample collected from a man in Kinshasa, Democratic Republic of Congo, later proved positive for HIV. Genetic analysis of his blood suggests that HIV-1 may have stemmed from a virus that existed in the early 1940s or even the late 1930s.

Researcher Beatrice Hahn at the University of Alabama, Birmingham (UAB), proved that HIV spread to humans from wild chimpanzees in southern Cameroon. HIV infected the blood of hunters there as they caught, killed, and cut up the chimpanzees for bushmeat.[3]

Around 1978, gay men in America, Sweden, and Haiti begin to show signs of AIDS. Between 1979 and 1981, Kaposi's sarcoma and *Pneumocystis carinii* pneumonia unexpectedly showed up in gay males in Los Angeles and New York.

On June 5, 1981, the Centers for Disease Control (CDC) announced the discovery of a mysterious "gay-related immune deficiency" (GRID) that had killed three gay men; only a month later, 108 cases of GRID were reported and 46 gay men were dead.

Three months after the first report of GRID in the summer of 1981, CDC announced that babies of drug-dependent women in New York City also had the disease. GRID was changed to *acquired immune deficiency syndrome* or *AIDS*.

In 1982, when physicians in New York and California had already seen hundreds of cases of AIDS, they still did not know its incubation period or causative agent. CDC guessed that incubation could be many years and that many thousands of people could be infected. No one then diagnosed with AIDS had lived more than two years, so AIDS frightened everyone.

In 1983, Luc Montagnier and the Institut Pasteur in France discovered that a virus, the *human immunodeficiency virus*, HIV, caused AIDS. Today, his virus is called HIV-1. In 1986, scientists discovered a second form, HIV-2, which may have been infecting residents for decades. HIV-2 develops more slowly, is milder than HIV-1, can be transmitted more easily heterosexually, and is rare outside West Africa.[4] HIV-1 has four sub-strains: M, N, O, and P. The first three strains came from chimpanzees, the last, a gorilla.[5] The virus existed in primates for at least 32,000 years and sometime between 1900 and 1959, "something allowed a human infection with a chimpanzee virus to spread widely enough to evolve into modern HIV-1, which could spread easily among humans."[6]

As early as 1982, the CDC warned that donated blood could carry the agent causing AIDS. Blood could have been screened for hepatitis, thereby indirectly screening for HIV, but officials deemed this too expensive and unfortunately did not do so.

In 1984, the FDA approved the ELISA test for antibodies to HIV. Now blood donated or otherwise obtained could be tested for HIV. However, authorities running blood banks did not immediately test blood using the ELISA test. Why?

First, various groups politicized every fact about HIV and AIDS. A little historical background shows how this occurred. This background may predict what would occur if SARS or a lethal bird flu became epidemic.

## AIDS AND IDEOLOGY

By the end of 1981, CDC epidemiologists realized that gay men were being killed by a new kind of infectious disease of unknown nature and transmission. CDC postulated that sex among gay men might be spreading the disease, especially sex with anonymous partners in bathhouses in cities such as New York and San Francisco.

These bathhouses constituted what epidemiologists call an *amplification system* for the spread of a disease. Because some of the men had many anonymous sexual partners, some of whom, in turn, traveled to other places for sex with multiple partners, the virus could spread quickly. Another such system was easy, cheap travel by plane around the world. At one point, a best-selling book identified a gay airline steward as Patient Zero, the first person to bring HIV from Africa to the United States and to introduce it to gay bathhouses (the publisher later admitted that Patient Zero was a publicity stunt to get attention for the book and HIV-infected patients).[7]

Sharing needles and syringes to inject drugs constitutes another amplification system. Blood withdrawn from a user's vein mixes both with a drug in the syringe and with viral particles from previous users.

A community's blood supply constitutes another amplification system. Blood banks pool both plasma and clotting factor for hemophiliacs from many sources. So, one infected donor can infect many recipients.

The CDC called upon federal and state governments to fund studies to see if a new lethal disease had appeared in the blood system, but none responded. At the time, medical experts believed that all lethal infectious diseases had been discovered, so no one then suspected that a new one had emerged.

By 1981, gay men and lesbians had won some freedom from prejudice: resistance against oppressive police round-ups began in 1969 at a bar called the Stonewall Inn in Greenwich Village in New York City. In the Stonewall Riots there, gay men resisted the harassment by police, fostering a new pride and encouraging men to come out of the closet.

During the 1970s, sexual freedom spread among heterosexuals, fueled by birth control, permissive attitudes towards non-marital sex, Woodstock, mind-altering drugs, and rebellion against authority. Gay men and lesbians then rode the crest of a larger wave of sexual change crashing through society. In medicine, psychiatrists removed homosexuality from their list of psychiatric illnesses.

But many people still despised gay men. Reverend Jerry Falwell blamed homosexuals for AIDS. In 1982, the secretary of Moral Majority, Greg Dixon, wrote, "If homosexuals are not stopped, they will in time infect the entire nation, and America will be destroyed—as entire civilizations have fallen in the past."[8] In 2001 when the World Trade Center was destroyed, Reverend Falwell and Pat Robertson blamed gays and atheists for the event, saying it was God's punishment on America, echoing earlier clergy who had scapegoated Jews for plague and the Irish for cholera.[9]

The head of the Southern Baptist Convention said that God had created AIDS to "indicate His displeasure with the homosexual lifestyle."[10] Monsignor Edward Clark of St. John's University in Queens, New York, claimed that, "If gay men would stop promiscuous sodomy, the AIDS virus would disappear from America."[11] Conservative Patrick Buchanan decried, "The poor homosexuals—they have declared war on nature and now nature is exacting an awful retribution."[12]

Reverend Falwell, who founded Moral Majority, a religious-political organization, advocated shutting down bathhouses where gay men engaged in anonymous sex. Owners of such bathhouses countered with ads in gay newspapers extolling freedom and calling Falwell a bigot. When gay activist Larry Kramer argued that shutting down bathhouses would save lives, gay men attacked him as a prude.

French philosopher Michel Foucault asserted that HIV did not cause AIDS and that HIV was not spread sexually. Foucault himself patronized bathhouses in the 1970s and died of AIDS in 1984, earning the ignominy of having his view refuted by the manner of his own death.

In the mid-1980s, the *New York Review of Books* contributing editor Jonathan Lieberson, a graduate student in philosophy at Columbia University, penned several influential articles about AIDS. In one such essay, he claimed that irrationality about AIDS was running wild, that only 10 percent of HIV-infected people would ever get AIDS, and that contact tracing should never be used to track down sex partners of infected men, because the new freedom of gay men was too important to sacrifice.[13] Around 1989, Lieberson himself died of AIDS.[14]

## TRANSMISSION OF HIV AND TESTING FOR HIV

HIV is transmitted in only three ways: through blood, through semen, or to babies during birth or breast-feeding.

Without treatment, HIV causes a progressive weakening of the immune system and hence decreases the ability to resist normal infections. Without anti-retroviral drugs, the average time between HIV-infection and full-blown AIDS in 2005 was 9.5 years, and 9.2 months between full-blown AIDS and death.

Cells called CD4 lymphocytes (or simply T4 cells) indicate the health of the immune system: the lower the number of cells, the worse it is doing. When the count of CD4 cells drops below 200, a person with AIDS usually gets *opportunistic infections* such as Kaposi's sarcoma, PCP, a fungal infection called oral thrush, or cervical cancer.

In 1984 and in the midst of the above controversies described earlier, authorities weighed whether to test America's blood supply for hepatitis as an indirect test for HIV. Those *against* testing won.

Some vocal gay men argued that their donations of blood should not be "quarantined" and that HIV had not really been proven to cause AIDS. Blood banks worried that if they screened blood they might lose income (although they do not charge for blood, they make money classifying, transferring, and storing blood).

In May 1984, Stanford University started screening blood for HIV. Two months later, defending a national decision *not* to screen, Health and Human Services Secretary Margaret Heckler famously said, "I want to assure the American people that the blood supply is 100 percent safe. . . ."[15]

Joseph Bove, M.D., who chaired the FDA's committee overseeing the safety of the nation's blood, also said that the "overreacting press" had caused hysteria about blood.[16] In March 1984, when the CDC counted 73 cases of deaths from AIDS caused by transfusion, Bove dismissed this danger: "More people are killed by bee stings."[17] Six months later, 269 people had died of AIDS from tainted blood.

In making these statements, Bove and Heckler either lied, were incompetent, or both. In March 1985, most American blood banks began using the ELISA test to screen blood, a full year after they should have begun. Because of this lag, thousands of Americans and hemophiliacs became infected with HIV. One of them was Ryan White, a hemophiliac who died at age 18 in 1990.

In 1985, a female prostitute and intravenous drug user tested positive for HIV. Now that Ryan White and a female prostitute had the disease, AIDS seemed to be no longer just a gay disease. It had infiltrated heterosexuals and the country's blood supply.

People hoped that HIV-infected people would not die. That changed dramatically in 1986, when researchers predicted that, without treatment, almost all HIV-infected people would develop AIDS and die.

The same year, a few gutsy people founded ACT-UP to help people with AIDS. Its demonstrations forced the FDA to shorten its process for approving new drugs by two years, and in 1987, AZT (zidovudine) became the first anti-HIV drug.

In 1996, a decade later, scientists discovered protease inhibitors. These drugs block the protease enzyme needed to create new, mature particles of HIV and allowed HIV-infected people to live somewhat normal lives.

At the start of AIDS, 25 percent of children born of infected mothers became infected. AZT blocks such *vertical transmission* to less than 1 percent.

Protease inhibitors plus AZT can cost $10,000 a year, and they cause severe complications. They do not cure HIV infection, but provide a way to survive it. The author knows professors, physicians, and administrators who were infected in the early 1980s, got these drugs early, and are still alive today.

In 2001, about 65,000 Americans over 50 lived with HIV, but in 2006, that number nearly doubled to 116,000.[18] At the NIH, the Mult-Site AIDS Cohort Study has been following the health of 2,000 subjects for the past 25 years. Although alive, many people with HIV in their late 50s suffer from Parkinson's or dementia, end-stage liver disease, diabetes, depression, and bouts of pneumonia. Despite these problems, as one person says, enduring such problems as a result of escaping AIDS is "better than the alternative."

## KIMBERLY BERGALIS'S CASE

In 1987, David Acer, a dentist in Jensen Beach, Florida, extracted two molars from 21-year-old Kimberly Bergalis, a junior at the University of Florida in Gainesville. After graduating in 1990, Kimberly tested positive for HIV.

A Caucasian male in his early 30s, Acer admitted to having had sexual relations during the previous decade with as many as 150 men. In 1987, he developed Kaposi's sarcoma, and two months later, treated Bergalis. In 1989, he sold his practice and his tools and destroyed his records. In 1990, he died of AIDS.

When his former patients got tested, six others tested HIV positive. By using DNA sequencing, CDC proved that Acer had infected all seven patients.

All seven felt betrayed by the health professions. In 1991, with little hair and weighing only 70 pounds, Bergalis testified before Congress, passionately urging that Congress make it a felony for HIV+ health professionals to interact with patients without revealing their HIV status. The law never passed, and Bergalis died publicly and painfully in December at age 23.

Exactly how or why Dr. Acer infected his patients remains a mystery. Some people believe that he deliberately infected heterosexuals so that Americans would no longer see AIDS as a disease of gay men. The truth will never be known. In some ways, it is better for public health if Dr. Acer deliberately infected Bergalis. Why is that? Because if he did, then she did not get infected through unsafe practices, and hence, no reason exists to test health professionals for HIV.

Retrospective analysis of cases of HIV+ dentists, surgeons, and internists reveal virtually no cases of accidental infection of patients. In general, probability of infection varies with the amount of blood injected, how deeply the injection goes, and how much virus the blood contains. Also, the same procedures (double-gloving, masking, and not re-using needles) that protect patients from infection also protect physicians and dentists from getting infected.

## THREE ETHICAL ISSUES IN STOPPING THE SPREAD OF AIDS

### Homosexuality

Some people believe that teaching gay men how to practice safe sex—a Harm Reduction strategy—condones such sex between men. The opposite view is that sex between men is sinful and should not be tolerated. As we shall see later, worldviews collide over homosexuality and stopping AIDS. Is conceptualizing homosexuality as an evil lifestyle *homophobia*? Part of the problem of stopping AIDS? Or is tolerance of homosexuality, drugs, and other immorality a root cause of the spread of AIDS?

Homosexuality has existed for thousands of years. In ancient Greece, bisexuality among men was popular, and leaders among Greek men such as Socrates preferred male lovers. Gay figures include Roman emperor Hadrian, King Frederick the Great of Prussia, playwright Tennessee Williams, and novelist Gore Vidal. According to the late Yale historian John Boswell, Christianity tolerated homosexuality more before the twelfth century than in later centuries.[19]

Although some people see homosexuality as a choice, most medical researchers today believe that sexual orientation is biologically determined. The lived experience of gay men and lesbians testifies to this biological view. Virtually every lesbian or gay man reports fighting against her/his sexual attraction and trying to accept the norm of heterosexuality. Because teenagers want to fit in, most gay and lesbian teenagers resist being attracted to members of the same sex and date heterosexually. Their final sexual orientation appears a resisted discovery rather than as a choice.

Many people harbor the false belief that state or federal laws protect sexual orientation. Only if Congress, a state, a city, or a county passed such a law would it be illegal to evict or fire someone because of homosexuality. Currently, except for San Francisco and two cities in Colorado, it is legal to do so almost everywhere.

Indeed, in *Bowers v. Hardwick*, the U.S. Supreme Court in 1988 allowed Georgia to keep a law making forms of anal and oral intercourse illegal between members of the same sex. Ironically, a footnote to the decision did *not* allow the state to criminalize the same behavior among heterosexuals. Obviously, this decision violates Mill's harm principle and cries out for an explanation of why such sexual behavior between members of the same sex is a crime, but not a crime when between members of different sexes.

Five years later in 2003, the U.S. Supreme Court admitted in *Lawrence v. Texas* that it had made a mistake, that the issue was not (as the *Bowers* court said) whether the Constitution conferred upon "homosexuals a right to engage in sodomy," but whether the Constitution conferred a liberty interest to all Americans broad enough to allow consenting sex among adults.[20]

In 2013, the U.S. Supreme Court overturned the Defense of Marriage Act (DOMA), thus upholding legislation in 13 states and the District of Columbia to legalize marriage between same-sex partners. In these states, married gay couples get the same rights as married, heterosexual couples to benefits of survivors for pensions in Social Security, time off for children under the Family and Medical Leave Act, and COBRA extension of medical coverage after termination of employment. In many national companies, the net effect will be to grant married gay couples the same rights as heterosexual couples because having different benefits for two different kinds of married couples in 13 states, plus Washington, D.C., versus the other 36 states is too complicated.

## HIV EXCEPTIONALISM

In the first decade of AIDS, authorities in public health caved in to pressure from AIDS activists and did not pursue contact tracing the way they had with other sexually transmissible diseases. Because of prejudice against gay men, they feared that tracing those exposed to HIV might lead to gay people losing their medical insurance or jobs. Besides, until AZT arrived in 1986, authorities could offer no treatment, so few reasons existed to identify. Thus, authorities then made an exception for contact tracing for HIV.

Today, with AZT and protease inhibitors, early notification can save lives by helping the infected get prompt treatment. Now, if an HIV+ person knowingly practices unsafe sex, he can be charged in many states with a crime. In 1997 in New York, Nushawn Williams knew he was HIV+ and infected 28 teenage girls; he went to jail for doing so. In this case, contact tracing prevented even more girls from becoming infected.

HIV exceptionalism is now generally regarded in public health as a mistake. It succumbed to pressure from gay activists and may have cost some of them their lives.

In 2006, the CDC recommended that physicians routinely test all patients for HIV. Of course this created controversy. Conservative religious groups retorted that no reason existed to test people in traditional marriages. In 2009, medical leaders repeated the call to make HIV testing part of routine medical exams.

## STOPPING THE WORLDWIDE SPREAD OF HIV: FOUR VIEWS

In the first edition of this book in 1990, it seemed shocking that by 1987, 60,000 Americans had died of AIDS—more than had died in the Vietnam War. Researchers guessed that 10 million people might have then been infected worldwide. Two years later, gay activist Larry Kramer wrote:

> When I first became aware of this disease, there were only 43 cases in the United States; now there are 12 million people infected with AIDS around the world; within the next eight years, this figure could rise to 40 million. From 43 to 40 million should be enough not only to cause some level of panic, but also to

make everyone ask: how is this plague spreading so quickly? Indeed, 1 million new people worldwide were infected with the AIDS virus last year alone.[21]

Twenty-five years after Larry Kramer wrote this, and after a quarter century of AIDS, we still argue about how to stop this disease. Meanwhile, the number of victims of AIDS keeps rising.

By 2001, AIDS had killed nearly a half a million Americans, but at least in America, HIV had become a chronic infection with which victims could live. However, in the developing world, AIDS seemed unstoppable.

In 2001, when the virus had killed 20 million people and infected another 40 million, Secretary-General Kofi Annan of the United Nations called for new efforts. Irish singer and activist Bono pressured America to give more aid, and under the George W. Bush administration, it did. Politicians aimed at universal access to treatment, costing $20 billion a year, and $10 billion of that idealistic number was actually donated.[22] In 2008, Bush signed PEPFAR (President's Emergency Plan for AIDS Relief), committing $48 billion over the next five years.[23]

In 2006, UN Secretary-General Kofi Annan lamented that, despite progress, AIDS still was "the single greatest reversal in the history of human development." Why was Annan so gloomy? Because after *25 years of the epidemic, AIDS had killed 25 million humans.*

| Year | Living HIV-Infected | Cumulative Deaths[24] |
|------|---------------------|-----------------------|
| 1981 | 600 | 200 |
| 1990 | 10,000,000 | 1,000,000 |
| 1999 | 30,000,000 | 10,000,000 |
| 2006 | 35,000,000 | 25,000,000 |
| 2008 | 33,000,000 | 29,000,000 |
| 2012 | 30,000,000 | 30,000,000 |

So how to stop AIDS is an urgent question. Over the next four decades, HIV could infect as few as 10 million or as many as a billion people. Useless approaches affect more people's lives than any other issue in bioethics, and thus, stopping the spread of HIV with proven strategies could save more lives than surgery, drugs, hospitals, and vaccinations combined.

From this perspective, *global bioethics* clamors for attention. If moral actions create the greatest good for the greatest number of humans, then moral people will fight to end AIDS. If past trends continue in the next decades, the 30 million people now infected could pass HIV on to another 30 million people.

Over the last 30 years, AIDS has changed whom it infects, from a disease of gay men and drug users to a disease of women and children. Women compose half of the world's HIV-infected population, 60 percent in sub-Saharan Africa. Young people under age 25 make up half of new infections worldwide.

The part of Africa south of the Sahara Desert has the greatest pool of HIV infection, 2.56 million. South Africa alone has 5.6 million infected.

China and India cause concern because of their blood-amplification systems and populations of a billion each; India has 2.4 million HIV-infected people, whereas China officially has 740,000 but probably has at least a million.

Eastern Europe and Central Asia (the Ukraine, Kazakhstan, etc.) with large numbers of intravenous drug-users, in 2011 had 1.5 million infected, up from 1 million in 2010.[25]

So how do we stop the spread of HIV around the globe? Part of the answer involves ethics. Should we attack behaviors or viruses? Use non-moralistic education or moralistic condemnation? Spend money on education? Buy cheap anti-AIDS drugs when the numbers infected keep doubling? When many lack clean water? Should we triage countries with masses of infected people that are hopelessly corrupt, concentrating where we can save the most lives? These questions will concern us for the rest of this chapter.

The following section sketches four views of how to stop AIDS, including exchanges between proponents of these different views.

## Educational Prevention

Ultimately, non-moralistic education is humanity's only hope of preventing HIV. Self-interested humans can learn to protect themselves against HIV by negotiating safe sex, using clean needles, avoiding infected blood, and taking anti-retroviral drugs to prevent infection of newborns.

Cynics deride education, but it has worked. Between 1990 and 2010, new infections in the developed world declined. Blood became safe in developed countries, people used condoms, and mothers stopped HIV from infecting their babies.

Needle exchange programs (NEPs) prevent the spread of HIV by giving drug users a clean needle and syringe each time they inject drugs, eliminating the need to share contaminated syringes. One study in New Haven, Connecticut, achieved a 33 percent reduction in HIV transmission by giving out clean needles to at-risk persons. A 1992 study by the CDC of 23 NEPs showed that they caused no increase in drug usage.

In the late 1980s, Thailand modeled how to arrest HIV. With a national campaign for 100 percent use of condoms, it advertised on television, hired outreach workers, ran testimonials by its royal family, and educated its sex workers, drug-users, and citizens in preventing HIV infection. Allowing free access to testing and counseling, it protected the infected against discrimination. Giving out free AZT, it allowed production of generic anti-AIDS drugs for the poor. Over the next decade, new infections dropped 80 percent, preventing 200,000 HIV infections.[26]

During the 1990s, similar efforts worked in Uganda. Led by President Yoweri Museveni, Uganda ran testimonials on television by famous Ugandans diagnosed with HIV. Infection rates among Uganda's youth dropped dramatically. In rural areas, rates dropped by half and by two-thirds among urban, pregnant women.

Brazil shows surprising success in using education to prevent HIV infection. Like Cuba, Brazil has a large commercial sex industry for both its citizens and tourists, so in 1990 its large cities had high rates of HIV infection. In 1996, the Brazilian government funded universal access to the best anti-AIDS drugs, creating a national system of out-patient centers, local manufacture of generic anti-AIDS drugs, sophisticated labs, and record keeping. As a result, Brazilian deaths from AIDS dropped by half, and rates of infection in São Paulo and Rio de Janeiro dropped 54 and 73 percent, respectively.[27] Cuba has free medical care, contact-tracing, virtually mandatory treatment programs, and, despite its sex industry, "the world's smallest epidemic" of HIV infection.[28]

Brazil's huge population means this program is a great success. Although both Brazil and South Africa have similar middle-class economies, Brazil's efforts at educational prevention fared much better. Education and prevention do work, given the will and funding. One country led, the other denied that HIV caused AIDS.

## Feminism

The key to stopping AIDS is empowering women to prevent themselves from getting infected. We must enable women to vote, to earn money, and to reject domestic violence.

HIV is a curse on millions of women and children. Nearly half the 33 million humans on the globe living with HIV are women of reproductive age, and almost all the 2 million children living with HIV were infected during pregnancy, birth, or breast-feeding.[29]

A noted physician-fighter against AIDS for 25 years concluded his 2006 review of this disease with these words: "The prime mover of the epidemic is not inadequate antiretroviral medications, poverty, or bad luck, but our inability to accept the gothic dimensions of a disease that is transmitted sexually. Only if we cease to dodge this fact will effective HIV-control programs be established. Until then, it is no exaggeration to say that our polite behavior is killing us."[30]

The "gothic dimensions" of AIDS include the fact that nasty behavior by men around the world infects millions of women and children, that soldiers use mass rape as a weapon, that women and children are sold into sexual slavery, and that poor, powerless women cannot refuse sex from their more powerful, infected husbands. The only name for this behavior is *evil*.

This evil is the kind caused by human decisions. AIDS is not a punishment from God, but a way that evil manifests itself. Consider the case of 13-year-old Rhaki in Rajasthan, India:

> From a poor, rural family, Rhaki had an arranged marriage at age 13 to a 23 year-old man who worked in the distant city of Mumbai for 11 months of the year. Once a year, her husband returned for a month, during which time he had sex with her. While he lived in Mumbai, he had sex with prostitutes and became HIV+. At age 19, she learned that she and her 2-year-old son were HIV+.
>
> Despite the fact that she remained faithful to her husband and used no drugs, she was blamed for bringing shame into her family. She feared she would be ejected from the family and forced to become a prostitute in a distant city.[31]

In Namibia, one study found that 95 percent of 1,000 women were forced in their first sexual encounter.[32] A third of women in Sierra Leone reported the same. In sub-Saharan Africa, with two-thirds of the world's HIV infections, 60 percent of those infected are women.[33] Of those newly infected and aged 15 to 24, a whopping 77 percent are women.

Bad motives cause this pattern. Some African men perceive that sex with a young girl is unlikely to infect them with HIV, and some believe that sex with a virgin will cure HIV. These practices ensure that many teenage females will become infected.

In South Africa, India, and around the world, an amplification system exists that involves truck drivers, mobile soldiers, and commuting workers. India's new diamond-shaped interstate allows millions of truck drivers to transport commodities from rural areas to cities and ports. Along the way, drivers patronize prostitutes, become infected, and then infect their wives at home, resulting in infected babies.

South Africa's migratory pattern built up over a century, with millions of men traveling to distant mines and being housed in dormitories. Such patterns dramatically increase non-marital sex. In Abidjan, the richest city in the Ivory Coast, migrants compose 40 percent of the city's population, and this city has the highest incidence of HIV in West Africa.[34]

Despite efforts of the United Nations and Christians to stop it, human slavery still exists in parts of northern Africa. In India, Eastern Europe, Mexico, and Korea, young women are tricked, kidnapped, and sold into distant brothels, where they become sex workers, living like slaves.

In Bosnia-Herzegovina, soldiers raped as many as 50,000 women to make them pariahs. In East Timor, the Congo, Rwanda, Azherbaiijan, and Uganda, rape became not only a spoil of war, but also a weapon in it. In Somalia and Darfur, marauders raped thousands of women and expelled them from their homes.

These are terrible human acts. To face a problem, you must name it. This is evil. To deal with it, we must confront it. This means that moral condemnation must be a weapon against AIDS. We cannot remain neutral against such appalling acts. We cannot merely pursue bland education and sanitized programs in public health.

Slavery of all kinds must end. Mass rape must end. Forced sex must end.

Tough love must be tougher. In Cuba, Nushawn Williams would have been executed. What if the government of Ethiopia hanged a man who infected his wife with HIV? It is time to take morally tough stands, or else millions of women and children will die.

## Triage

In some parts of the world, bad behavior is entrenched. Doctors cannot bring peace to warring countries; this is not a medical problem but a political one. Similarly, physicians cannot end slavery or famine; these are larger problems than medicine can solve. Some countries such as Angola have corrupt governments going back a hundred years. It is naïve to think that do-gooder missionaries and loving physicians can change much there.

We need to triage countries such as South Africa, where President Mbeki for a decade publicly resisted the fact that HIV causes AIDS and where he not only did not lead the fight against spread of HIV, but also helped to spread it by his poor example. Angola and Somalia are lost, failed states, so triage dictates ignoring them.

Pouring money and time into some countries is a waste. The point of triage is to intervene to change at-risk lives into saved lives. So, we should ignore countries that don't need our help (North America, Europe, Thailand, Uganda) and ignore countries where nothing we do will make a difference. We should focus on countries in the middle, perhaps India, where politicians lead and where people can change.

Similarly, if people don't care for their own safety, education and counseling will go only so far. After twenty-five years, most adults on the planet know that having unprotected sex, getting a blood transfusion, or sharing needles can get you infected with HIV. If your own self-interest doesn't protect you now from HIV, more education certainly won't.

Besides, as one expert gripes, most AIDS education is bland and generic, and hence, of little value in teaching teenagers. It doesn't teach them how to negotiate usage of condoms during sex or how to safely use hard drugs. "We lack the political will to implement these things," he says.[35]

Among large portions of the world, primal drives for sexual pleasure, fueled by poor judgment under the influence of alcohol and other drugs, lead people to practice unprotected sex. In Russia and Asia, despair over the conversion to capitalism has fueled widespread prostitution and use of alcohol.

All these forces swamp educational efforts to stop AIDS. Wisdom lies in recognizing that we can't control the private actions of most people. Wisdom lies in keeping a candle lit in the darkness.

Survivors will be fastidiously aware of what behaviors can kill them, and teach their children to be similarly aware. Maybe a billion people may die from AIDS, but the other 6 billion will go on. Plagues, flu, and floods have wiped out similar millions before, but humanity has survived. Sadly, such deaths involve humanity's Darwinian evolution.

## Structuralism

Activist groups such as Paul Farmer's Partners in Health emphasize that the cause of the spread of AIDS is not irresponsible personal behavior, but unjust *structures* of society. Education and prevention will never work until these structures change. Prevention is mere window dressing, feminism focuses wrongly on moralism, and triage just breeds despair.

As some structuralists lament, "Obviously it is simpler to blame the victims for the rapid spread of AIDS in poor countries than to analyze the socioeconomic and political structures that underlie, frame, and often predetermine such personal 'choices.' "[36]

What evil structures? For starters, poverty, colonialism, apartheid and its legacy, racism, class injustice, and imperialism. Anthropologist Philippe Bourgois argues that in poor communities, lack of good jobs emasculates men who want to be good providers, who then turn to self-destructive behaviors out of frustration—using drugs, selling them, addicting women, and using violence to control others. Feminism for Bourgois ignores the "objective, structural desperation of a population without a viable economy."[37]

Poverty is a major cause of the spread of HIV-infection. In the 1990s, thousands of dirt-poor farmers in China's Hena province sold their plasma each week. They did so because they could not earn a good living by farming but could do so by selling plasma. Plasma is collected by taking blood from the donor's body, separating the plasma, and returning the rest of the blood to the donor. In this way, donors can give weekly rather than once a month, with whole blood.

Because the province's blood supply became infected with HIV, most of the donors became infected. Whole villages were wiped out. Moreover, because of the secrecy of the Chinese government, we have no idea how many Chinese patients received infected blood, plasma, or clotting factors. Millions of Chinese could be infected and not suspect it.

Too much of the world adopts the approach of "it won't happen here." As Kent Sepkowitz bemoans, "For the past 25 years, the lessons learned about HIV prevention and control in one country have failed to inform decisions in others. As a result, the world has witnessed a slow-motion domino effect, as the disease overwhelms country after country."[38]

Leaders always deny that AIDS endangers the country (our blood is safe; we don't have prostitutes) and then, when cases of AIDS surface, those who are infected are blamed as deviant or foreign. Sepkowitz continues, "This sort of buck passing has delayed the control of AIDS in every country. By the time they finally appreciate the scale of the problem, they face a mature epidemic and the cost of lives and money has increased exponentially."

The connection between the spread of AIDS and structuralism may be put conceptually: *an unjust structure is an amplification system for HIV*. Women turn to prostitution to survive, male manual laborers use drugs to endure semi-slavery, and poor hygiene and public health lead to diseases creating sores and infections, making HIV easier to transmit.

## Replies and Rebuttals

**Feminism Replies**   The key to stopping AIDS is to create social structures that empower women.

Poor women around the world shoulder the burden of AIDS. Such women know they are at-risk, but often can do little to protect themselves. Bearing the paycheck, and hence, food and clothing and other goods of life, men control these women. We will only stop AIDS when we give these women more say over voting, jobs, and sex.

Vaccines, vaginal gels, and female condoms need technological breakthroughs to be effective, and one day may be so. In the meantime, women must be allowed to say "No" to abusive infection by males and forced sexual slavery. Unless structures are created to avoid infection, AIDS will continue to spread and kill.

Although unfashionable, isn't old-fashioned feminism better than triaging 20 million people and forgetting about them? At least, feminism directed at people says that someone *cares* about them (versus the *belle indifference* of triage).

Structuralism is partly correct in that many of the evil structures of the world lead to the abuse, rape, killing, and HIV infection of women, but we can help women without having a complete revolution in every society. Realistic change may need to be step-by-step rather than cataclysmic.

Thus, basic rights for mothers, daughters, and wives can be implemented in small, faith-based communities, such as where clergy wield power in African villages. Money, food, and supplies, combined with faith and goodwill, can model sex-only-within-marriage. Such an approach will also combat slavery and sexual exploitation of women and children and be compatible with conservative religions.

Secular public health proposals that emphasize education may be inappropriate for faith-based, poor communities, where many people are illiterate and ignorant of the most basic scientific facts. Because AIDS is lethal and because a person who gets infected only once gets this lethal disease, such populations cannot wait to be taught to read or to be taught basic science. They need a solution now, and feminism is the answer.

Finally, we do not know that moral censure has not worked. Without it, who knows how many more millions might have died or have been infected? Fear of moral condemnation motivates many people, and maybe that is not a bad thing.

AIDS kills. AIDS is caused by HIV. It's bad to infect someone with HIV. It's heinous to do so deliberately or with indifference. What other definition of a bad person do we need? Why not be a little moralistic here? After all, we're talking about *ethics*, not sanitation or legality.

**Educational Prevention Responds**    Educational prevention rejects the moralism of feminism and structuralism. First, what's wrong with feminism in public health is that it really serves the emotions of the moralizer, not the one condemned. Moralizing did nothing to stop gay men from having sex after AIDS was discovered, but fear of death did. Moralizing only made matters worse.

The key claim is that feminism can change behavior. Is that true? One argument that it won't is that a lot of tough love has already been directed against using drugs, much less intravenous drugs. Similarly, a lot of moralism has been directed toward not having sex outside marriage, but has it worked?

If we execute men who infect their wives, who will bring home a paycheck to feed the wives? And feed the children? Execution sounds like a good idea, but if thought through, it's not. Seeing what would happen to their men, wives would protect their husbands and not turn them in to authorities.

For workers in public health, triage is too pessimistic. Why not generalize that attitude and let everyone starve? Or go without penicillin? Why bother about the rest of the planet at all? Why not let the undeveloped world fight it out among itself and let the rich nations keep it at a distance? Just stay in your hot tub enjoying the scenery and sipping your wine.

But is this a *moral* point of view? What does the Golden Rule enjoin us to do? Triage does not offer the world a moral solution; it gives up on finding one.

The essence of medical morality is to fight pragmatically for the good of the many, especially the tools of medicine. If we give up on that assumption, we might as well give up on medicine.

**Triage Replies**    The champion of triage replies, "You're right. If there are 7 billion people now on the planet and if a billion of them die of AIDS, mostly on the other side of the planet and unknown to me, I don't care. The planet already has too many people and it could easily lose a billion. When stories about AIDS appear on the news, I change the channel. In fact, to avoid such stories, I don't even watch the news anymore."

"Yes, I may be morally deficient, but at least I have enough moral honesty to admit that I have no moral feelings of compassion, shame, or outrage about the mass of human deaths from AIDS. It's going to happen: it's a fact; it's accelerated Darwinian evolution; I don't think governments or missionaries can do anything about it; that's just the way it is."

Structuralists like economist Jeffrey Sachs argue that if Western nations transferred $150 billion a year to developing nations, by 2025 poverty could be wiped off the planet. Singer Bono has jumped on this approach. But will simply transferring money end poverty? And will ending poverty stop the spread of AIDS?

William Easterly, a senior research economist at the World Bank, in *White Man's Burden* criticizes humanitarian planners who impose their own solutions on developing countries, especially the idea that building infrastructure with foreign aid will end poverty.[39] Too many programs are funded top down, with no feedback from poor people. Paul Theroux agrees, criticizing celebrities such as Bono who fly in for dramatic quick fixes and ignore problems that Africans must solve themselves.[40]

With AIDS, Easterly argues that more life-years could be saved by not diverting money from anti-malarial programs and childhood vaccinations and by fighting ordinary scourges such as tuberculosis. A million people still die each year from malaria in Africa.

Second, Easterly urges the West to focus on prevention rather than cure, especially by giving out condoms rather than giving the infected expensive AIDS medicines.

Third, children starve while the parents get anti-retrovirals. HIV takes almost a decade to make people sick. One infected woman said she didn't need the medicines, but a job to feed her family.

Finally, some countries may be hopeless. Twenty years ago, LiveAid concerts raised $100 million for Ethiopia, but little changed, and today, Ethiopia is among the most ravaged countries on earth.

**Educational Prevention Once Again**    The champion of educational prevention also rejects the cynicism of triage. Both triage and feminism sound like solutions, but they are not. In fact, they serve the interests of those who espouse them, not the interests of the world's vulnerable women and children.

Triage would have us not offer expensive treatment to those infected but instead concentrate on preventing new infections. In 2006, the standard of care for HIV infection became *HAART*, Highly Active AntiRetroviral Therapy, which costs $10,000 a person per year in developed countries and which 90 percent of HIV-infected people in the world do not get. Studied initially in infected patients at UAB[41] and elsewhere, HAART helped change HIV infection from a death sentence to a chronic, livable condition.

The key argument for offering HAART treatment at all in certain countries is that *it gives people a reason to get tested*. When Brazil offered HAART free to all its citizens, testing for HIV accelerated and thousands came forth for treatment. Without the offer of free treatment, how many would have gotten tested?

Triage is not an option. Let's call it what it is: global medical apartheid. The racial system of apartheid should not be replaced with a medical one.

Triage acquiesces to hopelessness, and hopelessness allows countries to spiral downward in war, rape, famine, and infection.

## CONCLUSION

In the past five years, remarkable progress has occurred in slowing AIDS.

Whether the approach is feminism, educational prevention, or structuralism, and given different religious backgrounds, provincial leaders, and scientific understanding, some of these approaches work better in, say, Brazil than, say, Botswana. And some of them really have worked.

Since the last edition of this text, the number of infections worldwide has dropped from 33 to 30 million people. Since 2001, the Global Fund to Fight AIDS, Tuberculosis, and Malaria and the Doha Agreement, allowing poor countries to buy or make generic anti-AIDS drugs, have worked to support the most effective prevention and treatment.

Prevention *can* work. In North America, prevention has dropped mother-to-child transmission from 1,300 a year in 1992 to 100 a year in 2002 and needle-exchange programs and changing patterns have dropped infections by drug use 80 percent.[42] In Africa, the exponential growth of HIV infection has been checked, mother-to-child transmission has dramatically dropped, and the number of HIV-infected Africans getting anti-retroviral drugs has increased from 50,000 to over 5 million.[43]

To its credit, the administration of George W. Bush did a lot for victims of AIDS, and billions of U.S. aid poured forth. Seeing that otherwise huge economies might be destroyed, the World Bank also poured money into AIDS prevention. A similar threat to world security galvanized developed nations to respond. These efforts prevented millions of new infections and allowed millions of HIV-infected people to live, especially women, who in turn support millions of children.

In 2011, two new studies proved that uninfected women could be protected from acquiring HIV by taking a combination of daily, anti-retroviral drugs.[44] In "discordant" couples, where one was infected and the other not, those who took the pills faithfully had as high as 90 percent protection.

Today, the best approach combines treatment and prevention: HAART for those infected, and for those at-risk, anti-retrovirals drugs, education, and microbial gels. Using this approach, the rate of new HIV infections around the world between 2001 and 2008 fell by 17 percent.[45] It is encouraging news that people with early infections who immediately start anti-retroviral medicines are 96 percent less likely to pass on the virus.[46] Even more amazing, 14 patients and a baby who started such drugs immediately after infection have been virtually cured of the typical effects of HIV infection.[47] Several other HIV-infected patients receiving other treatments obtained "cures," defined as the point where HIV could no longer be detected in their bodies.[48]

Finally, some of the most impressive successes come in small packages: a stamp-sized paper test for HIV, usable in remote villages;[49] grouping HIV people in cohorts of six, allowing them to share trips to distant clinics for drugs and support one another;[50] the Mother-Baby Pack for HIV-infected pregnant women, which sends them home from clinics with anti-retrovirals and vitamins.[51] These interventions show that pragmatic, good people can save the lives of infected humans and, perhaps, prevent this deadly virus from infecting another 30 million.

## FURTHER READING

Randy Shilts, *And the Band Played On*, New York: St. Martin's, 1987.

Alexander Irwin, Joyce Millen, and Dorothy Fallows, *Global AIDS: Myths and Facts*, Cambridge, MA: South End Press, 2003.

Anton A. Van Niekerk and Loretta M. Kopelman, *Ethics and AIDS in Africa*, Walnut Creek, CA: Left Coast Press, 2006.

Alexander Irwin, Joyce Millen, and Dorothy Fallows, *Global AIDS: Myths and Facts: Tools for Fighting the AIDS Epidemic*, Cambridge, MA: South End Press, 2003.

## DISCUSSION QUESTIONS

1. Explain how each of the views on stopping the spread of HIV tends to see the other four views as part of the problem of spreading HIV.

2. How could blood screening have been screened early in America and France, where the most public scandals occurred and where these countries had the resources to screen prevented thousands of deaths from AIDS?

3. How much can education do to prevent the spread of HIV? Are some people just evil and incapable of being educated to practice safe techniques?

4. How has there always been a trend to blame the victim, whether it's cholera, syphilis, or AIDS?

5. Is being gay, lesbian, or intersex a choice or a matter of biology?

6. Do needle-exchange programs increase drug users or merely make using drugs safer?

7. Why is offering HAART important to motivate people to get tested for HIV?

8. What progress has recently been made in stopping the global spread of HIV?

# CHAPTER 18

# Ethical Issues of the Affordable Care Act

*T*his chapter discusses ethical, political, and historical issues surrounding finance of medical care in the United States and Canada. It discusses whether the new Affordable Care Act, intended to provide affordable medical care to all Americans, is good, just, and practical.

## ROSALYN SCHWARTZ

In 1987, Rosalyn Schwartz, age 47, lived in Ridgefield, New Jersey, and had one child, Andy. Divorced, she lost medical coverage she had previously held through her husband's job.[1] The gift-wrap company where she worked with five other employees, each making $19,000 a year, did not provide medical coverage,

Because she had a *preexisting condition*, an ulcer, when Rosalyn tried to buy coverage, companies offered her only policies that excluded treatment for ulcers and that still cost $4,000 a year, more than she could afford.

In 1988, physicians found a small lump in her breast that might have been cancerous and recommended its removal, but having no coverage, Rosalyn postponed its excision. Unfortunately, cancers are cells gone wild, so they must be excised and radiated immediately, before they spread to bone and organs.

In 1989, Rosalyn felt pain tear through her hip. By then her cancer had metastasized, making her bones fragile. When she fell to the floor, her hip socket shattered. In the ambulance, she sobbed. "Andy, you've just turned 18. Tell them [at the hospital] I have no insurance. But don't sign anything or you'll be responsible."

Hospitalized for 23 days, Rosalyn had three surgeries, costing $40,000, half paid by charity. Rosalyn owed the rest to 12 physicians and two hospitals, each of whom she paid $10 a month.

Unable thereafter to work, Rosalyn received disability under Medicare for $10,500 a year. Attempting again to get medical coverage, she found it would not cover her ulcers or cancer and would still cost her $4,000 a year. Declining such coverage, she then forewent physical therapy, as well as bone scans every six months to check whether her cancer had returned.[2] In 1999, Rosalyn died.[3]

# UNIVERSAL MEDICAL COVERAGE

*Universal medical coverage* supports basic medical care for all citizens. One form is a *single-payer system* administered by one organization. Many developed countries provide universal medical coverage, including Austria, Belgium, Denmark, Finland, France, Germany, the Netherlands, Norway, Portugal, Spain, Sweden, the United Kingdom, Australia, Canada, Cuba, Japan, New Zealand, South Africa, and Taiwan.

One form of universal medical coverage is *mandated multi-plan coverage,* where every citizen must purchase some form of medical coverage, either from a private or public plan. Usually, a government agency regulates all plans.

## 1962 to Present: Canada

Starting in 1962, Canada funded national medical care much like Social Security in America. Its plan covers every Canadian and all medically necessary services. It is universal, portable (transferable between jobs), and publicly administered.

General taxes fund the system, including stiff taxes on cigarettes, alcohol, and gasoline. As in England, each province regulates its supply of services, a situation that leads to frustration among physicians who get licensed easily in one province but never in another.

Canadian physicians can order routine tests for their patients. They do not need permission from a gatekeeper in a managed care plan.

Canadian physicians do not work for the government. Like American physicians, Canadian physicians work for themselves and bill on a fee-for-service basis. However, Canadian physicians cannot collude to raise fees.

Between 1990 and 2010, the Canadian system cost $4,445 American dollars per capita and covered all Canadians; the American system cost $8,233 per capita and left 46 million uncovered.[4]

Canadians live to about age 80, Americans to about 77. Every pregnant Canadian woman gets free care, so Canada has one of the lowest infant morality rates of developed countries. In the United States, only 17 percent of pregnant women have similar coverage.[5] All Canadians can purchase reasonable, long-term care in nursing homes. In the United States, few people can do so.

To control costs, Canada limits the number of specialists. Between referral and first appointment, Canadians wait weeks to see dermatologists, ophthalmologists, oncologists (5.5 weeks) and orthopedic surgeons (40 weeks).[6] Canada also limits the number of expensive machines, such as CT scanners.

The Canadian system doesn't cover everything. While paying most costs of hospitalization or physicians, it pays little for non-hospital drugs, dentistry, or vision care.

In 2005, Canada's Supreme Court overturned a crucial law that had allowed Canadians to buy (or physicians and private insurers to sell) essential medical services.[7] Before the Court struck it down, Vancouver's Cambie Surgery Center, without the usual two-year wait, performed knee surgeries for cash for wealthy patients.[8]

The Canadian system is not perfect. Because provinces possess so much power, physicians can be frustrated by inconsistencies between provinces, lack of national rules, and inefficient allocation of specialists and generalists.[9]

## The National Health Service in England

The National Health Service (NHS) of the United Kingdom is technically four different services (Northern Ireland, Wales, Scotland, and England), but we will use England's to stand for all four. Established in 1948 after victory in World War II and in gratitude to the suffering of the people during that war, the NHS began providing free medical services to all citizens. After a year of legal residence, immigrants also are covered. The NHS is funded through general taxation.

Private health insurance is available as a supplement to NHS, and 10 percent of citizens purchase it. Patients pay for long-term care, dentistry, eye care, and some prescriptions.

Beginning in 1972 and strengthened in 1984, Regional Health Authorities decided how many expensive machines and services to purchase.

The system is massive and has recently suffered problems. These problems involve waiting times, costs, and accountability for errors.

NHS limits medical services by gatekeepers, typically primary care physicians, and by priorities, rather than by price or kind of insurance. This leads to waiting lines in England to see specialists and for elective surgeries.

NHS can be expensive and has had cost overruns. Phase III of Guy's Hospital in London, budgeted around £30 million, ended up costing over £150 million.[10] Its attempt to make records digital, originally estimated to cost £2.3 billion in 2004, may cost £30 billion by 2014 before it is completed.[11]

Primary care physicians in the National Health Service in England, Scotland, and Ireland make substantially more than their American counterparts. Neither system has had great problems attracting physicians to primary care.[12]

## THE AMERICAN MEDICAL SYSTEM: 1962–2012

Because America lacked a unified system of medical finance for the last century, explaining how such finance worked is complex. America essentially stumbled into a patchwork system that covered most serious problems for most people most of the time.

In the early 1970s, Republican President Richard Nixon first tried to rein in costs in American medicine by establishing health maintenance organizations (HMOs) that would make insurance companies compete against one another to lower costs.[13] Under managed care, a gatekeeper would determine whether patients go forward to see a specialist or get admitted to a hospital. The gatekeeper, usually a physician in primary care, could also be a nurse or manager for the plan.

Since World War II, private insurance plans multiplied to more than 300 companies, each with its own rules, qualifications, reimbursement rates, and forms to be filled out by patients and physicians.[14] For the average physician, two full-time clerks deal with only billing and insurance.

## 1965: Medicare Begins

In 1965, Congress walked one step toward universal coverage when Texas Demo-crat Lyndon Johnson wrangled Medicare into law. Originally aimed at helping poor seniors during illness, Congress soon extended it to all seniors over 65, dropping any income requirements.

When Americans reach age 65, Medicare covers about 80 percent of their expenses for hospitals and physicians. Medicare is a single-payer system run by the federal government.

The creation of Medicare stemmed from the evaluative premise that healthy, young citizens should pay for the medical care of sick, elderly citizens. A related idea lay behind Johnson's creation of the Great Society legislation of the 1960s, which created Head Start, food stamps, VISTA, and Aid to Families with Depend-ent Children (AFDC).

Medicare gave the elderly a previously unknown medical security. Before 1965, many elderly Americans worried whether they could afford physicians and hospitalization. Before 1965, retired workers were on their own for medical cover-age. Before 1965 and for financial reasons, entering a hospital terrified the elderly.

Medicare also covers about 4 million people with disabilities under age 65, plus 100,000 people on dialysis under the End Stage Renal Disease Act (ESRDA). All of Medicare in 2013 covered about 43 million Americans.[15]

Medicare is financed from mandatory payroll taxes—indicated on paycheck stubs as FICA (Federal Insurance Corporation of America). Medicare in 2011 cost $554 billion.[16]

In 2006, a Republican Congress under George W. Bush surprised its critics by expanding Medicare to cover costs of drugs for seniors on both sides of a "donut hole," i.e., some initial costs, then a big gap, then all costs after the end of that gap. This expanded coverage increased the national debt and future medical costs.

## 1965: Medicaid Begins

In 1965, a second arm of American health care began as Medicaid, also part of Johnson's Great Society legislation. As a state program covering medical services, each Medicaid program operates differently (a fact that becomes important with the ACA), but federal matching funds guide states' efforts and enforce national guidelines.

Medicaid covers medical expenses only for poor people, especially those on public assistance, children of poor parents, poor seniors, people with disabilities, and adults with mental illness. (A memory aide: Medic*aid aids* the poor; Medic*are cares* for the elderly).

Eligibility for a state's Medicaid plan varies by each state. A citizen could qualify for Medicaid coverage with a higher income in California than in Alabama. In New York in 2013, a single parent with two children could not have resources more than $9,000 or income more than $750 a month and qualify for Medicaid.

What Medicaid covers also varies from state to state. Over the last two dec-ades, Medi-Cal, MassHealth, and TennCare have covered the most services, and hence, had the most problems with their budgets.

Medicare does not cover nursing homes or long-term care. Only Medicaid does. To qualify for such coverage, seniors must exhaust all personal wealth, including sale of personal homes. To avoid families sneaking around these rules and transferring assets to adult children, in the five years before application for a nursing home, Medicaid penalizes such transfers.

Medicaid pays for drugs of people with schizophrenia who do not work. Because most such people take their drugs for life, such drugs are expensive. Like the poor, people with schizophrenia face a dilemma between (a) not working and getting their drugs through Medicaid, and (b) working a job with poor coverage for mental health and getting no drugs.

The bailout of 2008 by the federal government of American banks oddly included the Mental Health Parity Act, requiring insurers to cover mental illnesses in the same way they cover physical illnesses.[17] This act reversed incentives for people with mental illness not to work, because their insurance would now be covered by employers.

An especially controversial aspect of American medical finance has been coverage for undocumented, immigrant workers. The Deficit Reduction Act of 2005 forbids Medicaid from covering services for them (more on this later).

## 1997: CHIP

Starting in 1997, the federal government began the State Children's Health Insurance Program (sCHIP, where the "s" is a placeholder for each state, e.g., Utah-CHIP). Designed for those who earn too much to qualify for Medicaid yet are unable to cover their children through employment or private insurance, sCHIP works with each state's Medicaid program. Under it, children can obtain check-ups, prescriptions, dental work, and eye care, as well as services at hospitals and by physicians. The first act of Congress under President Barack Obama expanded sCHIP to cover 4 million additional children (up from 7 to 11 million), paid for by increasing federal taxes on cigarettes.

Before sCHIP, poor working parents faced the dilemma of going to work, losing eligibility for Medicaid, and then losing coverage for their children. If they became unemployed, they (and, hence, their children) became eligible for Medicaid. SCHIP thus also reversed incentives for not working.

## Tricare and VA Hospitals

A different medical system covers military personnel, their families, and veterans. While on active duty, members of the armed services see physicians through Tricare (formerly called CHAMPUS), which allows them to see military or private physicians. Tricare is part of the Department of Defense Military Health System.

Veterans may utilize a national system of hospitals and clinics run by the Veterans Health Administration (VHA), which is not part of the Military Health System but part of the Department of Veterans Affairs. Founded after World War II in appreciation to America's veterans, the VHA is based on the moral premise that no one who served in the armed forces should later lack medical care.

The VA system is the second-largest department of the federal government. Caring for injuries of veterans of wars in Iraq and Afghanistan has doubled its budget from $70 billion in 2005 to $140 billion in 2013.[18] The VHA employs now more physicians and nurses than any other American institution. In recent decades, it has shed its old reputation for shoddy care and emerged as a national leader of good, efficient, electronic, medical care.[19]

The VHA covers veterans not only for surgery, drugs, and visits to physicians, but also for mental illness and long-term care in nursing homes. The Armed Services runs its own nursing and medical schools and, in return for later service, pays for students to attend those schools.

## 1985: COBRA

In 1985, Congress passed COBRA, allowing employees to continue medical insurance at group rates for *18 months* by paying their share plus the employer's share of their former premiums. COBRA also covers spouses after divorce and adult children.[20] Even with COBRA, many employees cannot afford it because they must now pay for the employer's former share, which may have paid for as much as 95 percent of their previous coverage.

## 1986: EMTALA

Part of America's medical system is the Emergency Medical Treatment and Active Labor Act (EMTALA) of 1986, which forbids emergency rooms from turning away patients who are medically unstable. All ER patients, regardless of coverage or ability to pay, must be stabilized before they are released.

This federal requirement means that emergency rooms serve as a national safety net for the uninsured and for illegal immigrants. States with large numbers of these patients face escalating costs for patients treated under EMTALA.

## 1993–1994: Clinton's Health Care Security Bill

In 1993, President Bill Clinton proposed his Health Care Security Act to expand Medicare for all Americans. This act assumed two tenets: (1) an *employer mandate*: all employers had to pay something toward medical insurance for their employees; (2) formation of large *managed care plans*. The act encouraged such plans to compete to lower costs.

Both assumptions faced opposition. Small businesses fought the employer mandate because they feared being made to pay. Many said they would rather not hire workers.

Second, many Americans, especially seniors, disliked managed care and gatekeepers. Seniors liked Medicare and wanted to keep it as it was. Because seniors vote in large numbers, politicians feared their power.

The act's greatest financial problem lay in trying to expand medical services while simultaneously reducing costs. After a year of national discussion, it failed to get to the floor of Congress for a vote.

## 1996: HIPPA

In 1996, the federal Health Insurance Portability and Accountability Act (HIPPA) required portability for workers between similar plans and banned excluding pre-existing conditions in such transfers (without this ban, workers with any medical problem would be trapped in their existing job). It also guaranteed privacy of medical records for patients.

## 1962–2012: Coverage at Work through Private Plans

Between 1962 and 2012, about half of Americans got medical coverage though employment.[21] This includes their spouses and children (including adult children up to age 26). Coverage in retirement varies according to the largesse of the employee's former employer.

As a benefit to employees, some employers provide medical coverage. Employers with many employees can negotiate lower rates than employers with few employees because they spread costs of illness over more people. So large employers with their discounts offer the best medical plans.

One disadvantage of employer-based coverage comes from small employers. Small businesses out to maximize profits do not provide medical coverage to their employees, in part because employers with fewer than 25 employees pay the highest rates.

A second disadvantage of employment-based plans is that when workers leave jobs, medical coverage often ceases. This happened to Rosalyn Schwartz.

A third disadvantage of employer plans is *cost shifting*. American hospitals are not reimbursed for providing medical care to the poor in emergency rooms, but EMTALA forbids them from turning patients away. To compensate for such losses, hospitals charge large employers more for services for insured patients. Large employers resent such cost shifting, because it forces them, but not small employers, to subsidize the indigent. For this reason in Oregon, Vermont, and Massachusetts, large employers there favored statewide, universal coverage.

A fourth disadvantage of employer plans is that American employers claim the cost of insuring their employees is too high. In 1990, over $675 of the cost of each new Ford vehicle went to pay for medical coverage for employees.[22]

In 2010–2012, small companies employing 20–50 employees often saw costs of medical coverage jump 20 percent a year.[23] In 2011 in New Hampshire, more than 90 percent of employers had fewer than 50 employees, and a single employee's monthly premium jumped to $550 from $384 the year before. Because of such high costs, some employers created a two-class system, with regular employees with good benefits and part-time employees with no benefits.

A fifth disadvantage of the employment-based system occurs when illness or injury dislodges workers into chronic unemployment. Many people become poor because of cancer, schizophrenia, or car accidents, which then makes them undesirable to employers, so chronic unemployment results, trapping them in poverty and making them dependent on Medicaid and public assistance.

People who are unemployed or who work for a small company that offers no medical insurance may buy individual policies. About 12 to 15 million Americans do so, including the self-employed, seasonal workers, adult students, and people between jobs. But as Rosalyn Schwartz discovered, individual policies are expensive and may exclude just what is needed. Keeping the same policy for such people with the same physician became a contested issue under the ACA.

## BLUE CROSS/BLUE SHIELD AND KINDS OF RATINGS

Prior to the ACA, private insurers used either community or experience rating. In *community rating*, they evaluate risk for a large employer, state, or area and charge the same to every policyholder in that group. Community rating favors ill people because they cannot be excluded and healthy people subsidize them. National, universal medical coverage spreads community rating over an entire country.

*Experience rating* charged an individual or small business based on previous illnesses or numbers of employees, and so dramatically increased costs for some policies. In extreme cases, insurers maximized profits by selling policies to healthy young people, who were unlikely to make claims and by avoiding people who were sick, old, disabled, or at high risk of accidents—that is, people likely to make expensive claims. For a small business with 35 employees, one employee needing a liver transplant could make premiums exorbitant for the rest.

During the 1930s, surgeons and physicians founded Blue Cross and Blue Shield to ensure that patients could pay them after hospitalization for catastrophic conditions. By state law, the "Blues" were nonprofit organizations. As such, they paid no state or federal taxes.

In return for their nonprofit status, Blue Cross Blue Shield (BCBS) companies had to adopt community rating, in other words, had to insure everyone who wanted to be insured. Between the 1930s and the 1960s, things worked reasonably well for everyone: BCBS insured everyone in a state who wanted insurance and rates remained reasonable.

In the early 1970s, changes in federal regulations allowed commercial medical coverage of a new kind to emerge. These companies used experience rating, and they *cherry-picked* the healthiest customers, leaving BCBS as the insurer of last resort for the unhealthiest and neediest customers.[24]

These factors explain what happened to Empire BCBS in New York in the 1980s: commercial companies left it with only the sickest customers, such as those with AIDS. As a result, Empire BCBS raised premiums for its remaining customers by 100 percent and nearly went bankrupt.

Another target of cherry-picking, Kentucky BCBS, between the early 1960s and the late 1970s saw its share of policies statewide drop from 90 to 30 percent. Some states later made cherry-picking illegal.

If a businessman wanted to make the most money, he would cherry-pick and cover only companies with healthy young people, e.g., those working for Google, who were unlikely to make claims and with employers who paid most of the premiums. He would not cover employees at pest-control companies.

People misunderstand "medical insurance," a misleading phrase. Thirty years ago, it meant simply insurance—a hedge against a dreaded but remote possibility. People then bought medical insurance hoping they'd that never use it. As such, policies covered catastrophes like automobile accidents or diagnoses of cancer.

Gradually, medical policies evolved into *prepaid group medical coverage.* They expanded to cover not just catastrophic but all "major medical" expenses. This was logical: if people would pay small premiums to protect themselves against catastrophic risks, why not pay somewhat more to protect against common risks? Thus, insurance grew until it included every medical service, and today, people complain when their "insurance" doesn't cover everything, as if that is what the term means.

Many people mistakenly believe that most Americans without medical coverage are *unemployed.* In fact, most Americans without medical coverage *work.*[25] Most waiters and waitresses lack employer-sponsored medical insurance, as do most workers in small businesses. Only the rare business that employs fewer than 10 people 1 in 10 provides medical coverage.[26]

## OREGON, VERMONT, AND MASSACHUSETTS COVER EVERYONE

In 1987, Oregon broadened its Medicaid plan to cover 30,000 Oregonians of 90,000 who applied through a lottery for a new Oregon Health Plan (OHP).

OHP did *not* fund some expensive medical services such as in vitro fertilization, experimental therapies for people with AIDS, or heart and liver transplants. In 1988, it refused to pay for a bone-marrow transplant of 7-year-old Coby Howard, despite his parents' appeals to the media, a rare failure of the rule of rescue.

In 1993, OHP had spent $84 million, but only $34 million had been allocated for it; overall, it faced a predicted $1.2 billion shortfall.[27] In 2003, OHP reduced benefits and required higher deductibles and co-payments.[28] Between 2003 and 2005, two-thirds of its members lost their insurance coverage, and over three-fourths went uninsured for more than six months. Despite a restoration of some coverage in 2004, many of those dropped continued to experience problems obtaining medical care. In short, OHP proved more expensive than Oregonians could pay for.

Importantly, OHP not only covered hospitalization but also mental, vision, and dental care, as well as some associated products. This expansion of services undoubtedly contributed to the rising costs of OHP.

In 2013, Oregon expected that OHP would need to cover an extra 600,000 people with its expansion of Medicaid for the ACA; the projected cost of this expanded Oregon Health Plan was $6.5 billion.[29] (The exact amount that OHP would cost is controversial and difficult to calculate.) It also found itself compelled to reduce reimbursement to providers by 11 percent.

In 2008, Massachusetts and Vermont cranked up their own systems of universal medical coverage. As is the case with car insurance, they required every citizen to have health insurance or lose a tax credit of $209 in 2008, but this lost credit (lost credit amount increased substantially between 2009 and 2012).[30]

Where Massachusetts penalized non-compliance, Vermont encouraged its uninsured residents to enroll in its Catamount Health. Under it, and for about $500 a month, families got the same coverage as Blue Cross Blue Shield, with tiered co-pays for drugs and the same deductibles.[31] On a sliding scale, Vermont subsidized families making up to 300 percent of the poverty level (about $30,000 for one parent and $60,000 for a family of four).[32]

Vermont's plan recognized that people with chronic conditions (diabetes, heart disease, obesity, high blood pressure) consumed 80 percent of the medical dollars. It covered screening, counseling, and prevention for people with these conditions to try to reduce more expensive interventions later. Employers with more than 10 employees that did not provide medical coverage had to pay the state medical fund $295 per employee.

In Massachusetts, the poorest residents (making under $10,000) got access to medical coverage with no premiums and no deductibles. Massachusetts/CHIP also expanded to cover all expenses of children in families up to 300 percent of the poverty level.[33] By 2011, 99.8 percent of children were covered and 98.1 percent of adults.[34] Some patients had trouble finding a primary care physician willing to treat new patients, some of whom had long postponed care.[35]

Already the state that was spending the most on medical care per resident, in 2009 Massachusetts experienced a budget deficit of $4 billion and sought to rein in medical costs. As a result of expanded coverage, Massachusetts spent far more than average on medical care, and by 2018, experts predict that it will spend $16,000 per person, $3,000 more than the national average.[36]

Both plans are costly. In Massachusetts, Medicaid payments for medical care went up to $90 million by 2009, about what private insurers formerly paid. One scholar predicted that working families (who will pay $14,000 a year) won't be able to afford it and that the Massachusetts plan will go bankrupt because, like Medicare, physicians and patients in the plan have no incentives to cut costs.[37]

Both plans put the lie to the idea that universal coverage must be a government-run, single-payer system. By cobbling together several plans, these states managed to provide coverage for all citizens.

## 2010: THE PATIENT PROTECTION AND AFFORDABLE CARE ACT

In 2010, President Barack Obama signed into law the Patient Protection and Affordable Care Act (PPACA), succinctly called the Affordable Care Act (ACA). ACA could be the greatest expansion of medical coverage in America since President Johnson's Great Society legislation of 1965. Through a combination of mandates, subsidies, and tax credits to both individuals and employers, the act's ultimate goal was covering all Americans and making medical costs reasonable.

Much drama and politics led up to this event, which eased with the re-election of President Obama in 2012, squashing attempts to delay implementation of the ACA. A few months later, the U.S. Supreme Court controversially upheld the constitutionality of the ACA, justifying it not as a *mandate* to buy coverage by individuals or as a mandate to provide it by employers, but as a *tax* that could be imposed on those choosing not to buy coverage. The Court, however, created an important opening by holding that states need not expand Medicaid to cover everyone, but instead could form exchanges where individuals could purchase coverage. In mid-2013, 21 states had elected not to expand Medicaid and 6 were debating it, so only 24 states had actually expanded their Medicaid programs.

The ACA required insurance companies to cover all applicants at the same rates and not to employ experience rating or to decline coverage for preexisting conditions. By 2013, it had already required employers to carry 6 million young adult children on family policies until the age of 26, shrunk the "donut hole" for prescription drug costs of Part D in Medicare, added 600,000 new Medicaid enrollees in seven states with expanded plans, and (it claimed) rebated more than $1 billion to 12.8 million consumers on insurance premiums.[38]

The ACA will be implemented in phases between 2013 and 2018. Various kinds of citizens (single, married, working, unemployed, retired, etc.) will pay more each year between 2013 and 2018 or pay more taxes/penalties. This has been the strategy in Massachusetts, which achieved 98 percent coverage.

Nevertheless, the young will vote with their dollars on the ACA. For example, in Oregon, for a person making $25,000 a year, penalties for not carrying health insurance will be, respectively, $150, $325, and $695 in 2014, 2015, and 2016. This rise in penalties parallels what officials did in Massachusetts, gradually raising the penalties until the point that 98 percent of citizens decided they might as well buy coverage.

## FOR AND AGAINST THE ACA

### Opposing the ACA #1: Illegal Immigrants

The elephant in the room of universal medical coverage is illegal immigrants. In the fall of 2013, America's population reached 313 million people, a growth of 100 million people since 1967. About 53 percent of the new Americans were recent immigrants, and about 11 million were illegal.

Forcing employers to provide medical coverage to illegal workers will break the bank. If such workers are covered, those with expensive diseases and disabilities will flock to America. This is what is known in the insurance industry as *adverse selection.*

In England, foreign visitors can obtain a National Health System Number when they need to see a physician. On subsequent visits with this identifying number, foreign patients can get treatment because English physicians do not want to be immigration officers and deny services to needy patients, so (according to one former finance officer for a regional health authority), "Word has gotten 'round in Nigeria, Ghana, India, and Pakistan that it is possible to receive treatment on the UK taxpayer without restraint."[39]

Whether hospitals admit illegal immigrants varies in America from hospital to hospital, state to state. Reimbursement figures show that the largest group of illegal immigrant patients is pregnant women.[40] Consider two hospitals in the Dallas-Ft. Worth area: Parkland Hospital in Dallas does not ask immigrants about their national status, and pregnant mothers from Mexico flock to it. The hospitals of the JPS Health Network in Dallas require proof of American citizenship, and hence, see few illegal pregnant women.[41]

In 2012, California spent over $1.25 billion on medical care for illegal immigrants. The other top states giving such care were Arizona, Texas, New York, and Illinois.

If children are born in America, hospitals have their births reimbursed by Medicaid. The child is then an American citizen, with K–12 public schooling available to him, as well as other benefits.

America cannot afford to open its borders and to give away medical coverage and jobs to everyone who wants to enter. This is the age-old story, played out long ago in England in the *tragedy of the commons*: the owner of each flock increased the number of sheep he grazed on town land—the commons—until it was so over-grazed that the grass disappeared and the commons was destroyed.[42]

Should we start illegal immigrants on chemotherapy for cancer or hemo-dialysis for kidney failure? Once such therapies begin, because of the rule of rescue, they are difficult to stop. Once they are started for some immigrants, it is difficult not to do the same for others. But the more such expensive medical services are bestowed, the greater the incentives for people to slip into America illegally to get them.

Vermont, Massachusetts, and Oregon, with their expanded coverage, do not model the rest of America. How many illegal workers do they have? Vermont is one of the whitest states (96 percent) in the country and has few jobs that attract immigrants. Oregon is 88 percent white. These are not two states experiencing massive problems with illegal immigrants and hence, it was easier for them to insure that all their citizens had coverage.

## Favoring the ACA #1: Illegal Immigrants

Myths abound about illegal workers. Most Americans do not believe that such workers pay FICA and income taxes, but these taxes are in fact deducted from their paychecks.[43] In 1996, the Internal Revenue Service began issuing identification numbers to illegal workers to take their taxes. Whether a gangster or an illegal worker, other authorities may delay dealing with you, but the IRS will not; it demands your taxes. Each year, half of the 7 million illegal workers use such ID numbers to file federal and state returns and pay the same tax rates as traditional Americans.[44]

Anti-immigration advocates claim that illegal workers burden hospitals and drain resources from traditional Americans. Starting in 1996, reforms to welfare disqualified illegal immigrants from receiving welfare, food stamps, subsidized housing, Medicaid, and Medicare.

In 2013, studies led by researchers at Harvard Medical School discovered that immigrants created a surplus in Medicare funds of $115 billion, whereas established Americans created a deficit of $28 billion.[45] This is because most immigrants, legal or illegal, are young and few legal immigrants are old enough to get Medicare.

The Obama administration promises that illegal immigrants will not break the bank of the new system. On the other hand, reforming immigration (allowing a legal pathway to citizenship) would help finance the ACA by adding millions of tax-paying young people and encouraging workers to be paid on the books. A recent study by the Pew Research Center showed that with controlled, regulated immigration, the U.S. population could grow by 2050 to nearly 400 million.[46] If so, that would add 75 million new people to pay premiums for decades for the ACA.

## Favoring the ACA #2: Greater Efficiency

The ACA could eliminate the overhead, profit, and waste of multiple private insurers. About 4 to 12 percent of health care costs represent fees and profits of private insurance plans, *$100 billion* in 2005.[47] By comparison, Medicare has maintained reasonable administrative expenses, about 2.5 percent of total expenditures.[48] The ACA could use that $100 billion to cover medical care for poor people.

Medicare and VA hospitals have been successful. Both employ technologically advanced systems. Moreover, both have done so while the number of people using them and the services offered have increased.

## Opposing the ACA #2: Federal Bureaucracy Is Inefficient

The ACA will create a bloated, unresponsive federal bureaucracy. During the 1960s and 1970s, the Veterans Administration became such a bureaucracy. The federal government cannot do certain things well, and one of them is health care.

The ACA does not eliminate private insurers, but merely manages them. It is not a single-payer system. Instead it offers every citizen the chance to purchase insurance (private or in a state-exchange) or pay a tax. Therefore, it is unclear what savings will be generated, if any, by the ACA.

The ACA will likely become another End Stage Renal Disease Program, with runaway costs. What everyone pays for, nobody pays for. In public systems, everyone will seek his own advantage to the detriment of the overall good. Again, this is the tragedy of the commons.

Despite lip service to greater efficiency, the huge federal government is not famous for its efficiency. Witness the Armed Services, where cost overruns are common for huge weapon systems. Without competition, there will be no accountability.

What is the proper role of the federal government in medical care? Consider federal funding for end stage renal disease, artificial hearts, and AIDS, which is politicized and occurs at the expense of other diseases, such as cancer. The American government is being asked to do too many things for too many people.

One-seventh of the American economy is at stake in health care, plus one-sixth of new jobs. The federal government already runs one-sixth of the economy connected to the Armed Services and national defense, not to mention another sixth controlled by other federal agencies, states, cities, and county governments. As said, the VA is already the second-largest branch of the federal government and runs all VA hospitals. Considering all this, we do not need another expansion of government.

Recent scandals in England at the National Health Service show what happens when government-run medical systems grow too large. Supposedly, 1,200 patients starved to death and all told, 3,000 deaths in NHS-trust hospitals are being investigated for suspicious surroundings. A similar scandal occurred at Walter Reed Naval Hospital in Washington, D.C.—right under the eyes of Congress—until courageous whistleblowers publicized the abysmal conditions and caused massive reforms.

The states resisting expansion of Medicaid are not callous but are fiscally conservative. Although the federal government pays for 90 percent of the expansion for the first three years, after that, each state must pay for all the new Medicaid patients. At present, many states must choose between fully funding universities, Medicaid, or prisons, but not all. Without massive new taxes, Medicaid cannot be prudently expanded.

It is unclear right now how much universal coverage will cost each state. Is it prudent to promise such care without knowing how to pay for it? Many governors say it is not.

Also, is the tax *enough* on individuals for not having coverage? For adults over 26, premiums will cost at least $3,000 a year, but the tax is only $100 (or loss of a tax credit in Massachusetts of $219). The Congressional Budget Office estimated in 2013 that 6 million people would opt to pay the $100 and forgo coverage.[49] That bodes ill for the ACA, which, starting in 2014, needs premiums of healthy, young people to subsidize costs of caring for the old.

### Favoring the ACA #3: Making Medicine Rational

Starting in 2013, the ACA banned experience rating by insurance companies. The ACA assumes that coverage is a moral enterprise of sharing risk to help those with bad genes or those who are victims of accidents. It rejects the idea that selling medical insurance should be a way to make profits.

Of importance, because physicians and surgeons created Blue Cross Blue Shield, it reimburses *procedures* well, but not *preventive services*. Specialists who do procedures receive far more than physicians in primary care who talk to patients: an ophthalmologist gets $2,000 for removing a cataract in an hour but a geriatric psychiatrist gets only $180 for talking to the same patient.

The ACA must emulate Canadian and English systems—pay more to primary care physicians and pay less for procedures (or limit access to them). It is outrageous that the physicians who directly care for so many people make only half as much as dermatologists and ophthalmologists.

One way that the ACA does try to control costs is by setting up systems to encourage evidence-based medicine. At present, Medicare reimburses physicians for almost any treatment that works, or that might work. The ACA sets up review panels to rationally evaluate whether surgery works best for diverticulitis at $100,000 or simple antibiotics plus dietary changes at a cost of $400.

### Opposing the ACA #3: Government Cannot Make Medical Finance Rational

Democracies try to balance two competing values: equality and liberty. A system once in equilibrium with perfect financial equality must forbid inheritance of money, unequal trades, or unequal pay, else the system will soon create citizens of unequal wealth.

We might conceive of equality and individual liberty as the X and Y axis of Cartesian coordinates, respectively. The more we move to perfect equality, the more individual liberty vanishes. For example, for many decades America had no income tax: citizens kept all the money they made. The programs of the Great Society transferred money from the working to the needy. The liberty of some to keep all their money was reduced to increase financial equality for all.

Transfers of income mean taxation, and all taxation is involuntary. Involuntary taxation to some is a kind of working slavery, where a certain portion of the year is required just to pay one's taxes, say, the first six months. The cost of the ACA is too high if everyone must work another month against their will to pay for it.

For universal coverage to work, patients cannot be allowed to opt out of the system. This is like having a situation of perfect equality and then allowing unequal trades. This problem undermined the Canadian system. Similarly, physicians would not be allowed to sell their services privately or avoid being in the ACA.

What we need in medicine is not socialized medicine but a real market of supply and demand. When consumers have choices among competing providers, price will reflect what people want and determine future supply. Markets regulate other goods and services without bloated bureaucracies and wasteful costs. Why not medicine, too?

## Opposing the ACA #4: Health Care Is Not a Right

The ACA would make access to health care a *right* of all American citizens.

Elderly Americans now think of Medicare as a right, and most Americans would come to think of the ACA as a right. Is that what we want?

Supporters of the ACA claim that citizens have a right to *basic* health care. The problem here is conceptual: America was founded on *negative rights of non-interference:* rights to be left alone, to pursue happiness, and to think, speak, assemble, and worship without interference from government. Such "freedom from" differs dramatically from "freedom to." The latter is *a positive right to some service* from others, i.e., an entitlement.

The modern state has moved too much from negative to positive rights, fostering life-long dependency among millions of people on government. This is, in effect, a transfer of money from the hard-working people who pay taxes to fund the government to the dependents. This is wrong.

After three years of Medicaid coverage of everyone in a state, both physicians and patients will develop a mentality of entitlement and expect coverage. States will then be in a bind, such as Illinois and California found themselves in around 2012, where voters refused to increase taxes but wanted more services. But why create this fiscally irresponsible expectation in the first place?

What this means is that there is no logical point after which we must stop providing health care and before which coverage is a right. It all blends together, and once you make one part of the continuum a right, soon the whole thing will be.

Besides, no one can agree on what is basic medical care. Basic care in America, like dialysis, is luxurious in Mexico or Kenya. When American physicians visit developing countries, they despair that they cannot provide the basic care of American medicine.

As medicine improves, what is minimal becomes normal, what is extraordinary becomes ordinary. So in 1962, kidney dialysis was extraordinary; now it is ordinary. In the 1970s, kidney transplants were extraordinary; now they are ordinary. And so on.

Problems at the margins would be difficult: who is a citizen and entitled to national care? A baby born here? An immigrant? How long must one live here before becoming eligible? Would it be right to let some move here and, say, after seven years, have the same medical benefits as someone who has paid into the system for 30 years?

## Favoring the ACA #4: Minimal Health Care Is a Right

Justice requires universal medical coverage, at least it does if "Justice is Fairness," as defined by philosopher John Rawls. Rawls argued that justice applies to the basic structure of society, and health care is part of that structure.

According to him, two main principles of justice exist. Imagine a social contract where citizens choose under *a veil of ignorance* about their own age, race, religion, sex, health, wealth, abilities, and talents, so they cannot bias their choices by considering their arbitrary personal characteristics. Under these conditions, Rawls believes that rational people would not gamble but would first choose those structures that gave people maximal equal liberty.

Rawls recognized that the world is naturally unfair: some people are born into rich families, some into poor ones; some are born healthy, others with spina bifida. Government can either worsen such inequalities or lessen them. For Rawls, just governments reduce natural inequality while preserving liberty.

So, and second, some liberty could be sacrificed to achieve greater equality. When? For Rawls, inequality is justifiable when it works to the advantage of those who are worst off. We would choose this under the veil of ignorance because, when it lifts, we might be the worst-off person. This is Rawls's second principle of justice, *the difference principle.*

How might Rawls's approach be applied to America now and the ACA? The last 40 decades have not been good for the poor in America. Between 1967 and 2010, the gap between the richest Americans and poorest Americans vastly widened, as the former jumped from a median salary of $86,000 to $139,000, while the latter only inched from $9,300 to $11,900. Worse, in 2012, the top 10 percent of Americans owned 80 percent of the financial assets of America.

Over these years, more and more workers had to work longer hours just to keep what they had. Jobs that once paid $20 an hour now paid $7. Before, people could graduate from high school and get a good job for life in a unionized auto plant, but that is no longer possible. If, as Rawls assumes, a just society is egalitarian, then American society became more unjust.

Prior to the ACA, more than 46 million Americans lacked coverage, which is an unjust, structural inequality at a level where life-and-death decisions are made. We know that inherited genes cause many diseases and no one is responsible for the genes he or she inherits. Why allow the structure of medical finance to intensify injustices of fate?

According to Rawls's difference principle, an unequal medical structure would be just only if the poor were better off under it than under an egalitarian system. In the present, unequal American medical system, that is obviously false.

Underlying Rawls's approach to justice is the ability to imagine ourselves as worst off—to see ourselves as sick, hurt, poor, and uninsured; to imagine how bad it would be to have a serious accident and how much worse it would be to have no way to pay for the care we need.

As for using capitalistic markets to control medical finance, let's analyze this idea in some depth. In a true market, people would buy health care, such as an operation on their knee, with their own money. There would be no medical insurance and thus no reimbursement from insurers. Because people would have to pay for their care themselves, prices would tumble.

For a routine eye examination, patients might choose a nurse practitioner charging $10, a primary care physician charging $30, or an ophthalmologist charging $300. Given these alternatives, most would not choose the ophthalmologist, and so ophthalmologists would lower their fees to compete, unless they could somehow demonstrate that their services were worth more. On the other hand, if covered by their medical plan, most Americans would go to an ophthalmologist.

Such a true market would lower costs, but a market in medicine also has burdens, especially for sick and elderly patients. When people have just discovered they have cancer or multiple sclerosis, they do not always make good decisions. As one expert group concluded:

> The elderly are less equipped to deal with a marketplace of health care than younger, working persons. . . .[they] suffer from physical and mental impairments (including eyesight, hearing, and memory), have more trouble . . . comprehending the increasingly complex insurance arrangements . . .[and] lack the counsel of the purchasing agents and benefits representatives who serve younger, employed populations. . . . . many [retired persons] will not fare well in the rough and tumble of a health care marketplace.[50]

In a true market, medical professionals would become hardboiled, doing wallet biopsies before helping anyone. A real market in medicine would be a harsh, cruel system where patients and professionals no longer worked together to overcome illness, but where each bargained with the other for financial gain.

It is also true that if health care were like other commodities—rather than being subsidized as it now is—many people who could afford care would make foolish decisions (right now, half of applicants for Social Security take it at age 62 rather than waiting until 70, when benefits nearly double). If they had to choose between a new car and a hip replacement, some would choose the car. Moreover, some people might be tempted, or pressured, to sacrifice health care for the sake of their families; a parent might give up a hip replacement and put the money toward a house for her family. In this regard, a true market is exactly what people lacking insurance face today.

Some libertarians call the ACA "socialized medicine." Lest that emotional phrase freeze our thought, consider exactly what "socialized" means. "Socialized" could mean simply "publicly owned." If so, that is not necessarily a bad thing, or even, unusual. In America, highways and waterways, public schools, state colleges and universities, the armed forces, airwaves, the air, the skies, and national parks are publicly owned

When Congress debated Medicare in 1965, the American Medical Association (AMA) opposed it as socialized medicine. In 2009, the AMA opposed President Obama's plans for universal coverage (although only one-third of American physicians joined the AMA). American physicians in 1965 then feared that government-administered care financed by taxes would mean government-controlled care[51] and that all physicians would soon be employees of the federal government. To placate these physicians, a crucial decision was then made: under Medicare, physicians would be reimbursed on a fee-for-service basis. Eventually, this arrangement made physicians rich and gave them the best of both worlds: freedom to work independently rather than as government employees and freedom to order infinite services for their patients—services paid for by government through higher Medicare taxes.

## Opposing the ACA #5: Health Care Is Not a Right

Rawls does not own the only theory of justice. His next-door neighbor at Harvard, Robert Nozick, championed a libertarian theory of justice that advocates a minimal, not a maximal, state. For libertarians, the *last* thing the federal government should do is enter the business of providing medical care. Not only is government inefficient in providing medical care, but it is also too expensive when it does so too bureaucratic and too intrusive to privacy. More important, it's morally wrong for big government to do so. Providing medical care is the job of physicians, medical practices, and hospitals, but not the State.

The more health care is seen as a right, the more life becomes medicalized, that is, people tend to seek medical care in more and more circumstances. That happened in Australia, whose system once covered payments for in vitro fertilization. Furthermore, people now live much longer—partly because of the care Medicare provides—and people who live to be old cost the most.

As said, Massachusetts is on track, by 2018, to spend $16,000 per person, $3,000 more than the national average.[52] What if every state has the same problem?

The National Health Service in the United Kingdom is struggling to rein in costs, as is the Canadian system. An axiom of medical finance is that increasing access while expanding services increases costs.

Our experience with Medicare has taught us an important lesson: the system cannot expand the number of patients covered and the range of services offered and simultaneously decrease costs. Coverage for mental illness in the ACA will be on the same level as coverage for physical illness. This parity alone will cost billions.

Each increase in services provided to all Americans costs more money. The increases in services that are most commonly mentioned are long-term care in nursing homes, home health care, hospice care, transportation to medical facilities, coverage for pregnancy and birth control, and dental services for children.

Initially, the ACA was to offer voluntary long-term care insurance, but this had to be scuttled when few people indicated a willingness to buy such coverage and at the very time when private insurers were dropping such coverage.[53]

Backing up such coverage would have incurred exorbitant costs by the federal government.

In 2013, the trustees of Medicare and Social Security announced that, without changes, Medicare will run out of money in 2026 and Social Security in 2033.[54] Despite this announcement, in 2006, Congress passed a new drug benefit for Medicare recipients.[55] This only increases the likelihood that the system will go bankrupt.

Libertarian University of Chicago law professor Richard Epstein emphasized that the cost of the ACA dramatically increases as the system moves from insuring each smaller segment of the 46 million uninsured Americans.[56] Covering most children is relatively cheap. Covering most of the adult, working poor is not exorbitant. But covering the last 10, 5, or 1 percent is expensive because such percentages represent the real cost-busters that all private systems avoid. These patients suffer diabetes, schizophrenia, or congestive heart failure. If a national system entitles them to the best care, no one can say when a just limit of care has been reached.

Libertarians such as Epstein believe Clinton's Health Security Act previewed exactly what would go wrong when the government mandated medical coverage. Clinton's act first ran into trouble with libertarians over its vague estimates of cost. Even the act's advocates said it might entail an extra tax on income of 10 percent.

Libertarians just do not believe that the American government should control costs and provide universal coverage, as happened in Canada, Germany, and Australia. They fear that government will limit freedoms of physicians, businesses, and mandate expensive services requiring higher taxes.

Finally, the End Stage Renal Disease Program stands as a shining example of a federally run, medical entitlement that has cost billions more than expected. Generalizing, it will be impossible not to fund more and more services, running risks of bankrupting the country yet that is what the ACA tries to do.

Medicaid presently gobbles a large share of state budgets. In 2011 and according to the National Association of State Budget Officers, Medicaid cost about 25 percent of state budgets, competing with funding of prisons, highways, K–12 education, higher education, and pensions for state employees.

Between 2014 and 2016, the ACA will pay for the cost of expanding Medicaid to all people under age 65 with family incomes below 138 percent of the federal poverty level. But in 2017, states will begin to shoulder a larger and larger share of these benefit costs, ending at 10 percent in 2020.

Importantly, the ACA does not pay for the administrative costs of expanding Medicaid rolls. The conservative think tank the Heritage Foundation writes:

> Texas recently concluded that the Medicaid expansion may add more than 2 million people to the program and cost the state up to $27 billion in a single decade. The Florida Agency for Health Care Administration estimated in April that the ACA's Medicaid expansion would require an additional $5.2 billion in spending between 2013 and 2019 and more than $1 billion a year beginning in 2017. In California, the Legislative Analysts Office concluded that the ACA's Medicaid expansion will likely add annual costs to the state budget in the low billions of dollars. Mississippi . . . retained Milliman, Inc., a national health care

econometrics firm, to perform a fiscal analysis . . . For Mississippi, . . . between 206,000 and 415,000 people will be added to Medicaid, with a 10-year impact on the state budget of between $858 million and $1.66 billion.

The seven-year cost of the Medicaid expansion in Indiana is estimated to be between $2.59 billion and $3.11 billion, with 388,000 to 522,000 people joining the state's Medicaid rolls. Finally, Milliman estimates that the ACA will result in nearly one of five Nebraskans being covered by Medicaid at a cost of $526 million to $766 million over the next decade.[57]

One way to put the crunch is this: voters in Illinois, California, and Alabama consistently refuse to raise taxes, so legislators have a zero-sum budget (funding one thing more means less for what's left). If funding for Medicaid is 24 percent and higher education is 15 percent of a state's budget, and both are funded equally, then funding Medicaid at 34 percent means funding higher education at 5 percent.

## Favoring the ACA #5: Costs Can Be Controlled

According to the American Heritage Foundation, "New taxes on drug companies ($27 billion) and medical device makers ($20 billion), as well as new reporting requirements and regulations imposed on physicians, will make access to health care and services more costly and difficult for seniors under the ACA."

This is deceptive. In 2007, the top 10 pharmaceutical companies made more profits than the other 490 Fortune 500 companies.[58] Manufacturers of medical devices, such as LVADs, dialysis machines, and stents, also made huge profits. Taxing such companies to fund more medical services for more patients is not unreasonable.

On July 1, 2013, a new federal sunshine law begins, requiring physicians to report gifts over $10 to a watchdog agency, which will publish the results a year later. Drug companies in Minnesota, one of the only states to previously have a sunshine law, paid some physicians $800,000 a year to push their brand-name drugs. It is hard to agree with the Heritage Foundation that either of these developments will "make access to health care more costly and difficult for seniors."

Fixing Medicare and Social Security is not as difficult as alarmists predict. Incremental changes will produce big long-term results. Because people are living longer, the age of eligibility for Social Security has been raised to 67 (for those born after 1960) and later, will perhaps rise to 70. The Medicare payroll tax has increased from 1.45 to 2.35 percent for a married, employed couple.

Likewise, to pay for the ACA, the amount that can be sheltered from taxes in flexible spending accounts has dropped from $10,000 to $5,000 to $2,500 for employees of companies offering such plans—a net increase in taxes. In 2018, the most generous medical plans will be under a new tax. For the wealthy, the ACA raised the tax for Medicare for hospitals from 2.9 to 3.8 percent. It also raised the taxes on capital gains, royalties, and dividends from 15 to 18.8 percent.

Despite the lamentations of those opposed to the ACA, none of these new taxes are earthshaking. The new taxes are incremental, and they tax the very people who have gained so much wealth and income over the last two decades (one-sixth of whom work in health care).

Under the ACA, state regulators can reject "unreasonable" increases in premiums by insurers. In Massachusetts in 2010, they rejected 90 percent of such requests, resulting in 7.7 percent increases in premiums rather than the national average of 20 percent.[59] This ability to regulate increases in premiums by private insurers should help consumers (it saved people in Massachusetts $8 million in 2010).

Given the power of government to regulate increases in premiums and to study rational medical care, it may be possible to expand coverage and reduce costs. Without change, Medicare would have continued to increase its costs exponentially, so the opportunity cost of a future without the ACA is millions more Americans without any medical coverage at all and workers paying more costly premiums each year for lesser coverage. Something had to be done.

## Opposing the ACA #6: Intergenerational Injustice

Financing the ACA will create a massive battle of intergenerational justice. The Baby Boomer generation now retiring is no "Greatest Generation": it did not experience world wars or the Great Depression, but instead experienced relatively good times and relatively luxurious medical care. These entitled seniors will not give up their perks easily and will want every dime of their Social Security checks and Medicare coverage.

One popular book about Medicare benefits states, "The most fundamental point is that Medicare is not a gift. You paid for it while you were working. Medicare owes you services in just the same way that a health insurer to whom you have paid premiums owes them to you."[60]

In fact, and as shown by the FICA taxes on their paychecks, today's young workers pay for the Medicare benefits going to today's elderly.[61] After the first few years on Medicare, most beneficiaries receive benefits amounting to far more than they paid in.

Richard Lamm, Colorado governor from 1978–1987, wrote that, "Dr. Thomas Starzl recently gave a liver transplant to a 76-year-old woman. It cost $240,000. Dr. Starzl should understand that with the average U.S. family making $24,000 a year, he has sentenced 10 U.S. families to work all year so that he could transplant a 76-year-old woman."[62]

The ACA will sentence not just 10 U.S. families, but Generation Xers, Millennials (Generation Y), and the Silent Generation (Generation Z) to tax slavery to pay for (1) more and more medical care for (2) more and more seniors who are (3) living longer and longer. According to the Social Security Administration, 10,000 Americans a day become eligible for its benefits, and between 2007 and 2027, 80 million new beneficiaries will receive Social Security entitlements.

Will anything be left for young people after the Baby Boomers eat through all medical care possible and live into their 90s? This is also assuming no expensive, major war or depression occurs, which—given the state of world affairs—is optimistic.

States that do not expand Medicaid to cover everyone may be doing the young a favor, because once an entitlement is created for universal medical coverage, the young will be yoked to this tax burden forever.

Already the act is hurting people aged 20–30. Some universities have limited the hours that adjunct professors and graduate students work to under 30 to avoid providing medical coverage. Many employers are doing the same. So the first effect of the ACA on many young adults is to ask them to pay for medical coverage when they've just lost thousands of dollars.

In selling the ACA to Americans, President Obama often said: "If you like your plan, you can keep your plan" (e.g., in St. Charles, Missouri, on March 10, 2010). He also said citizens could keep their physician. But the ACA hurt some of the 12 to 15 million Americans who previously had bought individual policies, especially healthy citizens who took risks and who thus chose cheap policies that did not cover pregnancy or mental illness and that had high deductibles. Because of mandated, more extensive coverage in the ACA (e.g., for mental illness) and because the healthy must subsidize the sick, people holding these policies often saw their premiums increase under the ACA. In late 2013, Congress was considering allowing such people to pay the same rates as before, which might undermine the ACA, especially if people only signed up for the ACA who were likely to make medical claims.

### Favoring the ACA #6: No Intergenerational Injustice

No intergenerational injustice exists under the ACA. First, under the veil of ignorance, everyone would choose to insure themselves against being injured in a car accident and having no coverage.

Second, many young people without insurance are now free riders, paying nothing into the system, yet being cared for when sick or injured.

Some seniors need to pay more. Seniors making over $250,000 a year should not get free Medicare. There should be some means testing.

Justice has different meanings. It will be unjust if 20 states don't expand Medicaid. They are violating the idea that the whole country is creating a pool for community rating.

### FURTHER READING

Ezekiel Emanuel, *The Ends of Human Life: Medical Ethics in a Liberal Polity*, Cambridge, MA: Harvard University Press, 1992.

Richard Epstein, *Mortal Peril: Our Inalienable Right to Health Care?* New York: Basic Books, 1997.

Thomas Bodenheimer and Kevin Grumbac, *Understanding Health Policy,* 5th ed., New York: McGraw-Hill, 2008.

"Sicko,"(2008), a documentary film by Michael Moore on the American medical system, in contrast with England, Canada, France, and Cuba.

### DISCUSSION QUESTIONS

1. How is community rating generally Rawlsian in nature, and how is experience rating more libertarian?
2. How did Canada's system work for many years by forbidding physicians and patients from contracting with each other for money outside the national system? Why was this necessary?

3. Does a just society offer its citizens some minimal level of medical care? How would that minimal level be defined?

4. Should illegal immigrants be entitled to medical care? If not, should physicians work for the INS and report illegal immigrants in the ER?

5. What are some of the common misconceptions about medical coverage in America?

6. What are likely costs of the Affordable Care Act to states?

7. Will young people today really benefit from Affordable Care Act, or are they going to be tax slaves to pay for it?

8. What's the best thing about the Affordable Care Act? The worst thing?

9. What happens to states if a president who dislikes the Affordable Care Act is elected and fails to fund it?

# CHAPTER 19

# Ethical Issues in Medical Enhancement

*T*his chapter explores ethical issues of medical enhancement, including the following cases. In the summer of 2012, South African Oscar Pistorius, born with deformed feet, amazed the world with how fast he could run on his Cheetahs, special carbon blades that surgeons attached to his leg bones. Similarly, Sara Reinersten, a single-leg-amputee, runs marathons using a Cheetah instead of a foot. But Cheetahs are graphite—stronger and more flexible than bone. Should they have been allowed to compete? Did medicine make them go from *dis*-abled to *too*-abled?

In 2007, psychiatrist Peter Kramer described the transformation of his 30ish patient Tess, who, after her father died when she was 12 lived in public housing and cared for her nine siblings and elderly mother, rendering her depressed, withdrawn, fearful, and unable to form a relationship. After taking Prozac, an anti-depressant and serotonin re-uptake inhibitor, Tess overcame her fears, started to date, left public housing, and became independent.

Critics such as bioconservative Leon Kass claim that Tess's happiness is ersatz and manufactured, that she would have been better off fighting through her paralysis to the same ends. Now she depends on a drug manufacturer for her happiness, must find a way to pay for the drug, and hopes that its effects don't wane over time. In sum, critics say, Tess has fake happiness, not the real thing.

In the 1980s, professional cyclists began secretly taking the hormone erythropoietin (EPO), a hormonal growth factor that the body creates to stimulate production of red blood cells. As a medical treatment, EPO was approved for patients with anemia. At some point during these years, professional cyclists began storing their own blood, then secretly injecting themselves with the stored blood, both before and during races.

*Doping* may have originated from "doop," a Dutch word Americanized as slang for a way of drugging victims, or from the South African "dop," a potent alcohol/stimulant combination. Regardless, doping now means secret use of performance-enhancing substances to gain advantage over competitors.

Doping with red blood cells gives an advantage in sports that require heavy use of oxygen, such as cycling and cross-country skiing. Training at high altitudes in the Rocky Mountains achieves the same effect because the lower concentration of oxygen stimulates the blood to create more red blood cells. Some athletes naturally possess genes that give them more red blood cells.

An athlete may also transfuse himself with others' blood with high counts of red blood cells. Any transfer of blood runs risk of infections, mix-ups, and contamination. If such transfusions are done to avoid detection, then the blood must be transported and given discretely and then all equipment secreted away.

From 2006 through 2008, random testing in the Tour de France revealed that leading contestants had high levels of hematocrit, or the percentage of blood volume occupied by red blood cells—a sign of doping. Such high levels caused these cyclists to be kicked out of the race.[1] Several cyclists later claimed that every competitor in the race used similar methods.

Psychiatrists estimate that attention deficit hypersensitivity disorder (ADHD) affects approximately 4 percent of school-age children, 75 percent male. ADHD follows two-thirds into adolescence and 40 percent into adult years.[2] Such kids need to be maintained either on methylphenidate (Ritalin) or dextroamphetamine (Adderall), which allow them to function well. By 1998, Ritalin had been prescribed for 5 million American children.[3] For both adults and children between 2003 and 2006, and for these two drugs, American doctors wrote 80 million prescriptions.[4]

The active ingredient of dextroamphetamine is an amphetamine salt, and amphetamines are highly addictive. Is it a good thing that millions of American children function well only on Adderall? Are physicians complicit in this massive drug dependency? Are they engaged in an unprecedented experiment, risking creation of millions of life-long addicts?

Finally, over the past decades, personal body shaping has become more acceptable among males and females. To create lean, muscular physiques, males combine extensive exercise with injections of anabolic steroids and human growth hormone. To create more youthful bodies and faces, women use exercise, surgery, and injections of botox.

Is such body modification just personal taste or a perversion? Is there anything morally wrong with it? Are the physicians who provide it sleazy?

These topics about enhancement occupy a major, expanding area of modern medicine and create unique ethical issues. The rest of this chapter explores them.

## ETHICAL ISSUES OF MEDICAL ENHANCEMENT

### What Counts as an Enhancement?

Consider running a race, say, a half-marathon. What is an acceptable way to increase performance? Taking mega dosages of caffeine before the race? Wearing an expensive running shoe? Hiring a team to provide water and energy bars at 1-mile intervals? Using a music player with songs with a good beat? A GPS device that beeps when your pace slows below your target?

In any competitive sport, coaches are enhancers. As such, the early years of the Olympics banned coaches. Anyone with special knowledge about physiology, training, equipment, endurance, muscles, metabolism, and mental focus helps any athlete to run faster, jump higher, and win. A wealthy athlete who need not work has an enhancement. Is it fair for him to compete against athletes who must train after work? Ideally, everyone starts from a level playing field.

A college kid with ADHD taking Adderall does not seem like an enhancement but a remedy. On the other hand, his natural state is lack of concentration, so Adderall changes this state for the better. We think of things that bring people up to normal as *therapy*, whereas the same things, when they take normal people higher, we think of as *enhancements*.

This makes for a lot of gray areas. One medical dean claims that by prescription, a third of medical students take Ritalin, Adderall, or modafinil (a stimulant that counters narcolepsy). To gain prescriptions for mentally enhancing drugs, have savvy medical students learned to fake the symptoms of ADHD or sleep disorders? Many such students discover that what worked to get them there—intelligence and hard work—aren't enough to compete well in medical school. To excel, they need something more.

## Positional Advantage

If everyone used steroids, there would be no benefit to doing so. If every cyclist doped, there would be no advantage to doping. Right now, only a small percentage of athletes take steroids, so a shot-putter who injects steroids can gain more muscle mass than others and gain a *positional advantage*. A positional advantage confers on the beneficiary an asset in a contest relative to others, but vanishes if everyone else has the same asset.

In competitive sports, even gaining a slight positional advantage over opponents can make the difference between a good performance and an average one. Even when competing against oneself in marathons, runners go to great lengths to gain small improvements: training at high altitudes before big races at lower altitudes, eating special meals before races, running behind a pacer, buying better shoes, and so on.

## An Arms Race

If athletes suspect that competitors dope or take steroids, they realize that, by not doing the same, they are at a competitive *dis*advantage. This suspicion motivates them to take even more enhancements, often secretly.

For example, taking several steroids together is known as *stacking* and carries special dangers. Physicians have reported several cases where young male bodybuilders took massive amounts of steroids and damaged their livers or hearts, or became violent. In American professional wrestling, which is really body building and acting, several cases of "roid rage" have occurred, as when professional wrestler Chris Benoit in 2007 strangled his wife, suffocated his 7-year-old son, and hanged himself with a weight-machine pulley.[5]

The life and death of Lyle Azado, who played 15 seasons for several professional football teams, shows the dangers of stacking. In college in 1969, he began taking anabolic steroids to become bigger and never stopped.[6] At his peak, Alzado spent $30,000 a year on steroids and human growth hormones, often buying them at gyms around the country. Alzado admitted the steroids made him so crazy that at times he couldn't deal with social stress. His second wife blamed the breakup of their marriage on his mood swings that steroids caused, a pattern also seen in wrestler Chris Benoit.

After years of denying that he used steroids and three months after being diagnosed with brain cancer, Alzado confessed, "It was addicting, mentally addicting," Alzado wrote of his steroid use. "I just didn't feel strong unless I was taking something." After receiving radical chemotherapy and contracting pneumonia, Alzado died at age 43 in 1992. Officially, he died from brain lymphoma, a rare form of cancer. Use of steroids cannot be medically proved to have caused Alzado's lymphoma, but Alzado himself believed this.

## End Secrecy; Legalize Enhancements

Citing the myriad problems of the Tour de France, British bioethicist Julian Savulescu believes that rather than prohibiting use of banned substances in sports, we should legalize them. For him, the enormous rewards of winning, coupled with the minimal consequences of cheating and the low chance of being caught, make doping irresistible to athletes.

Savulescu thinks that drug use in elite sport is wrong only because it violates the rules, so we should change the rules to make it permissible. He argues that doing so will not lead to an arms race of drug taking: "We should not think that allowing cyclists to take EPO would turn the Tour de France into some kind of 'drug race,' any more than the various training methods available turn it into a 'training race' or a 'money race.'"[7]

Savulescu thinks the only limit of drugs in sport should be safety. His opponents think the safety of athletes is a good reason for prohibiting enhancing drugs in sports, but Savulescu counters that many sports carry risks of permanent injuries: racecar driving, ski jumping, boxing, diving, jumping horses, pole vaulting, gymnastics, and competitive group cheerleading. Yet we tolerate these activities and lionize their champions.

Furthermore, banning a substance may carry its own harms. Just as prohibition of alcohol in the 1920s increased deaths due to the unregulated quality of bootleg alcohol, banning drugs in sport leads to similar problems. If it's out in the open and medically supervised, everyone will be better off.

## Inauthentic

Perhaps the case where enhancement seems most troubling involves taking drugs that change mood and personality, e.g., Peter Kramer's patient Tess. In *Better than Well*, physician-bioethicist Carl Elliott laments that millions of people create drug-dependent, new versions of themselves that may be fake and ill advised.[8]

Wake Forest English professor Eric Wilson, in *Against Happiness: In Praise of Melancholy,* goes even further, arguing that Prozac simulates a living death, blocks our creativity, hinders our spiritual growth-through-suffering, and should be avoided.[9] For Wilson, creativity, success, ambition, and vision actually *conflict* with happiness. Settling for happiness leads to "half-lives, to bland existences, to wastelands of mechanistic behavior."[10] To immunize oneself inside a shell of Prozac, while millions die each year from AIDS is to be "inauthentic." Sorrow is "sweet," he says, but happiness is "self-satisfied smiles" (smugness), "treacly expressions . . . painted on our faces" like botoxed lips and rouge. To be happy is to have "an essential part of [our] hearts sliced away and discarded like so much waste." For Wilson, this world is so evil and awful that, if one does not hide from it inside some drug-induced fog, one cannot possibly face it and be happy.

## Cheating

Perhaps most cyclists in the Tour de France dope. Does that make it ethical? Isn't that the ad populum fallacy? Even if only one cyclist does not cheat, an honorable man still exists. American cyclist Lance Armstrong was a hero for years because he beat cancer and claimed he did not cheat and "lived strong" without doping. Now we know he did cheat.

If the majority of athletes do not cheat, then the sport maintains a good, dominant ethos. But when most athletes cheat—as appears to be the case in the Tour de France—then the entire sport becomes unworthy of competition. The history of the Tour de France does not explain why we should legalize enhancements, but explains what happens when a culture of cheating and self-medication *corrupts a sport*. That the Tour de France has become synonymous with doping, that everyone assumes a winner to be a cheater, that sponsors decline now to endorse athletes because of tarnished images is the end of honorable, professional cycling.

In all sports, whether professional, college, or high school, taking steroids to compete is cheating, plain and simple. Anything not legally open to all competitors should be banned. Here, the controversy among users and non-users about the long-term safety of using steroids is moot. Steroids are used to gain an unfair advantage in these sports—and that is wrong.

Of even greater importance, the casual acceptance of cheating through doping and use of steroids, not the use of enhancements in itself, undermines the spirit of fair competition. The casual acceptance inside body building, cycling, and weight lifting of taking anabolic steroids and other enhancers is not a good thing. The attitude of blatantly cheating to win is destroying many sports. Certainly when we see a large-muscled man in body building, football, or other contact sports, we just assume he's taken steroids or growth hormones. Over the last decade, the average weight of NFL linemen in football has increased about 80 pounds, and a lot of it is muscle. Only steroids could do that.

As athletes stack more and more drugs, it is inevitable that cheaters get caught. When East German female swimmers started to look like American football players, everyone knew what was going on. It was also only a matter of time before everyone knew what was occurring in the Tour de France and in professional baseball in America.

Trite as it may sound, winning isn't everything in sports. It's how you win, and taking banned drugs isn't the way we want children and friends to win. We shouldn't harangue high school athletes about the dangers of using steroids.

They will hear the opposite from older, successful athletes. Rather, we should emphasize that it's cheating to use steroids or to dope.

If we don't ban but allow steroids, doping, and other supplements, as Savulescu argues, what happens? Given the pervasive culture of cheating in cycling, athletes will not suddenly stop cheating. If a *whole culture* is secretly injecting enhancement drugs to gain positional advantage, then that culture is not going away overnight. Legal drugs will become the baseline; new drugs for positional advantage will be sought.

Okay, so secret use of enhancers is wrong in sports where they are banned, but what about use of enhancers provided by physicians? What about Tess, college students on Adderall, and people getting botox injections every other month for wrinkle-free faces? Are they all *cheating*?

Here it's important to do two things. First, we must define "cheating" carefully and distinguish its different meanings. Second, we must separate kinds of cases and ethical analysis of each.

First, we don't think it's cheating to defy what occurs naturally. Death in childbirth from unwashed hands, lifelong pain after automobile accidents, and unchecked spread of leukemic cells are natural, but reversible by modern medicine.

As said, when medicine restores someone to normal functioning, or when it brings someone below normal functioning at birth up to normal functioning, we consider it therapy, not enhancement.

Cheating is best defined when the rules say competitors can't do X and someone secretly does X. As several infamous runners have done, it's cheating to sneak out early of a marathon; hop on a car, bike, or subway; and then rejoin the leaders at the end. Likewise, it's cheating to compete in cycling or baseball and secretly inject banned enhancers.

So we need to separate two quite different kinds of cases: (1) where enhancement is explicitly banned and participants secretly use banned enhancers, and (2) where use of the enhancers is a personal, mainly self-regarding decision.

What about an 80-year-old person who is trying to present her face to the world as if it's 30 or 40 years old? Here, someone is "cheating" in a different sense. Insofar as the deception succeeds, the person cheats other people of knowledge of the person's true age. But no one is breaking any rules here.

What about anti-depressants? Is it cheating to end depression and feel normal? After all, what's so great about feeling lousy? What about taking the same drugs to go from feeling normal to "better than well"?

Of course, we suspect overnight transformations caused by taking drugs as transient. Surely there is something admirable about struggling with relationships, building virtues in facing existential crises, and gaining insights by talking about previous mistakes. Maybe there is a sense here, which Kant would like, where taking anti-depressants is "cheating oneself."

The movie *Limitless* portrays Eddie Mora who, after taking a potent, modafinil-like drug, suddenly acquires amazing intellectual powers and boundless energy for short-term projects. Eddie regards the drug as helping him harness his whole brain, not just the small part of his brain that he normally uses. As such, Eddie regards his work on the drug as his true self.

One way in which Eddie would be cheating would be if he entered intel-lectual contests where use of the drug gave him positional advantages. In fair contests, everybody should have access to the same enhancers.

Similarly, Tess regards herself on Prozac as finding her true self. Critics believe that the new selves of Tess and Eddie are fake selves that are not built on their real characters and, hence, are fragile and ultimately, not worth having. Which is the real self? The best self? Here we enter deep issues in the philosophy of mind best left to other philosophers to solve.

Consider also Wilson's claim about real selves and the suffering of the world. Let's accept the premise that anti-depressants insulate people against the suffering of millions of starving, AIDS-stricken people. If so, what's so special about drugs? Isn't a person who spends all his life playing games on an X-box or chatting on Facebook equally insulated? Or people spending all their free time at country clubs playing golf and tennis? Why single out anti-depressants?

## Not Dangerous

Some athletes believe that the dangers of using steroids are exaggerated and, in particular, that if steroids are used correctly and in moderation, they pose few risks to health. Such athletes also believe that ideology biases the public's view. They liken it to medical marijuana, where people may be pro or con before they learn the real facts.

Although it's *possible* that low dosages of steroids by older adults aren't harm-ful, the way most athletes take steroids and growth hormone for positional advan-tage is not in such low dosages. And such athletes secretly stack and are surely not carefully monitored by physicians.

Many enhancements are not studied first in randomized controlled trials, and as a result, problems often emerge later. For example, in the early 1960s, surgeons began implanting in women silicone-filled rubber bags, either between the chest wall and the pectoral muscles or between pectoral muscles and the breast. Dow Corning manufactured these bags. A decade later, surgeons used a less viscous silicone gel and a thinner sac, resulting in more ruptures.

In 1995 and after three decades of such implants, 400,000 women registered as potential claimants in 20,000 lawsuits against Dow Corning.[11] In 1998, because of costs of defending itself against these lawsuits, Dow Corning filed for bankruptcy reorganization. To settle all claims against it, Dow agreed to compensate women for removal of breast implants or for ruptures of silicone in the implants.

After these lawsuits, surgeons started to use saline-filled bags. However, even this procedure led to major complications, including capsular contractures, when the rubber sac tightens and squeezes the saline, causing leakage from the capsule.

All the class action suits in federal courts came to a head under the late fed-eral judge Sam C. Pointer in Birmingham, Alabama, who in 1998 appointed four independent experts to review claims that the implants harmed women. These court-appointed masters concluded that medical evidence did not show that the saline implants caused any serious diseases. In 1999, the Institute of Medicine concluded the same, stating that although implants caused local scarring and hardening of surrounding tissues, they did not cause serious disease.[12] Other large studies around the world came to the same conclusions.

Even if breast implants don't cause disease, many women didn't know enough before they got them. In one survey in 2007, 40 percent of women with implants believed that, before they had their surgeries, they should have learned more about their complications.[13]

In one study of 100 women who had their implants removed, rheumatologists diagnosed autoimmune or rheumatic disease in 18 of them. In this class of women, 75 percent had lost some sensitivity in their nipples, and 25 patients had lost all sensation.[14] These women had 186 implants removed, and of these, 57 percent had failed by rupturing or leaking, and bacteria had infected 42 percent.

All implants eventually need to be replaced. Even with the best, third-generation implants, after 10 years 15 percent of women have implants replaced.[15] Did most women who had implants years ago get informed consent about this? Did they know that women who smoke have twice the rate of complications as non-smokers?[16] That for women getting experimental or premarket implants at discounted fees, after three years, the rate of repeat operations runs as high as 20 percent?[17]

## Bad Effects of Legalization

There is an *exposure effect* in legalizing banned drugs in sport. Yes, maybe 10 percent of football players in America use steroids, but if steroids were allowed, 90 percent would use them. And with that greater public exposure, and probably stacking, many more problems would occur.

Legalization will ramp up the arms race. When medical marijuana was legalized in Colorado hundreds of vendors sprang up overnight, including vending machines that dispensed marijuana to those with prescriptions. Liquor stores are ubiquitous in many poor communities, competing with shops offering Pay Day Loans, EZ Pawn, and Fast Cash for Car Titles. Do we want the poor similarly victimized by marijuana head shops on every other corner?

In sports, instead of a few athletes becoming addicted and injured, most athletes would become so. This makes us raise an even deeper question: What is the true purpose of sport? To win at all costs? Or to exercise, compete, have fun, and enjoy fellowship with others?

## THE ROLE OF PHYSICIANS

Another issue in enhancement concerns the role of the physician. If athletes' taking enhancers is cheating then physicians providing enhancers to athletes is also corrupting, both of medicine and sports.

Although medicine is too elastic to rigidly uphold any distinction between therapy and research—where one is a proper, the other, an improper goal—it is not too elastic to ignore the distinction between what is in the rules and what is not.

In 2010 in New Jersey, 45-year-old physician Joseph Colao wrote prescriptions for anabolic steroids for 248 police officers and firefighters.[18] Although less than 1 percent of men suffer from any hormonal condition requiring steroids, Dr. Colao colluded with these men to get group medical coverage to pay. (He also quickly transformed himself into a hulk by taking steroids, but suddenly died in 2010 of heart failure.)

Arne Lundqvist, chairman of the International Amateur Athletic Federation's doping commission, writes that providing prescription drugs to healthy adults, drugs meant for therapeutic purposes, is "medical malpractice."[19] That statement is too strong for most drugs, e.g., Viagra, but not for purposes of breaking the rules in competitive sports to gain positional advantage.

Second, given the medical dangers discussed in this chapter, physicians who enable such men to bulk up are corrupt. Fake bodily enhancement is a two-way illicit street, bringing down both those who prescribe and those who get steroids, growth hormones, and other muscle-producing substances.

## CONCLUSIONS

Enhancement medicine is an expanding, profitable area of medicine rife with ethical challenges. For some, its providers and customers will be seen as sleazy, and if things go wrong, people will get what they deserve. Proponents of enhancement, both patients and physicians, see themselves on the cutting-edge of a new patient-controlled, autonomous world, where *caveat emptor* rules, and medicine has developed a true, cash-and-carry marketplace.

## FURTHER READING

Ronald Bailey, *Liberation Biology: The Scientific and Moral Case for the Biotech Revolution*, Amherst, NY: Prometheus Books, 2005.

Elliot, Carl, and Peter Kramer, *Better than Well: American Medicine Meets the American Dream*, New York: Norton, 2004.

Evans, John, *Playing God: Human Genetic Engineering and the Rationalization of Public Debate*, Chicago: University of Chicago, 2002.

Fukuyama, Francis, *Our Posthuman Future: Consequences of the Biotechnology Revolution*, New York: Farrar, Straus & Giroux, 2002.

Green, Ronald, *Babies By Design: The Ethics of Genetic Choice*, New Haven, CT: Yale University Press, 2007.

Habermas, Jürgen, *The Future of Human Nature.*

Harris, John, *Enhancing Evolution: The Ethical Case for Making Better People*, Princeton, NJ: Princeton University Press, 2007.

Harris, John, *Wonderman and Wonderwoman: The Ethics of Human Biotechnology*, New York: Oxford University Press, 1992.

Hughes, James, *Citizen Cyborg*, Boulder, CO: Westview Press, 2004.

Kramer, Peter D., *Listening to Prozac*, New York: Viking, 1993.

Pence, Gregory, *How to Build a Better Human: An Ethical Blueprint*, Lanham, MD: Rowman & Littlefield, 2012.

President's Council on Bioethics, *Beyond Therapy: Biotechnology and the Pursuit of Happiness*, Washington, DC: Dana Press, 2003.

Sandel, Michael, *The Case Against Perfection: Ethics in the Age of Genetic Engineering* Cambridge, MA: Harvard University Press, 2007..

Stock, Gregory, *Redesigning Humans: Our Inevitable Genetic Future*, New York: Houghton Miflin, 2002.

Savulescu, Julian, B. Foddy and M. Clayton, "Why We Should Allow Performance Enhancing Drugs in Sport," *British Journal of Sports Medicine*, 38 (2004), pp. 666–670.

Wilson, Eric, *Against Happiness* Farrar, Straus & Giroux, New York, 2008.

## DISCUSSION QUESTIONS

1. Is enhancement always cheating? What if no one else is affected? Does it make sense to say one can "cheat oneself" when one is fully aware of the consequences and freely chooses them?

2. Is there such a thing as natural norms or natural limits that should not be transgressed? Does cosmetic surgery do this? What about a person who wanted his face remade to look like a cat or dog? Would it be ethical for a plastic surgeon to do this?

3. If doping and steroids are legalized, won't athletes just search for other enhancements to gain positional advantage? In other words, would legalization really solve the problem of cheating in sports?

# Notes

## Chapter 1

1. R. M. Hare and Louis Pojman (eds.), *Ethical Theory: Classical and Contemporary Readings*, Wadsworth: California, 2007, pp. 480–481.

2. James Rachels may have invented this example. See Stuart Rachels, introduction to *The Legacy of Socrates*, ed. Stuart Rachels. Columbia Univesity Press, New York, 2008, p. IX–X.

## Chapter 2

1. Associated Press, October 16, 1983.

2. Robert Steinbock and Bernard Lo, "The Case of Elizabeth Bouvia: Starvation, Suicide, or Problem Patient?" *Archives of Internal Medicine* 146 (January 1986), p. 161.

3. Quoted in George Annas, "When Suicide Prevention Becomes Brutality: The Case of Elizabeth Bouvia," *Hastings Center Report* 14, no. 2 (April 1984), p. 20.

4. Associated Press, in *Birmingham Post-Herald*, December 14, 1984, p. A2.

5. Quoted in Arthur Hoppe, *San Francisco Examiner*, December 20, 1983.

6. Steinbock and Lo, "The Case of Elizabeth Bouvia," p. 161.

7. *Bouvia v. County of Riverside*, California Superior Court, December 16, 1983.

8. Richard Scott, in "Patient's Suicide Wish Troubles Hospital MDs," *American Medical News*, January 20, 1984, p. 5.

9. Hoppe, *San Francisco Examiner*.

10. Annas, "When Suicide Prevention Becomes Brutality," p. 46.

11. George Annas, "Elizabeth Bouvia: Whose Space Is This Anyway?" *Hastings Center Report* 16, no. 2 (April 1986), p. 20.

12. Steinbock and Lo, "The Case of Elizabeth Bouvia," p. 162.

13. Annas, "Elizabeth Bouvia," pp. 24–25.

14. Derek Humphrey and Ann Wickett, *The Right to Die: Understanding Euthanasia*, Harper and Row, New York, 1986, p. 150.

15. Paul Longmore, "Elizabeth Bouvia, Assisted Suicide, and Social Prejudice," in *Issues in Law and Medicine*, no. 2 (Fall 1987), p. 158.

16. The hospital's rationale in its brief to Judge Deering is quoted in Annas, "Elizabeth Bouvia," p. 24.

17. *Bouvia v. Glenchur*, Los Angeles Superior Court, *California Reporter* 225 (1986), pp. 296–308.

18. *Bouvia v. Superior Court* (Glenchur), *California Reporter* 297, California Appellate 2 District, 1986.

19. In *Bartling v. Superior Court* (1984), California court recognized the constitutional right of a competent patient to refuse life-sustained treatment, as id did in a 1983 criminal case, *Barber v. Superior Court*. A Florida court in 1978 recognized a competent patient's right to remove a life-sustaining device in *Satz v. Perlmutter* 362 So.2nd 160. Thanks to Bonnie Steinbock and Alicia Ouellette for these references.

20. Jeff Wilson (AP), "Precedent-Setter Lives On after Plea to Die," *Indianapolis Star*, December 19, 1993, p. H7.

21. Elaine Woo, "Obituary: Harlan Hahn; USC Professor Fought for Disability Rights, Sued University to Improve its Access," May 10, 2008, *Los Angeles Times*.

22. B. D. Colen, "His Life, to Take or Not," *Newsday*, September 25, 1989, pp. 5–19.

23. Susan Schindehette and Gail Wescott, "Deciding Not to Die," *People*, January 18, 1993, p. 86.

24. Ibid.

25. Russ Fine, *UAB Report*, September 4, 1992, p. 4.

26. Ibid.

27. Associated Press, "Thousands Retiring without Social Security," February 16, 1993.

28. Russ Fine, personal communication to author, May 16, 1994.

29. Cowart's case became the topic of famous videotape, "Please Let Me Die," and a later film, *Dax's Case*. See also L. Kliever, *Dax's Case—Essays in Medical Ethics and Human Meaning*, SMU Press, Dallas, TX, 1989.

30. Dax Cowart, personal communication to author at meeting of American Association of Medical Colleges, Chicago, IL, October 1989.

31. Personal communication to author, August 12, 2012.

32. Quotations are from Phaedo, in E. Hamilton and H. Cairns, eds., *Plato: The Collected Dialogues*, Princeton University Press, Princeton, NJ, 1961.

33. Epictetus, Dissertations, 1.9, p. 16. Quoted by James Rachels, "Euthanasia," in T. Regan, ed., *Matters of Life and Death*, 3d ed., McGraw-Hill, New York, 1993, p. 35.

34. Seneca, *De Ira*, quoted in Rachels, "Euthanasia."

35. Jean Paul Sartre, *Existentialism Is a Humanism*, Philosophical Library, New York, 1947.

36. Frederick Russell, *The Just War in the Middle Ages*, Cambridge University Press, Cambridge, England, 1975.

37. Quoted in James Gutman, "Death and Dying in Western Culture," *Encyclopedia of Bioethics* 1, Free Press, New York, 1978, p. 240.

38. Baruch Spinoza, *Ethics*, William White and Amelia Stirling, trans., Hafner, New York, 1949.

39. Quoted in Derek Humphrey and Ann Wickett, *The Right to Die: Understanding Euthanasia*, Harper and Row, New York, 1986, pp. 8–9.

40. David Hume, "On Suicide" (1755), in Eugene Miller, ed., *Collected Essays of David Hume*, Liberty Classics, Indianapolis, IN, 1986.

41. Ibid.

42. Immanuel Kant, "On Suicide" (1755–1780), *Lectures on Ethics*, L. Enfield, trans., Harper and Row, New York, 1963, pp. 148–154.

43. Ibid.

44. Immanuel Kant, *The Metaphysical Principles of Virtue*, trans. J. Ellington, Bobbs-Merrill, Indianapolis, IN, 1959, p. 84.

45. John Stuart Mill, *On Liberty* (1859), Appleton-Century-Crofts, New York, 1974.

46. Quoted in Humphrey and Wickett, *The Right to Die*, p. 16.

47. Art Kleiner, "Life after Suicide," *High Wire*, Summer 1982, p. 30.

48. Tad Friend, "Jumpers" *New Yorker*, October 13, 2003.

49. H. Hendin, "Suicide in America," *Miami News*, August 30, 1982, p. B1.

50. T. Woody, "Was His Act of Mercy Also Murder?" *New York Times*, November 7, 1988.

51. Quoted in Humphrey and Wickett, *The Right to Die*, p. 152.

52. Ibid., p. 155.

53. Ibid., p. 154.

54. Kevin D. O'Rourke, "Value Conflicts Raised by Physician-Assisted Suicide," *Linacre Quarterly* 57, no. 3 (August 1990), pp. 38–49.

55. SUPPORT Principal Investigators, "A Controlled Trial to Improve Care of Seriously Ill Hospitalized Patients. The Study to Understand Prognoses and Preferences for Outcomes and Risks of Treatment (SUPPORT), *Journal of the American Medical Association* 274 (1995), pp. 1591–1598.

56. John Shuster, talk at UAB Medical School, August 14, 1995.

57. *The Economist*, July 17, 2010, p. 65.

58. Paul Longmore, column in *Electric Edge*, January/February 1997.

59. Paul Longmore, "Elizabeth Bouvia, Assisted Suicide, and Social Prejudice," *Issues in Law and Medicine* 2, no. 2 (Fall 1987), p. 158.

60. Fine, *UAB Report*, p. 12.

61. Ibid., p. 4.

62. Douglas Martin, "Disability Culture: Eager to Bite the Hands That Would Feed Them," *New York Times*, June 1, 1997, p. A1.

# Chapter 3

1. Johannes J. M. van Delden et al., "The Remmelink Study: Two Years later," *Hastings Center Report* 23, no. 6 (November–December 1993), p. 24.

2. http://www.euthanasia.cc/dutch.html#remm

3. Tara Burgh art, Associated Press, "1 in 18 Opt Out of Assisted Suicide," August 18, 2005, *Birmingham News*, p. A11.

4. Veronica English et al., "Ethics Briefings," *Journal of Medical Ethics*, 32 (2006), pp. 371–372.

5. Isabel Wilkerson, "Physician Fulfills a Goal: Aiding a Person in Suicide," *New York Times*, June 7, 1990.

6. Timothy Quill, "Death and Dignity: A Case of Individualized Decision Making," *New England Journal of Medicine* 327 (1992), pp. 1380–1384.

7. Susan Okie, "Dr. Pou and the Hurricane: Implications for Patient Care During Disasters," *New England Journal of Medicine*, no. 1 (January 3, 2008), pp. 1–5.

8. Okie, "Dr. Pou and the Hurricane," p. 1.

9. Susan Tolle, "Care of the Dying: Clinical and Financial Lessons from the Oregon Experience," *Annals of Internal Medicine* 128, no. 7 (April 1, 1998).

10. Ibid.

11. Ezekiel Emanuel and Margaret Battin, "What Are the Potential Cost-Savings of Legalizing Physician-Assisted Suicide?" *New England Journal of Medicine*, 339 (1998), pp. 167–172.

12. Susan Tolle et al., *The Oregon Death with Dignity Act: A Guidebook for Health Professionals*, (PDF document), p. 7: http://www.ohsu.edu/ethics/toc.pdf#search=%22Susan%20Tolle%20Guidebook%20Oregon%22.

13. J. Prokopetz and L. Lehmann, "Redefining the Physicians' Role in Assisting Dying," *New England Journal of Medicine* 367, no. 2 (July 12, 2012), p. 98.

14. *Seventh Annual Report on Oregon's Death with Dignity Act,* Office of Disease Prevention and Epidemiology, Department of Human Services, State of Oregon, March 10, 2005, 800 N.E. Oregon Street, Portland, OR 97232.

15. Tolle et al., *A Guidebook*, p. 23–25.

16. Dave Parks, "Study: Ill Oregonians Refuse Food to Die, Rejecting Suicide Law, *Birmingham News*, July 24, 2003, p. A12.

17. Ludwig Edelstein, *Ancient Medicine: Collected Essays of Ludwig Edelstein*, O. Temkin and L. Temkin, eds., Johns Hopkins University Press, Baltimore, MD, 1967.

18. G. E. R. Lloyd, *Hippocratic Writings*, trans. Chadwick and W. N. Mann, Penguin, New York, 1950, p. 13.

19. Leo Alexander, "Medical Science under Dictatorship," *New England Journal of Medicine* 42 (July 14, 1949).

20. Robert Jay Lifton, *The Nazi Doctors*, Basic Books, New York, 1986.

21. J. C. Wilke, *Assisted Suicide and Euthanasia: Past and Present, Hayes Publications*, 1998, p. 9. I am indebted to Stephen W. Poff, M.D., for this reference and for points made in this paragraph.

22. Timothy Egan, "Sucide Law Placing Oregon on Several Uncharted Paths," *New York Times,* November 25, 1994.

23. "Excerpts from Court's Decision," *New York Times*, June 27, 1997, p. A18.

24. Gina Kolata, "'Passive Euthanasia' in Hospitals Is the Norm, Doctors Say," *New York Times*, June 28, 1997, p. A1.

25. Christine Cassell, quoted in Michael Specter, "Suicide Device Fuels Debate," *Washington Post*, June 8, 1990.

26. James Rachels, "Active and Passive Euthanasia," *New England Journal of Medicine* 29 (January 9, 1975), pp. 78–80.

27. Baruch Brody, "Ethical Questions Raised by the Persistent Vegetative Patient," *Hastings Center Report* 18, (February-March, 1988) no. 1, p. 35.

28. Bonnie Steinbock, "The Intentional Termination of Life," in *Killing and Letting Die*, ed. B. Steinbock, Englewood Cliffs, NJ: Prentice-Hall, 1980.

29. Jean Davies, "Raping and Making Love Are Different Concepts: So Are Killing and Voluntary Euthanasia," *Journal of Medical Ethics* 14 (1988), pp. 148–149.

30. Quoted in Barnard White Stack, "Doctors Divided Over the Very Ill, *Pittsburgh Post Gazette*, June 11, 1990.

31. Timothy Quill and Margaret Pabst Battin, "Excellent Palliative Care as the Standard, Physician-Assisted Dying as a Last Resort," in Timothy Quill and Margaret Pabst Battin, eds., *Physician-Assisted Dying: The Case for Palliative Care and Patient Choice*, Johns Hopkins Press, Baltimore, MD, pp. 323–330.

32. Quoted in Alan Parachini, "A Dutch Doctor Carries Out a Death Wish," *Los Angeles Times*, July 5, 1987, sec. 6, p. 9.

33. Quoted in Barnard White Stack, "Doctors Divided Over the Very Ill," *Pittsburgh Post Gazette*, June 11, 1990.

34. Margaret Battin, "The Least Worst Death," *Hastings Center Report* 13. no. 2 (April 1983), pp. 13–16

35. Douglas Walton, *Slippery Slope Arguments*, Oxford University Press, New York, 1992.

36. Alexander, "Medical Science Under Dictatorship," p. 47.

37. Ibid., p. 44.

38. Yale Kamisar, quoted in Earl Ubell, "Should Death Be a Patient's Choice?" *Parade Magazine*, February 9, 1992, p. 27.

39. T. Curiel, "Murder or Mercy? Hurricane Katrina and the Need for Disaster Training," *New England Journal of Medicine*, 355, no 20 (November 16, 2006), p. 2067.

40. Michael Specter, "Suicide Device Fuels Debate," *Washington Post*, June 8, 1990.

41. Quoted in Peter Steinfels, "Dutch Study Is Euthanasia Vote Issue," *New York Times*, September 20, 1991.

42. Nat Hentoff, "The Deadly Slippery Slope," *Village Voice*, September 1, 1987.

43. L. Ganzini, et al., "Prevalence of Depression and Anxiety in Patients Requesting Physicians Aid in Dying: Cross Sectional Survey," *British Medical Journal* 337 (2008), pp. 973–975.

44. Timothy Egan, "Assisted Suicide Comes Full Circle in Oregon," October 26, 1997. . . ."

45. Nat Hentoff, "The Coat Hanger of Assisted Suicide," *Washington Post*, December 12, 1997.

46. Christiaan Barnard, *One Life*, Macmillan, New York, 1965.

47. Joan Teno and Joanne Lynn, "Voluntary Active Euthanasia: The Individual Case and Public Policy," *Journal of the American Geriatrics Society* 39 (1991), pp. 827–830.

48. Quill and Pabst Battin, "Excellent Palliative Care," p. 325.

49. Alto Charo, quoted by Okie, "Dr. Pou and the Hurricane," p. 4.

50. Sheri Fink, "Deadly Choices at Memorial," *New York Times Magazine*, August 27, 2009. Co-published with Pro Publica: Journalism in the Public Interest. See also, Sheri Fink, *Five Days at Memorial*, Crown, New York, 2013.

## Chapter 4

1. Robert Morse, in *In the Matter of Karen Quinlan: The Complete Legal Briefs, Court Proceedings, and Decisions in Superior Court of New Jersey*, vols. 1 and 2, University Publications of America, Frederick MD, 1982, p. 236 (hereafter, *Proceedings 1, Proceedings 2*). The later court transcript contradicts itself about the exact drugs Karen consumed. Attending physician Robert Morse testified that, "She had some barbiturates, which was normal, 0.6 milligrams; toxic is 2 milligrams, and the toxic dose is about 5 milligrams percent" [sic]. Julius Korein, in *Proceedings 1*, pp. 34–35. Consulting neurologist Julius Korein, whom the Quinlans hired, testified that Karen's drug screen "was positive for quinine, negative for morphine, barbiturates and other substances. A subsequent test for Valium and Librium was positive."[3] (No one else mentioned Librium.) Court prosecutor George Daggett testified that Karen had taken tranquilizers with alcohol shortly before becoming unconscious.[4] George Daggett, *New York Times*, September 20, 1975, New Jersey sec. The Quinlans denied that the drug screen showed barbiturates: "The early urine and blood samples, taken on the day Karen was brought to the hospital, revealed only a 'normal therapeutic' level of aspirin and the tranquilizer Valium in her system."[5] Joseph and Julia Quinlan with Phyllis Battelle, *Karen Ann: The Quinlans Tell Their Story*, 1977, New York, Doubleday Anchor, p. 22.

2. Joseph and Julia Quinlan with Phyllis Battelle, *Karen Ann: The Quinlans Tell Their Story*, Doubleday Anchor, New York, 1977, p. 27.

3. Daniel Coburn, in *Proceedings 1*, p. 17.

4. Julius Korein, in *Proceedings 1*, p. 329.

5. Fred Plum, in Quinlan and Quinlan, *Karen Ann*, p. 198.

6. Robert Morse, in Quinlan and Quinlan, *Karen Ann*, pp. 188–189.

7. Quinlan and Quinlan, *Karen Ann*, pp. 272–273 (the nun is not named).

8. Gino Concetti, quoted in Quinlan and Quinlan, *Karen Ann*, p. 284.

9. Quoted in Quinlan and Quinlan, *Karen Ann*.

10. Nat Hentoff, "The Deadly Slippery Slope," *Village Voice*, September 1, 1987.

11. Ibid.

12. *Cruzan v. Director, Missouri Dept. of Health*, 110 S. Ct. 2841, 1990.

13. George Annas, "Nancy Cruzan and the Right to Die," *New England Journal of Medicine* 323, no. 10 (September 6, 1990), p. 670.

14. "Love and Let Die," *Time*, March 19, 1990, pp. 62ff.

15. Andrew M. Malcolm, "Nancy Cruzan: End to Long Goodbye," *New York Times*, December 29, 1990, p. A3. See also, "A Conversation with Mr. and Mrs. Cruzan," *Midwest Medical Ethics: The Nancy Cruzan Case* 5, nos. 1–2 (Winter/Spring 1989).

16. Ronald Cranford, lecture at UAB Medical School, January 19, 1991.

17. Joanne Lynn and Jacqueline Glover, "Cruzan and Caring for Others," *Hastings Center Report* 20, no. 5 (September–October 1992), p. 11.

18. Annas, "Nancy Cruzan and the Right to Die," p. 672.

19. Timothy E. Quill, "Terri Schiavo—A Tragedy Compounded," *New England Journal of Medicine* 352 (April 21, 2005), pp. 1630–1633.

20. According to Kenneth Goodman, M.D, of the Department of Bioethics at the University of Miami. Personal communication, November 14, 2004.

21. Arian-Camp-Flores, "The Legacy of Terri Schiavo," *Newsweek*, April 4, 2005, p. 26.

22. Austrian physician Semmelweis correctly charged his colleagues with spreading child-birth fever by not washing their hands and going from birth to birth; he was subsequently regarded by his fellow physicians as crazy.

23. Arian-Camp-Flores, "The Legacy," p. 26.

24. Quoted from William Colby, *The Long Goodbye: The Deaths of Nancy Cruzan*, Hay House Publishing, Carlsbad, CA, 2002.

25. Manuel Roig-Franzia, "Florida High Court Overrules Governor in Schiavo Case," *Washington Post*, September 24, 2004, p. A3.

26. Manuel Roig-Franzia, "Court Lets Right-to-Die Ruling Stand," *Washington Post*, January 24, 2005, A12.

27. Ibid.

28. Charles Babington and Mike Allen, "Congress Passes Schiavo Measure," *Washington Post*, March 2, 2005, p. A1.

29. Democrat Jim Jordan, quoted by Charles Babington, "Viewing Videotape, Frist Disputes Fla. Doctors' Diagnosis of Schiavo," *Washington Post*, March 20, 2005, p. A3.

30. Tamara Lipper, "Between Life and Death," *Newsweek*, March 28, 2005, p. 30.

31. Manuel Roig-Franzia, "Schiavo's Parents Take 'Final Shot' to Keep Her Alive," *Washington Post*, March 26, 2005, p. A4.

32. Nancy Weaver Teichert, "Experts: Lack of Food, Water, Does Not Cause Pain for Dying," *Sacramento Bee*, March 28, 2005; *Birmingham News*, March 29, 2005, p. A6.

33. "Report of Autopsy," Medical Examiner, District Six, Pasco and Pinellas Counties, 10900 Ulmerton Road, Largo, FL 33778, Autopsy date: April 1, 2005. p. 8.

34. President's Commission for the Study of Ethical Problems in Medicine and Biomedical and Behavioral Research, *Defining Death*, Superintendent of Documents, Washington D.C., 1981, p. 14.

35. Ad Hoc Committee of the Harvard Medical School to Examine the Definition of Brain Death, "A Definition of Irreversible Coma," *Journal of the American Medical Association* 205, no. 337 (1968).

36. The characteristics listed by the philosopher Mary Anne Warren in Chapter 5 (with regard to whether an aborted fetus is a person) might be used in a similar way to define the higher person standard: If all these characteristics are lacking we do not have a person.

37. Robert Morrison, "Death: Process or Event?" *Science* 173 (1971), pp. 694–698.

38. Lance Stell, "Let's Abolish 'Brain-Death,'" *Community Ethics* (University of Pittsburgh Center for Medical Ethics) 4, no. 1 (Winter 1997).

39. David Hammer, "Different Cases Cast Light on U.S. right-to-die cases," Associated Press, *Birmingham Post-Herald*, November 10, 2003, p. C5; Associated Press, "Arkansas Man Wakes After 19 Years in Coma," July 9, 2003; Benedict Carey, "Man Recovering from Brain Injury after 19 Lost Years," *New York Times*, July 4, 2006, reprinted in *Birmingham News*, July 4, 2006, p. A1.

40. Associated Press, "Policeman who Briefly Emerged from Coma-like State in '96 Dies," *Birmingham News*, April 16, 1997, p. 7A.

41. Benedict Carey, "Inside the Injured Brain, Many Kinds of Awareness," *New York Times*, April 5, 2005.

42. Multi-Society Task Force on PVS, "Medical Aspects of the Persistent Vegetative State," parts 1 and 2, *New England Journal of Medicine* 330, no. 22 (May 26, 1994; June 2, 1994), pp. 1572–1579.

43. S.I. Dubroja, et al., "Outcome of Post-traumatic Unawareness Persisting for More than a Month," *Journal of Neurological Neurosurgery Psychiatry* 58, no. 4 (1995), pp. 465–66; R. Chen et al., "Prediction of Outcome in Patients with Anoxic Coma: A Clinical and Electrophysiologic Study," *Critical Care Medicine* 24, no. 4 (April 1996), pp. 672–678; Associated Press, "Policeman who Briefly Emerged from Coma-like State in '96 Dies."

44. Dubroja, et al., "Outcome of Post-traumatic Unawareness Persisting for More than a Month."

45. R. Chen et al, "Prediction of Outcome in Patients with Anoxic Coma: A Clinical and Electrophysiologic Study," *Critical Care Medicine* 24, no. 4 (April 1996), pp. 672–678.

46. Carey, "Inside the Injured Brain."

47. Carl Zimmer, "What If There's Something Going On in There?" *New York Times Magazine*, September 29, 2003.

48. Ibid.

49. M. Monti et al., "Willful Modulation of Brain Activity in Disorders of Consciousness," *New England Journal of Medicine* 362, no. 7 (February 18, 2010), pp. 579–590.

50. Owen, Adrian, "Using Functional MRI Imaging to Detect Covert Awareness in the Vegetative State," *Archives of Neurology* 64, no. 8 (August 2007), p. 1098.

51. Morgan Peck, "Brain-Wave Test Challenges Vegetative-State Diagnosis," August 6, 2008, *IEEE Inside Technoogy Spectrum*, p. 1. http://www.spectrum.ieee.org/biomedical/diagnostics/brainwave-test-challenges-vegetativestate-diagnosis; Rita Jenkins, 8 September, 2006, "Vegetative Woman Displays Intelligent Brain Activity," daily News Central, http://health.dailynewscentral.com/content/view/0002414/55/; Gary Greenberg, "Back from the Dead," *WIRED*, September 2006, pp. 114–118.

52. Kate Connolly, *The Guardian*, November 23, 2009.

53. Her CT scan is on the Web site of University of Miami Department of Bioethics at http://www.miami.edu/ethics2/schiavo/CT%20scan.png.

54. Rita Rubin, "Doctors Work to Understand Vegetative States," *USA Today*, March 21, 2005, 3A.

55. Cathy Lynn Grossman, "Pope Declares Feeding Tubes a 'Moral Obligation,'" *USA Today*, April 2, 2004, A1.

56. John Paris, quoted by Lisa Greene, "At Pope's Word, New Schiavo Cases?" *St. Petersburg/Tampa Bay Times*, May 1, 2004, http://www.sptimes.com/2004/05/01/Tampabay/At_pope_s_word__new_S.shtml

57. Manuel Roig-Franzia, "Catholic Stance on Tube-Feeding Is Evolving," *Washington Post*, March 27, 2005, p. A7.

58. Kirk Johnson, "Hospital Mergers Resent Abortion-Access Battle," *New York Times*, May 12, 2013, p. A1.

59. Harriet McBryde Johnson, "Overlooked in the Shadows," *Washington Post*, March 25, 2005.

60. Lisa Belkin, "As Family Protest, Hospital Seeks End to Woman's Life Support," *New York Times*, January 10, 1991, pp. A1–2.

61. Steven Miles, "Interpersonal Issues in the Wanglie Case," *Kennedy Institute of Ethics Journal* 2, no. 1 (March 1992), pp. 61–72.

62. For a review of these cases, see *Law, Medicine, and Health Care* 20 (1993), pp. 310–315.

63. R. Knox, "Americans' New Way of Dying: Don't Fight It," *Boston Globe*, June 5, 1994.

64. Ibid., app. B, p. 288.

65. Daniel Callahan, "On Feeding the Dying," *Hastings Center Report* 13, no. 5 (October 1983), p. 22; Gilbert Meillander, "On Removing Food and Water: Against the Stream," *Hastings Center Report* 14, no. 6 (December 1984), pp. 11–13.

66. American Medical Association, *Opinions of the Judicial Council*, Chicago, IL, 1973.

67. SUPPORT Principal Investigators, "A Controlled Trial to Improve Care of Seriously Ill Hospitalized Patients. The Study to Understand Prognoses and Preferences for Outcomes and Risks of Treatment (SUPPORT)," *Journal of the American Medical Association* 274 (1995), pp. 1591–1598.

68. R. F. Uhlmann, R. A. Pearlman, and K. C. Cain, "Physicians and Spouses' Predictions of Elderly Patients' Treatment Preferences," *Journal of Gerontology* 43 (1988), pp. 115–121.

69. Rick Weiss, "Patients' Surrogates Often Wrong about Preferred Treatment," *Washington Post*, March 14, 2006, p. A3.

# Chapter 5

1. Maggie Scarf, "The Fetus as Guinea Pig," *New York Times Magazine*, October 19, 1975, pp. 194–200.

2. Ibid.

3. A. Philipson et al., "Transplacental Passage of Erythomycinan Clindamycin," *New England Journal of Medicine* 288, no. 23 (June 7, 1973), pp. 1219–1221.

4. Paul Ramsey, *The Ethics of Fetal Research*, Yale University Press, New Haven, CT, 1975.

5. William Nolen, *The Baby in the Bottle*, Coward, McCann, and Geoghegan, New York, 1978, p. 203.

6. Ibid.

7. "The Edelin Trial," transcript of a WBGH re-creation of Edelin's trial for a television documentary by Bill Moyers. Project of Legal-Medical Studies, Inc., Box 8219, John F. Kennedy Station, Government Station, Boston, MA 12134.

8. *Commonwealth v. Kenneth Edelin*, Mass. Supreme Court 359, N.E. 2d, 1976.

9. Kenneth Edelin, quoted in *Ob. Gyn. News*, January 1, 1977, p. 1.

10. Quoted from Ramsey, p. 94.

11. Nolen, *The Baby in the Bottle*, p. 174.

12. Ibid.

13. John Hurder and Trip Grabrial, "Philadelphia Abortion Doctor Guilty of Murder of Late-Term Procedures," *New York Times*, May 13, 2013.

14. Paul Badham, "Christian Beliefs and the Ethics of In Vitro Fertilization," *Bioethics News* 6, no. 2 (January 1987), p. 10.

15. Michael Luo, "On Abortion, It's the Bible of Ambiguity," *New York Times*, November 13, 2005, Ideas and Trends Section, pp. 1, 3.

16. Paul Johnson, *A History of Christianity*, Atheneum, New York, 1983, Ch. 3.

17. John Connery, "Abortion: Roman Catholic Perspectives," *Encyclopedia of Bioethics* 1, Macmillan, New York, 1978.

18. Robert W. Mulligan, S. J., Jesuit Community at St. Louis University, personal letter to author.

19. *Roe v. Wade*, Supreme Court Reporter 93, 410 US 151, pp. 709–762.

20. Barbara Ehrenreich and Deirdre English, *For Her Own Good: 150 Years' of Experts' Advice to Women*, New York, Doubleday, 1987, pp. 319–320.

21. Alan Guttmacher Institute, http://www.guttmacher.org/statecenter/spibs/spib_MWPA.pdf.

22. Allan F. Guttmacher Institute, *Abortion and Women's Health*, New York and Washington, D.C., 1990, p. 27.

23. Centers for Disease Control, http://www.cdc.gov/mmwr/preview/mmwr html/ss6015a1.htm?s_cid=ss6015a1_w.

24. *A Private Affair*, a 1992 movie about this case, starred actress Sissy Spacek as Sherry Finkbine.

25. Peter Steinfels, "Papal Birth-Control Letter Retains Its Grip," *New York Times*, July 29, 1993, p. A1, 13.

26. Fact Sheet: Abortion Surveillance, June 7, 2002, Centers for Disease Control, Atlanta, Ga. For updates, see: www.cdc.gov/mmwr/preview/mmwrhtml/ss5407a1.htm.

27. Mary Anne Warren, "On the Moral and Legal Status of the Fetus," *Monist* 57 (1973), pp. 43–61.

28. Peter Singer, *Rethinking Life and Death: The Collapse of Our Traditional Ethics*, Text Publishing, Melbourne, Australia, 1994.

29. Don Marquis and Warren Quinn, "Why Abortion Is Immoral," *Journal of Philosophy* 86 (1989), pp. 183–202.

30. John T. Noonan, Jr., "An Almost Absolute Value in History," in John T. Noonan, Jr. ed., *The Morality of Abortion: Legal and Historical Perspectives*, Harvard University Press, Cambridge, MA, 1970, pp. 51–59.

31. Judith Jarvis Thomson, "A Defense of Abortion," *Philosophy & Public Affairs* 1, no. 1 (Fall 1971), pp. 47–66.

32. Francis Kamm, *Creation and Abortion*, Oxford University Press, New York, 1992.

33. Connery, "Abortion: Roman Catholic Perspectives," pp. 9–13.

34. Ellen Willis, "Harper's Forum on Abortion," *Harper's Magazine*, July 1986, p. 38.

35. Ross Douthat, "160 Million and Counting," *New York Times*, June 27, 2011, p. A10; "Gendercide," *The Economist*, March 6, 2010, p. 13.

36. "Explosions Over Abortion," *Time*, January 14, 1985, p. 17.

37. Jeff Lyon, "Doctor's Dilemma: When Abortion Gives Birth to Life, Physicians Become Troubled Saviors," *Chicago Tribune*, August 15, 1982, Sec. 12, pp. 1, 3. (A 2.5 pound baby may be viable; jockey Willie

Shoemaker, born prematurely, weighed this much and was kept warm in a shoebox in an oven.)

38. Linda Villanova, "Newest Skill for Future OB/GYN's Abortion Training," *New York Times*, June 11, 2002.

39. Susan Lee et al., "Fetal Pain: A Systematic Review of the Literature," *Journal of the American Medical Association*, 294 (2005), pp. 947–954.

40. Consultants to the Advisory Committee to the Director, National Institutes of Health, *Report of the Human Fetal Tissue Transplantation Research Panel*, 1, National Institutes of Health, Bethesda, MD, 1988.

41. For costs and various kinds of pills, Google "Planned Parenthood" and "Emergency Contraception."

42. Kenneth Jost, "Mother versus Child," *American Bar Association Journal*, April 1989 p. 86.

43. E. Abel and Robert Sokol, "Fetal Alcohol Syndrome Is Now the Leading Cause of Mental Retardation" (letter), *Lancet* 8517, November 22, 1986, pp. 898–899.

44. Associated Press, "Mother Gets 6 Years for Drugs in Brest Milk," *New York Times* October 28, 1992. p. A11.

45. Harold Morowitz, "Roe v. Wade Passes a Lab Test," *New York Times*, November 25, 1992, p. A13.

46. *Planned Parenthood v. Casey*, excerpts quoted from *New York Times*, June 30, 1992, p. A8.

47. "Restrictions on Young Women's Access to Reproductive Services," Center for Reproductive Rights, June 2006, Item F010, www.crlp.org/tools.

48. Hadley Arkes, "Courts Strike Down Laws Against Partial-Birth Abortion," *Wall Street Journal*, December 17, 1998, p. A31.

## Chapter 6

1. Patrick Steptoe and Robert Edwards, *A Matter of Life*, Morrow, London, 1980.

2. *Time*, August 7, 1978, p. 68.

3. Richard Blandau, quoted in *Time*, November 13, 1978, p. 89.

4. Walter Kornberg, "Playing God in Laboratory: Question of Man's Wisdom, *Los Angeles Times*, March 16, 1969, p. G3.

5. Audrey Smith, quoted in Steptoe and Edwards, *A Matter of Life*, p. 48.

6. Nicholas Bakalar, "First Mention: In Vitro Fertilization," *New York Times*, March 22, 2011, p. D7.

7. Sheryl Gay Stolberg, "For the Infertile, a High-Tech Treadmill of Despair," *New York Times*, December 14, 1997.

8. Centers for Disease Control, *Assisted Reproductive Technology Success Rates in the United States: 1996 National Summary and Fertility Clinic Reports*. (CDC Web site)

9. For one such account, see Holly Finn, "My Fertility Crisis," *Wall Street Journal*, July 23, 2011.

10. Seale Harris, *A Women's Surgeon: The Life Story of J. Marion Sims*, Macmillan, New York, 1950, p. 245; Barron Lerner, "Scholars Argue over Legacy of Surgeon Who Was Lionized, Then Vilified," *New York Times*, October 28, 2003, p. D7.

11. Elaine Tyler, *Barren in the Promised Land: Childless Americans and the Pursuit of Happiness*, Cambridge, MA, Harvard University Press, 1995, pp. 65–69.

12. Sheryl Gay Stolberg, "Quandary on Donor Eggs: What to Tell the Children," *New York Times*, January 18, 1998.

13. Gina Kolata, "New Pregnancy Hope: A Single Sperm Injected," *New York Times*, August 11, 1993, p. B7.

14. Peggy Orenstein, "Your Gamete, Myself," *New York Times*, July 15, 2007.

15. K. Sauer, Richard Paulson, and Rogerio A. Lobo, "Reversing the Natural . . . of Pregnancy," *New England Journal of Medicine* 322 (1990), pp. 659–644.

16. B. Luke et al., "Cumulative Birth Rates with Linked Assisted Reproductive Technology Cycles," *New England Journal of Medicine* 366 no. 26 (June 28, 2102), p. 2483.

17. Gina Kolata, "Successful Births Reported with Frozen Human Eggs," *New York Times*, October 17, 1997, A1.

18. David Colker, "It's a Boy—Embryo Is Viable after 1990 Freezing," *Los Angeles Times*, February 17, 1998.

19. Kirsty Horsey, "Twins Born 16 Years Apart," *Daily Mail* (England), May 30, 2006, A1.

20. Richard Jerome, "In the Band," *People*, July 1, 2002, pp. 48–50.

21. Sylvia Westphal, "New Way to Extend Fertility," *Wall Street Journal* April 20, 2007, p. A1.

22. Denise Grady, "Parents Torn Over Extra Frozen Embryos from Fertility Procedures," *New York Times*, December 4, 2008, p. A22.

23. Nancy Snyderman, "New IVF Technology Offers Dramatic Results," *NBC Nightly News*, May 13, 1013.

24. The Ethics Committee of the American Society for Reproductive Medicine, American Society for Reproductive Medicine, "Financial Compensation of Oocyte Donors," 2006.

25. Gina Kolata, "Soaring Price of Donor Eggs Sets Off Debate," *New York Times*, February 25, 1998, p. A1; Adrienne Knox, "Brokers and Fertility Clinics in Bidding War for Women Willing to Sell Eggs from Ovaries," *Birmingham News*, March 15, 1998, p. A3.

26. Laura Mansnerud, "The Baby Bazaar: How Bundles of Joy Not for Sale Are Sold," *New York Times*, October 26, 1998.

27. Ibid.

28. U.S. State Department, quoted from *New York Magazine*, February 4, 2013, p. 7.

29. The American Surrogacy Center, "Legal Overview of Surrogacy Laws by State," 2002, www.surrogacy.com

30. Elizabeth Cohen, "Surrogate Offered $10,000 to Abort Baby," CNN Health, http://www.cnn.com/2013/03/04/health/surrogacy-kelley-legal-battle.

31. Richard Jerome, "Mortal Choices," *People*, October 7, 1996, pp. 96–102.

32. Ann Curry, "After 10 Years, New Adventures for Septuplets," *Dateline*, December 12, 2007, http://www.nbcnews.com/id/22223331/#.USAS0hzB-AE.

33. Robert Samuels, "Nine Years After Birth of Sextuplets, Now-Single Mom Struggles," *Washington Post*, 1 October 2006.

34. "Grandmother," *People*, June 28, 2006.

35. Reproductive Health and Early Life Changes," http://www.unfpa.org/modules/intercenter/cycle/earlylife.htm.

36. Henry Chu, "China: Too Many Men, Too Few Women," *The Birmingham News*, February 23, 2001.

37. "Text of Vatican's Statement on Human Reproduction," *New York Times*, March 11, 1987, pp. 10ff.

38. Laurie Goodstein and Elisabeth Povoledo, "Vatican Issues Instructions for Bioethics," *New York Times*, December 12, 2008.

39. Paul Ramsey, *Fabricated Man*, Yale University Press, New Haven, CT, 1970.

40. Steptoe and Edwards, *A Matter of Life*, p. 113.

41. Paul Ramsey, *The Ethics of Fetal Experimentation*, Yale University Press, New Haven, CT, 1975.

42. Joseph Fletcher, *Ethics of Genetic Control: Enduring Reproductive Roulette*, Doubleday Anchor New York, ; reprinted by Prometheus, Buffalo, NY, 1984, p. 36.

43. Joseph Fletcher, "Ethical Aspects of Genetic Controls," *New England Journal of Medicine* 285, no. 14 (1971), pp. 776–781.

44. *Time*, November 13, 1978, p. 89.

45. John Marlow, quoted in *U.S. News and World Report*, August 7, 1978, p. 24.

46. John Marshall, quoted in *Time*, July 31, 1978, p. 59.

47. Leon Kass, "The New Biology: What Price Relieving Man's Estate?" *Journal of the American Medical Association* 174 (November 19, 1971), pp. 779–788.

48. James Watson, "Moving towards the Clonal Man," *Atlantic*, May 1971, p. 53.

49. Max Perutz, quoted in Steptoe and Edwards, *A Matter of Life*, p. 117.

50. Daniel Callahan, *New York Times*, July 27, 1978. A16.

51. M. Hansen et al., "The Risk of Major Birth Defects after Intracytoplasmic Sperm Injection and in Vitro Fertilization," *New England Journal of Medicine* 346 (March 7, 2002), pp. 725–730.

52. Ibid.

53. Examination of leftover embryos created by IVF reveals a good deal of genetic abnormalities, such as mosaicism and morphological problems [Yamada Shita, "ART and Birth Defects," *Congenital Abnormalities* 45 (2005), 39–43]. IVF may contribute to aberrant imprinting and DNA methylation, or epigenetic changes in the embryo's DNA. Scientists need to study whether different methods of stimulating superovulation or culturing embryos, as well as different times of transferring embryos to the uterus, affect epigenetic alternations [M. Hansen, "ART and Risk of Birth Defects—A Systematic Review," *Human Reproduction* 20 (2005), 328–338].

54. Amy Docker Marcus, "A Registry for Test-Tube Babies," *Wall Street Journal*, September 16, 2003, D1, D9.

55. M. Davies et al., "Reproductive Technologies and the Risk of Birth Defects," *New England Journal of Medicine* 366, no. 19, (May 10, 2012).

56. Jeremy Rifkin and Ted Howard, *Who Shall Play God?* Dell, New York, 1977, p. 115.

57. Hans Tiefel, "In Vitro Fertilization: A Conservative View," *Journal of the American Medical Association* 247, no. 23 (June 18, 1982), pp. 3235–3242.

58. Jeff Minerd, "ESHRE: Birth Defect Risk Preferable to Childlessness in IVF Survey," *MedPage Today*, June 23, 2005.

59. Stolberg, "Quandary on Donor Eggs."

60. Cynthia Cohen, "Parents Anonymous," Cynthia Cohen, (ed.) *Egg Donation*, Johns Hopkins University Press, Baltimore, MD, 1997.

61. Susan Schindelhette, "My Life as a Sperm Donor," *People*, June 5, 2006, pp. 135–37.

62. For example, see Wesley J. Smith, "Eggs for Sale?" *The Weekly Standard*, May 20, 2013; David Tuller, "Payment Offers to Egg Donors Prompt Scrutiny," *New York Times*, May 11, 2010, p. D5.

63. Helen Ragone, *Conception from the Heart*, Indiana University Press, Bloomington, IN, 1994.

64. Gina Kolata, "With Help of Science, Infertile Couples Can Even Pick Traits," *New York Times*, November 23, 1997, p. A1.

65. Frederic Golden, "Good Eggs, Bad Eggs," *TIME*, January 11, 1999, p. 58.

66. Mary Rutz, "Selling Eggs: Cost and Consent in the Bull Market," *Bulletin of the University of Illinois at Chicago Department of Medical Education* 5, no. 2 (January 1999), p. 3.

67. Dina Kraft, "Where Families Are Prized, Help Is Free," *New York Times*, July 18, 2011, p. A5.

68. Tamara Audi and Arlene Chang, "Assembling the Global Baby," *Wall Street Journal*, December 11–12, 2010, p. C1–2.

69. Scott Carney, "Cash on Delivery," *The Red Market: On the Trail of the World's Organ Brokers, Bone Thieves, Blood Farmers and Child Traffickers*, William Morrow, New York, 2011, p. 142.

70. Rick Weiss, "Bioethics Panel Calls for Ban on Radical Reproductive Procedures," *Washington Post*, January 16, 2004

71. *Time*, August 7, 1978; *Newsday*, February 8, 2009, p. A46

# Chapter 7

1. Maggie Scarf, "The Fetus as Guinea Pig," *New York Times Magazine*; October 19, 1975, pp. 194–200; Paul Ramsey, *The Ethics of Fetal Research*, Yale University Press, New Haven, CT, 1975.

2. Associated Press, "Ex-Husband Has Embryos Destroyed," June 16, 1993.

3. "The Science and Application of Cloning," National Bioethics Advisory Commission, *Cloning Human Beings: Report and Recommendations of the National Bioethics Advisory Commission*, Rockville, MD, June 1997, p. 20.

4. I. Wilmut et al., "Viable Offspring Derived from Fetal and Adult Mammalian Cells," *Nature* 385 (February 27, 1997), pp. 810–813.

5. Arnold Kriegstein, Director, University of California Institute of Regenerative Medicine, quoted in Nancy Gibbs and Alice Park, "What A Bush Veto Would Mean for Stem Cells," *Time*, July 24, 2006, p. 36.

6. Douglas Melton, quoted in Gibbs and Park, "What a Bush Veto Would Mean for Stem Cells."

7. Justin Gillis and Rick Weiss, "NIH: Few Stem Cell Colonies Likely Available for Research," *Washington Post*, March 3, 2004, A3.

8. Chee Yoke Heong, "Malaysia New Dream: Biovalley," *Asia Times*, 2003.

9. "China, a Cloning Paradise," *Asia Times*, February 24, 2005.

10. "State Cloning Laws," The National Conference of State Legislators, April 18, 2006, http://ncls.org/programs/health/Genetics/rt-shcl.htm.

11. "State Human Cloning Laws," April 18, 2006, The National Conference of State Legislatures, http://www.ncls.org/rorams/health/Genetics/rt-shel.htm.

12. Gautam Nak, "Human Cloning Moves Small Step Closer," *Wall Street Journal*, May 15, 2013, p. A3.

13. Rick Weiss, "Mature Human Embryos Cloned," *Washington Post*, February 12, 2004, p. A28.

14. Gina Kolata, "Koreans Report Ease in Cloning for Stem Cells," *New York Times*, May 20, 2005, p. A1.

15. David Stout, "In First Veto, Bush Blocks Stem Cell Bill," *New York Times*, July 19, 2006, p. A1.

16. Paul Basken, "NIH Pleases Scientists with New Rules for Stem Cell Research," *Chronicle of Higher Education*, July 7, 2009 (web edition).

17. Rob Stein, "Researches May Have Found the Equivalent of Embryonic Stem Cells," *Washington Post*, July 24, 2009, p. A5.

18. Rob Stein, "Lab Produces Monkeys with Two Mothers," *Washington Post*, August 27, 2009.

19. Stein, "Researchers May Have Found Equivalent of Embryonic Stem Cells."

20. "Undifferentiated Ethics," *Scientific American*, September 2010, p. 18.

21. Nicholas Wade, "After Setbacks in Harvesting Stem Cells, a New Approach Shows Promise," *New York Times*, October 6, 2011, p. A20.

22. Rob Stein, "First Test of Human Embryonic Stem Cell Therapy in People Discontinued," *Washington Post*, November 14, 2011, p. A1; Andrew Pollack, "Noncontroversial Type of Stem Cells Failed a Key Test, Researchers Report," *New York Times*, May 14, 2011, p. A14; E. Snyder et al., "Stem Cells and Spinal Cord Repair," *New England Journal of Medicine*, 366:20, May 17, 2012, pp. 1940–1942.

23. Richard McCormick, "Who or What Is a Preembryo?" *Kennedy Journal of Ethics* 1, no. 1 (March 1991), p. 5.

24. Ibid. It is also true that some Catholic theologians hold out for personhood as beginning some short time after conception. For our purposes here, and since their view has been de-emphasized of late, that view will not be discussed.

25. http://www.snowflakes.org/.

26. McCormic, "Who or What Is a Preembryo?" p.12

27. Bonnie Steinbock, "Moral Status, Moral Value and Human Embryos: Implications for Stem Cell Research," ed. Bonnie Steinbock, *Oxford Handbook of Bioethics* Oxford University Press, New York, 2007.

28. Brian Leiberman, "Use of In-Vitro Fertilisation Embryos Cryopreserved for 5 Years or More," *Lancet* 15, no. 4 (October 4, 2000).

29. "Committee Decides 'Therapeutic Cloning' Can Go Ahead," *BioNews* 147 (May 3, 2002), p. 2.

30. David Ozar, "The Case for Not Unthawing Frozen Embryos," *Hastings Center Report* 15, no. 4 (August 1985), pp. 7–12.

31. Gene Outka, "The Ethics of Human Stem Cell Research," *Kennedy Institute Journal of Ethics*, 12 (2002), pp. 175–213

32. Lee Silver, *Re-Making Eden: Cloning and Beyond in a Brave New World*, Avon, New York, 1997.

33. Leon Kass, "Cloned Embryos," *First Things*, June 2002.

# Chapter 8

1. A famous movie in medical ethics follows a case that is a collage of these three cases: *Who Should Survive?* Produced by the Joseph P. Kennedy Foundation, Film Service, 999 Asylum Avenue, Hartford, CT 10605.

2. James Gustafson, "Mongolism, Parental Desires, and the Right to Life," *Perspectives on Biology and Medicine* 16 (Summer 1973), p. 529.

3. R. Duff and A. Campbell, "Moral and Ethical Dilemmas in the Special-Care Nursery," *New England Journal of Medicine* 289, no. 17 (October 25, 1973), pp. 890–894.

4. John Lorber, "Results of Treatment of Myelomeningocele: An Analysis of 524 Unselected Cases, with Special Reference to Possible Selection for Treatment," *Developmental Medicine and Child Neurology* 13, no. 2 (1971), pp. 279–303.

5. Laura J. Williams, "Decline in the Prevalence of Spina Bifida and Anencephaly by Race/Ethnicity, 1995–2002, *Pediatrics,* 116, no. 3, (September 1, 2005), pp. 580–586.

6. Mary Tedeschi, "Infanticide and Its Apologists," *Commentary*, November, 1984, p. 34.

7. John Boswell, *The Kindness of Strangers: The Abandonment of Children in Western Europe from Late Antiquity to the Renaissance*, Pantheon, New York, 1989; Robert Weir, *Selected Nontreatment of Handicapped Newborns*, Oxford University Press, New York, 1984.

8. William Lecky, *A History of European Morals from Augustus to Charlemagne II*, Braziler, New York, 1955, pp. 25–56 (originally published 1869).

9. Shari Staaver, "Siamese Twins' Case Devastates MDs," *American Medical News*, October 9, 1981, pp. 15–16.

10. Bonnie Steinbock, "Whatever Happened to the Danville Siamese Twins? *Hastings Center Report* 17, no. 4 (August–September 1987), pp. 3–4. See also John Robertson, "Dilemma in Danville," *Hastings Center Report* 11, no. 5 (October 1981), p. 7.

11. U.S. Commission on Civil Rights, *Medical Discrimination Against Children with Disabilities*, Washington, D.C., September 1989, p. 391.

12. Ibid.

13. C. Everett Koop, "The Seriously Ill or Dying Child: Supporting the Patient and the Family," in D. Horan and D. Mall, eds., *Death, Dying and Euthanasia*, University

Publications of America, Frederick, MD, 1977, pp. 537–539.

14. Adrian Peracchio, "Government in the Nursery: New Era for Baby Doe Cases," *Newsday*, November 13, 1983. Reprint, *The Bay Jane Doe Story: Winner of the 1984 Pulitzer Prize for Local Reporting*, Newsday, 1983.

15. Kathleen Kerr, "An Issue of Law and Ethics," *Newsday*, October 26, 1983; B. D. Colen, "A Life of Love—and Endless Pain," *Newsday*, October 26, 1983. (Available from *Newsday* in the reprint "The Bay Jane Doe Story: Winner of the 1984 Pulitzer Prize for Local Reporting"); "Baby Jane Doe," *Wall Street Journal*, November 21, 1983.

16. Kathleen Kerr, "Legal, Medical Legacy of Case," *Newsday*, December 7, 1987.

17. Ibid.

18. Bonnie Steinbock, "Baby Jane Doe in the Courts," *Hastings Center Report* 14, no. 1 (February 1984), p. 15; *Hastings Center Report* 14, no. 4 (August 1984).

19. Kerr, "Legal, Medical Legacy of Case" *Newsday*, December 7, 1987, p. 2.; see also Kathleen Kerr, "Reporting the Case of Baby Jane Doe. *Hastings Center Report*, Vol. 14, No. 4, August, 1984, pp. 7–9."

20. "Baby Jane Doe Has Surgery to Remove Water from Brain," *New York Times*, April 7, 1984, p. 28.

21. Ibid.

22. Kerr, "Legal, Medical Legacy of Case."

23. *Hastings Center Report* 24, no. 3 (May–June 1984), p. 2.

24. Rhoda Amon, "A Long-Running Morality Play," www.lihistory.com/9/hs9 oral.htm.

25. Jamie Talan, "A Fighter's Spirit: 20-year-old Keri-Lynn—Baby Jane Doe—Beat the Odds," *Newsday*, October 13, 2003, pp. A3, A22.

26. From a photo of the family posted online.

27. Steven Baer, "The Half-Told Story of Baby Jane Doe," *Columbia Journalism Review*, November–December 1984, pp. 35–38; Mary Tedeschi, "Infanticide and Its Apologists," *Commentary*, November 1984, p. 34.

28. Gustafson, "Mongolism, Parental Desires."

29. C. Everett Koop, "The Slide to Auschwitz," *Whatever Happened to the Human Race?* Revell, Old Tappan, NJ, 1979.

30. *Who Should Survive?*

31. Kerr, "Legal, Medical Legacy of Case."

32. Fred Bruning, "The Politics of Life," *MacLean's*, December 12, 1983, p. 17.

33. James Rachels, "Active and Passive Euthanasia," *New England Journal of Medicine* 292 (January 9, 1975), pp. 78–80.

34. Koop, "The Slide to Auschwitz."

35. R. McCormick, "To Save or Let Die: The Dilemma of Modern Medicine," *Journal of the American Medical Association* 229, no. 8 (July 1974), pp. 172–176.

36. Peter Singer, *Practical Ethics*, Cambridge University Press, New York, 1979, p. 137; Tristam Engelhardt, "Ethical Issues in Aiding the Death of Young Children," in Marvin Kohl, ed., *Beneficent Euthanasia*, Prometheus, Buffalo, NY, 1975; Michael Tooley, "Abortion and Infanticide," *Philosophy and Public Affairs* 2, no. 1 (Fall 1972), pp. 37–65.

37. Robert Weir, *Selected Nontreatment of Handicapped Newborns*, Oxford University Press, New York, 1984.

38. R. B. Zachary, "Life with Spina Bifida," *British Medical Journal* 2 (1977), p. 1461.

39. David Gibson, "Dimensions of Intelligence," in *Down Syndrome: The Psychology of Mongolism*, Cambridge University Press, New York, 1978, pp. 35–77; Janet Carr, "The Development of Intelligence," in David Lane and Brian Stafford, eds., *Current Approaches to Down Syndrome*, New York, Praeger, 1985, pp. 167–186.

40. Carr, "The Development of Intelligence.

41. Tom Regan, *The Case for Animal Rights*, University of California Press, Berkeley, CA, 1985.

42. Mathew Rarey, "Wrongful-birth Lawsuits Put doctors in Ethical Dilemma," *Washington Times*, August 5, 1999, p. A20.

43. "High Court Rules 'Wrongful Birth' Suits Invalid," *Atlanta Journal-Constitution*, July 7, 1999, p. E1.

44. John Robertson, "Extreme Prematurity and Parental Rights After Baby Doe," *Hastings Center Report* (July/August 2004), p. 33.

45. Brenda Coleman, "Moral Floodgates Opened by Father Pulling Plug on Son," Associated Press, May 1, 1989; Gregg Levoy, "Birth Controllers," *Omni*, August 1987, p. 31.

46. *In the Matter of Baby K*, U.S. District Court, E. D. Virginia, July 7, 1993, no. Civ. A. 93-104-A; see also "The Case of Baby K," *Trends in Health Care, Law, and Ethics* 9, no. 1 (Winter 1994), pp. 1–48.

47. Gina Kolata, "Parents of Tiny Infants Find Care Choices Are Not Theirs," *New York Times*, September 30, 1991, p. A1.

48. Bill Bartholomene, personal communication, who also read an earlier version of this chapter and who was a resident at the time and narrated the movie, *Who Should Survive?* Also, John Freeman, "On Learning Humility: A Thirty-Year Journey," *Hastings Center Report* (May–June, 2004), pp. 13–16.

49. A. Gallo, "Spina Bifida: The State of the Art of Medical Management," *Hastings Center Report* 14, no. 1 (February 1984), pp. 10–13.

50. Ibid.

51. Spina Bifida Association, *Brief Amicus Curiae of the Spina Bifida Association of America, Weber v. Stony Brook Hospital*, New York State Supreme Court, Appellate Division, 2d Department, *New York Law Journal*, October 28, 1983; quoted in Steinbock, "Baby Jane Doe in the Courts," p. 19.

52. Bob Meadows and Lorna Grisby, "Precious Child, Impossible Choice, *People*, May 15, 2006, p. 123.

53. Francis Kamm "What is and What is Not Wrong with Enhancement," July 7, 2006, KSG Working Papers, No. RWPOG-20, Harvard-Kennedy School. http://papers .ssrn.com/sol3/papers.cfm?abstract_ id=902372 (accessed December 22, 2013).

54. Anita Silvers, "Rights Are Still Rights: The Case for Disability Rights," *Hastings Center Report* (November/December 2004), pp. 39–40.

# Chapter 9

1. In this chapter, "animals" refers to "non-human animals."

2. http://en.wikipedia.org/wiki/Unnecessary_ Fuss.

3. Quoted from the tape by W. Robbins, "Animal Rights: A Growing Movement in the U.S.," *New York Times*, June 15, 1984, p. A16.

4. *Evaluation of Experimental Procedures Conducted at the University of Pennsylvania Experimental Head-Injury Laboratory 1981–1984 in Light of the Public Health Science Animal Welfare Policy*, Office for Protection of Research Risks, National Institutes of Health, 1985, p. 37.

5. Robbins, "Animal Rights."

6. Robert Marshak, quoted in *New York Times*, July 29, 1984, p. A12.

7. Donald Abt, quoted in *New York Times*, August 12, 1984, p. B1.

8. *New York Times*, December 10, 1984, p. A10.

9. Ibid.

10. "Of Pain and Progress," *Newsweek*, December 26, 1988, p. 53.

11. Quoted in J. Duschek, "Protestors Prompt Halt in Animal Research," *Science News*, July 27, 1985, p. 53.

12. Edward Taub, "The Silver Spring Monkey Incident: The Untold Story," *Coalition for Animals and Animal Research Newsletter*, 4, no. 1 (Winter–Spring 1991), pp. 1–8.

13. Tony Dajer, "Monkeying with the Brain," *Discover*, January 1992, p. 70–71. See also Warren E. Leary, "Sharp Brain Healing Found in Disputed Monkey Tests," *New York Times*, June 28, 1991, p. A9.

14. Joachim Liepert, Heike Bauder, Wolfgang H. R. Miltner, Edward Taub, and Cornelius Weiller, "Treatment-Induced Cortical Reorganization After Stroke in Humans," *Stroke: The Journal of the American Heart Association*, pp. 31 (June 2000) 1210–1216.

15. Edward Taub, *Topics in Stroke Rehabilitation*, Vol. 3, pp. 38–61. "Constraint-Induced Movement Therapy: A New Family of Techniques," *Journal of Rehabilitation Research and Development*, Vol. 36, No. 3, July, 1999.

16. Sandra Blakeslee, "Pushing Injured Brains and Spinal Cords to New Paths," *New York Times*, August 28, 2001, p. D6.

17. "Stroke Rehab Therapy Shows Benefits in 2-year Follow-up," *UAB Reporter*, April 12, 2006. "Right after a stroke, a limb is paralyzed," he says. "Whenever the person tries to move an arm, it simply doesn't work." But often the cells that represent the arm are still alive. The patient assumes the arm is permanently dead, expects failure from trying to use it, and does not. "We call it learned non-use," Taub said.

The more the patient relies on the good arm, the less likely recovery becomes in the bad arm. Timing is critical. Immediately after a stroke, if movement is induced in the bad limb, damage increases to the brain. But in the second or third week, therapy can begin.

Requiring rehabilitation therapists trained in the new techniques, the therapy goes six to seven hours every weekday for ten consecutive weeks. Patients move around with good limbs tightly bandaged.

To meet the demand, in 2001 UAB opened the Taub Clinic for CI therapy. Although neither private insurance nor

Medicare pays for CI therapy, which runs $6,000 to $13,000, over 5,000 stroke patients now wait for it. Demand for CI therapy has also created ethical problems similar to that of Seattle's God Committee in 1962.

18. "Taub Wins American Psychological Association Scientific Award," *UAB Synopsis*, February 16, 2004.

19. Edward Taub, Gitendra Uswatte, Danna Kay King, David Morris, Jean E. Crago, and Anjan Chatterjee, "A Placebo-Controlled Trial of Constraint-Induced Movement Therapy for Upper Extremity After Stroke," *Stroke: The Journal of the American Heart Association*, 37 (April 2006), pp. 1045–1049.

20. John Durant, quoted in John Hargrove, "Bush Signs Heflin Bill to Protect Researchers," *Birmingham Post-Herald*, August 28, 1992.

21. Biomedical Research Education Trust, http://www.bret.org.uk/num.htm.

22. Bernard Rollins, *Animal Rights and Human Morality*, Prometheus, Buffalo, NY, 1981, pp. 97–99.

23. D. Carvajal, "A New Science, at First Blush," *New York Times*, November 20, 2007. pp. C1, 4.

24. http://www.bret.org.uk/num.htm.

25. Press Release, National Academies of Science, May 29, 2009, http://www8.nationalacademies.org/onpinews/newsitem.aspx?RecordID=12641.

26. Office of Technology Assessment, *Animal Usage in the United States*, Superintendent of Documents, Washington, D.C., 1986, p. 12; *Newsweek*, December 26, 1988, p. 51; Andrew Rowan, *Of Mice, Models, and Men: A Critical Evaluation of Animal Research*, State University of New York Press, Albany, NY, 1984, pp. 67–70.

27. Nicholas Fontaine, Memoires pour servir Ö l'histoire de Port-Royal, vol. 2, originally published in Cologne in 1738; quoted in L. Rosenfield, *From Best-Machine to Man-Machine: The Theme of Animal Soul in French Letters from Descartes to La Mettrie*, Oxford University Press, New York, 1940, pp. 52–53; also quoted in Peter Singer, "*Animal Liberation*," *New York Review of Books*, 1975.

28. C. S. Lewis, *How Human Suffering Raises Almost Intolerable Intellectual Problems*, Macmillan, New York, 1940, pp. 131–133.

29. David Hume, *A Treatise of Human Nature*, 1789, Dover Publications, Mineola, NY, 2003 ed.

30. Singer, "Animal Liberation." New York, NY.

31. Shelly Kagan, quoted from

32. Quoted in S. Isen, "Laying the Foundation for Animal Rights: Interview with Tom Regan," *Animals Agenda*, July–August, 1984, pp. 4–5.

33. Tom Regan, *The Case for Animal Rights*, Berkeley, CA, University of California Press, 1983.

34. Quoted in "Animals in the Middle," in the television series *Innovation*, sponsored by Johnson and Johnson on the A & E Network, September 5, 1987.

35. Ibid.

36. Carl Cohen, "The Case for Animal Rights,' *New England Journal of Medicine* 315, no. 14 (October 4, 1986), pp. 865–870.

37. Wise Young, quoted by Niall Shank, Ray Greek, Nathan Nobis, and Jean Swingle-Greek, "Animals and Medicine: Do Animal Experiments Predict Human Responses?" *The Skeptic*, 13, no. 3 (2007), p. 1.

38. http://emice.nci.nih.gov/aam/mouse/how-and-why-mouse-cancer-models-are-used.

39. http://www.nature.com/news/2011/110608/full/news.2011.356.html.

40. http://science.education.nih.gov/animal-researchfs06.pdf.

41. Shank et al., "Animals and Medicine."

42. Lawrence Hansen, "Noxious Groupthink," *Chronicle of Higher Education*, November 12, 2010, pp. B6–7.

43. Roscoe Bartlett, "Stop Using Chimps as Guinea Pigs," *New York Times*, August 10, 2011.

# Chapter 10

1. Eugene Kogon, *The Theory and Practice of Hell*, Berkley Trade, New York, 1998.

2. Vera Alexander, *The Search for Mengele*, HBO movie, October 1985; interviewed by Central Television (London) and quoted in Gerald Posner and John Hare, *The Complete Story*, Cooper Square Press, New York, 2000, p. 37.

3. William Curran, "The Forensic Investigation of the Death of Joseph Mengele," *New England Journal of Medicine* 315, no. 17 (October 23, 1985), pp. 1071–1073.

4. David Rothman, "Ethics and Human Experimentation," *New England Journal of Medicine* 317, no. 19 (November 5, 1987), p. 1198.

5. Robert Bazell, "Growth Industry," *New Republic*, March 15, 1993, p. 14.

6. Constance Pechura, "From the Institute of Medicine," *Journal of the American Medical Association* 269, no. 4 (January 27, 1993), p. 453.

7. Rothman, "Ethics and Human Experimentation."

8. Dan Stober, Knight-Ridder Newspapers, "Dr. Hamilton Was Enthusiastic Experimenter in Radiation," *Birmingham News*, February 20, 1994, p. 10A; "America's Nuclear Secrets," *Newsweek*, December 27, 1993, p. 15.

9. Keith Schneider, "Scientists Are Sharing the Anguish over Nuclear Experiments on People," *New York Times*, March 2, 1994, p. A9.

10. Robert Burns, "Radiation Experiments Were Far-Reaching," Associate Press, *Birmingham Post-Herald*, August 18, 1995, p. E6.

11. Dennis Domerzalski, Scripps-Howard News Service, "Radiation 'Guinea Pigs' Tell Stories," *Birmingham Post-Herald,* February 3, 1994, p. A8.

12. Philip J. Hilts, "U.S. Is Urged to Repay Some in Radiation Tests," *New York Times*, July 17, 1995, p. A9. See also *Final Report*, Advisory Committee on Human Radiation Experiments, U.S. Government Printing Office, Washington, D.C.

13. H. Beecher, "Ethics and Clinical Research," *New England Journal of Medicine* 274 (1966), pp. 1354–1360.

14. H. Pappworth, *Human Guinea Pigs*, Beacon, Boston, MA, 1968.

15. Arthur Caplan, "Rethinking the Cost of War," *Due Consideration*, Wiley, New York, 1998, pp. 123–124.

16. Molly Selvin, "Changing Medical and Societal Attitudes toward Sexually Transmitted Diseases: A Historical Overview," in King K. Holmes et al., eds., *Sexually Transmitted Diseases*, McGraw-Hill, New York, 1984, pp. 3–19.

17. Alan Brandt, "Racism and Research: The Case of the Tuskegee Syphilis Study," *Hastings Center Report* 8, no. 6 (December 1978), pp. 21–29.

18. Paul de Kruif, *The Microbe Hunters*, Harcourt Brace, New York, 1926, p. 323.

19. J. E. Bruusgaard, "öber das Schicksal der nichtspezifischbehandeltenLuetiker" ("Fate of Syphilitics Who Are Not Given Specific Treatment"), *Archives of Dermatology of Syphilis* 157 (April 1929), pp. 309–332.

20. H. H. Hazen, "Syphilis in the American Negro," *Journal of the American Medical Association* 63 (August 8), 1914, p. 463.

21. James Jones, *Bad Blood,* Free Press, New York, 1981, p. 74.

22. Ibid.

23. Ibid.

24. Quoted in E. Ramont, "Syphilis in the AIDS Era," *New England Journal of Medicine* 316, no. 25 (June 18, 1987), pp. 600–601.

25. R. A. Vonderlehr, T. Clark, and J. R. Heller, "Untreated Syphilis in the Male Negro," *Journal of the American Medical Association* 107, no. 11 (September 12, 1936), pp. 856–860.

26. Jean Heller, "Syphilis Victims in U.S. Study Went Untreated for 40 Years," *New York Times*, July 26, 1972, pp. 1, 8.

27. Or worse: in 1988, a malpractice suit brought against a hospital in Vermont was settled out of court for $2.7 million on behalf of a 28-year-old woman who had gone into a coma after being incompetently tapped by a resident. "Malpractice Suit Settled for $2.7 Million," *Burlington Free Press* (Alabama), December 21, 1988.

28. Archives of National Library of Medicine; quoted in Jones, *Bad Blood*, p. 127.

29. W. J. Brown et al., *Syphilis and Other Venereal Diseases*, Harvard University Press, Cambridge, MA, 1970, p. 34.

30. Heller, "Syphilis Victims in U.S. Study."

31. Ibid.

32. Allison Mitchell, "Survivors of Tuskegee Study Get Apology from Clinton," *New York Times*, May 17, 1997, p. A1.

33. Carol Yoon, "Families Emerge as Silent Victims of Tuskegee Syphilis Experiments," *New York Times*, May 9, 1998, P. A1.

34. Marcia Angell, "The Ethics of Clinical Research in the Third World," *New England Journal of Medicine* 337, no. 12 (September 18, 1997), pp. 847–849.

35. R. H. Kampmeier, "The Tuskegee Study of Untreated Syphilis" (editorial), *Southern Medical Journal* 65, no. 10 (October 1972), pp. 1247–1251.

36. Thomas Benedek, "The 'Tuskegee Study' of Untreated Syphilis: Analysis of Moral Aspects versus Methodological Aspects," *Journal of Chronic Diseases* 31 (1978), pp. 35–50. I have drawn considerably on this excellent article.

37. Kampmeier, "The Tuskegee Study of Untreated Syphilis."

38. "The Deadly Deception" (with George Strait), *Nova*, January 28, 1992.

39. Benedek, "The 'Tuskegee Study' of Untreated Syphilis," p. 44.

40. Personal correspondence, April 25, 1985. Benjamin Friedman is Professor Emeritus of Medicine, UAB.

41. Benedek, "The 'Tuskegee Study' of Untreated Syphilis."

42. G. W. Hayes et al., "The Golden Anniversary of the Silver Bullet," *Journal of the American Medical Association* 270, no. 13 (October 6, 1993), p. 1610.

43. R. H. Kampmeier, "Final Report of the 'Tuskegee Study' of Syphilis," *Southern Medical Journal* 67, no. 11 (1974), pp. 1349–1353. Kampmeier advances a fourth argument that is somewhat more technical. Penicillin achieves seroreversal in latent syphilis, but Kampmeier insists that such seroreversal has never been proved to be associated with decreased morbidity or mortality. A related point is possible uncertainty over diagnosis and thus over therapeutic effects. [S. Edberg and S. Berger, *Antibiotics and Infection*, Churchill Livingstone, New York, 1983, pp. 141–142; K. Holmes et al., *Sexually Transmitted Diseases*, McGraw-Hill, New York, 1984, p. 1352; John Hotson, "Modern Neurosyphilis: A Partially Treated Chronic Meningitis, *Western Journal of Medicine* 135 (September 1981), pp. 191–200; Sarah Polt, Professor of Pathology, UAB, personal correspondence.]

44. Benedek, "The 'Tuskegee Study' of Untreated Syphilis."

45. Ibid.

46. Sheryl Gay Stolberg, "U.S. Ends Overseas HIV Studies Involving Placebos," *New York Times*, February 19, 1998.

47. Marcia Angell, "Tuskegee Revisited," *Wall Street Journal*, October 28, 1997.

48. Ruth Macklin, "Ethics and International Collaborative Research, Part I," *American Society for Bioethics and Humanities Exchange* 1, no. 2, p.1. Reprinted in Ruth Macklin, *Ethics in Global Health*, Oxford University Press, 2012.

49. Ellen Goodman, 2006. "Is Tuskegee Study OK Abroad?" *The Boston Globe*. September 25, 1997.

50. Ibid.

51. D. Bagenda and P. Musoke-Mudido, "We're Trying to Help Our Sickest People, Not Exploit Them," *Washington Post*, September 28, 1997, p. C3.

52. Macklin, "Ethics and International Collaborative Research."

53. Marcia Angell, "Tuskegee Revisited," *Wall Street Journal*, October 28, 1997.

54. Goodman, "Is Tuskegee Study OK Abroad?"

55. Stolberg, "U.S. Ends Overseas HIV Studies."

56. Manuel Roig-Franzia, "Probe Opens on Study Tied to Johns Hopkins," *Washington Post*, August 23, 2001, p. B1.

57. Tamar Levin, "U.S. Investigating Johns Hopkins Study of Lead Paint Hazard," *New York Times*, August 24, 2001.

58. *Grimes v. Kennedy-Krieger Institute*. 782 F2d 807 (Ct App Md 2001). [Maryland Court of Appeals. 2001; No. 128, September Term, 2000.

59. Ronald McNeil, "Panel Hears Grim Details of V.D. Test on Inmates," *New York Times*, August 31, 2011, p. A21, *A Study Guide to "Ethically Impossible" STD Research in Guatemala from 1946 to 1948*, Presidential Commission for the Study of Biomedical Issues, November 2012. http://www .bioethics .gov

60. Rick Weiss, "Research Volunteers Unwittingly at Risk," *Washington Post*, August 1, 1998, p. A1. See also this article from the online journal *Target Health: Target Health*, June 14, 1998. http://www.targethealth.com/.

61. Institute of Medicine, *Responsible Research: A Systems Approach to Protecting Research Participants*, National Academy Press, Washington, D.C., 2002.

62. For psychiatrists who abused patients in psychiatric research on schizophrenic patients, see Robert Whitaker, "Lure of Riches Fuels Testing," *Boston Globe*, November 17, 1998, p. A1; for another story about abuse of subjects and fraud in medical research, see Douglas M. Birch and Gary Cohn, "How a Cancer Drug Trial Ended in Betrayal," *Baltimore Sun*, June 24, 2001.

63. Steve Stecklow and Laura Johannes, "Drug Maker's Relied on Clinical Researchers Who Now Await Trial," *Wall Street Journal*, August 15, 1997, p. A1.

64. *The Olivieri Report: The Complete Text of the Report of the Independent Inquiry Commissioned*, Canadian Association of University Teachers, Lorimer, 2001, Miriam Shuchman, *The Drug Trial: Nancy Olivieri and the Science*

*Scandal that Rocked the Hospital for Sick Children*, Random House, New York, 2005.

65. *The Olivieri Report.*

66. Harold Shapiro and Eric Meslin, "Ethical Issues in the Design and Conduct of Clinical Trials in Developing Countries," *New England Journal of Medicine* 345 (July 12, 2001), pp. 139–142.

67. George Annas, "Global Clinical Trials and Informed Consent," *New England Journal of Medicine* 360, no. 20 (May 14, 2009).

68. See author's *Elements of Bioethics*, Chapter 8.

69. Carl Elliot, *White Coat, Black Hat*, Beacon Press, Boston, MA, 2010, p. 60.

70. Personal communication to author from Michael Saag, MD, head of UAB AIDS research unit.

71. Ilesh Jani and Treveror Peter, "How Point-of Care Testing Could Drive Innovation in Global Health," *New England Journal of Medicine* 368, no. 24 (June 13, 2013), pp. 2319–2324.

72. Footnote on real authors of this model.

73. http://www.recerca.uab.es/ceeah/docs/CIOMS.pdf.

74. Richard Jerome, "Death by Research," *People*, February 21, 2000, p. 123.

75. Deborah Nelson and Rick Weiss, "Hasty Decisions in the Race to a Cure? Gene Therapy Proceeded Despite Safety, Ethics Concerns," *Washington Post*, November 21, 1999, p. A1.

76. Arthur Caplan is quoted extensively in "Complaint for Civil Action" filed by John Gelsinger for the estate of Jesse Gelsinger against Trustees of University of Pennsylvania et al., www.sskrplaw.com/links/healthcare2.html.

77. Nelson and Weiss, "Hasty Decisions."

## Chapter 11

1. Obituary of Norman Shumway, *The Independent* (London, England), February 16, 2006.

2. Thomas Starzl, *The Puzzle People: Memoirs of a Transplant Surgeon*, Pittsburgh University Press, Pittsburgh, PA, 1992, p. 151.

3. Christiaan Barnard and Curtiss Bill Pepper, *One Life*, Macmillan, New York, 1969, p. 372.

4. Ibid.

5. "The Ultimate Operation," *Time*, December 15, 1967, p. 65; "Heart Transplant Keeps Man Alive in South Africa," *New York Times*, December 4, 1967, p. A1.

6. Barnard and Pepper, *One Life*, p. 444.

7. Quoted in Connie Chung, "Knife to the Heart," television documentary on heart transplant surgery, January 27, 1997.

8. Donald McRae, *Every Second Counts: The Race to Transplant the First Human Heart*, Putnam, New York, 2006, p. 272.

9. Erica Goode, "Dr. Francis Moore, 88, Dies; Innovative Leaders in Surgery," *New York Times*, November 29, 2001.

10. Francis Moore, M.D., quoted in interview with Connie Chung, "Knife to the Heart."

11. Andre Courmand, *New York Times*, December 6, 1967.

12. Norman Staub, quoted in Peter Hawthorne, *The Transplanted Heart*, Keartland Publishing, Johannesburg, South Africa, 1968, p. 188.

13. Denise Grady, "Summary of Discussion of Ethical Perspectives," in Margery Shaw, ed., *After Barney Clark*, University of Texas Press, Austin, TX, p. 52.

14. *Time*, December 9, 1982, p. 43.

15. *Time*, March 14, 1983, p. 74.

16. Thomas Preston, "Who Benefits from the Artificial Heart?" *Hastings Center Report* 15, no. 1 (February 1985), p. 5; *New York Times*, December 5, 1988, p. A2.

17. *Washington Post*, May 1, 1983, p. A2.

18. William A. Check, "Lessons from Barney Clark's Artificial Heart," *Health*, April 1984, pp. 22, 26.

19. Gideon Gill, "Burcham Dies After Blood Accumulates in Chest," *Louisville Courier-Journal*, April 26, 1983.

20. ibid.

21. Michael Vitez, "Marriage of Two Minds: 'World's Smartest Couple' Nears First Anniversary," Knight-Ridder Newspapers, July 3, 1988.

22. Steve Ditlea, "Robert Jarvik Returns," *Red Herring*, October 11, 2002.

23. Thomas H. Maugh II, "Dr. Willem Kolff Dies at 97; Dutch Physician Built First Kidney Dialysis Machine," *Los Angeles Times*, February 14, 2009.

24. David Benatar and Don A. Hudson, "A Tale of Two Novel Transplants Not Done: The Ethics of Limb Allografts,"

*British Medical Journal* 324 (April 20, 2002), pp. 971–975.

25. http://www.thesun.co.uk/sol/homepage/news/1784671/Transplant-man-Karl-Merk-feels-like-a-teenager.html.

26. http://www.brighamandwomens.org/about_bwh/publicaffairs/news/handtransplant/katyhayes.aspx.

27. According to Dr. Nadey Hakim of London, interviewed by Lawrence K. Altman, "A Pioneering Transplant, and Now an Ethical Storm," *New York Times*, December 6, 2005.

28. Marco Lanzetta et al., "International Registry on Hand and Composite Tissue Transplantation," *Transplantation* 79, no 9 (May 15, 2005).

29. Susan Okie, "Brave New Face," *New England Journal of Medicine* 354, no. 9 (March 2, 2006).

30. Ariane Bernard and Craig S. Smith, "French Face-Transplant Patient Tells of Her Ordeal," *New York Times*, February 7, 2006.

31. Craig S. Smith, "As a Face Transplant Heals, Flurries of Questions Arise," *New York Times*, December 14, 2005, p A1.

32. Lawrence K. Altman, "A Pioneering Transplant, and Now an Ethical Storm," *New York Times*, December 6, 2005, p. D1.

33. Personal communication to author, September 7, 2006.

34. Jean-Michel Dubernard, "Outcomes 18 Months after the First Human Partial Face Transplantation," *New England Journal of Medicine*, December 13, 2007, pp. 2451–2460.

35. Reuters, "China Performs Its First Human Face Transplant," April 14, 2006.

36. Jeff Truesdell and Alex Tresniowski, "A New Face, A New Life," *People*, August 15, 2011, pp. 57–60.

37. "Boston Hospital Completes World's Seventh Face Transplant." *Red Orbit* , April 11, 2009, Web.

38. Nichole Egan, "Love that Heals," *People*, June 24, 2013, pp. 61–68.

39. Donald McRae, *Every Second Counts: The Race to Transplant the First Human Heart*, Putnam, New York, 2006.

40. Lawrence K. Altman, "A Pioneering Transplant, and Now an Ethical Storm," *New York Times*, December 6, 2005.

41. Werner Forssmann, quoted in Barnard and Pepper, *One Life*, p. 360.

42. Starzl, *The Puzzle People*, p. 148.

43. McRae, *Every Second Counts*, p. 192.

44. William Pierce, "Permanent Heart Substitution: Better Solutions Ahead," editorial, *Journal of the American Medical Association* 259, no. 6 (February 12, 1988), p. 891.

45. *New York Times*, editorial, December 16, 1982, p. A26.

46. "The Dracula of Medical Technology," Editorial, *New York Times*, May 16, 1988.

47. National Heart Transplant Life Expectancy Statistics, NazihZuhdi Transplant Institute, Oklahoma City, OK, http://integrisok.com/nazih-zuhdi-transplant-institute-oklahoma-city-ok/heart-transplant/heart-transplant-life-expectancy-statistics.

48. Stacy Burling, "Widow Sues Artificial-Heart Maker," *Philadelphia Inquirer*, October 17, 2002; Sheryl Gay Stolberg, "On Medicine's Last Frontier: The Last Journey of James Quinn," *New York Times*, October 8, 2002.

49. Lauran Neegaard, "FDA Advisers Reject Abiomed's Artificial Heart," Associated Press, *Birmingham News*, June 24, 2005, p. A14.

50. Norman Shumway, quoted in *Transplant News*, July 13, 2001, from an interview in the *San Francisco Chronicle*.

51. Rob Stein, "Heart Pump Creates Life-Death Ethical Dilemma," *Washington Post,* 24, April 24, 2008.

52. Sandeep Jauhar, "The Artificial Heart," *New England Journal of Medicine*, February 5, 2004, pp. 542–544.

53. Denise Grady, "Researchers Find Poor Use of Pumps for Ailing Hearts," *New York Times*, November 6, 2008, p. A19.

54. H. J. Eisen and S. R. Hankins, "Continuous Flow Rotary Left Ventricular Assist Device," *Journal of the American College of Cardiology* 54, no. 4 (2009), pp. 322–324. doi:10.1016/j.jacc.2009.04.028. PMID 19608029.

55. Alan Moskowitz, "The Cost of Long-Term LVAD Implantation," *Annals of Thoracic Surgery* 71 (2001), pp. S195–S198.

56. Transplant Living, UNOS, http://www.transplantliving.org/before-the-transplant/financing-a-transplant/the-costs/.

57. D. P. Lubeck and J. P. Bunker, Office of Technology Assessment, *Case Study 9, The Artificial Heart: Costs, Risks, and Benefits*, U.S. Government Printing Office, Washington, D.C., 1982.

58. *Progressive*, February 1983, pp. 12–13.

59. Lawrence K. Altman, "Patient Opted for Transplant as Method to Mend Face," *New York Times*, December 12, 2005, p. A6.

60. Rene Fox and Judith Swazey, *The Courage to Fail: A Social View of Organ Transplants and Dialysis*, 2nd ed., rev., University of Chicago Press, Chicago, 1974, 1978.

61. P. M. Park, "The Transplant Odyssey," *Second Opinion* 12, November 1989, pp. 27–32; quoted in Rene Fox and Judith Swazey, *Spare Parts: Organ Replacement in American Society*, Oxford University Press, New York, 1992, p. 202.

62. "Norman Shumway, Heart Transplantation Pioneer, Dies at Age 83," Press Release, February 10, 2006, Stanford Medical Center.

## Chapter 12

1. James Childress, "Who Shall Live When Not All Can Live?" *Soundings* 53, no. 4 (Winter 1970).

2. Belding Scribner, unpublished manuscript, quoted in Renée Fox and Judith Swazey, *The Courage to Fail: A Social View of Organ Transplants and Dialysis*, 2d ed. rev., University of Chicago Press, Chicago, IL, 1974, 1978, p. 227.

3. Fox and Swazey, *The Courage to Fail*, p. 235.

4. One of the first organized interdisciplinary conferences to discuss such issues took place in 1967, funded by a company called CIBA.

5. H. M. Schmeck, Jr., "Panel Holds Life-or-Death Vote in Allotting of Artificial Kidney," *New York Times*, May 6, 1962, pp. 1, 83.

6. Shana Alexander, personal communication to author, "The Birth of Bioethics" conference, Seattle, WA, University of Washington Medical School, September 24, 1992.

7. Shana Alexander, "They Decide Who Lives, Who Dies: Medical Miracle Puts a Burden on a Small Committee," *Life* 53, no. 102, (November 9, 1962).

8. Fox and Swazey, *The Courage to Fail*, p. 209.

9. Judith Swazey at "The Birth of Bioethics" conference, Seattle, WA, University of Washington Medical School, September 24, 1992.

10. David Sanders and Jesse Dukeminier, "Medical Advance and Legal Lag: Hemodialysis and Kidney Transplantation," *UCLA Law Review* 15 (1968), pp. 357–412.

11. http://www.cms.hhs.gov/ESRD GeneralInformation/Downloads/2004 ProgramHighlights.pdf.

12. Dale H. Cowan, ed., *Human Organ Transplantation: Social, Medical-Legal, Regulatory, and Reimbursement Issues*, Health Administration Press, Ann Arbor, MI, 1987, p. 60.

13. Fox and Swazey, *The Courage to Fail*, p. 232.

14. Sanders and Dukeminier, "Medical Advance and Legal Lag."

15. George Annas, "The Prostitute, the Playboy, and the Poet: Rationing Schemes for Organ Transplantation," *American Journal of Public Health* 75, no. 2 (1985), pp. 187–189.

16. Fox and Swazey, *The Courage to Fail*, chapter 9.

17. Ibid., p. 234.

18. Herbert Fingarette, *Heavy Drinking*, Berkeley, University of California Press, 1988.

19. Alvin Moss and Mark Seigler, "Should Alcoholics Compete Equally for Liver Transplantation?" *Journal of the American Medical Association* 265, no. 10 (March 13, 1992), p. 1295.

20. C. Cohen and M. Benjamin, "Alcoholics and Liver Transplantation," *Journal of the American Medical Association* 265, no. 10 (March 13, 1992), pp. 1295–1301.

21. Nicholas Rescher, "The Allocation of Exotic Medical Lifesaving Therapy," *Ethics* 79 (April 1969).

22. Tracy E. Miller, "Multiple Listing for Organ Transplantation: Autonomy Unbounded," *Kennedy Institute of Ethics Journal* 2, no. 1 (March 1992) pp. 43–57.

23. Ronald Munson, *Raising the Dead*, Oxford University Press, New York, 2002, pp. 26–45.

24. Ibid., p. 29.

25. Ibid., p. 30.

26. Ibid., p. 36.

27. Ibid., p. 45.

28. Miller, "Multiple Listing for Organ Transplantation."

29. M. Michaels et al., "Ethical Considerations in Listing Fetuses as Candidates for Neonatal Heart Transplantation," *Journal of the American Medical Association* 269, no. 3 (January 20, 1993), pp. 401–402.

30. Renée Fox and Judith Swazey, *Spare Parts: Organ Replacement in American Society*, Oxford University Press, New York, 1992.

31. Albert R. Jonsen, "Bentham in a Box," *Law, Medicine and Health Care* 14 (1986), pp. 172–174.

32. http://www.cnn.com/2013/08/26/health/sarah-murnaghan-update/.

33. Newsroom Fact Sheets," United Network for Organ Sharing, November 21, 2005, http://www.unos.org/inthenews/factsheets.asp, July 10, 2006.

34. Michael Stoll, "A New Waiting Game for Hearts," *Philadelphia Inquirer*, February 7, 2000.

35. Jeffrey Kahn and Susan Parry, "Organ and Tissue Procurement," *Encyclopedia of Bioethics*, 3rd ed., Macmillan, New York, 2004; see also, "A Science Odyssey: People and Discoveries: First Successful Kidney Transplant Performed," http://www.pbs .org/wgbh/aso/databank.entries/dm54ki .html.

36. A. Bass, "New Liver Transplants; Pressure on Parents," *Boston Globe*, December 17, 1989, pp. 1, 75; quoted in Fox and Swazey, *Spare Parts*.

37. Norman Fost, "Conception for Donation," *Journal of the American Medical Association* 291 no. 17 (May 5, 2004), p. 2126.

38. Charles B. Huddleston, et al., "Lung Transplantation in Children," *Annals of Surgery* 236, no. 3 (September 2002), pp. 270–276.

39. S. Quattrucci et al., "Lung Transplantation for Cystic Fibrosis: 6-Year Follow-Up," *Journal of Cystic Fibrosis* 4, no. 2 (May 2005), pp. 107–114.

40. V. Fourbister, "Living Donors Dramatize Risk vs. Need," *American Medical News*, September 20, 1999, p. 1.

41. Dr. Jean Edmond in V. Fourbister, "Living Donors Dramatize Risk vs. Need," *American Medical News*, September 20, 1999, p. 1, confirmed the death.

42. Debra Shelton's update is "Donor Has Physical Pain, But Peace About Decision," and "Man's Second Chance Hasn't Turned Out Like He Expected," *St. Louis Post-Dispatch*, December 21, 2003.

43. Mary Ellison et al. "Living Kidney Donors in Need of Kidney Transplants," *Transplantation*, November 15, 2002, pp. 1349–1351. These 56 patients were out of 140,00 patients. Also, UNOS elevates anyone who previously donated a kidney—but now needs one—to the top of the list.

44. Carole Tarrant, "For Family, Selfless Act Goes Awry," *New York Times*, March 12, 2002.

45. HN Ibrahim et al., "Long-term Consequences of Kidney Donation," *New England Journal of Medicine* 360 (2009), pp. 459–469.

46. http://www.transplantliving.org/before-the-transplant/financing-a-transplant/the-costs/.

47. Richard D. Lamm, "Health Care as Economic Cancer," *Dialysis and Transplantation* 16, (1987), p. 433.

48. Fox and Swazey, *Spare Parts*, p. 10.

49. Robert Arnold and Stuart Younger, "Back to the Future: Obtaining Organs from Non-Heart Beating Cadavers," Kennedy Institute of Ethics Journals, Vol. 3, no. 2, p. 106.

50. Ibid.

51. Interview, *Good Morning America*, July 9, 1993.

52. http://srtr.transplant.hrsa.gov/annual_reports/2011/.

53. Walter Robinson, *Medical Ethics, Lahey Clinic Medical Ethics Newsletter* 11, no. 2 (Spring 2004), p. 8.

54. Ibid., p. 6.

54. Peter Landers, "Longer Dialysis Offers New Hope But Poses a Dilemma," *Wall Street Journal*, October 2, 2003, p. A1.

# Chapter 13

1. Rene Fox and Judith Swazey, *The Courage to Fail: A Social View of Organ Transplants and Dialysis*, 2d ed., rev., University of Chicago Press, Chicago, 1974, 1978; Harmon Smith, "Heart Transplantation," *Encyclopedia of Bioethics*, Free Press, New York, 1978.

2. Richard Howard and J. Najarian, "Organ Transplantation—Medical Perspective," *Encyclopedia of Bioethics* 3, Free Press, New York, 1978, pp. 1160–1165.

3. *Animals Voice* 2, no. 3 (December 1984).

4. Charles Krauthammer, "The Using of Baby Fae," *Time*, December 3, 1984, p. 14.

5. Quoting Kenneth P. Stoller, M.D., "The Baby Fae: The Unlearned Lesson," *Perspectives on Medical Research* 2 (1990), www.curedisease .com/Perspectives/vol.2_1990/BabyFae .html.

6. "Baby Fae Stuns the World," *Time*, November 12, 1984, p. 72.

7. Debra Berger, "The Infant with Anencephaly: Moral and Legal Dilemmas," *Issues in Law and Medicine* 5, (1989), p. 68.

8. Medical Task Force on Anencephaly, "The Infant with Anencephaly," *New England Journal of Medicine* 332, no. 10 (March 8, 1990), p. 669.

9. Robert D. Trough and John D. Fletcher, "Can Organs Be Transplanted before Brain Death? *New England Journal of Medicine* 321, no. 6 (1989), p. 388.

10. Associated Press, "Hospital Sets Policy on Organ Donor Use," February 23, 1988.

11. Joan Heilman, "Tiny Gabriel's Gift of Life," *Redbook*, December 1988, p. 162. (Article given to author by Lynn Bondurant.)

12. "Gift of Life Surrounded by Controversy," *Windsor Star* (Canada), April 3, 2011.

13. J. Peabody et al., "Experience with Anencephalic Infants as Prospective Organ Donors," *New England Journal of Medicine* 321, no. 6 (August 10, 1989), pp. 344–350.

14. A. Kantrowitz et al., "Transplantation of the Heart in an Infant and an Adult," *American Journal of Cardiology* 22, no. 782 (1968).

15. Associated Press, "Ethicists Debate Death and Baby's Lacking Brain," *Birmingham News,* March 31, 1992, p. A1.

16. Brian Udell, quoted in *USA Today*, March 30, 1992, p. 3A.

17. *In Re T. A. C. P., Southern (Law) Reporter,* 2d Series, Supreme Court of Florida, November 12, 1992, pp. 588–595.

18. Alice Dregger, *One of Us*: *Conjoined Twins and the Future of Normal,* Harvard University Press, Cambridge, MA, 2004, p. 93.

19. Ibid., pp. 125, 127.

20. Alice Dregger, "Jarring Bodies: Thoughts on the Display of Unusual Anatomies," *Perspectives in Biology and Medicine* 43, no. 2, (Winter 2000), pp. 161–172.

21. Ben Carson, *Gifted Hands: The Ben Carson Story*, Zondervan Press, Grand Rapids, MI, 1990.

22. Press Release, "Conjoined Twin Fact Sheet," Johns Hopkins Children's Center, www .hopkinschildrens.org/pages/news/twins_factsheet.html.

23. Press Release, "Hopkins Team Separates Conjoined Twins," Johns Hopkins International, September 16, 2004.

24. "Baby Fae Stuns the World," p. 70.

25. Tom Regan, "The Other Victim," *Hastings Center Report* 15, no. 1 (February 1985), pp. 9–10.

26. Thomasine Kushner and Raymond Belotti, "Baby Fae: A Beastly Business," *Journal of Medical Ethics* 11 (1985), pp. 178–183.

27. Denise Breo, "Interview with 'Baby Fae's' Surgeon," *American Medical News*, November 16, 1984, p. 18.

28. "Interview with Dr. Jack Provonsha," *U.S. News and World Report*, November 12, 1984, p. 59.

29. Dan Chu and Eleanor Hoover, "Helped by a Baboon Heart, An Imperiled Infant, 'Baby Fae,' Beat the Medical Odds," *People,* November 18, 1984.

30. Breo, "Interview with," p. 18.

31. Chu and Hoover, "Helped by a Baboon Heart," p. 74.

32. Ibid.

33. Thomas Starzl, *The Puzzle People: Memoirs of a Transplant Surgeon,* University of Pittsburgh Press, Pittsburgh, PA, 1992, p. 123.

34. Breo, "Interview with," p. 18.

35. David Wasserman, "Killing Mary to Save Jodie: Conjoined Twins and Individual Rights," *Philosophy and Public Affairs Quarterly* 21, no. 1 (Winter 2001), pp. 9–14.

36. Dregger, *One of Us*, p. 63.

37. T. P. Votteler and K. Lipsky, "Long-Term Results of 10 Conjoined Twin Separations," *Journal of Pediatric Surgery* 40, (April 2005), pp. 618–629.

38. Paul Ramsey, "The Enforcement of Morals: Nontherapeutic Research on Children," *Hastings Center Report* 6, (August 1976), pp. 21–30.

39. Richard McCormick, "Proxy Consent in the Experimentation Situation," *Perspectives in Biology and Medicine* 18, no. 1 (Autumn 1974), pp. 2–20.

40. Alexander Capron, "When Well-Meaning Science Goes Too Far," *Hastings Center Report* 15, no. 1 (February 1985), pp. 8–9.

41. George Annas, "The Anything Goes School of Human Experimentation," *Hastings Center Report* 15, no. 1 (February 1985), pp. 15–17.

42. Dregger, *One of Us*, p. 66, quoting Rowena Spencer, *Conjoined Twins: Developmental Malformations and Clinical Implications*, Johns Hopkins University Press, Baltimore, MD, 2003, pp. 310–311.

43. Dregger, *One of Us,* p. 67.

44. "Celebrity surgery" was a term coined in a *New Republic* editorial, December 17, 1984.

45. Keith Reemtsma, *Hastings Center Report*, February 1985, p. 10.

46. Alex Capron, *Hastings Center Report*, February 1985, p. 8.

47. Charles Krauthammer, "The Using of Baby Fae," *Time*, December 3, 1984, pp. 87–88.

48. Breo, "Interview with," p. 18.

49. Ibid., p. 13.

50. Starzl, *The Puzzle People*, p. 123.

51. "Baby Fae Stuns the World," p. 70.

52. Jacques Loman, *Journal of Heart Transplantation* 4, no. 1, (November 1984), pp. 10–11.

53. Annas, "The Anything Goes School."

54. *Nature* 88, no. 312 (November 8, 1984), p. 5990.

55. Krauthammer, "The Using of Baby Fae."

56. "Judicial Council Offers New Guidelines," *American Medical News* 27 (December 14, 1984), p. 46.

57. D. Shewmon, "Anencephaly: Selected Medical Aspects," *Hastings Center Report* 18, no. 5 (1988), pp. 11–9.

58. Laurie Abraham, "The Use of Anencephalic Infants as Organ Sources," *American Medical News* 261, no. 12 (March 24–31, 1989), pp. 1773–1781.

59. Debra H. Berger, *Issues in Law and Medicine* 67 (1989), pp. 84–85; quoted by Estella Moriarty in *In Re T. A. C. P.*, p. 595.

60. D. Medearis and L. Holmes, "On the Use of Anencephalic Infants as Organ Donors," *New England Journal of Medicine* 321, no. 6 (August 10, 1989), p. 392.

61. Beth Brandon, "Anencephalic Infants as Organ Donors: A Question of Life and Death," *Case Western Law Review* 40 (1989–199), p. 781; quoted by Estella Moriarty in *In Re T. A. C. P.*

62. *In Re T. A. C. P.*, p. 590.

63. A. Capron, "Anencephalic Donors: Separate the Dead from the Dying," *Hastings Center Report* 17, no. 1 (February 1987), pp. 5–8; John Arras, "Anencephalic Newborns as Organ Donors: A Critique," *Journal of the American Medical Association* 259, no. 15 (April 15, 1986), pp. 2284–2285.

64. S. L. Boulet,"Trends in the Postfortification Prevalence of Spina Bifida and Anencephaly in the United States," National Center for Birth Defects and Developmental Disabilities, CDC, Atlanta, July 7, 2008, pp. 527–532.

65. Shewmon, "Anencephaly: Selected Medical Aspects."

66. Dregger, *One of Us*, p. 65.

# Chapter 14

1. John Colapinto, *As Nature Made Him: The Boy Who Was Raised as a Girl*, Harper Collins, New York, 2000, p. 22.

2. Mel Grumbach, pediatric endocrinologist at the University of California, San Francisco, quoted in *As Nature Made Him*, p. 75.

3. Colapinto, *As Nature Made Him*, p. 180.

4. L. Sax, "How Common Is Intersex? A Response to Ann Fausto-Sterling," *Journal of Sex Research* 39, August, 2002 no. 3, pp.

5. Consortium on the Management of Disorders of Sex Development, *Clinical Guidelines of the Management of Disorders of Sex Development in Childhood*, Intersex Society of North America, 2006.

6. "What's the Difference between Being Transgender or Transsexual and Having an Intersex Condition?" Intersex Society of North America, http://www.isna.org/faq/transgender.

7. Maureen Dowd, "Between Torment and Happiness," *New York Times*, April 26, 2011, p. A23.

8. Associated Press, "Runner Reported to Have Internal Male Sex Organs," September 12, 2009, *Birmingham News*, Section D, p. 2.

9. "Ex GI Becomes Blond Beauty," *New York Daily News*, December 1, 1952, p. A1.

10. "Letter of Concern from Bioethicists"(see following): http://www.fetaldex.org/letter_bioethics.html.

---

Dear Sir or Madam:

We write to express our grave concern over possible non-IRB-approved clinical research on pregnant women that has been conducted under the auspices of Mount Sinai Medical Center and Weill Cornell Medical College, Cornell University, under the direction of Dr. Maria New.

This work involves off-label administration of dexamethasone to pregnant women who may give birth to girls with Congenital Adrenal Hyperplasia (CAH). It is our understanding that Dr. New has long prescribed dexamethasone for purposes of preventing genital virilization associated with CAH in 46,XX females. This indication is not approved by the FDA. Genital virilization is a cosmetic issue, one that has been recognized within Dr. New's field as independent of the genuine medical concerns—often serious and life-threatening in some forms of CAH—*unaddressed by prenatal dexamethasone treatment*. That is to say, prenatal treatment with dexamethasone is intended to avoid a cosmetic issue associated with CAH, rather than to treat the medical issues that should be the primary concern of physicians.[1] Furthermore, use of prenatal dexamethasone has been demonstrated to bear significant iatrogenic risk.[2]

Off-label use of prescription medication is a long-time practice of medicine that has not been understood to constitute research requiring IRB oversight. We do not take issue here with the practice of off-label prescribing in general. We are concerned instead with a particular instance of what appears to constitute a de facto clinical trial involving many hundreds of patients now among the targeted "subjects" of long-term research. In clear violation of established bioethical protocols, these pregnant women appear to have been recruited (and perhaps are still being recruited) without the benefit of IRB oversight.[3]

In professional contexts among her peers, Dr. New has publicly resisted discussion of the details of the information pregnant women and their partners are provided. One online promotion of the treatment with dexamethasone administered by Dr. New's clinic nevertheless promised that follow-up with hundreds of children treated prenatally over 20 years "has found no adverse developmental consequences. . . . the treatment appears to be safe for mother and child."[4]

Human studies have demonstrated, on the contrary, that prenatal dexamethasone treatment results in detrimental changes to the brains of children,[5] over 90% of whom will receive no benefit from this treatment. (Only 1 in 8 fetuses started on this treatment are actually 46,XX CAH, and of the 1/8 who are, 20% will not benefit from the treatment.) Children exposed prenatally to dexamethasone for CAH show problems with working memory, verbal processing, and anxiety.[6] Animal studies have also indicated reason to be very concerned about prenatal dexamethasone's effect on fetal brains.[7] Therefore, contrary to the apparent claims aimed at prospective patients, dexamethasone treatment cannot responsibly be characterized as benign.[8]

Despite knowledge of risks to fetal development, it does not appear that physicians prescribing this drug to hundreds of women have sought IRB approval for clinical trials of dexamethasone for the purposes of minimizing genital virilization in 46,XX females at risk for CAH *in utero*. Pregnant women who have been prescribed

dexamethasone external to IRB-approved trials may not have provided fully informed consent as would happen formally under an IRB-approved trial. Public descriptions of this drug as safe and effective may have misled some women to believe the use is FDA-approved, when it is not.

Given the well-established risks to fetal development, physicians should initiate treatment of this type only through structured clinical trials with human subjects research protections in place. Registered clinical trials ensure that women and their families make fully informed decisions with respect to the risks they assume for themselves and on behalf of their future children. Studies such as these also ensure that adverse effects will be noticed as soon as possible, and that any harm that comes to women and their children provide the benefit of increased scientific knowledge that can subsequently protect other women and babies from the same harms.

We call for rigorous investigation into possible regulatory violations in this matter. We also believe that women who have been treated without the protection of IRBs should now be advised of the information that may not have been made available to them at the time of treatment, and that they should be given the most recent information from studies indicating long-term risks to women and children. Finally, we agree with Dr. Walter Miller, Distinguished Professor of Pediatrics and Chief of Endocrinology at the University of California San Francisco, who has written that "this experimental treatment is not warranted and should not be pursued even in prospective clinical trials."[9]

Citations:

[1] Miller W. L. "Dexamethasone treatment of Congenital Adrenal Hyperplasia in utero: an experimental therapy of unproven safety." J Urol 1999; 162: 537–40.

[2] National Institutes of Health Consensus Development Panel, "Antenatal Corticosteroids Revisited: Repeat Courses. National Institutes of Health Consensus Development Conference Statement, August 17–18, 2000." ObstetGynecol 2001; 98:144–50.

[3] Kitzinger E. (Weill Medical School of Cornell University). "Prenatal Diagnosis

& Treatment for Classical CAH." CARES Foundation, Winter 2003.

[4] Ibid.

[5] French NP, Hagen R, Evans SF, Mullan A, Newnham JP. "Repeated antenatal corticosteroids: effects on cerebral palsy and childhood behavior."Am J ObstetGynecol 2004: 190:588–95.

[6] See, for example: [a]Hirvikoski T, Nordenstrom A, Lindholm T, et al. "Cognitive functions in children at risk for congenital adrenal hyperplasia treated prenatally with dexamethasone."J ClinEndocrinolMetab. 2007; 92:542–8; and [b]Trautman, PD, Meyer-Bahlburg HF, Postelnek J, New MI. "Effects of early prenatal dexamethasone on the cognitive and behavioral development of young children: results of a pilot study."Psychoneuroendocrinology 1995; 20: 439–449.

[7] Uno H., Eisele S., Sakai A., et al. "Neurotoxicity of glucocorticoids in the primate brain." HormBehav 1994; 28: 336–48.

[8] Lajic S, Nordenstrom A, Hirvikoski, "Long-term outcome of prenatal treatment of congenital adrenal hyperplasia." In Fluck, C. E. and Miller W.L. (eds): Disorders of the Human Adrenal Cortex. Endocr Dev. Basel: Karger, 2008, vol. 13: 82–98.

[9] Miller W. "Prenatal treatment of classic CAH with dexamethasone: pro vs. con." Endocrine News Tri-Point Series 2008: 16–18. [Part 1 and Part 2.]

List of signers at: http://www.fetaldex.org/letter_bioethics.html

———

11. L. B. McCullough, F. A. Chervenak, R. L. Brent, and B. Hippen, "A Case Study in Unethical Transgressive Bioethics: 'Letter of Concern from Bioethicists' about the Prenatal Administration of Dexamethasone," American Journal of Bioethics 10 September 2010, no. 9, pp. 35–45.

12. http://fetaldex.org/AJOB_Sept_2012.html.

13. Sheri Groveman and Cheryl Chase, quoted in Benatar, ed., Cutting to the Core.

14. Lindsay Beyerstein, "Federal Regulators Vindicate Dr. Maria New," BigThink, September 28, 2010, http://bigthink.com/focal-point/federal-regulators-vindicate-dr-maria-new.

15. This sentence is indebted to Margaret Talbots, "About a Boy," New Yorker, March 18, 2013, p. 59.

16. Louis Gooren, "Care of Transsexual Persons," New England Journal of Medicine 364, no. 13 (March 3, 2011), p. 1256; See also, Letter, "Care of Transsexual Persons," Walter Booking, 346 (June 30, 2011), p. 26.

17. Dowd, "Between Torment and Happiness."

18. Cheryl Chase, 1998, interviewed by Robin Whites (November 28, 1997). Intersexuals (interview with Chase). All Things Considered, NPR. See also Elizabeth Weil, What if It's (Sort of) a Boy and (Sort of) a Girl?" New York Times Magazine, September 2006.

19. Alice Dregger, One of Us: Conjoined Twins and the Future of the Normal, Harvard University Press, Cambridge, MA, 2005.

20. American Academy of Pediatrics (2000).

21. "I'm Finally Myself," People, May 23, 2011, pp. 65–67.

22. Nancy Jeffrey, "Becoming Nikki," People, July 8, 2013, pp. 48–52.

23. Ellen Wittlinger, Parrotfish, Simon & Schuster, New York, 2011; Julie Ann Peters, Luna, Little Brown, Boston, 2006; Chris Beam, I am J, Little Brown, Boston, 2011.

24. Talbot, "About a Boy," pp. 56–65.

25. Ibid., pp. 61ff.

26. Milton Diamond discovery, cited in Coliptano, As Nature Made Him.

27. In particular, Colapinto mentions two male twins with botched circumcisions born in Atlanta in 1985 and cases cited by Toronto child psychiatrist Kenneth Zucker, in As Nature Made Him, pp. 249, 274.

28. Ken Kipnis and Milton Diamond, "Pediatric Ethics and the Surgical Assignment of Sex," Journal of Clinical Ethics, 9, no. 3 (1998).

29. Gooren, "Care of Transsexual Persons," p. 1256.

30. Linda Geddes, "Puberty Blockers Recommended for Transsexual Teens," New Scientist, December 10, 2008.

31. Peter Lee, et. al, "Consensus Statement on Management of Intersex Disorders," Pediatrics, 188, no. 2 (August 2006), pp. e488–e500.

# Chapter 15

1. New York Times, November 6, 1987, p. B1.

2. Ibid.

3. New York Times, November 13, 1987, p. B21.

4. Ibid.

5. Ibid., p. A1.

6. Ibid.

7. "Brown versus Koch," *60 Minutes*, interview with Ed Bradley, 1988.

8. "Court Backs Treatment of Woman Held under Koch Plan," *New York Times*, December 19, 1987, p. A1.

9. "Brown versus Koch," *60 Minutes*.

10. "Brown versus Koch," *60 Minutes*.

11. *New York Times*, January 20, 1988, p. A16.

12. "Participants Laud Drug Treatment Program," *New York Daily News*, May 2, 2000.

13. Julian Jaynes, *The Origin of Consciousness and the Breakdown of the Bicameral Mind*, Houghton Mifflin, Boston, 1976.

14. Thomas Szasz, "Involuntary Mental Hospitalization: A Crime against Humanity," in *Ideology and Insanity*, Doubleday, New York, 1970.

15. D. L. Rosenhan, "On Being Sane in Insane Places," *Science* 179 (1973), pp. 250–258.

16. *O'Connor v. Donaldson*, 422 U.S. 563. 95 S. Ct. 2486, June 26, 1975.

17. John Petrilia, "Mental Health Therapies," *BioLaw*, University Publications of America, Frederick, MD, 1986, pp. 177–215.

18. Quoted in Charles Krauthammer, "How to Save the Homeless Mentally Ill," *New Republic*, February 8, 1988, p. 24.

19. Saul Feldman, "Out of the Hospitals, into the Streets: The Overselling of Benevolence," *Hastings Center Report* 13, no. 3 (June 1983), pp. 5–7.

20. C. Dugger, "Judge Orders Homeless Man Hospitalized," *New York Times*, December 23, 1992, p. B1.

21. See "Kendra's Law" in Wikipedia, http://en.wikipedia.org/wiki/Kendra's_Law.

22. Treatment Advocacy Center, "State Standards for Assisted Treatment: State by State Chart," *New York Times*, December 12, 2004; www.psychlaws.org.

23. E. Rosenthal, "Who Will Turn Violent? Hospitals Have to Guess," *New York Times*, April 7, 1993, p. A1.

24. *Tarasoff v. Regents of University of California*, 17 Cal. 3d 425, 551 P.2d 334, 131 *California Reporter* 14 (Cal. 1976).

25. Virginia Abernethy, "Compassion, Control, and Decisions about Competence," *American Journal of Psychiatry* 141, no. 1 (1984), pp. 53–58.

26. Ibid.

27. *New York Times*, November 13, 1987, p. A1.

28. Robert Levy and Robert Gould, "Psychiatrists as Puppets of Koch's Round-Up," *New York Times*, November 27, 987.

29. Paul Chodoff, "The Case for Involuntary Hospitalization of the Mentally Ill," *American Journal of Psychiatry* 133, no. 5 (May 1976).

30. Ellen Goodman, "Before They Die with Their Rights On," *Washington Post*, November 21, 1987.

31. J. Livermore, C. Malmquist, and P. Meehl, "On the Justification of Civil Commitment," *University of Pennsylvania Law Review* 117 (November 1968), pp. 75–96.

32. Alice Baum and Donald Burnes, *A Nation in Denial: The Truth about Homelessness*, Westview, Boulder, CO, 1993.

33. Clifford J. Ivy, "The State Is Failing the Mentally Ill in Adult Homes, Pataki Administration Study Says," *New York Times*, September 15, 2002, p. 21.

34. David Kopel, "Guns, Mental Illness, and Newtown," *Wall Street Journal*, December 18, 2012, p. A17.

35. Livermore, Malmquist, and Meehl, "On the Justification of Civil Commitment," p. 75.

## Chapter 16

1. Angelina Jolie, "My Medical Choice," *New York Times*, May 14, 2013.

2. Michele Tauber et al., "Angelina Jolie: I Made a Strong Choice," *People*, May 27, 2013, pp. 67–73.

3. Benjamin A. Pierce, *Genetics: A Conceptual Approach*, 2nd ed., W. H. Freeman, New York, 2006, p. 123.

4. Natalie Angier, "Team Reports Genetic Cause of Huntington's," *New York Times*, March 24, 1993, p. A1.

5. Rita Rubin, "Ray of Hope for Huntington's," *USA Today*, p. A1–2.

6. Daniel Kevles, *In the Name of Eugenics: Genetics and the Uses of Human Heredity*, Knopf, New York, 1985, pp. 3–19.

7. Ibid., pp. 93–94.

8. Robert Lacey, *Ford: The Man and the Machine*, Little, Brown, New York, 1987.

9. Kevles, *In the Name of Eugenics*, p. 97.

10. Kim Severson, "Payment Set for Those Sterilized in Program," *New York Times*, January 11, 2012, p. A13.

11. Kevles, *In the Name of Eugenics,* p. 97.

12. Here is a start about the mistakes of the Eugenics Movement: (1) *The reductionist assumption that each trait identified by social distinctions.* Prostitution, retardation, poverty, and criminality were each supposedly caused by a single gene. (2) *The reductionist assumption* that each gene causes a disease in a simplistic, one-gene-to-one way. A few genetic diseases do work this way, but most do not. (3) *Ignorance about recessive inheritance.* Two unaffected carriers can each pass a gene for a recessive trait to a child, who will then be homozygous for the trait. (4) *Ignorance of environmental effects on expression of genes.* How a gene, or a combination of genes, is expressed depends partly on what happens during gestation, in early childhood, and in the environment. Genes have a fan-like range of expression (their norm of reaction). (5) *Naiveté about the ease of controlling reproduction* in couples. Humans are driven to have sex, and if they aren't careful, children result. When informed of risk of a child with genetic disease, few humans can or will prevent birth of children, especially without access to contraception. (6) *Ignorance of mutations and chromosomal breakage.* Not knowing about these aspects of genetics, eugenicists mistakenly believed that if all mentally challenged people could be prevented from reproducing, their conditions could be eliminated from the gene pool. (7) *Ignorance of population genetics.* Eugenicists hoped to perfect humanity through selective breeding, but population genetics have since shown that there will be a regression to the mean. (8) *Regression to the mean* is the inherent tendency in stable populations to return to an average value over time; in population genetics, the underlying causes creating a mean value will eventually normalize any deviant values.

13. Herman Muller, *Out of the Night: A Biologist's View of the Future,* Vanguard, New York, 1935, quoted in Kevles, *In the Name of Eugenics,* p. 164.

14. Ronald W. Clark, *The Life and Work of J. B. S. Haldane,* Coward-McCann, New York, 1968, p. 70, quoted in Kevles, *In the Name of Eugenics,* p. 127.

15. B. S. Haldane, "Toward a Perfected Posterity," *The World Today* 45 (December 1924), quoted in Kevles, *In the Name of Eugenics,* p. 127.

16. "Maria Lopez" is a composite, based on a 4-part series in the *New York Times* on the emerging epidemic in diabetes, January 9–12, 2006.

17. N. R. Kleinfield, "Diabetes and Its Awful Toll Quietly Emerge as a Crisis," *New York Times,* January 9, 2006, p. A1.

18. World Health Organization, Department of Noncommunicable Disease Surveillance, *Definition, Diagnosis and Classification of Diabetes Mellitus and its Complications.* World Health Organization, Geneva, 1999.

19. Marc Santora, "East Meets West, Adding Pounds and Peril," *New York Times,* January 12, 2006, p. A1.

20. Kleinfield, "Diabetes and Its Awful Toll."

21. N. R. Kleinfield, "Living at the Epicenter of Diabetes, Defiance and Despair," *New York Times,* January 10, 2006, p. A1.

22. "Diabetes Gene Detected," *Sydney Morning Herald,* January 19, 2006.

23. Gina Kolata, "Two Tests Could Aid in Risk Assessment and Early Diagnosis of Alzheimer's, *New York Times,* January 19, 2011.

24. Katherine Greider, "Diagnosing Alzheimer's," *AARP Bulletin,* October 2011, p. 10.

25. D. Blacker, "ApoE-4 and Age at Onset of Alzheimer's Disease: The NIMH Genetics Initiative," *Neurology* 48, no. 1 (January 1997), pp. 139–147.

26. R. Caselli, et al., "Longitudinal Modeling of Age-Related Memory Decline and the APOE-4 Effect," *New England Journal of Medicine,* July 16, 2009, p. 256.

27. Alzheimer's Association, "Genetic Testing," http://www.alz.org/documents_custom/statements/genetic_testing.pdf.

28. Pam Belluck, "New Guidelines Offered to Diagnose Alzheimer's," *New York Times,* April 19, 2011, p. A13.

29. http://www.alz.org/alzheimers_disease_stages_of_alzheimers.asp.

30. Denise Grady, "Study Shows Few Women Rue Preventive Breast Operation," *New York Times,* April 17, 1999, p. A14.

31. Timothy Rebbeck et al., "Bilateral Prophylactic Mastectomy Reduces Breast Cancer Risk in *BRCA1* and *BRCA2* Mutation Carriers: The PROSE Study Group," *Journal of Clinical Oncology* 22 no. 6 (March 15, 2004)

32. Paul Recer, "Studies May Have Exaggerated Breast Cancer Risk," *Birmingham News,* August 21, 200, p. 5A.

33. Justin Lowenthal et al., "The Ethics of Early Evidence—Preparing for a Possible Breakthrough in Alzheimer's Disease," *New England Journal of Medicine* 367 (August 9, 2012), pp. 488–490.

34. Denise Grady, "The Ticking of a Time Bomb in the Genes," *Discover*, June 1987, p. 34.

35. G. Meissen et al., "Predictive Testing for Huntington's Disease with Use of a Linked DNA Marker," *New England Journal of Medicine* 318, no. 9 (March 3, 1988), pp. 538ff.

36. Ibid.

37. Danish Council of Ethics, *Ethics and Mapping of the Human Genome*, 1993.

38. John Hardwig, "A Duty to Die?" *Hastings Center Report* 27, no. 2 (March–April 1997), pp. 34–42.

39. Catherine Hayes, "Genetic Testing for Huntington's *New England Journal of Medicine*, Vol. 327, 1992, pp. 1449–51. Disease," Natalie Angier, "Vexing Pursuit of Breast Cancer Gene," *New York Times*, July 12, 1994.

40. C. Muir, *Cancer Incidence in Five Continents*, International Agency for Research on Cancer, Lyon, 1987, Table 12–2.

41. "Diabetes and Its Awful Toll."

42. L. R. Vartanian et al., "Effects of Soft Drink Consumption on Nutrition and Health: A Systematic Review and Meta-analysis," *American Journal of Public Health* 97, no. 4 (2007).

43. "Cancer Genetics," in Pierce, *Genetics*, pp. 627–637.

44. C. Bloss et al., "Effect of Direct-to-Consumer Genomewide Profiling to Assess Disease Risk," *New England Journal of Medicine*, February 10, 2011, pp. 524–533.

45. Ronald Bailey, "Bioethicists Can't Handle the Truth," *Reason*, February 1, 2011. See also Gregory Pence, "Should We Test for Disease That Can't Be Cured?" *Birmingham News*, January 9, 2011, http://blog.al.com/birmingham-news-commentary/2011/01/viewpoints_should_we_test_for.html.

46. D. Craufurd and R. Harris, "Ethics of Predictive Testing for Huntington's Disease: The Need for More Information," *British Medical Journal* 293 (July 26, 1986), pp. 249–251.

47. M. Waldoz, "Probing the Cell: The Diagnostic Power of Genetics Is Posing Hard Medical Choices," *Wall Street Journal*, April 1986, p. A1.

48. Grady, "The Ticking of a Time Bomb."

49. Arthur Beaudet of Baylor College of Medicine, quoted in Waldoz, "Probing the Cell."

50. President's Commission for the Study of Ethical Problems in Medicine and Biomedical and Behavioral Research, *Screening and Counseling for Genetic Conditions: The Ethical, Social, and Legal Implications for Genetic Screening, Counseling, and Educational Problems*, U.S. Government Printing Office, Washington, D.C.,1983.

51. C. Norton, "Absolutely Not Confidential," *Hippocrates*, March–April 1989, pp. 53–59; see also *Medical Records: Getting Yours*, Public Citizen, Washington DC., 1986.

52. Genetic Information Nondiscrimination Act (GINA) of 2008: Information for Researchers and Health Care Professionals, http://www.genome.gov/24519851.

53. Ian Urbina, "In the Treatment of Diabetes, Success Often Does Not Pay," *New York Times*, January 11, 2006, p. A1.

54. Ibid."

55. Nicholas Wade, "Gene Identified as Risk Factor for Heart Ills," *New York Times*, May 4, 2007, p. A1.

56. Sharon Begley, "Reading the Book of Jim," *Newsweek*, June 4, 2007, p. 50.

57. Natalie Angier, "Gene for Mental Illness Proves Elusive," *New York Times*, January 13, 1993, p. B3.

58. Miron Baron, quoted in Angier, "Gene for Mental Illness Proves Elusive."

59. James P. Evans et al., "Preparing for a Consumer-Driven Genomic Age," *New England Journal of Medicine* 363, no. 12 (September 16, 2010), p. 1101.

60. Adam Liptak, "Justices, 9-0, Bar Patenting Human Genes," *New York Times*, June 13, 2013, P. A1.

61. https://www.23andme.com/?utm_source=google&utm_medium=cpc&utm_campaign=Search-Beta-Genetic&utm_term=mid237&gclid=CI_mouHXkbgCFed-Z7AodqD4AqA.

62. Begley, "Reading the Book of Jim."

63. "New Research Shows Secondhand Smoke Raises Diabetes Risk," *British Medical Journal*, April 17, 2006.

64. Judith Fradkin et al., "What's Preventing Us from Preventing Type 2 Diabetes?" *New England Journal of Medicine* 367, no. 13 (September 27, 2012), p. 1177.

65. Melinda Beck, "In Search of Alcoholism Genes," *Health Journal*, February 8, 2011.

66. Begley, "Reading the Book of Jim," p. 48.

## Chapter 17

1. AMFAR, "Statistics Worldwide," http://www.amfar.org/about-hiv-and-aids/facts-and-stats/statistics--world wide/.

2. Barbara Tuchman, *A Distant Mirror,* Knopf, New York, 1978, p. 119.

3. B, Hahn, G. Shaw, and F. Gao, "Origin of HIV–1 in the Chimpanzee *pan troglodytes troglodytes,*" *Nature* 397 (February 4, 1999), pp. 436–441. The authors also offered proof that the three major phylogenetic groups of HIV-1 (M, N, and O) arose from three independent transmissions to man of simian immunodeficiency virus, SIVcpz, which they hypothesized had existed in chimps for hundreds of thousands of years.

4. Centers for Disease Control, "Overview of HIV/AIDS" and "Human Immunodeficiency Virus Type 2," www.cdc.gov/hiv/hivinfo.

5. Donald McNeil, "Study Dates HIV Ancestor to at Least 32,000 Years Ago," *New York Times,* September 17, 2010, p. A4.

6. Ibid.

7. Phil Tiemeyer, *Plane Queer: Labor, Sexuality, and AIDS in the History of Male Flight Attendants,* University of California Press, Berkeley, CA, 2013.

8. Greg Dixon, "Stop Homosexuals before They Infect Us All," *USA Today,* January 16, 1983.

9. "Television evangelists Jerry Falwell and Pat Robertson, two of the most prominent voices of the religious right, said liberal civil liberties groups, feminists, homosexuals and abortion rights supporters bear partial responsibility for Tuesday's terrorist attacks because their actions have turned God's anger against America." From John F. Harris, "God Gave U.S. 'What We Deserve,' Falwell Says," *Washington Post,* September 14, 2001, p. C3.

10. Charles Stanley, quoted in Scripps-Howard News Service, *Birmingham Post-Herald,* January 21, 1986.

11. Interviewed on *Cross Fire,* CNN, November 16, 1987.

12. Quoted in Randy Shilts, *And the Band Played On,* St. Martin's, New York, 1987, p. 311.

13. Jonathan Lieberson, "The Reality of AIDS," *New York Review of Books,* January 16, 1986.

14. This periodical never apologized for these inaccurate pieces or to giving so much editorial power to an ideological graduate student.

15. Margaret Heckler, quoted in Shilts, *And the Band Played On,* p. 345.

16. Joseph Bove, quoted in Shilts, *And the Band Played On,* p. 345.

17. Ibid.

18. Jane Gross, "AIDS Patients Face Downside of Living Longer," *New York Times,* January 6, 2008.

19. John Boswell, *Christianity, Social Tolerance, and Homosexuality; Gay People in Western Europe from the Beginning of the Christian Era to the Fourteenth Century,* University of Chicago Press, Chicago, 1980.

20. 539 U.S. 558 (2003), http://www.law.cornell.edu/supct/html/02-102.ZS.html.

21. Larry Kramer, "Who Says AIDS Is Hard to Get?" *Newsweek,* 1992.

22. Nick Wadhams, "World Falls Short on AIDS Goals, U.N. Warns," *Birmingham News,* June 2, 2006, p. 4A.

23. Robert Steinbrook, "The AIDS Epidemic: A Progress Report from Mexico City," *New England Journal of Medicine* 359, no. 9 (August 28, 2008), pp. 886–887.

24. Figures on AIDS in Africa and worldwide are notoriously vague and political. See Alan Whiteside, "AIDS in Africa: Facts, Figures and the Extent of the Problem," pp. 1–15; Anton A. Van Niekerk and Loretta M. Kopelman, *Ethics and AIDS in Africa,* Left Coast Press, Walnut Creek, CA, 2006. According to the World Health Organization, 33 million people live with HIV as of July 4, 2009; http://www.who.int/hiv/en/.

25. "A Global Menace," *Newsweek,* May 15, 2006, p. 52.

26. Alexander Irwin, Joyce Millen, and Dorothy Fallows, *Global AIDS: Myths and Facts,* South End Press, Cambridge, MA, 2003, p. 52.

27. Ibid., p. 55.

28. Donald McNeil, "A Regime's Tight Grip on AIDS," *New York Times,* May 8, 2012, pp. D1–4.

29. Marc Lallemant, "Preventing Mother-to-Child Transmission of HIV—Protecting this Generation and the Next," *New England Journal of Medicine* 363, no. 16 (October 14, 2010), p. 1570.

30. Kent Sepkowitz, "One Disease, Two Epidemics—AIDS at 25," *New England Journal of Medicine* 354, no. 23 (June 8, 2006), pp. 2413–2414.

31. The case is taken from Irwin, Millen, and Fallows, *Global AIDS*, pp. 21–22.

32. Ibid.

33. Michael Merson, "The HIV-AIDS Pandemic at 25—The Global Response," *New England Journal of Medicine* 354, no. 23 (June 8, 2006), p. 2414.

34. J. Decosas et al., "Migration and AIDS," *Lancet* 346, no. 8978 (1995), pp. 826–228; quoted in Irwin, Millen, and Fallows, *Global AIDS*.

35. Jeffrey Fisher, quoted in L. A. McKeown, "Preventing AIDS in the Next Generation," *WebMD Medical News*, December 1, 1999.

36. Quoted in Irwin, Millen, and Fallows, *Global AIDS*, pp. 21–22.

37. Philippe Bourgois, "In Search of Horatio Alger: Culture and Ideology in the Crack Economy," in *Crack in America: Demon Drugs and Social Justice*, eds. B. Rienarman and H. Levine, University of California Press, Berkeley, CA, 1997.

38. Sepkowitz, "One Disease, Two Epidemics," p. 2413.

39. William Easterly, *White Man's Burden: Why the West's Efforts to Aid the Rest Have Done So Much Ill and So Little Good*, Penguin, New York, 2006.

40. Paul Theroux, *Dark Star Safari*, Houghton Mifflin Harcourt, New York, 2003; Paul Theroux, *Last Train to Zona Verde*, Houghton Mifflin Harcourt, New York, 2013.

41. S. K. Ghosh , M. E. Taylor , V. A. Johnson, E. Emini, P. Deutsch, J. D. Lifson, . . . G. M. Shaw, "Viral Dynamics in Human Immunodeficiency Virus Type 1 Infection," *Nature* 373 (1995), pp. 117–122.

42. Donald McNeil, "New HIV Cases Remain Steady Over a Decade," *New York Times*, August 4, 2011, p. A16.

43. Sheryl Gay Stolberg, "College Campuses Are Producing a New Style of AIDS Activist," *New York Times*, December 1, 2000, p. A14.

44. Donald McNeil, "Two Studies Show Pills Can Prevent HIV Infection," *New York Times*, July 14, 2011, p. A15.

45. "Waltzing with Death," *The Economist*, July 24, 2010, p. 77.

46. Donald McNeil, "Early Therapy for HIV Said to Cut Spread," *New York Times*, May 13, 2011, pp. A1–3.

47. Editorial Board, "A Cure, in Essence, for H.I.V. in Some Adults," *New York Times*, March 18, 2013.

48. Andrew Pollack, "New Hope for a Cure of H.I.V.," *New York Times*, November 29, 2011, pp. D1–2; David Brown, "Baby Born with HIV Is Apparently Cured with Aggressive Drug Treatment, " *Washington Post*, March 3, 2013, p. A1.

49. Donald McNeil, "Far from Any Lab, Paper Bits Find Illness," *New York Times*, September 27, 2011, p. D1.

50. Celia Dugger, "Sharing Burden of Living with AIDS," *New York Times*, September 27, 2011, p. D1.

51. Nicholas Bakalar, "Drugs to Curb a Deadly Inheritance," *New York Times*, September 27, 2011, p. D6.

# Chapter 18

1. Lisa Belkin, "Twice a Victim: Of Both Cancer and Care System," *New York Times*, March 26, 1993, p. B12.

2. Personal communication from Lisa Belkin to author, June 17, 2006.

3. This case stemmed from a 1993 story by Lisa Belkin. In 2006, an e-mail to her revealed that one of her children said that Rosalyn had died "several years before."

4. "International Profiles of Health Care Systems: 2012," *OECD Health Data*, June 2012.

5. Allan Guttmacher Institute, quoted in Associated Press, December 15, 1987.

6. Clifford Krauss, "In Blow to Canada's Health System, Quebec Law Is Voided," *New York Times*, June 10, 2005, A3.

7. Ibid.

8. Ibid.

9. Personal communication to author, from former UAB alumnus who practices as a physician in Canada.

10. Geoffrey Rivett, *From Cradle to Grave: 50 Years of the NHS*, Kings Fund, 1998, p. 437. ISBN 1-85717-148-9.

11. Graeme Wearden, October 12, 2004, "NHS IT Project Costs Soar," *ZDNet*,

12. Ian Morrison, "The Primary Care Problem," Hospitals and Health Network, September 6, 2011, http://www.hhnmag.com/hhnmag/HHNDaily/HHNDailyDisplay.dhtml? id=2800001976.

13. Paul Starr, *The Social Transformation of American Medicine*, Basic Books, New York, 1982, p. 381.

14. This has been repeatedly claimed by members of Physicians for a National Health Program; see, e.g., John V. Walsh, *Providence Journal* (Scripps-Howard), column, July 14, 1993. See also Paul Krugman, May 1, 2006, *New York Times*. "Death By Insurance."

15. Medicare Enrollment Reports," http://www.cms.hhs.gov/MedicareEnrpts/, 2013.

16. http://www.kaiserhealthnews.org/Daily-Reports/2013/June/04/end-of-life-care.aspx.

17. Robert Pear, "Bailout Provides More Mental Health Coverage," *New York Times*, October 6, 2008, p. A1.

18. "VA Budget Fast Facts," http://www.va.gov/budget/docs/summary/Fy2014_Fast_Facts_VAs_Budget_Highlights.pdf.

19. Paul Krugman, "Health Care Confidential," *New York Times*, January 26, 2006, p. A23.

20. The act allows both workers and their immediate family members who had been covered by a health care plan to maintain their coverage if a "qualifying event" causes them to lose coverage. Among the qualifying events listed in the statute are loss of benefits coverage due to (1) the death of the covered employee; (2) a reduction in hours (which can be the result of resignation, discharge, layoff, strike or lockout, medical leave, or simply a slowdown in business operations) that causes the worker to lose eligibility for coverage; (3) divorce, which normally terminates the ex-spouse's eligibility for benefits; or (4) a dependent child reaching the age at which he or she is no longer covered. COBRA imposes different notice requirements on participants and beneficiaries, depending on the particular qualifying event that triggers COBRA rights. COBRA also allows for longer periods of extended coverage in some cases, such as disability or divorce, than others, such as termination of employment or a reduction in hours. COBRA does not apply, on the other hand, if employees lose their benefits coverage because the employer has terminated the plan altogether. Consolidated Omnibus Budget Reconciliation Act of 1985, Wikipedia, http://en.wikipedia.org/wiki/Consolidated_Omnibus_Budget_Reconciliation_Act_of_1985.

21. Robert Steinbrook, "Health Care Reform in Massachusetts—A Work in Progress," *New England Journal of Medicine* 543, no. 20 (May 18, 2006), p. 2095.

22. Jack K. Shelton and Julia Mann Janosi, "Unhealthy Health Care Costs," *Journal of Medicine and Philosophy* 17, no. 1 (February 1992), p. 8.

23. Robert Pear, "Health Care Premiums Soar as Coverage Shrinks," *New York Times*, March 5, 2011, p. A13.

24. Consumers Union, "The Crisis in Health Insurance," *Consumer Reports*, August 1990, p. 543.

25. "Key Facts about the Uninsured Population," Henry Kaiser Foundation, September 26, 2013, http://kff.org/uninsured/fact-sheet/key-facts-about-the-uninsured-population/.

26. Consumers Union, "Wasted Health Care Dollars," *Consumer Reports*, July 1992, p. 436.

27. Courtney S. Campbell, "Gridlock on the Oregon Trail," *Hastings Center Report* 23, no. 4, (July–August 1993), p. 6.

28. Matthew J. Carson, "Results of Oregon Health Plan Study Released," The Commonwealth Fund, July 29, 2005, http://www.cmwf.org/newsroom/newsroom_show.htm?doc_id=288798, July 10, 2006.

29. Oregon Health Authority, "2011–2013 Budget Reductions."

30. Steve LeBlanc, "Mass. Health Care Plan Riles Some Liberals," Associated Press, April 7, 2006.

31. Patricia Barry, "Coverage," *AARP Bulletin*, July–August, 2006, pp. 8–10.

32. Stuart Altman and Michael Doonan, "Can Massachusetts Lead the Way in Health Care Reform?" *New England Journal of Medicine*, 354, no. 20, (May 18, 2006), p. 2094.

33. Ibid.

34. Alan Raymond, "Massachusetts Health Care Reform: A 5-Year Progress Report," Blue Cross-Blue Shield Foundation of Massachusetts, p. 4, https://www.mahealthconnector.org/portal/binary/com.epicentric.contentmanagement.servlet.ContentDeliveryServlet/Health%2520Care%2520Reform/Overview/BlueCrossFoundation5YearRpt.pdf.

35. Kevin Sack, "In Massachusetts, Universal Coverage Strains Care," *New York Times*, April 5, 2008, p. A1.

36. Raymond, "Massachusetts Health Care Reform."

37. Olga Pierce, "Analysis: Can Mass. Plan Stay Solvent?" United Press International Story, July 6, 2006.

38. John McDonough, "The Road Ahead for the Affordable Care Act," *New England Journal of Medicine*, 367, no. 3 (July 19, 2012), p. 200.

39. Cal Thomas, "NHS Lessons for The ACA," *Tuscaloosa News*, July 12, 2013, Tribune News Service, p. A6.

40. Julia Preston, "Texas Hospitals' Separate Paths Reflect the Debate on Immigration," *New York Times*, July 18, 2006, p. A18.

41. Ibid.

42. Garrett Hardin, "The Tragedy of the Commons," *Science* 162, (1968), pp. 1243–1248.

43. Shikha Dalmia, "Who's Milking Who? *"Reason*, August/September 2006, p. 44.

44. Eduardo Porter, "Here Illegally, Working Hard and Paying Taxes," *New York Times*, June 19, 2006, pp. A1–14.

45. Sabrina Tavernise, "For Medicare, Immigrants Offer Surplus, Study Finds," *New York Times*, May 29, 2013, p. A1.

46. Jeffrey Passel, "Pew Research Center: Immigration to Play Lead Role in Future U.S. Growth," February 11, 2008, pewresearch .org.

47. Consumers Union, "Medicare for All Americans," *Consumer Reports*, September 1992, p. 592.

48. Ibid.

49. Kelli Kennedy, "Health Insurers Fear Young People Will Opt Out," Associated Press, *Tuscaloosa News*, July 6, 2013, p. 3A.

50. David Blumenthal et al., "The Future of Health Care," *New England Journal of Medicine* 314, no. 11 (March 13, 1986), p. 723.

51. Paul Starr, *The Social Transformation of American Medicine*, Basic Books, New York, 1982.

52. Raymond, "Massachusetts Health Care Reform," p. 29.

53. LTC coverage increasingly looks like a bad deal for everyone: consumers face rising premiums and not enough young people are buying (or keeping) LTC policies.

54. Amy Goldstein, "Forecast Dire for Medicare Fiscal Health," *Washington Post*, May 2, 2006, reprinted in *Birmingham News*, "Medicare Remains on Fast Track to Bankruptcy," p. 3A, http://www.rpc.senate.gov/policy-papers/medicare-remains-on-fast-track-to-bankruptcy.

55. Robert Pear, "In Medicare Debate, Massaging the Facts," *New York Times*, May 23, 2006, A19.

56. Richard Epstein, remarks made at UAB, Conference on the Ethics of Managed Care, April 12, 1997. See also his *Mortal Peril*, Addison-Wesley Reading, MA, 1997, especially chapters. 7 and 8.

57. Heritage Foundation, "How Much Will The ACA Cost Your State?" http://www .askheritage.org/how-much-will-the ACA-cost-your-state/.

58. Carl Elliott, *White Coat, Dark Hat*, Beacon, New York, 2010.

59. Kevin Robillard, "A Health Care Showdown in Massachusetts," *Newsweek*, July 26, 2010, p. 8.

60. David Orentlicher, "Rationing and the Americans with Disabilities Act," *Journal of the American Medical Association* 271, no. 4 (January 26, 1994), pp. 308–314.

61. Ibid.

62. Richard Lamm, "St. Martin of Tours in a New World of Medical Ethics," *Cambridge Quarterly of HealthCare Ethics* 3 (1994), pp. 159–167. Reprinted in *Classic Works in Medical Ethics*, ed. Gregory Pence, McGraw-Hill, New York, 1998.

# Chapter 19

1. Jamey Keaten, "Tour Rocked Again by Doping," Associated Press, *Birmingham News*, July 18, 2008, p. 8D.

2. "ADD: Help is On the Way," St Louis Psychologists and Counseling Information and Referral, http://www.psychtreatment. com/adhd.htm.

3. Lawrence Diller, *Running on Ritalin: A Physician Reflects on Children, Society and Performance in a Pill*, Random House, New York, 1998.

4. Center for Drug Evaluation and Research, Food and Drug Administration, "One Year Post-Pediatric Exclusivity Post-Marketing Adverse Event Review Drug Utilization Analysis," June 20, 2007, http://www.fda .gov/ohrms/dockets/ac/07/briefing /2007-4325b_04_06_Modafinil%20Use%20 Review.pdf.

5. Associated Press, "Cops Eye 'Roid Rage in Wrestler's Murder-Suicide," June 27, 2007.

6. http://espn.go.com/classic/biography/s/ Alzado_Lyle.html.

7. Julian Savulescu, J. Foddy, and M. Clayton, "Why We Should Allow Performance-Enhancing Drugs in Sport," *British Journal of Sports Medicine*, 38 (2004), pp. 666–670.

8. Carl Elliott, *Better than Well: American Medicine Meets the American Dream*, Norton, New York, 2004.

9. Eric Wilson, *Against Happiness: In Praise of Melancholy*, Farrar, Straus and Giroux, New York, 2008.

10. Ibid., p. 6.

11. Robert J. Fenstershelb, "Breast Implant Lawsuits," http://www.breastimplantlawsuits.com/.

12. *Safety of Silicone Breast Implants*, Institute of Medicine, 1999.

13. Harris Interactive, "Patients Agree They Should Have Done More Homework Before Surgery, ASPS Survey Reveals," March 5, 2007.

14. W. Peters, "An Outcome Analysis of 100 Women after Explanation of Silicone Breast Implants," *Annals of Plastic Surgery* 39, no. 1 (July 1997), pp. 9–19.

15. J. K. McLaughlin, "The Safety of Silicone-Gel Breast Implants: A Review of the Epidemiological Evidence," *Annals of Plastic Surgery* 59, no. 5 (November 2007), pp. (5): 569–80.

16. C. M. McCarthy, et al., "Predicting Complications Following Expander/Implant Breast Reconstruction: An Outcome's Analysis Based on Preoperative Clinical Trials," *Plastic Reconstructive Surgery* 121, no. 6 (June 2008), pp. 1886–1892.

17. J. B. Tebbets, "Achieving a Zero Percent Reoperation Rate at 3 Years in a 50-Consecutive-Case Augmentation Mammoplasty Premarket Approval Study," *Plastic Reconstructive Surgery* 118, no. 6 (November 2006), pp. 1453–1457.

18. Amy Brittan and Mark Mueller, "New Jersey Doctor Supplied Steroids to Hundreds of Law Enforcement Officers, Firefighters," *New Jersey Star-Ledger*, March 9, 2010.

19. Arne Lundquist, statement at a UNESCO Social and Human Sciences Conference to examine the future of the fight against doping, October 21, 2009.

# Name Index

Abernethy, Virginia, 289–290
Acer, David, 320–321
Adkins, Janet, 40, 55
Admiraal, Peter, 50
Alexander, Leo, 45
Alexander, Shana, 230–231
Allwood, Mandy, 114
Altman, Lawrence K., 220
Alzado, Lyle, 358–359
Ambrose, 29
Amen, Denise, 115
Anderson, Jack, 20
Angell, Marcia, 200
Annan, Kofi, 323
Annas, George, 21, 22–23, 234,
    258–259
Antinori, Severino, 131
Aquinas, Thomas, 13–14, 29,
    88, 136
Aristotle, 152
Armstrong, Lance, 360
Asch, Ricardo, 111
Ashworth, Alan, 296
Augustine, 28–29, 88, 96
Aurelius, Marcus, 28
Ayala, Marissa and Anissa,
    168, 241

Bacchus, Habeeb, 20
Badham, Paul, 87
Baer, Ted D., 215
Bailey, Leonard, 249–253,
    255–262, 266
Bailey, Ron, 308
Baker, John, 153
Barnard, Christiaan, 71, 78,
    208–212, 219–224, 250,
    251, 253
Barnard, Marius, 208, 221
Barnes, Donald, 173
Bartlett, Roscoe, 184
Battin, Margaret, 50, 51, 56

Battiste, Christopher, 288
Beatty, Warren, 275
Beaumont, William, 186
Beecher, Henry, 189
Benedek, Thomas, 196, 198
Benjamin, Martin, 235
Benning, Annette, 275
Benoit, Chris, 358–359
Bentham, Jeremy, 9
Bergalis, Kimberly, 320–321
Bernard, Claude, 192
Bernat, James, 75
Bertrand, Marcheline, 296
Bijani, Ladan and Laleh, 259
Blaiberg, Phillip, 211, 220–221
Block, Lee and Tabea, 255
Bloomberg, Michael, 307
Boeck, Caesar, 191, 198
Bono, 323, 330
Bono, Chaz, 275
Bopp, James, 52
Boswell, John, 321
Bourgois, Philippe, 327
Bousada, Maria Carmen del, 116
Bouvia, Elizabeth, 19–25, 31,
    32–36
Bouvia, Richard, 20
Bove, Joseph, 319
Bradley, Ed, 159
Brandt, Karl, 45
Brinkley, Christie, 110
Britton, John, 99
Broelsch, Christoph, 241
Brown, John, 107–109
Brown, Joyce, 280–284, 288,
    290–293
Brown, Lesley, 107–109, 117
Brown, Louise, 107–109, 116–118,
    128, 130
Brown, Natalie, 108
Brown, William J., 195
Brownback, Sam, 132
Bruning, Fred, 161

Bruusgaard, J. E., 191, 193, 198
Buchanan, Patrick, 318
Buck, Carrie, 299–300
Bunker, Eng and Chang, 257, 273
Burcham, Jack, 216
Bush, George H. W., 26
Bush, George W., 67, 69, 118,
    132–134, 323, 331, 336
Bush, Jeb, 67–68, 70
Buxtun, Peter, 194–195
Buyukmichi, Nedim, 172
Buzzanca, Jaycee, 113

Callahan, Daniel, 52–53, 118
Campbell, A., 151
Campo, Laura, 253–254
Canal, Danny, 238–239
Caplan, Arthur, 206
Capron, Alexander, 258,
    260, 264
Carder, Angela, 102
Carr, Elizabeth, 109, 128
Carson, Ben, 254–255, 259
Casey, Robert, 237
Cates, Judy, 115
Cathell, Dale R., 201
Ceaucescau, Nicolae, 99
Charlton, Eda, 189
Charo, Alto, 56
Chase, Cheryl, 273, 274
Chodoff, Paul, 292
Christerson, Tom, 223
Chukwu, Nkem, 115
Claire-King, Mary, 296
Clark, Barney, 213–215,
    220–223, 260
Clark, Edward, 318
Clark, Una Loy, 215
Clinton, Bill, 101, 131, 195, 338
Clinton, Hillary, 202
Cohen, Carl, 180, 235
Colao, Joseph, 363

Colby, William, 68
Coler, Pascal, 219
Collins, Francis, 184
Compton, Carolyn, 180
Constantine, 152
Coolidge, Calvin, 300
Cornelson, Ronald, 100
Costello, Catherine, 289
Courmand, Andre, 212
Cowart, Dax (Donald), 27, 33, 35
Cranford, Ronald, 68, 78
Cronkite, Walter, 86
Crowfeather, Ernie, 234, 239, 246
Cruzan, Joe and Joyce, 64–66
Cruzan, Nancy, 59, 75, 76
Culp, Connie, 219
Curren, William, 90

Darvall, Denise, 71, 209, 221
Darvall, Edward, 209, 221
Darwin, Charles, 299
Davis, Emma, 111
Davis, Geena, 110
Davis, Mary Sue and Junior, 129
Davis, Nancy. See Cruzan, Nancy
Davis, Niamh, 111
Deering, Warren, 23
Delahunty, James, 165
DeLury, George, 37
Descartes, Rene, 72, 176–177
DeSillers, Ronnie, 238
Devauchelle, Bernard, 218
DeVries, William, 213–216, 220, 222–223, 251, 260
Diamond, Milton, 276
Dickinson, Robert Latou, 110
Dinoire, Isabelle, 218–222, 225
Dion, Celine, 110
Dixon, Greg, 318
Dockery, Gary, 73
Doerflinger, Richard, 133
Donaldson, Kenneth, 286
Donne, John, 29
Dreger, Alice, 254, 257, 259, 266, 272, 275
Dubernard, Jean-Michel, 217, 218, 221–223
Duff, R., 151
Duff-Fraker, Leilani, 168

Easterly, William, 330
Edelin, Kenneth, 83–87, 91, 94–95, 98
Edmond, Jean, 242
Edwards, Robert, 107–108, 109, 117, 128
Eisen, Howard, 241

Elbe, Lili, 271
Elliott, Carl, 359
Engelhardt, Tristam, 163
Epstein, Richard, 351
Erlich, Paul, 191
Everett, Emmett, 57

Falwell, Jerry, 318
Farfel, Marc, 201
Farmer, Paul, 327
Felos, George, 70
Fine, Russ, 26–27, 36
Fingarette, Herbert, 235
Fink, Sheri, 56–57
Finkbine, Sherri, 90
Fins, Joseph, 73
Fisher, Donald, 20
Fiske, Charles, 239
Fiske, Jamie, 239
Flanagan, Newman, 85–87, 94, 161
Fleming, Alexander, 198
Fletcher, John, 160
Fletcher, Joseph, 117–118
Fontaine, Nicholas, 176–177
Ford, Henry, 299
Forssmann, Werner, 221
Foucault, Michel, 318
Fox, Michael J., 133
Fox, Michael W., 173
Fox, Renée, 226, 233
Freud, Sigmund, 268
Friedman, Benjamin, 198
Frist, Bill, 69
Frustaci, Patti and Sam, 114

Galen, 284
Galton, Francis, 299
Gearhart, John, 130–131
Gelsinger, Jesse, 205–207
Gennarelli, Thomas, 170–172, 179
Giacino, Joseph, 73
Gianelli, Paul, 158
Giffords, Gabby, 294
Gilgunn, Caroline, 78
Gill, Carol, 33
Gilligan, Carol, 13
Gillman, Charlotte Perkins, 31
Giminez, Enrique, 84–85
Girsh, Faye, 37
Giuliani, Rudolph, 294
Glazer, Shep, 231
Glick, Seymour, 55
Gonzalez, Juan, 288
Goodall, Jane, 184
Goodman, Ellen, 200, 292
Gosnell, Kermit, 87
Gosselin, Kate and Jon, 105–106, 114, 119

Gould, Robert, 291
Grawitz, Ernst, 186–187
Gray, Fred, 195
Grayton, Jaheem, 289
Greek, Ray, 182
Greer, George, 67, 69, 70
Groveman, Sheri, 273
Gunn, David, 99
Gusella, James, 298
Gustafson, James, 151, 160

Hahn, Beatrice, 316
Haldane, J. B. S., 300
Hallam, Clint, 217, 218, 220
Hamilton, Joseph, 189
Hamilton, Pamela, 161
Hammesfahr, William, 68
Hardin, Garrett, 243
Hardwig, John, 306
Hardy, James, 251, 258–259
Hare, R. M., 3
Harris, Reuben, 288–289
Hartke, Vance, 231
Hata, S., 191
Hatch, Orrin, 134
Haydon, Murray, 216
Hayes, Catherine, 306
Hayes, Katy, 217
Hearst, William, 299
Heckler, Margaret, 319
Heller, Jean, 195, 197
Helms, Ron and Roz, 114
Hensel, Abigail and Brittany, 273
Hentoff, Nat, 53, 54
Herrick, Richard and Ronald, 241
Hews, John, 20–21
Higgins, Catina, 201
Hill, Paul, 99
Hippen, Ben, 272
Hippocrates, 43–44, 284
Hirsch, Joy, 73
Hirschfield, Mangus, 271
Hogue, Larry, 288
Holc, Alice and Gordon, 252–253
Holc, Paul, 252–253, 265
Holmes, Oliver Wendell, 300
Holtrop, Hugh, 84–85
Homans, William Perkins, Jr., 85–87, 94–95
Hoppe, Arthur, 21
Houben, Rom, 74
Howard, Coby, 341
Hughes, Marl, 129–130
Hughes, Viola, 201
Hume, David, 29, 177
Humphrey, Derek, 22–23, 46, 50, 51
Hunter, Holly, 110

Hurewitz, Mike, 242–243
Hutzler, Alice, 57
Huxley, Aldous, 2, 109
Hwang Woo-suk, 132–133

Iliescu, Adriana, 115, 116

Jacobsen, Cecil, 111
Jarvik, Robert, 213, 216, 229
Javed, Arshad, 61, 62, 80
Jaynes, Julian, 284
Jefferson, Mildred, 84
Jobs, Steve, 236–237
John Paul II (pope), 76, 136
Johnson, Edward, 26
Johnson, Frank, 286
Johnson, Harriet McBryde, 77
Johnson, Lyndon, 154, 336, 342
Jolie, Angelina, 110, 296–297, 303,
    305, 310, 311
Jones, Howard and
    Georgeanna, 128
Jones, James, 196
Jonsen, Albert, 90, 239
Jorgensen, Christine, 271
Jorgensen, George, 271

Kagan, Shelly, 179
Kamisar, Yale, 52
Kamm, Francis, 96, 168
Kampmeier, R. H., 196, 197,
    198, 199
Kamrava, Michael, 105, 125
Kant, Immanuel, 11–12, 29–30,
    199, 200, 233–234
Kantrowitz, Adrian, 219, 253
Kass, Leon, 118, 141, 148, 356
Keh, Arceh, 115
Kelley, Crystal, 113–114
Kennedy, James, 70
Kennedy, John F., 287–288
Kepner, Jeff, 217
Kerr, Kathleen, 156, 158
Keuskamp, Arjen, 155
Kevorkian, Jack, 37, 38, 39–41,
    53, 55
Kipnis, Kenneth, 277
Kirklin, John, 212
Klein, Martin, 102
Klein, Nancy, 101–102
Koch, Ed, 280–284, 291
Kolff, Willem, 212–213, 215, 216,
    229, 231
Koop, C. Everett, 154, 157, 159,
    160, 162
Koop, James, 100
Korein, Julius, 61
Kornberg, Warren, 108–109
Kramer, Larry, 322

Kramer, Peter, 356, 359
Krauthammer, Charles,
    260–261, 262
Kübler-Ross, Elisabeth, 46

Lakeberg, Angela and Amy,
    254–255
Lamm, Richard, 243–244, 353
Lanza, Robert, 135
Latimer, Robert, 37
Laughlin, Harry, 299
Laureys, Steven, 74
Lay, Ken, 134
Lee, Naeeham, 289
Lee, W. P. Andrew, 217
Levy, Robert, 291
Lewis, C. S., 177
Lieberson, Jonathan, 318–319
Lifton, Robert Jay, 45
Linares, Dan, 166
Linares, Rudy, 166
Lippman, Robert, 281–283, 292
Longmore, Paul, 22–23, 34–36
Lopez, Maria, 300–302, 304
Lorber, John, 151–152, 164, 167
Lower, Richard, 208–209, 233
Lucas, James, 193
Lundqvist, Arne, 364
Lynn, Joanne, 55
Lyons, Emily, 99

Mahoney, Patrick, 69–70
Mantle, Mickey, 237
Marquis, Don, 93–94
Martinez, Mel, 81
Marx, Karl, 16
Mayfield, William, 68
Mbeki, Thabo, 326
McAfee, Larry, 25–27, 31, 33, 35,
    36, 294
McArdle, Charles, 180
McArdle, John, 173
McCanus, Wilda, 57
McCaughey, Bobbi and
    Kenny, 115
McCormick, Richard, 136–137,
    139, 162, 258, 265
McCorvey, Norma, 90–91
McCullough, Larry, 272
McFarlane, Robert, 32
McGuire, James, 85–86
McKiever, Keven, 288
McRae, Donald, 211
Meese, Edwin, 157
Mengele, Josef, 187–188
Meredith, James, 36
Merk, Karl, 217
Mill, John Stuart, 9, 17, 30, 51
Millar, J. D., 195
Money, John, 267–270, 273, 276

Montagnier, Luc, 317
Montaigne, Michel de, 29
Moore, Francis, 212
Moriarty, Estella, 254, 264
Morse, Robert, 61, 62, 80
Moss, Alvin, 235
Mueller, Pamela and Robert,
    152–153
Mullen, Nancy, 32–33
Muller, Hermann J., 300
Murnaghan, Sarah, 239
Murray, Joseph, 241

Najarian, John, 261
Napoleon, 152
Nash, Jamie, 219
Nehlsen-Cannarella, Sandra,
    250, 261
Neidner, Matthew, 121–122
New, Maria, 272
Newkirk, Ingrid, 171, 174
Newman, Edwin, 230
Newman, George, 155, 156, 159
Nixon, Richard, 20, 335
Nolen, William, 85–87
Noonan, John, 94
Norwood, William, 257
Nozick, Robert, 15, 350

O'Connor, J. B., 286
O'Connor, Sandra Day, 102
O'Rourke, Kevin, 33, 76
Obama, Barack, 134, 342–343, 354
Olivieri, Nancy, 203
Orlans, Barbara, 175
Osler, William, 192
Outka, Gene, 138
Owens, Walter, 153–154
Ozar, David, 138

Pacheco, Alex, 173
Palin, Sarah, 161
Pappworth, Henry, 189
Pariente, Barbara, 68
Paris, John, 76
Patel, Nayna, 124
Paul VI (pope), 90
Pearson, Justin, 253–254
Pearson, Theresa Ann Campo,
    253–254
Pelosi, Nancy, 134
Perutz, Max, 118
Picoult, Jodi, 241
Pinel, Philippe, 284
Pistorius, Oscar, 356
Pitt, Brad, 296, 305
Pius IX (pope), 88, 136
Pius XII (pope), 78
Pizzo, Philip, 226

Plato, 26–27, 152, 211, 284
Plum, Fred, 61
Poddarin, Prosenjit, 289
Pointer, Sam C., 362
Pons, Timothy, 173
Pou, Anna, 38, 41–42, 44, 49–52,
    55–57
Preston, Thomas, 215
Proxmire, William, 195
Pythagoras, 43

Quill, Timothy, 41, 50, 55, 56
Quinlan, Joseph, 60–63
Quinlan, Julia, 60–63
Quinlan, Karen, 49, 52, 59–63, 75,
    78–80
Quinn, James, 223
Quinn, Warren, 93–94

Rachels, James, 49, 162
Ramsey, Paul, 84, 117, 258
Randall, Tony, 116
Rascher, Sigmund, 187
Raskind, Richard, 271
Rawls, John, 15–16, 18, 148,
    348–349
Reagan, Ronald, 20, 154
Reemtsma, Keith, 249, 258, 260
Regan, Tom, 179–180, 255
Reich, Warren, 90
Reimer, Bruce/Brenda,
    267–270, 276
Reimer, David, 267–270, 274
Reimer, Ron and Janet, 267
Rescher, Nicholas, 236
Reverby, Susan, 202
Rhoads, Cornelius, 188
Richards, Rene, 271
Richey, Charles, 174
Richter, Rudolf, 271
Rifkin, Jeremy, 118, 119
Rios, Mario and Elsa, 129
Rivers, Eunice, 193, 194
Roberts, Edward V., 36
Robertson, Pat, 318
Robinson, William, 299
Roche, Ellen, 201
Rodríguez, Nilda, 242
Roosevelt, Franklin, 188
Roosevelt, Theodore, 299
Rosenhan, D., 286
Rosier, Robert, 32
Rothman, David, 188
Rudolph, Eric, 99–100
Russell, Frederick, 29

Sachs, Jeffrey, 330
Saint James, Aleta, 115–116
Sanchez, Thomas, 96

Sandburg, David E., 272
Sanderson, Robert, 99
Santorum, Rick, 161
Sartre, Jean-Paul, 28
Saunders, Cicely, 46, 50
Savoie, Rose, 57
Savulescu, Julian, 359, 361
Scantlin, Sarah, 73
Schiavo, Michael, 66–71, 77
Schiavo, Scott, 70
Schiavo, Terri, 39, 53, 59, 66–71,
    74–81
Schiff, Nicholas, 73
Schindler, Bobby, 77
Schindler, Robert and Mary,
    66–71, 77
Schouten, Karen and Fred,
    252–253, 265
Schroeder, William, 215–216
Schwartz, Rosalyn, 333, 339
Scott, Kenneth, 189
Scott, Matthew, 217
Scott, Richard, 24
Scott, Rodney, 57
Scribner, Belding, 229–232,
    234, 239
Scrushy, Richard, 134
Seed, Dick, 131
Seigler, Mark, 235
Seimionow, Maria, 217–219, 226
Seligman, Martin, 173
Semenya, Caster, 271
Seneca, 28
Sepkowitz, Kent, 328
Sewell, James and Barbara, 242
Seymour, Jane, 110
Shanks, Niall, 182
Shewmon, Alan, 73–74,
    252, 263
Shriver, Sargent, 117
Shumway, Norman, 208–209, 219,
    223, 226
Siegel, Norman, 291
Silver, Lee, 144
Sims, J. Marion, 109–110
Singer, Peter, 9, 37, 163,
    178–179
Slepian, Barnett, 100
Smith, Roy, 302–303, 309
Smith, Teri and Alyssa, 241
Snow, John, 316
Socrates, 13, 26–27, 43, 211
Song Sin, 288–289
Sorkow, Harvey, 113
Spinoza, Baruch, 29
St. Aubert, Maryline, 218, 221
Stahl, Lesley, 159
Starnes, Vaughn, 242
Starzl, Thomas, 218, 221, 244,
    249, 251, 256, 261, 353
Staub, Norman, 212
Steinbeck, John, 197

Steinbock, Bonnie, 49, 137–138
Stell, Lance, 72
Steptoe, Patrick, 108, 128
Stern, Bill, 113
Stern, Elizabeth, 113
Stern, Melissa, 113
Stevens, Paul, 153
Suleman, Nadya, 105, 114,
    119, 126
Swain, Rosee, 115–116
Swango, Michael, 52
Swazey, Judith, 226, 231, 233
Szasz, Thomas, 285–286

Talbot, Margaret, 275–276
Talbot, Simon, 217
Tannenbaum, Melvyn, 156
Tarasoff, Tatiana, 289
Tarrant, Barbara, 243
Taub, Edward, 170, 173–174,
    182, 183
Teich, Steve, 84–85
Teraski, Paul, 256, 261
Terry, Randall, 69–70, 99
Theile, John, 57
Theroux, Paul, 330
Thogmartin, Jon, 70
Thomas, Griffith, 25
Thompson, Jacqueline, 115
Thomson, James, 131
Thomson, Judith Jarvis, 96
Thurmond, Strom, 116
Tiefel, Hans, 119
Tiller, George, 100
Tong, Paul, 90
Tooley, Michael, 163
Tools, Robert, 223
Trepanier, Angela, 312
Trutt, Stephanie, 172
Tuchman, Barbara, 315–316
Tucker, Bruce, 111, 233

Udobi, Iyke Louis, 115

van Zyl, Dirk, 223
Ventura, Mary, 289
Vonderlehr, Raymond, 192
Vos Savant, Marilyn, 216

Waddill, William, 100
Wade, Henry, 90
Waithe, Mary Ellen, 246
Wallace, George, 70
Wallis, Terry, 73
Walsh, Alexis, 288
Wangansteen, Owen, 208
Wanglie, Helga, 77–78
Warren, Mary Ann, 92

Warren, Petra, 152
Washburn, Lawrence, 156
Washkansky, Louis, 71, 208–211, 220–221, 223, 224
Watson, James, 118
Webdale, Kendra, 288–289
Weber, William, 156, 159
Weins, Dallas, 219
Weisbard, Alan, 245
Weldon, Dave, 69
Weller, Barbara, 70
Westhusin, Mark, 133
Wexler, Leonard, 157

Wexler, Nancy, 297–298, 305, 308, 309
White, Ryan, 319
White Bull, Patricia, 73
Whitehead, Mary Beth, 113
Whitner, Comelia, 102
Whittemore, James, 69
Wilkes, J. C., 45
Williams, Nushawn, 322, 326
Wilmut, Ian, 130
Wilson, E. O., 6
Wilson, Eric, 359–360
Wilson, James, 206–207

Winners, Michael and Brenda, 253
Wood, Walter, 242–243
Woods, Carl, 110, 115

Yamanaka, Shinya, 134–135
Youk, Thomas, 41

Zachary, R. B., 164
Zavos, Pamayiotis, 131

# Subject Index

Abnormal harm, 120, 165
Abortion, 83–105
  culture of death and, 38, 97–98
  doctrine of double effect and, 14, 88
  Edelin case, 83–87, 91, 94–95, 98
  feminist views of, 96–97
  fetal tissue research and, 100–101
  Finkbine case, 90
  gender selection and, 98–99
  genetic defects and, 97
  illegal, experience of, 89
  vs. infanticide, 161–162
  language of, 87
  legal developments and fine-tuning on, 103
  limited pro-choice view of, 96
  live birth, 100
  marginal cases, 95–96, 102
  maternal vs. fetal rights, 101–102
  partial birth, 104
  personhood/potentiality and, 86, 91–94
  procedures of, 100
  protests and violent acts against, 99–100
  religious views on, 76, 84, 87–89, 90, 97, 98
  Roe v. Wade decision, 62, 89, 90–91, 94, 95
  state restrictions on clinics, 104
  statistics on, 91, 97
  surrogacy contract and, 113–114
  as three-sided issue, 99
  viability and, 85, 94–95, 102–103
Absolute risk, 119, 301–302
Ad hominem ("to the man"), 5
Adoption, payment for, 112–114

Ad populum, 7, 360
Adult stem cells, 131–132
Advance directives, 80
Affordable Care Act (ACA), 42, 310, 342–354
  arguments for and against, 343–354
  costs under, 350–353
  efficiency vs. bureaucracy under, 345–346
  illegal immigrants and, 343–345
  intergenerational justice under, 353–354
  rationality and, 346–347
Against Happiness: In Praise of Melancholy (Wilson), 359–360
AIDS. See HIV/AIDS
Akanksha Infertility Clinic, 124
Alcoholism, genetics of, 312–313
Alcohol-related end-stage liver disease (ARESLD), 234–235
Alcohol use, 2, 59, 234–236
Allocation of resources, 228–248
Alzheimer's disease, 40, 302–303
American Medical Association (AMA), 47, 61, 79–80, 101, 134, 191, 192
Americans with Disabilities Act (ADA), 35, 77, 166–167
Amplification system, 317–318, 328
Anencephaly, 249, 251–254, 263–265
Animal cloning, 81, 130, 132–133
Animal Liberation (Singer), 178–179
Animal Liberation Front (ALF), 170–172
Animal research, 170–185
  arguments against, 182–183
  as bad science, 182–183

Cartesianism and, 176–177
  committees overseeing, 172, 174–175
  cost vs. benefit of, 183
  equivalence and, 182
  laws on, 174–175
  numbers and kinds of, 175–176
  Official View of, 181–182
  pain of animals in, 176–178
  philosophy of mind and, 177–178
  speciesism and, 178–181
  value of animal life and, 179–181
Animal-to-human transplants, 249–251, 254–262
Annie Hall (movie), 35
Antidepressants, enhancement with, 356, 359–360, 362
Appeals to feelings and upbringing, 7
Appeal to authority, 6
Argument, 1–2
Argument from marginal cases, 95–96, 102
Arm transplants, 217
Artificial feeding, 78–79. See also Feeding tubes
Artificial heart, 212–216
Artificial insemination, 109–110
Artificial kidney. See Kidney dialysis
As Nature Made Him: The Boy Who Was Raised as a Girl (Colapinto), 270
Assisted reproduction, 106–127
  commercialization (payment) in, 112–114, 122
  confidentiality in, 121
  and embryonic research, 128
  first IVF baby in U.S., 109, 128
  first test-tube baby, 107–108, 128

gender selection in, 116
genetic screening in, 122–123
harm in, 114–115, 118–122, 125
international use and
    tourism, 124
later developments in, 109–111
media coverage on, 108–109
mistakes and scandals in, 111
multiple births in, 106–107,
    114–115, 125
older parents in, 115–116, 125
regulation of fertility clinics,
    125–126
religious views on, 116–118
"Snowflake" children in,
    134, 136
Assisted suicide, 31–37. *See also*
    Physician-assisted dying
Attention deficit hyperactivity
    disorder (ADHD), 357, 358
Authority, appeal to, 6
Autonomy, 12, 16–17
    *vs.* involuntary psychiatric
        commitment, 289–290
    and physician-assisted dying,
        50–51
    and requests to die, 33–34, 50–51
Ayala case, 168, 241

Baboons
    medical research on, 170–172
    organs from, 249–251, 254–262
Baby(ies). *See also* Impaired
    babies
    costs and opportunity costs of
        procedures on, 265–266
    definition of, 87
    designer, 123–124
    informed consent for
        procedures on, 258–259
    as organ donors, 249, 251–254,
        262–266
    as research subjects, 257–258,
        260–262
Baby Doe rules, 150, 154–155
Baby Fae case, 249–251, 254–262
Baby Gabriel case, 251–253, 265
*The Baby in the Bottle* (Nolen), 86
Baby Jane Doe case, 150, 155–160
Baby K case, 166
Baby M case, 113
Baby S case, 114
Baby Theresa case, 249,
    253–254, 265
*Bad Blood* (Jones), 196
Baseline harm, 120, 165
Bayh–Dole Act, 202
Begging the question, 8
Beneficence, 17
Best interests of patients, 65
*Better than Well* (Elliott), 359

Beyond a reasonable doubt, 64
Bioethics
    birth of, 232
    four principles of, 16–18
    global, 323
    good reasoning in, 1–4
    mistakes in reasoning, 4–8
    politics and, 80–81
Biogenetic child, 110–111
Biological inequality, 144
Biological sex, 268, 273
Birth(s). *See also* Assisted repro-
    duction; Impaired babies
    multiple, 106–107, 114–115, 125
    wrongful, 120, 165–166
Black Death, 315–316
Blood supply, HIV transmission
    via, 317, 318
Blue Cross/Blue Shield, 340–341
Body shaping, 357
*Bowen v. American Hospital
    Association*, 157
*Bowers v. Hardwick*, 321
Brain death
    in anencephalic babies,
        253–254, 263–265
    in organ donors, 221–222, 233,
        244, 265
    standards for, 60, 71–72
*Brave New World* (Huxley), 2, 109
Breast cancer genes, 296–297
Breast implants, 362–363
Bubonic plague, 315–316
*Buck v. Bell*, 299–300

*Colautti v. Franklin*, 103
Canadian health-care system,
    334–335
Cancer, genetic testing in,
    296–297
Cardinal virtues, 13
Care, Ethics of, 12–13
Cartesianism, 176–177
Catholic Church
    on abortion, 84, 87–89
    on assisted reproduction,
        116–117
    on comatose patients, 62, 76
    on embryos, 136
    on suicide, 33
Cheating, medical enhancement
    and, 360–362
Cherry-picking, 340
Child Abuse Amendments, 166
Children's Health Insurance
    Program (CHIP), 337
Chimpanzees
    medical research on, 183–184
    organs from, 249–250, 258–259
Cholera, 316
Christian Defense Coalition, 69

Civility, 4
Clear and convincing evidence,
    64, 80
Cloning
    animal, 81, 130, 132–133
    fraudulent claims on research,
        131, 133–134
    history of, 130–135
    legal restrictions on, 132
    link between embryonic and
        reproductive, 148–149
    reproductive, 140–149
    sheep (Dolly), 81
COBRA, 338
Cognitive criterion
    of brain death, 71–72
    of personhood, 92, 163
Collaborative model, 204–205
Coma
    best interest of patients, 65
    chances of regaining con-
        sciousness from, 72–75
    compassion for patients in,
        75–76
    Cruzan case, 59, 63–66, 76, 79
    definition of, 60
    disability issues in, 77
    extraordinary *vs.* ordinary
        treatment in, 78
    futile *vs.* non-futile care in,
        77–78
    intentional behavior *vs.*
        reflexes in, 72
    Quinlan case, 49, 52, 59–63
    Schiavo case, 39, 53, 59, 66–71,
        75, 76–77, 80–81
    substituted judgment for
        patients, 63, 65, 76
    traumatic *vs.* anoxic causes of,
        73–74
    withdrawing *vs.* forgoing
        treatment, 79–80
Commercialization of assisted
    reproduction, 112–114, 122
*The Constant Gardener*
    (movie), 204
Common Rule, 202–203
Community rating, 340
Compassion, for comatose
    patients, 75–76
Compassion and Choices
    (Hemlock Society), 22–23,
    37, 50, 51, 53–54
Competence. *See also*
    Incompetent patients
    and involuntary psychiatric
        commitment, 289–290
    and requests to die, 32–33
Complete androgen insensitivity
    syndrome (CAIS), 277
Conceptual slippery slopes,
    51–53

Congenital adrenal hyperplasia (CAH), 271–273, 276
Conjoined twins, 152–153, 249, 254–255, 257, 259, 273
Consciousness. *See also* Persistent vegetative state
 chances of comatose patients regaining, 72–75
 as gradient, 74
 minimally conscious state, 71, 73–74
 sentience *vs.*, 177
Consequentialism, 9–10
Consistency, 2
Constraint-Induced Movement Therapy, 173–174
Contraception, emergency, 101
Contractarianism, Rawlsian, 15
Cost-plus reimbursement, 232
Cost shifting, 339
Council for International Organizations of Medical Sciences (CIOMS), 205
Counseling, genetic, 309–310
Cries for help, requests to die as, 55–56
Culture of death, 38, 97–98
Cycling, doping in, 356–357, 360
Cyclosporine, 222–223, 226

Death. *See also* Physician-assisted dying; Requests to die; Suicide
 of anencephalic babies, 253–254, 263–265
 criteria of, 59–60, 71–72
 culture of, 38, 97–98
 discovery *vs.* decision, 72
 medicalization of, 31
 of organ donors, 221–222, 233, 244–246, 265
 physician–patient discussion on, 51
"Death counseling," 42
Death with Dignity Act (Oregon), 42
Deception, of research subjects, 192–193, 196
Defense of Marriage Act (DOMA), 322
Deficit Reduction Act of 2005, 337
Deinstitutionalization, 287–288, 294
Depression, and request to die, 34, 53, 56
Deprivation argument, and abortion, 93–94
Designer babies, 123–124
Dexamethasone, prenatal use of, 272–273

Diabetes, genetic testing in, 300–302
Diagnostically Related Groups (DRGs), 232
Dialysis. *See* Kidney dialysis
Dickey Warner Amendment, 129
Difference principle, 16, 348–349
Disabilities, persons with. *See also* Impaired babies
 comatose patients as, 77
 culture of, 36–37
 legal rights of, 35
 Nazi killing of, 44–46
 prejudice and discrimination against, 34–37, 77
 requests to die, 19–37
Distributive justice, 18
 and allocation of medical resources, 228–248
Doctrine of double effect, 14, 88
Dolly (cloned sheep), 81, 130, 132
Donation after cardiac death (DCD), 244–246
Donor Sibling Registry, 121
Doping, 356–357, 360
Double effect, doctrine of, 14, 88
Down syndrome, 150–151, 153–154, 161–166, 167
Draize tests, 175
Durable power of attorney, 80
Duty, in Kantian ethics, 11

Egalitarianism, 18
Egg donors, payment for, 112, 122
Egg transfer, 110–111
*Eisenstadt v. Baird*, 103
"Either-or" fallacy, 7
*The Elephant Man* (movie), 35
Embryos. *See also* Abortion; Assisted reproduction
 Bush (George W.) policy on, 132–134
 Davis case, 129–130
 definition of, 87
 fraudulent claims on research, 131, 133–134
 frozen, 111, 129, 134, 136
 genetic screening of, 122–123, 241
 historical perspective on research, 128–135
 hybrid (human cells in cow eggs), 131
 induced pluripotent stem cells *vs.*, 134–135, 140
 interest view of, 137–138
 legal restrictions on use, 132
 Obama policy on, 134
 opportunity cost of missed research on, 139

 personhood/potentiality and, 136, 139
 religious views of, 136
 respect for, 138–139
 Rios case, 129
 slippery slope and, 136–137
EmbryoScope, 111
Emergency contraception, 101
Emergency Medical Treatment and Active Labor Act (EMTALA), 338
Empirical slippery slopes, 51–53
Employer mandate, for health care, 338
End-Stage Renal Disease Act (ESRD), 231–232, 336, 351
Enhancement. *See* Medical enhancement
Ensoulment, 88
Enthymeme, 2
Environmental inequality, 144
Epidemics, 315–316. *See also* HIV/AIDS
Equivocation, 7–8
Erythropoietin (EPO), 356
Ethical reasoning
 good reasons in, 1–4
 mistakes in, 4–8
Ethical theories, 8–15
 Ethics of Care, 12–13
 Kantian ethics, 11–12
 moral relativism, 8–9
 natural law, 13–15
 Thomistic, 13–15
 utilitarianism, 9–11
 virtue ethics, 13
Ethics Advisory Board, 128
Ethics of Care, 12–13, 240
Eugenics, 122–123, 299–300
Euthanasia, 31, 163. *See also* Physician-assisted dying
"Euthanasia by omission," 76
Evidence, 1–2, 64, 80
Existentialism, 28
"Exit Bag," 54
Experience rating, 340
Exposure effect, 363
Extraordinary *vs.* ordinary treatment, 78, 155

Face transplants, 217–218, 224, 226
Fair Benefits Model, 205
Fair-minded, 4
False dichotomy, 7
Fame, desire for, 208–237
Farm and Animal Research Facilities Protection Act, 174
Feeding tubes, 78–79
 Cruzan case, 63–66

extraordinary *vs.* ordinary
treatment, 78
futile *vs.* non-futile care, 77–78
impaired babies, 150
Quinlan case, 60
refusal of, 20–25
Schiavo case, 66–71
Feelings, appeals to, 7
Feminism
abortion views, 96–97
Ethics of Care, 12–13, 240
HIV/AIDS views and action,
325–326, 328–329
*vs.* paternalistic ethics, 17
Fetal dex, 272–273
Fetal tissue research, 100–101
Fetus. *See also* Abortion
to be aborted, experiments on,
83–85
definition of, 87
listing for heart transplants,
237–238
personhood and potentiality
of, debate over, 86, 91–94
rights of, maternal rights *vs.*,
101–102
viability of, 85, 94–95,
102–103
Finger transplant, 217
Focal incompetence, 290
Food. *See also* Feeding tubes
refusal of, 20–25
Frozen embryos, 111, 129,
134, 136
Futile *vs.* non-futile care, 77–78

Gamete intrafallopian transfer
(GIFT), 110
Gamete material, freezing
of, 111
*GATTACA* (movie), 308, 313
Gay-related immune deficiency
(GRID), 316–317
Gender identity, 268, 273
Gender presentation, 273
Gender reassignment
John/Joan case, 267–270
surgical, 270, 271, 276
Gender role, 268
Gender selection, 98–99, 116
Gene, 297
Gene therapy, death in, 205–207
Genetic criterion of
personhood, 94
Genetic defects, and abortion, 97
Genetic diseases, 297. *See also*
Genetic testing
Genetic identity, 141–142
Genetic Information
Nondiscrimination Act
(GINA), 310

Genetic testing, 296–314
Alzheimer's disease,
302–303
cancer, 296–297
counseling required with,
309–310
diabetes, 300–302
disease prevention through,
303, 312–313
eugenics and, 299–300
family issues in, 305–307
financial interests in,
311–312
good news sought in,
304–305
Huntington's disease,
297–298
insurance effects of, 310
personality responsibility for
disease in, 307–308
premature news and
oversimplification in,
310–311
prenatal, 97, 122–123, 241
self-interest in, 303–304
sick identity from, 308
suicide risk from results, 309
Genitalia, ambiguous. *See*
Intersex persons
Gingerbread Person, 273
Global bioethics, 323
God Committee, 228–232, 234,
246–247
Godwin's Law, 46
Golden Rule, 16, 75–76, 329
Gradient view of personhood,
92–93, 162–163
Great Ape Protection and
Savings Act, 184
Greece, ancient
death and suicide in, 27–28
Hippocratic Oath in, 43–44
infanticide in, 152
mental illness in, 284
natural law in, 13–15
virtue ethics in, 13
*Griswold v. Connecticut*, 61–62, 63,
90, 145
Groningen protocol, 39
Guardian *ad litem*, 153, 156
Guatemalan syphilis study, 202

HAART, 331
Hand transplants, 217
Harm
abnormal, 120, 165
assisted reproduction and,
114–115, 118–122, 125
baseline, 120, 165
involuntary psychiatric
commitment and, 292–293

medical enhancement and,
362–363
paradox of, 119–120
total, 165
Tuskegee Study and,
197–198
wrongful birth and wrongful
life, 120, 165
wronging *vs.*, 120–121
Harm principle, 17
Harm Reduction Movement,
10, 190
Harrison Act of 1914, 31
*Harris v. McRae*, 103
Harvard criteria of brain death,
71, 222, 244
Health care, 333–355. *See also*
Affordable Care Act
American system of
(1962–2012), 335–340
Canadian system of,
334–335
Clinton plan, 338, 351
cost shifting in, 339
costs in, 350–353
employer and private plans,
339–340
genetic testing and, 310
intergenerational justice in,
353–354
preexisting conditions and,
333, 343
prepaid group medical
coverage, 341
ratings and cherry-picking in,
340–341
as right, debate over,
347–352
United Kingdom system
of, 335
universal coverage, 334–335
Health Insurance Portability and
Accountability Act
(HIPPA), 339
Health maintenance
organizations (HMOs), 335
Heart, artificial, 212–216
Heart transplant
fetuses listed for, 237–238
first, 208–212
LVADs as bridge to, 223,
239–240
number and results of,
211–212
as therapeutic procedure, 226
Hemlock, 28
Hemlock Society, 22–23, 37, 50,
51, 53–54
Hemodialysis. *See* Kidney
dialysis
Hippocratic Oath, 17, 40,
43–44

HIV/AIDS, 315–332
  amplification system for,
    317–318, 328
  Bergalis case, 320–321
  causative agent of, 317
  education on, 324–325, 329,
    330–331
  exceptionalism in, 322
  feminist perspective and action
    on, 325–326, 328–329
  historical perspective on,
    315–319
  ideology and, 317–319
  placebo study in Africa,
    199–201, 204
  prevention of, 322–331
  structuralism and, 327–328
  suicide and assisted suicide
    in, 53–54
  testing for, 317, 319–320
  transmission of, 319–320
  triage in, 326–327, 330
Holland
  intersex persons in, 277
  physician-assisted dying in,
    38–39, 53, 55
Homeless persons
  deinstitutionalization and,
    287–288, 294
  housing for, 293–294
  involuntary psychiatric
    commitment of, 280–284,
    290–293
Homophobia, 321
Homosexuality, 316–319,
  321–322
Hospice movement, 49, 50
*Humanae Vitae*, 90
Human cloning. *See*
  Reproductive cloning
Human Cloning Prohibition
  Act, 132
Human Embryo Research
  Panel, 129
Humane Society, 184
Human Genome Project, 297
Human research subjects,
  186–207
  babies as, 257–258, 260–262
  collaborative model for,
    204–205
  Common Rule on, 202–203
  deception of, 192–193, 196
  Fair Benefits Model of, 205
  financial conflicts and, 202–203
  gene therapy death
    (Gelsinger), 205–207
  Guatemalan syphilis study
    on, 202
  harm to, 197–198
  HIV study in Africa on,
    199–201, 204

  informed consent from,
    188, 196
  international ethical standards
    of, progress toward, 203–207
  Kantian ethics on, 199, 200
  Krieger lead paint study on,
    201–202
  Nazi experimentation on,
    186–187
  Nuremberg code on, 188
  therapy *vs.* experimentation
    on, 226, 260–262
  Tuskegee Study on, 190–199
Huntington's disease, 297–298
Hydration, artificial, 78–79. *See
  also* Feeding tubes


Illegal abortion, 89
Illegal immigrants, health-care
  coverage for, 343–345
Immediate animation, 88
Immigrants, illegal, health-care
  coverage for, 343–345
Immigration Restriction Act of
  1924, 300
Immortalized stem cell lines,
  130–131
Immunosuppression, post-
  transplant, 222–223, 226
Impaired babies, 150–169
  abortion *vs.* infanticide,
    161–162
  ancient societies and, 152
  assisted reproduction and,
    114–115, 118–119, 125
  Baby Doe rules, 150, 154–155
  Baby Doe squads, 150, 154–155
  Baby Jane Doe case, 150,
    155–160
  Baby K case, 166
  conceptual dilemma on, 168
  degrees of defects, 163–164
  disability advocates and,
    167–168
  euthanasia in Holland, 39
  Infant Doe case, 150, 153–154
  Johns Hopkins cases, 150–151
  killing *vs.* letting die, 162
  legislation on, 166–167
  media coverage on, 154, 156,
    157, 158, 159–160, 161
  medically reasonable options
    for, 156
  Mueller case (conjoined twins),
    152–153
  Nazi killing of, 45
  pediatric intensivists on,
    151–152
  personal *vs.* public cases,
    160–161
  personhood of, 162–163

  reproductive cloning and,
    143–144
  selfishness and, 160
  wrongful birth *vs.* wrongful
    life, 165–166
Impartiality, 3
Incompetent patients. *See also*
  Coma; Mentally ill persons
  compassion for, 75–76
  substituted judgment for, 63,
    65, 76
Indeterminancy, of embryos, 139
Induced pluripotent stem (IPS)
  cells, 134–135, 140
Inequality, reproductive cloning
  and, 144
Infant(s). *See* Baby(ies); Impaired
  babies
Infant Doe case, 150, 153–154
Infanticide, 152, 161–162
Institutional Animal Care and
  Use Committees (IACUCs),
  172, 174–175
Institutional review boards
  (IRBs), 195
Insurance. *See* Health insurance
Interest view, of embryos,
  137–138
Intergenerational justice, 353–354
Intersex persons, 267–279
  civil rights of, 275–276
  conservative view of, 276
  Dutch approach to (delaying
    puberty), 277
  John/Joan case, 267–270
  Kipnis' proposals on, 277
  medical exceptions for
    treating, 276–277
  nature-nurture debate about,
    268, 276
  normalcy definition and, 273
  secrecy, in child's best
    interest, 274
  secrecy and shame,
    overcoming, 274–275
  transgender *vs.*, 271
Intracytoplasmic sperm injection
  (ICSI), 110
In vitro fertilization (IVF),
  107–108. *See also* Assisted
  reproduction
Involuntary psychiatric
  commitment, 280–295
  Brown case, 280–284, 288,
    290–293
  deinstitutionalization *vs.*,
    287–288, 294
  harm *vs.* benefit in, 292–293
  legal victories for patients,
    286–287
  *O'Connor* criteria for, 282, 284,
    286–287

overt act and, 287
paternalism and, 289
patients' rights *vs.*, 285–286
psychiatry and, 291–292
*Wyatt* decision on, 286
Irreversibility, in brain death, 72

Jarvik-7 artificial heart,
    213–216
Jaycee case (surrogacy), 113
Johns Hopkins cases, 150–151
Judicious neglect, 61
Justice
    in allocation of medical
        resources, 228–248
    as bioethical principle, 18
    in health care, 348–354
    Rawls on, 15–16, 18, 148,
        348–350
    theories of, 15–16
Justification, 1
*The Just War in the Middle Ages*
    (Russell), 29

Kantian ethics, 11–12
    and allocation of medical
        resources, 228, 233–236,
        238, 240
    and human research subjects,
        199, 200
    and suicide, 29–30
    utilitarianism *vs.*, 9–10
Kendra's Law, 289
Kidney dialysis
    allocation of resources,
        228–232, 246–247
    End-Stage Renal Disease Act
        and, 231–232
    Rogosin or nocturnal, 247
Krieger lead paint study, 201–202

*Lawrence v. Texas*, 321
LD-50 (lethal dosage) tests, 175
Lead paint study, 201–202
Least restrictive environment,
    287
Left ventricular assist devices
    (LVADs), 223, 239–240
Leprosy, 316
Libertarianism, 15
Lifeboat Test, 180
Life support. *See* Ventilators
Limb transplants, 217
*Limitless* (movie), 361–362
Live birth abortions, 100
Living organ donors, 2–3,
    232–233, 241–243
Living will, 80
Logic, 2

Malpractice, 61, 364
Managed care, 232, 338
Mandated choice, for organ
    donation, 233
Mandated multi-plan
    coverage, 334
Marginal cases, argument from,
    95–96, 102
Marxism, 16
Massachusetts health-care plan,
    341–342
Mass shootings, 294–295
Maximization, 9–11
Media coverage
    abortion, 99
    assisted reproduction,
        108–109, 114
    babies as organ donors, 251
    Baby Fae case, 259–260
    conjoined twins, 254
    Edelin case, 86
    impaired babies, 154,
        156–161
    organ transplantation, 211,
        220, 226, 239–240
    Schiavo case, 69–70, 81
    Tuskegee Study, 195, 197
Medicaid, 336–337
Medical enhancement, 356–365
    cheating and, 360–362
    defining, 357–358
    exposure effect in, 363
    harm in, 362–363
    legalization of, 360, 363
    positional advantage in, 358
    role of physicians in,
        363–364
Medicalization of death, 31
Medically reasonable
    options, 156
Medicare, 336
Mental Health Parity Act, 337
Mentally ill persons
    deinstitutionalization of,
        287–288, 294
    housing for, 293–294
    insanity of, ideology and,
        284–285
    involuntary psychiatric
        commitment of, 280–295
    rights of, 285–286
    violence of, 288–289, 294–295
Mercy, in physician-assisted
    dying, 49–50
*Million Dollar Baby* (movie), 35
Mind, philosophy of, 177–178
Minimally conscious state (MCS),
    71, 73–74
Mitochondria, 130
Mitochondria swapping, 135
Monkeys, medical research on,
    173–174

Moral relativism, 8–9
Multiple births, 106–107,
    114–115, 125
Multiple listings, for transplants,
    236–238
Myriad Genetics, 311
*My Sister's Keeper* (Picoult), 241

National Bioethics Advisory
    Commission (NBAC), 131
National Health Service (United
    Kingdom), 335
National Transplantation
    Act, 236
Natural law, 13–15
Nature *vs.* nurture, 268, 276
Nazi Germany, 8–9, 44–46,
    186–187, 299
Neonatal intensive care units
    (NICUs), 150. *See also*
    Impaired babies
Neurological criterion of
    personhood, 94
*New England Journal of Medicine*,
    49, 73, 84
Nocturnal dialysis, 247
Non-heart-beating cadaver
    donors (NHBCD),
    244–246
Nonmaleficence, 17–18
Norm of reaction, 297
Nuremberg Code, 188
Nutrition, artificial. *See*
    Feeding tubes

Obama health-care plan. *See*
    Affordable Care Act
*O'Connor v. Donaldson*, 282, 284,
    286–287
Octamom case, 105
*Oklahoma vs. Skinner*, 62, 90
*One Flew over the Cuckoo's Nest*
    (movie), 285
One-hit, two-hit model, 303
*On Liberty* (Mill), 17, 30, 51
Ontario Protocol, 251–253,
    263, 264
Onus of proof, 3
Operation Rescue, 99
Opportunistic infections, 319
Opt-out *vs.* opt-in policy, for
    organ donation, 233
Oregon
    health-care plan in, 341
    physician-assisted dying in, 38,
        42–43, 53, 54
Organ transplantation. *See*
    Transplantation
Organ-utilitarians, 238
Other-regarding acts, 30

Pain
  animal, 176–178
  suffering *vs.*, 50
Pain relief
  medicalization of dying
    and, 31
  palliative care and, 49
  physician-assisted dying and,
    49–50
  requests to die and, 34
Palliative care, 48, 50, 56
Paradox of harm, 119–120
*Parens patria,* 157
Parental age, in assisted
  reproduction, 115–116, 125
Parental consent, for
  abortion, 103
Parents, biological, harm in not
  knowing, 121–122
Partial birth abortions, 104
Paternalism, 17, 289, 309
Patient Protection and Affordable
  Care Act (PPACA). *See*
  Affordable Care Act
Patient rights movement, 17, 33,
  285–286
Payment, in assisted
  reproduction, 112–114, 122
People for the Ethical Treatment
  of Animals (PETA), 170,
  173–174, 175, 255
Persistent vegetative state (PVS)
  chances of regaining
    consciousness from, 72–75
  Cruzan case, 63–66
  definition of, 60
  misdiagnosis of, 74
  Quinlan case, 59–63
  Schiavo case, 66–71
Personhood
  and abortion, 86, 91–93
  cognitive criterion of, 92, 163
  and embryo research, 136, 139
  genetic criterion of, 94
  gradient view of, 92–93,
    162–163
  and impaired babies, 162–163
  neurological criterion of, 94
Physician-assisted dying, 38–58
  cries for help and, 55–56
  direct arguments about, 47–51
  financial issues/motivation
    in, 54
  Hippocratic Oath and, 40,
    43–44
  historical perspective on, 43–46
  Holland and, 38–39, 53, 55
  indirect arguments about,
    51–54
  inefficient means in, 53–54
  Kevorkian and, 38, 39–41,
    53, 55

  killing *vs.* letting die, 48–49
  "least worth death" in, 51
  legalization in U.S., 38, 42–43
  mistakes and abuses in, 55
  modern developments
    in, 46–47
  Nazi argument and, 44–46
  palliative care *vs.,* 49, 50, 56
  patient autonomy and, 50–51
  Pou and (Hurricane Katrina),
    38, 41–42, 44, 49–52, 55–57
  Quill and, 41, 55
  recent legal decisions on, 46–47
  relief of suffering in, 49–50
  role of physicians in, 54–55
  slippery slope argument on,
    38–39, 51–53
Pittsburgh protocol, for organ
  donation, 244–245
Plague, 315–316
Plan B contraceptive, 101
*Planned Parenthood v. Casey,* 103
*Planned Parenthood v.*
  *Danforth,* 103
Pneumonic plague, 315
Positional advantage, 358
*Post hoc, ergo propter hoc* ("after
  this, therefore, because of
  this"), 6
Potentiality, 93–94, 136, 139,
  162–163
Power of attorney, durable, 80
Preexisting conditions, 333, 343
Prepaid group medical
  coverage, 341
Preponderance of evidence, 64
Principle, 2
Privacy, right to
  abortion decisions, 62,
    90–91, 103
  *Griswold* decision, 61–62, 63, 90
  Quinlan case, 61–62, 63
Pro-choice view, limited, 96
Proof, onus of, 3
Psychiatric commitment. *See*
  Involuntary psychiatric
  commitment
Puberty, delaying, for intersex
  persons, 277


Quality of life, post-transplant,
  222–223
Question-begging mistakes, 8


Racism
  and involuntary psychiatric
    commitment, 282
  and Tuskegee Study,
    191–192, 196
Raelians, 131, 134

Rationality
  in Affordable Care Act,
    346–347
  in Kantian ethics, 12
  in suicide, 31, 32–33
Rawlsian justice, 15, 148, 348–350
Reasonableness, 3–4
Red Herring, 5–6
*Reductio ad absurdum,* 83,
  93–94, 137
Relative risk, 119, 301–302
Relativism, moral, 8–9
Relevance, 1
Religious views
  on abortion, 76, 84, 87–89,
    97, 98
  on assisted reproduction,
    116–118
  on comatose patients, 62, 76
  on embryos, 136
  on HIV/AIDS, 318
  of killing, 47–48
  on reproductive cloning, 141
  of suicide, 28–29, 33
Remmelink Commission, 38
Reproduction, assisted. *See*
  Assisted reproduction
Reproductive cloning, 140–149
Reproductive tourism, 124
*Republic* (Plato), 211
Requests to die. *See also*
  Physician-assisted dying
  autonomy and, 33–34, 50–51
  Bouvia case, 19–25
  competence and, 32–33
  Cowart case, 27
  cries for help *vs.,* 55–56
  intended action in, 31
  McAfee case, 25–27
  non-terminal patients, 19–37
  rationality and, 32–33
  terminal cases, 38–58
Required request, for organ
  donation, 233
Rescue, Rule of, 239–241
Research. *See* Animal research;
  Human research subjects
Respect
  for embryos, 138–139
  for impaired babies, 168
Respirators. *See* Ventilators
Retransplants, 238–239
Risk, absolute and relative, 119,
  301–302
*Roe v. Wade,* 62, 89, 90–91, 94, 95
  and Edelin case, 83, 85
  and embryonic research, 128
Rogosin dialysis, 247
Role-defined ethics, 13
Roman Catholic Church. *See*
  Catholic Church
Rome, ancient

death and suicide in, 27–28
infanticide in, 152
mental illness in, 284
natural law in, 13–15
Rule of Rescue, 239–241

Sacrifice surgeries, on conjoined
twins, 249, 254–255, 257, 259
*St. Elsewhere* (television series), 84
Savior siblings, 11, 168, 241
Scapegoats, 316
Scope-of-morality premise, 9–10
Sedating, terminal, 49
Self-regarding acts, 30
Sentience, 177
Sexual (gender) identity, 268, 273.
*See also* Intersex persons
Sexual orientation, 273, 321
Ship of fools, 284
Sickest first, for transplants,
240–241
Sick identity, 308
Single-payer system, 334
Slippery slope, 4–5
in anencephaly, 263–264
conceptual, 51–53
in embryo research, 136–137
empirical, 51–53
in physician-assisted dying,
38–39, 51–53
in Quinlan case, 62
"Snowflake" children, 134, 136
Social Darwinism, 299
"Socialized medicine," 349–350
Social worth criteria, 230,
233–234, 236
Somatic cell nuclear transfer
(SCNT), 130
Souls, 88, 176, 177
Spare embryos, 129
Speciesism, 178–181
Sperm transfer, 109–110
Spina bifida, 151–152, 155–159,
161, 163–164, 167–168
Sports, medical enhancement in,
356–365
Stacking, steroid, 358–359
Standards for Laboratory
Animals Act, 174
Stem cells, 128–135
acceptance, *vs.* tissue rejection,
139–140
adult, discovery of, 131–132
Bush (George W.) policy on,
132–134
ethical issues involving
embryos, 135–140
fraudulent claims on research,
131, 133–134
immortalized lines, creation of,
130–131

induced pluripotent,
134–135, 140
legal restrictions on, 132
Obama policy on, 134
opportunity cost of missed
research on, 139
setbacks to research, 135
Sterilization, 299–300
Steroid use/abuse, 358–364
Stoicism, 13, 28
Straw Man, 4, 5–6
Structuralism, and HIV/AIDS,
327–328
Substituted judgment, 63, 65, 76
Suffering
pain *vs.*, 50
relief of, 49–50, 292–293
Suicide. *See also* Physician-
assisted dying; Requests
to die
assisted, 31–37
autonomy and, 33–34
competence and, 32–33
failed attempts at, 31–32
genetic testing and risk of, 309
historical perspective on,
27–31
intended action in, 31
major philosophers on, 28–30
rationality and, 32–33
SUPPORT study, 33, 80, 305
Surgeons. *See also*
Transplantation
desire for fame, 208–237
Surrogacy, 113–114, 122
Sustenance. *See also* Feeding
tubes
refusal of, 20–25
*The Switch* (television movie), 26
Symptom relief, request to die
for, 34
Synergism, drug, 59
Syphilis
Guatemalan study of, 202
historical perspective on, 316
nature and history of, 190–191
Tuskegee Study on, 190–199

*Tarasoff* decision, 289
Task Force on Organ
Transplantation, 236
Temporal priority *vs.* causality, 6
Temporary incompetence, 289
Terminal sedating, 49
Terri's Law, 68–70
Test-tube babies, 107–108,
128. *See also* Assisted
reproduction
Therapy *vs.* experimentation,
226, 260–262
Thomistic ethics, 13–14

Torts, 120, 165
Total harm, 165
Totality, principle of, 14–15
Tragedy of the commons,
243–244, 344
Transgender persons, 271. *See
also* Intersex persons
Transplantation
allocation of organs for, 228
animal-to-human (xenografts),
249–251, 254–262
babies as donors, 249, 251–254,
262–266
costs *vs.* benefits of, 224–225,
243–244
death criteria for donor,
221–222, 244–246, 265
experimental *vs.*
therapeutic, 226
first, defense of, 224
first heart transplant, 208–212
good reasoning in, 2
informed consent for,
225–226
living donors for, 2–3, 232–233,
241–243
multiple listings and
favoritism in, 236–238
personality responsibility for
health and, 2, 234–236, 241
quality of life after, 222–223
retransplants in, 238–239
Rule of Rescue in, 239–241
sickest first in, 240–241
supply and demand of organs
for, 232–233
surgeon's desire for fame and,
208–237
Triage, 10
in HIV/AIDS, 326–327, 330
Tricare, 337
Trolley Problem, 10
*Tu quoque,* 5
Tuskegee Study, 190–199
Twins, conjoined, 152–153, 249,
254–255, 257, 259, 273

United Kingdom, health-care
system in, 335
United Network for Organ
Sharing (UNOS), 222,
236–241, 252
Universalization, 2–3
Universal medical coverage,
334–335
Upbringing, appeals to, 7
Utilitarianism, 9–11
and allocation of medical
resources, 228, 238, 240
virtue or Kantian ethics
*vs.*, 9–10

Value, theory of, 9–10
Values inventory, 80
Vegetative state. *See* Persistent
  vegetative state
Veil of ignorance, 15–16,
  148, 348
Ventilators
  extraordinary *vs.* ordinary
    treatment, 78
  futile *vs.* non-futile care, 77–78
  impaired babies on, 150
  pulling the plug *vs.* weaning,
    62–63
  Quinlan case, 59–66
  religious views of withdrawal
    of, 62, 76

Vermont health-care plan,
  341–342
Vertical transmission, 320
Veterans Health Administration
  (VHA), 337–338
Viability of fetus, 85, 94–95,
  102–103
Virtue ethics, 13
  utilitarianism *vs.,* 9–10
Vivisectionists, 176–177


*Webster v. Reproductive Health
  Services,* 103
*White Man's Burden*
  (Easterly), 330

*Whitner v. South Carolina,* 102
*Whose Life Is It, Anyway?* (movie),
  32, 35
*Who Shall Live* (television
  documentary), 230
*Who Shall Play God?* (Rifkin), 118
Withdrawing and forgoing
  treatment, 79–80
Wrongful birth *vs.* wrongful life,
  120, 165–166
Wronging *vs.* harming,
  120–121
*Wyatt v. Stickney,* 286


Xenografts, 249–262, 254–256